To my wife Sharon with love,
and for a debt I cannot repay.

E. Albert Reece

To all the physicians, teachers, and students
who are passionate about improving women's health
throughout the world.

Robert Barbieri

Obstetrics and Gynecology
The Essentials of Clinical Care

E. Albert Reece, MD, PhD, MBA
Vice President for Medical Affairs
University of Maryland
The John Z. and Akiko K. Bowers Distinguished Professor of Obstetrics,
Gynecology and Reproductive Sciences, and Dean
University of Maryland School of Medicine
Baltimore, Maryland
USA

Robert L. Barbieri, MD
Chairman
Department of Obstetrics, Gynecology and Reproductive Biology
Brigham and Women's Hospital
Kate Macy Ladd Professor
Harvard Medical School
Boston, Massachusetts
USA

With contributions by
Robert L. Barbieri, Daniela Carusi, Jon I. Einarsson, Jenifer O. Fahey,
Alberto Fernández, Vanina S. Fishkel, Tanya S. Ghatan, Carolina Ghia, Avi Harlev,
Melody Y. Hou, Julieta E. Irman, Natasha R. Johnson, Arie Koifman, Jan Kriebs,
Gustavo F. Leguizamón, Hugh E. Mighty, Felicitas von Petery, Benjamin Piura,
Fernenda Peres, Luciana Prozzillo, Jill A. RachBeisel, E. Albert Reece,
Shimrit Yaniv Salem, Ruthi Shako-Levy, Eyal Sheiner, Adi Y. Weintraub,
Arnon Wiznitzer, Natalia P. Zeff

240 illustrations

Thieme
Stuttgart · New York

Library of Congress Cataloging-in-Publication Data is available from the publisher.

Illustrator: Dr. med. Katja Dalkowski, Buckenhof, Germany

© 2010 Georg Thieme Verlag,
Rüdigerstrasse 14, 70469 Stuttgart, Germany
http://www.thieme.de
Thieme New York, 333 Seventh Avenue,
New York, NY 10001, USA
http://www.thieme.com

Cover design: Thieme Publishing Group
Typesetting by medionet, Berlin, Germany
Printed by L.E.G.O. S.p.A., Vicenza, Italy
ISBN   978-3-13-143951-2

1 2 3 4 5 6

Important note: Medicine is an ever-changing science undergoing continual development. Research and clinical experience are continually expanding our knowledge, in particular our knowledge of proper treatment and drug therapy. Insofar as this book mentions any dosage or application, readers may rest assured that the authors, editors, and publishers have made every effort to ensure that such references are in accordance with **the state of knowledge at the time of production of the book.**

Nevertheless, this does not involve, imply, or express any guarantee or responsibility on the part of the publishers in respect to any dosage instructions and forms of applications stated in the book. **Every user is requested to examine carefully** the manufacturers' leaflets accompanying each drug and to check, if necessary in consultation with a physician or specialist, whether the dosage schedules mentioned therein or the contraindications stated by the manufacturers differ from the statements made in the present book. Such examination is particularly important with drugs that are either rarely used or have been newly released on the market. Every dosage schedule or every form of application used is entirely at the user's own risk and responsibility. The authors and publishers request every user to report to the publishers any discrepancies or inaccuracies noticed. If errors in this work are found after publication, errata will be posted at www.thieme.com on the product description page.

Contributors

Robert L. Barbieri, MD
Chairman
Department of Obstetrics,
Gynecology and Reproductive
Biology
Brigham and Women's Hospital
Kate Macy Ladd Professor
Harvard Medical School
Boston, MA, USA

Daniela Carusi, MD, MSc
Instructor of Obstetrics, Gynecology
and Reproductive Biology
Harvard Medical School
Brigham and Women's Hospital
Boston, MA, USA

Jon I. Einarsson, MD, MPH
Director of Minimally Invasive
Gynecologic Surgery
Brigham and Women's Hospital
Boston, MA, USA

Jenifer O. Fahey, CNM, MPH
Assistant Professor of Obstetrics,
Gynecology and Reproductive
Sciences
University of Maryland Medical
Center
Baltimore, MD, USA

Alberto Fernández, MD
High Risk Pregnancy Unit
Department of Obstetrics
and Gynecology
Center of Medical Education
and Clinical Research
(C.E.M.I.C.) University
Buenos Aires, Argentina

Vanina S. Fishkel, MD
Department of Obstetrics
and Gynecology
Center of Medical Education
and Clinical Research
(C.E.M.I.C.) University
Buenos Aires, Argentina

Tanya S. Ghatan, MD
Instructor, Harvard Medical School
Brigham and Women's Hospital
Department of Obstetrics
and Gynecology
Boston, MA, USA

Carolina Ghia, MD
Department of Obstetrics
and Gynecology
Center of Medical Education
and Clinical Research
(C.E.M.I.C.) University
Buenos Aires, Argentina

Avi Harlev, MD
Instructor, Department of Obstetrics
and Gynecology
Soroka University Medical Center
Ben-Gurion University of the Negev
Beer-Sheva, Israel

Melody Y. Hou, MD, MPH
Department of Obstetrics
and Gynecology
Boston University School
of Medicine
Boston, MA, USA

Julieta E. Irman, MD
Department of Pediatrics
British Hospital
Buenos Aires, Argentina

Natasha R. Johnson, MD
Instructor, Harvard Medical School
Brigham and Women's Hospital
Department of Obstetrics
and Gynecology
Boston, MA, USA

Arie Koifman, MD
Instructor, Department of Obstetrics
and Gynecology
Faculty of Health Sciences
Soroka University Medical Center
Ben-Gurion University of the Negev
Beer-Sheva, Israel

Jan Kriebs, CNM
Assistant Professor of Obstetrics, Gynecology and Reproductive Sciences
University of Maryland Medical
Center
Baltimore, ML, USA

Gustavo F. Leguizamón, MD
High Risk Pregnancy Unit
Department of Obstetrics and
Gynecology
Center of Medical Education
and Clinical Research
(C.E.M.I.C.) University
Buenos Aires, Argentina

Hugh E. Mighty, MD, MBA
Associate Professor of Obstetrics,
Gynecology and Reproductive
Sciences
Chairman, Obstetrics, Gynecology
and Reproductive Sciences
University of Maryland Medical
Center
Baltimore, ML, USA

Felicitas von Petery, MD
High Risk Pregnancy Unit
Department of Obstetrics
and Gynecology
Center of Medical Education
and Clinical Research
(C.E.M.I.C.) University
Buenos Aires, Argentina

Benjamin Piura, MD, FRCOG
Professor, Unit of Gynecologic
Oncology
Soroka Medical Center and Faculty
of Health Sciences
Ben-Gurion University of the Negev
Beer-Sheva, Israel

Fernenda Peres, MD
Head of Adolescent Gynecology Unit
Department of Obstetrics
and Gynecology
Faculty of Health Sciences
Soroka University Medical Center
Ben-Gurion University of the Negev
Beer-Sheva, Israel

Luciana Prozzillo, MD
High Risk Pregnancy Unit
Department of Obstetrics
and Gynecology
Center of Medical Education
and Clinical Research
(C.E.M.I.C.) University
Buenos Aires, Argentina

Jill A. RachBeisel, MD
Associate Professor of Psychiatry
Director, Community Psychiatry
University of Maryland School
of Medicine
Baltimore, ML, USA

E. Albert Reece, MD, PhD, MBA
Vice President for Medical Affairs
University of Maryland
The John Z. and Akiko K. Bowers
Distinguished Professor of
Obstetrics, Gynecology and
Reproductive Sciences, and Dean
University of Maryland School
of Medicine
Baltimore, ML, USA

Shimrit Yaniv Salem, MD
Instructor, Departments
of Obstetrics and Gynecology
Faculty of Health Sciences
Soroka University Medical Center
Ben-Gurion University of the Negev
Beer-Sheva, Israel

Ruthi Shako-Levy, MD
Lecturer, Institute of Pathology
Soroka Medical Center and Faculty
of Health Sciences
Ben-Gurion University of the Negev
Beer-Sheva, Israel

Eyal Sheiner, MD, PhD
Senior Lecturer, Departments
of Obstetrics and Gynecology
Faculty of Health Sciences
Soroka University Medical Center
Ben-Gurion University of the Negev
Beer-Sheva, Israel

Adi Y. Weintraub, MD
Instructor, Departments
of Obstetrics and Gynecology
Faculty of Health Sciences
Soroka University Medical Center
Ben-Gurion University of the Negev
Beer-Sheva, Israel

Arnon Wiznitzer, MD
Professor of Obstetrics
and Gynecology
Faculty of Health Sciences
Soroka University Medical Center
Ben-Gurion University of the Negev
Beer-Sheva, Israel

Natalia P. Zeff, MD
Diabetes in Pregnancy Unit
Department of Obstetrics
and Gynecology
Center of Medical Education
and Clinical Research
(C.E.M.I.C.) University
Buenos Aires, Argentina

Foreword

All too often "handbooks" are dismissed as not providing the necessary and essential information required to practice OB/GYN medicine in the real world. This is a common complaint among both professors and clinicians.

This handbook is an exception to that rule. It is well organized and devotes extensive discussion to the major expected topics (e.g., labor and delivery). However, where appropriate it delves deeply in subtopics that are of current clinical interest and/or where controversies exist. For example, it presents an extensive discussion of the management and prevention of infectious diseases and also discusses the ethical issues involved in recommending specific preventive vaccines, such as the HPV vaccine. Most importantly, it clearly addresses all the major sub-specialties, including gynecologic oncology, reproductive endocrinology, and maternal–fetal medicine.

Most importantly, the information contained in these almost 60 chapters is clinically relevant and concisely presented. The sections devoted to breast disease, ethics, human sexuality, and preventive care should be read by all clinicians, not just obstetrics and gynecology medical students and trainees. Most importantly, the information contained in these comprehensive chapters is clinically relevant and concisely presented.

As the title of this book—Obstetrics and Gynecology: The Essentials of Clinical Care—suggests, what it presents are the evidence-based essentials of high-quality OB/GYN practice; not speculations or possibilities, but the tried and true approaches. Most importantly, in many sections it discusses what the minimum standards are for safe, professional, and ethical clinical care under often difficult circumstances.

Indeed, the sections devoted to ethics, psychiatric issues, legal issues, and patient-provider communications is a must read for all clinicians and healthcare workers, not just obstetrics and gynecology practitioners and medical students. Thus, it is a valuable resource for the students, trainees, practicing physicians, and other healthcare professionals who manage women of reproductive age. I hope all groups get as much out of reading it as I did.

Norman F. Gant, Jr, MD

Preface

The volume of information that today's OB/GYN practitioner needs to know is staggering and growing rapidly because of new basic research and clinical discoveries made daily. There is a critical need for both medical students and practicing physicians to have easy access to relevant information in a concise and carefully organized manner. This goal is difficult to achieve because 21st century medicine is characterized by a vast quantity of clinically relevant information. That is why the goal of this textbook is to clearly and concisely present the *essential* knowledge needed to practice state-of-the art obstetric and gynecologic medicine.

Women's health and the field of obstetrics and gynecology are critically important to the overall health of every society. Indeed, the health of women and their newborn children are key determinants of the potential of a society for advancing. The Association of Professors of Gynecology and Obstetrics has developed consensus learning objectives for medical students on clinical rotations in obstetrics and gynecology. These objectives, modified to focus on the most important and common clinical problems, are the basis for the extensive amount of material presented in this handbook.

Each chapter is presented in a clear, consistent manner and, where appropriate, begins with the definition of a particular condition, its common manifestations, and how it is routinely diagnosed. This is followed by a discussion of the prevalence and epidemiology of the condition, its etiology and pathophysiology, detailed information about the methods and protocols for its screening and/or detection, and the most recent, evidence-based information about its management. Each chapter uses photographs, tables, and other figures to present critical data and ideas, and ends by emphasizing the key clinical points. Within most chapters, an "Evidence" box is included to provide readers with exposure to how high-quality research information is used to guide clinical diagnosis and treatment. These "Evidence" boxes provide the kind of clinical information that inform the modern practice of OB/GYN medicine.

Medical students do not learn by a bolus infusion of a massive quantity of information. Rather, they learn through a continuous cycle of reading, thinking, talking, and doing. The purpose of this handbook is to assist the student and practitioner in this constant cycle of life-long learning and, more importantly, to offer the most evidence-based approach to the diagnosis and treatment of real OB/GYN patient problems.

E. Albert Reece, MD, PhD, MBA
Robert L. Barbieri, MD

Acknowledgements

The editors are deeply indebted to all of those who contributed so generously to the conceptualization, research, and writing of this project. Thanks to their enormous energy and creative input, we have developed an extremely informative, up-to-date handbook on the essentials of practicing modern OB/GYN medicine.

We greatly appreciate the efforts of Mr. Jim Swyers, MA, Director of Academic Outreach and Special Programs at the University of Maryland School of Medicine, office of the dean, who assisted in coordinating the entire project and was instrumental in helping to locate evidence-based studies and guidelines for many of the chapters as well as relevant photographs, figures, and tables.

We also are deeply indebted to our project editors at Thieme Publishing, Stephan Konnry and Rachel Swift, who kept us on task and on schedule and provided extremely valuable insights and recommendations throughout every stage of this project. Without their superior organizational skills and expert input, our task would have been much greater and taken significantly longer to complete.

Finally, we would like to express our sincere appreciation to all of the contributors to the various chapters of this book. The quality of this handbook is a testament to their commitment, selflessness, and outstanding scholarship. We are forever indebted to them.

E. Albert Reece, MD, PhD, MBA,
Robert Barbieri, MD

Table of Contents

Part I Patient Care

1 Life-Long OB/GYN Care for Women

E. Albert Reece and Robert L. Barbieri

The health of women and children is the foundation for the wellbeing and economic prosperity of a society. Quality obstetric and gynecologic (OB/GYN) health care is critical not only to a woman's health, but is absolutely essential to giving the children she bears a healthy start in life.

OB/GYN care includes the entire spectrum of a woman's life and life style, not just pregnancy and childbirth. When it comes to health care, women face a myriad of unique health and wellness issues compared to men. In addition to their unique gynecologic and reproductive challenges, women grow and mature physically and emotionally in different ways from men.

Women often have different responses to drugs than do men; the amount of drug getting to their cells can vary and their metabolism of drugs is often different from a man's. They also are at greater risk for certain mental illnesses, such as depression and generalized anxiety, compared with men. Finally, certain medical problems, such as osteoporosis, can impact women differently from men.

If physicians are not acutely aware of these sex differences,[*] some serious medical issues, such as cardiac disease or a heart attack, may be overlooked because their symptoms in many women are not as clear-cut as they are in men. Additionally, although women get some cancers, such as lung cancer, at lower rates than men they have a much higher mortality rate than men, for unknown reasons. Therefore, their care has to be more intensive.

There are also health disparities among different groups of women. For example, Black women in many developed countries live fewer years and acquire life-threatening conditions, such as heart disease and breast cancer, at younger ages than do White women. The majority of women and children infected with human immunodeficiency virus throughout the world, for example, are Black.

---

[*] The Institute of Medicine of the US National Academy of Sciences recommends the term "sex difference" to describe biological processes that differ between genetic males and females and the term "gender difference" to describe differences largely influenced by the social environment.

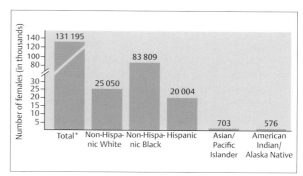

Fig. 1.1 Human immunodeficiency virus (HIV) infection takes a significantly larger toll on Black women compared with all other groups of women in the United States. This bar diagram shows the numbers of adolescent and adult females living with HIV/AIDS by race/ethnicity, and includes persons with diagnosis of HIV infection (not AIDS), diagnosis of HIV infection and AIDS, or concurrent diagnoses of HIV infection and AIDS for 33 States in the year 2006. (Data do not reflect improved estimates of HIV incidence released in August 2008). *Includes 1051 females of unknown race/ethnicity. Adapted from the Centers for Disease Control and Prevention HIV/AIDS Surveillance Report.

This is particularly true in the United States (**Fig. 1.1**), where Black women also have higher rates of other sexually transmitted infections and pelvic inflammatory disease than do women of other ethnic groups.

Thus, it is essential for physicians specializing in women's health to have an in-depth understanding of the unique sets of medical challenges faced by most women. They must also be well versed in the new sets of medical and psychological challenges that often occur in each phase of a woman's life, as well in her living environment. More importantly, physicians must be knowledgeable regarding the important, and often life-saving, preventive measures to follow at each life stage of a woman's life, or any dramatic changes in her environmental situation (e.g., a divorce) in order to be able to detect and prevent any potential medical risks.

From Birth to Adolescence

From birth to their teenage years, major health issues for young girls involve optimal physical and sexual growth, including the psychological aspects of puberty and gender identification within and outside the family.

Puberty

Puberty is the stage in life when a female first becomes capable of reproducing and is marked by maturation of the genital organs, development of secondary sex characteristics, acceleration in growth, and the occurrence of menarche.

The pubertal process is important in the transition from childhood to adolescence. Three important aspects of the pubertal process are adrenarche, somatarche, and menarche. Milestones in the pubertal process include the onset of breast development (average age 10–11 years), growth of pubic hair (average age 11–12 years), and first menses (average age 12–13 years) (**Fig. 1.2**).

Adrenarche is often referred to as the "awakening of the adrenal glands," where the hypothalamic–pituitary–adrenal (HPA) axis is activated. The HPA axis usually begins to mature in girls between the ages of 6 and 8 years. During adrenarche, there is an increase in the concentrations of three adrenal androgens: dehydroepiandrosterone (DHEA), its sulfate (DHEAS), and androstenedione.

In the early part of adrenarche, there are typically no external physical changes. However, as the concentrations of adrenal androgens increase, pubic hair becomes evident along with body odor, and often acne. These are first physical signs of the onset of puberty.

Although both girls and boys go through puberty, girls reach puberty and sexual maturity at earlier ages than do boys. Starting at around age 9 years, girls experience a significant growth spurt and weight gain. Breast development is an early sign of puberty in girls. This can happen before age 9 years in some girls, but later in others.

Although for most girls, breast development is the first sign of puberty, others might first notice pubic hair. An increase in hair on the arms and legs, in the armpits, and around the pubic area happens to girls early in puberty.

Soon after they develop breasts, most girls have their first period. This usually happens between ages 12 and 13 years, but menstruation can start earlier or later. During a menstrual period, there are 2–3 days of heavier bleeding, then 2–4 days of lighter flow.

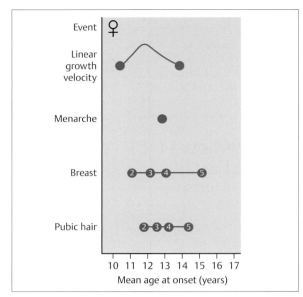

Fig. 1.2 Age range of pubertal milestones in young girls. From Semin Reprod Med © 2003 Thieme Medical Publishers.

Preventive Vaccinations

In addition to the normal vaccinations that children receive as part of routine pediatric care (e.g., mumps, measles, rubella), there is an ongoing controversy about whether young girls also should be vaccinated against the human papilloma virus (HPV).

Recent studies suggest that half of all sexually active women between 18 and 22 years of age in the United States are infected with HPV. Although most cases clear up on their own, sometimes infection persists and can cause cervical cancer decades later. The US Centers for Disease Control and Prevention predicts that deaths worldwide from cervical cancer could jump fourfold—to a million a year—by 2050.

The US Food and Drug Administration (FDA) recently licensed an HPV vaccine for use in girls/women of age 9–26 years. The vaccine is given through a series of three shots over a 6-month period. The HPV vaccine is recommended for 11–12-year-old girls, and can be given to girls as young as 9 years. The vaccine is also recommended for 13–26-year-old girls/women who have not yet received or completed the vaccine series.

Females who are sexually active may also benefit from the vaccine. But they may receive less benefit from HPV vaccination, since they may have already acquired one or more HPV type(s) covered by the vaccine. Few young women are infected with all four of these HPV types and would still get protection from those types they have not acquired. Currently, there is no test available to tell whether a girl/woman has had any or all of these four HPV types.

The HPV vaccine, nevertheless, is controversial. Many groups object to it on moral grounds, suggesting that it will encourage promiscuity among young people. Many parents are reluctant to immunize their preteen daughters against a sexually transmitted disease. Others believe the risk has been overstated and the vaccine over-marketed by pharmaceutical companies. There also is a common misconception that the HPV vaccine protects against all types of HPV.

Physicians need to be aware of these controversies and discuss them in a frank and open manner with parents of young girls. Chapter 23 contains a detailed discussion of the control and management of infectious diseases during pregnancy, including sexually transmitted diseases, such as HPV.

Exercise, Nutrition, and Weight Control

Proper weight control is particularly important for women. Compared to men, women suffer a disproportionate burden of disease attributable to overweight and obesity. Health-related drops in quality of life are nearly four times steeper for overweight women than for overweight men, and more than twice as great for obese women as for obese men.

Statistics indicate that 39% of boys and 58% of girls aged 7–18 years do not achieve the recommended levels of exercise; that is, spending at least an hour each day in a physical activity of at least moderate intensity. Furthermore, nearly two-thirds of US women are overweight and more than one-third are obese. This puts them at significantly higher risk of a range of acute and chronic diseases, including hypertension, heart disease, stroke, diabetes, and cancer. Women who are obese and diabetic and become pregnant are also at significantly higher risk of having a child with a serious birth defect compared with nonobese, nondiabetic women.

Obesity also has an important relationship with early puberty in girls. A recent study published in the in the journal *Pediatrics* found that 6–9-year-old girls who had started developing breasts or pubic hair were significantly more overweight than girls of the same age who had not. It also found that this association was stronger for White girls than for Black girls; however, it could not account for the finding that Black girls started puberty, on average, 1 year earlier than white girls.

Another study of 354 girls from 10 different regions in the United States found that increased body fat in girls as young as age 3 years and large increases in body fat between age 3 and the start of first grade schooling were associated with earlier puberty, defined as the presence of breast development by age 9 years.

Based on these findings, physicians should anticipate that overweight girls are more likely to show signs of early puberty. Physicians should take obesity and racial status into account when deciding how to manage early-maturing 6–9-year-old girls.

The Reproductive Years

The reproductive age span of a woman is typically assumed for statistical purposes to be 15–49 years of age. When a woman reaches the reproductive age, many more health care issues come into play including: reproductive health matters, such as childbearing, infertility problems, and pregnancy; depressive illnesses as well as anxiety disorders; sexually transmitted diseases; and autoimmune disorders. Furthermore, if she becomes pregnant at too early an age, she may face a whole new set of issues.

Thus, it is an important time period in a woman's life, and clinicians caring for young women must be able to recognize and reduce risk-taking and other unhealthy behaviors, such as smoking or unprotected sexual intercourse, and discuss contraceptives when is appropriate to protect from unplanned pregnancy.

Contraception

Nearly 15 million teenage women worldwide give birth each year, accounting for up to 10% of all births globally. The figure may be even higher as the number of mothers under 15 years of age is not recorded. Childbearing in adolescence is known to be a considerable health risk. Teenage mothers have more complications of pregnancy and delivery, including toxemia, iron deficiency anemia, premature delivery, prolonged and obstructed labor, hypertensive disorders of pregnancy, and even death. One quarter of the 500 000 women who die every year from causes related to pregnancy and childbirth are teenagers. Thus, the use of highly effective methods of contraception by teenagers at risk for unintended pregnancy may significantly decrease the number of other co-morbidities among this group.

The World Health Organization (WHO) has developed "eligibility" criteria for the population most likely to benefit from a particular method of contraception without unnecessary side effects (**Table 1.1**). Specifically, the WHO assigns categories to each contraceptive method for use in women under the age of 20 years. Category 1 is for methods for which there is no restriction on use. Category 2 is for methods where the advantages generally outweigh the risks. Category 3 is for methods where the risks usually outweigh the advantages. Category 4 is for methods that represent an unacceptable health risk to adolescent girls. Thus, these latter two categories are not listed in **Table 1.1.**

Although the use of contraceptives by adolescents is extremely controversial in most countries, scientific evidence suggests that condoms and long-acting contraceptives, including condoms, implants, and intrauterine devices (IUDs), are highly effective in preventing pregnancy. Use of these methods by adolescents has the potential to significantly decrease the rate of unintended pregnancy and its complications in this age group.

Endocrine and Autoimmune Disorders

Autoimmune disorders can cause great morbidity and have the highest prevalence in the reproductive years. Many of these diseases are influenced by changes in estrogen levels, particularly during pregnancy.

Thyroid disorders are the second most common endocrinologic disorder found in pregnancy. Overt hypothyroidism is estimated to occur in 0.3–0.5% of pregnancies. Subclinical hypothyroidism appears to occur in 2–3%, and hyperthyroidism is present in 0.1–0.4%.

Autoimmune thyroid dysfunctions remain a common cause of both hyperthyroidism and hypothyroidism in pregnant women. Graves disease accounts for more than 85% of all cases of hyperthyroid, whereas Hashimoto thyroiditis is the most common cause of hypothyroidism.

Postpartum thyroiditis (PPT) reportedly affects 4–10% of women. PPT is an autoimmune thyroid disease that occurs during the first year after delivery. Women with PPT present with transient thyrotoxicosis, hypothyroidism, or transient thyrotoxicosis followed by hypothyroidism. This presentation may be unrecognized, but is important because it predisposes the woman to develop permanent hypothyroidism.

Of interest, symptoms of autoimmune thyroid diseases tend to improve during pregnancy. A postpartum exacerbation is not uncommon and perhaps occurs because of an alteration in the maternal immune system during pregnancy. The improvement in thyroid autoimmune diseases is thought to be due to the altered immune status in pregnancy.

Table 1.1 World Health Organization Guidelines/Information for contraceptive use in adolescent girls

Contraceptive type	WHO category	Additional WHO recommendations/information
Barrier methods • Condoms • Diaphragm • Cervical cap • Sponge	1	Women with conditions that make pregnancy an unacceptable risk should be advised that barrier methods for pregnancy prevention may not be appropriate for those who cannot use them consistently and correctly because of their relatively higher typical-use failure rates
Combined estrogen–progestin	1 (no restrictions for women up to the age of 40 years)	WHO guidelines specifically state "theoretical concerns about the use of combined hormonal contraceptives among young adolescents have not been substantiated."
Depot medroxyprogesterone acetate	2	The advantages of using the method generally outweigh the theoretical or proven risks of the method, for up to 17 years of age. However, for women ages 18–45 years, this is a WHO category 1 (no restrictions) contraceptive
Other progestin-only hormonal • Progestin-only pills • Etonogestrel implant	1	Although it should be considered as a safe and highly effective method for this age group, more research is nevertheless needed on the use of the etonogestrel inplant in adolescents.
Intrauterine device	2	WHO does state that there is concern about expulsion and increased risk of sexually transmitted infections in nulliparous and younger women, respectively. However, the advantages of using the method generally outweigh the theoretical or proven risks of the method) for use in women younger than 20 years of age

Endometriosis

Endometriosis occurs in roughly 5–10% of women of reproductive age. Endometriosis in postmenopausal women is rare. Symptoms vary depending on where the cells implant outside the uterine cavity, but its main symptom is pelvic pain. Some women will have little or no pain despite having extensive endometriosis affecting large areas, or having endometriosis with scarring. On the other hand, women may have severe pain even though they have only a few small areas of endometriosis.

Endometriosis is commonly found in women with infertility. The link between infertility and endometriosis is still not fully understood. However, as the complications of endometriosis include internal scarring, adhesions, and cysts, it is believed that infertility is related to the scar formation and other anatomical distortions caused by endometriosis. It also has been postulated that endometriosis interferes with fertility by releasing cytokines and other chemical agents that interfere with reproduction.

A thorough history and a physical examination can lead to a suspected diagnosis of endometriosis in many patients. However, further tests are needed to confirm the diagnosis. The two most common imaging tests are ultrasonography and magnetic resonance imaging (MRI). Normal results on these tests do not eliminate the possibility of endometriosis—areas of endometriosis are often too small to be seen by these tests.

Laparoscopy is the only way to confirm a suspected endometriosis diagnosis. The diagnosis is based on the characteristic appearance of extrauterine growth and, if necessary, a tissue biopsy. Laparoscopy also allows for surgical treatment of endometriosis. **Figure 1.3** shows the potential management options for endometriosis following laparoscopy.

In women of reproductive age, the goal of management is to provide pain relief, to restrict progression of the process, and to relieve infertility, if needed. In younger women, surgical treatment tends to be conservative, with the goal of removing endometrial tissue and preserving the ovaries without damaging normal tissue. In women who do not want to preserve their reproductive potential, hysterectomy and/or removal of the ovaries may be an option. A hysterectomy, however, will not guarantee that the endometriosis and/or the symptoms of endometriosis will not come back. Indeed, surgery may induce adhesions, which can lead to further complications.

Uterine Leiomyomas

Uterine leiomyomas, or fibroids, are common, benign, smooth muscle tumors of the uterus. They are found in nearly half of women over the age of 40 years. Fibroids tend to grow under the influence of estrogen, and regress when the estrogen levels are reduced. Thus, after the onset of menopause, fibroids generally regress.

Most women with uterine fibroids have no symptoms, but some do. Symptoms that might be experienced include:

- heavy menstrual flows
- bleeding between periods
- pain
- infertility
- pelvic pressure
- stress urinary incontinence
- ureteral obstruction

In women with fibroids, the uterus is irregularly enlarged and usually somewhat asymmetrical. It may be tender and, unlike the soft uterus containing a pregnancy, the fibroid uterus is very firm.

The diagnosis is usually based on the clinical findings of an enlarged, irregularly shaped, firm uterus that may or may not be tender. Sometimes, the diagnosis is unclear and diagnostic tests are used to delineate the fibroids and rule out other problems. These include:

- ultrasonography
- MRI and computed tomographic scanning

Because fibroids often regress after menopause, in most cases no treatment is necessary. Fibroids often regress at menopause. Thus, the conservative approach is to measure and observe fibroids over time. For women with significant symptoms or very large or rapidly growing fibroids, a number of treatments can be considered.

Hysterectomy is the only permanent cure for fibroids. It provides definitive treatment, but requires major abdominal, vaginal, or laparoscopic surgery. For women who wish to preserve their childbearing capacity, removal of just the fibroids (myomectomy), with conservation of the rest of the uterus, is an option to be considered. Unfortunately, myomectomy is often a more complicated procedure than hysterectomy, involving a longer recovery period and an increased risk of needing a blood transfusion or developing an infection.

Good results have been reported with embolization in a limited number of cases. This procedure involves threading a catheter through the uterine arteries and injecting a bolus of tiny plastic pellets, which lodge in the small arterioles leading to the fibroids, reducing their blood flow and causing necrosis. Serious complications have been associated with this procedure, however, leading to emergency surgery and life-threatening problems.

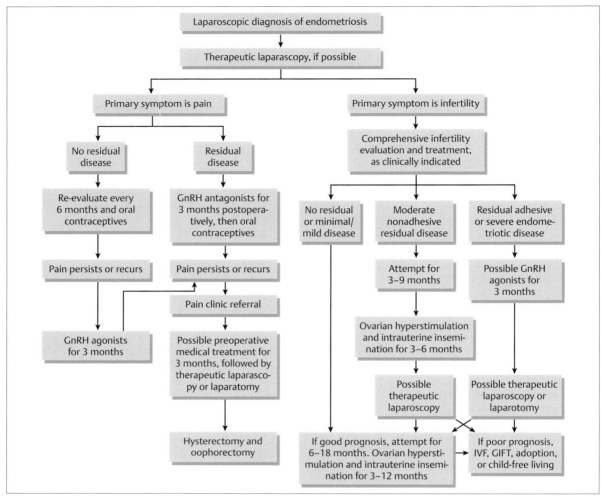

Fig. 1.3 Management scheme for cases of endometriosis positively identified via laparoscopic visualization. GnRH, gonadotropin-releasing hormone; IVF, in vitro fertilization; GIFT, gamete intrafallopian transfer. Modified with permission from Johnson N. Laparoscopic treatment of endometriosis. In: Adamson GD, Martin DC, eds. Endoscopic management of Gynecologic Disease. Philadelphia, Pa: Lippincott-Raven; 1996:147–187.

Whether this approach will prove to be widely accepted remains to be seen.

In some cases, progestins may be useful in controlling the aberrant growth of uterine cells until the patient reaches menopause, at which time the fibroids usually resolve on their own. Substances that suppress the release of gonadotropins have been shown to actually shrink fibroids. However, they can only be given for short periods, after which the fibroids rapidly regrow. On the other hand, this method may be useful for reducing the size of fibroids in women who require surgery. Important factors in deciding which therapy to administer are the severity of the symptoms, associated symptoms, age, and whether there is a need to preserve fertility.

Mental Health Issues

Mental illnesses affect women and men differently—some disorders, such as depression, are more common in women. Some express themselves with different symptoms in women compared to men.

Research is only just beginning to tease apart the contributions of various biological and psychosocial factors to mental health and mental illness in both women and men. In addition, researchers are currently studying the special problems of treatment for serious mental illness during pregnancy and the postpartum period.

Depression

Major depression is the leading cause of disease burden among females aged 5 years and older worldwide, and it affects females at twice the rate of men (12% women and 6% men). The reasons for this disparity are still unclear, but it is believed to be due to a number of factors, including the multiple roles women must assume at home and work, poverty, their increased risk for violence and abuse, the stress of raising children alone (single-mothers), and postpartum depression.

There is a direct correlation for this increased risk of depression and a higher rate for suicide ideation among women compared with men. Although men are more likely to die from a suicide attempt, a higher rate of women attempt suicide compared with men. Girls are more vulnerable to depression during periods of transition such as entering puberty or changing schools, and family changes, such as separation and divorce.

Clinical depression affects twice as many women as men, both in the United States and in many societies around the world. It is estimated that one out of every seven women will suffer from depression in their lifetime. Additionally, women experience higher rates of seasonal affective disorder and dysthymia (chronic depression). Although the rates of bipolar disorder (manic depression) are similar in men and women, women have higher rates of the depressed phase of manic depression and rapid-cycling bipolar disorder.

The gender gap in depression is most evident during the female reproductive years. Some women experience behavior and mood changes premenstrually. As many as 10–15% experience a clinical depression during pregnancy or after the birth of a baby (i.e., postpartum depression).

Postpartum depression, which is major episode of depression occurring within 4 weeks of delivering a baby, strikes one to two of 10 pregnant women. Scientists believe that hormonal changes involved in childbirth combined with psyschosocial stresses combine to make women particularly vulnerable to depression during this time.

Symptoms of postpartum depression include anxiety, a worsening mood in the evening, irritability, phobias, feelings of inadequacy, inability to cope, not feeling loving or caring enough for the baby, and excessive worry about the wellbeing of the baby.

Anxiety Disorders

Women also outnumber men in rates of anxiety and panic disorders, except for obsessive compulsive disorder (OCD) and social phobias. Female risk of post traumatic stress disorder (PTSD) following trauma is twice that of the male. The impact of these disorders is enormous. The economic cost, for example, of anxiety disorders in the United States has been estimated at $47 billion per annum. Fortunately, anxiety disorders are highly treatable conditions for the majority of sufferers.

There are also many medications, both prescription and over the counter, that can precipitate anxiety. The patient's nutrition should also be considered. Look carefully at the amount of caffeine in coffee, soda, diet soda, chocolate, and some aspirin preparations (e.g., Excedrin) likely to be circulating in her system. Even small amounts of caffeine in some at-risk individuals can precipitate or exaggerate anxiety.

Eating disorders are a type of anxiety disorder, and research has shown that anxiety caused by social and cultural factors contribute to the increasing prevalence of dieting and eating disorders in this group. However, there really is no single cause for an eating disorder. Anyone can have an eating disorder, though they most often affect girls and women. Eating disorders such as anorexia nervosa and bulimia are prevalent in up to 10% of adolescent girls.

Most girls who develop anorexia do so between the ages of 11 and 14 years (although it can start as early as age 7), and there are many reasons why. Some kids just don't feel good about themselves on the inside and this makes them try to change the outside. They might be depressed or stressed about things and feel as though they have no control over their lives. They see what they eat (or don't eat) as something that they can control.

Sometimes girls involved in certain sports, like ballet, gymnastics, and ice-skating, might feel they need to be thin to compete. Girls who model also might be more likely to develop an eating disorder. All of these girls know their bodies are being watched closely, and they may develop an eating disorder in an attempt to make their bodies more "perfect."

Eating disorders also may run in families. Therefore, if someone in a girl's family has an eating disorder, she might be at risk for developing one too. A girl may be more likely to develop an eating disorder if a parent is overly concerned with appearance, or if the parent isn't comfortable with his or her own body.

The person with an eating disorder may need to see a dietitian and a counselor or therapist in addition to her doctor. Together, the team can help the person achieve the goals of reaching a healthy weight, following a nutritious diet, and feeling good about herself again. Chapter 25 contains a detailed discussion about treatment approaches for depression and other psychiatric disorders during pregnancy.

Nutrition

Women are more likely to suffer from a variety of nutritional deficiencies than are men, for reasons including women's reproductive biology, low social status, poverty, and lack of education. Adequate nutrition, a fundamental cornerstone of any individual's health, is especially critical for women because inadequate nutrition wreaks havoc not only on their own health, but also on the health of their children. Children of malnourished women are more likely to face cognitive impairments, short stature, lower resistance to infections, and a higher risk of disease and death throughout their lives (**Fig. 1.4**).

After pregnancy, women's energy requirements remain high, especially when they are breast-feeding. Women require approximately 50 % more calories while breast-feeding than they need during pregnancy. Maintaining adequate levels of vitamin A is particularly important for nursing mothers, since vitamin A is passed on to the infant through breast milk and can help reduce the risk of maternal and infant illness and death. Nursing mothers should receive supplements of vitamin A, if necessary.

Menopause

Menopause is a natural process that happens to every woman as she grows older. Although it is not a medical problem, disease, or illness, many women have a difficult time adjusting to it because of the changes in hormone levels. The changes leading up to menopause happen over several years. The average age for menopause is 52 years. But menopause commonly happens anytime between the ages of 42 and 56 years. A woman can say she has begun her menopause when she has not had a period for a full year.

There are many possible signs of menopause, and each woman feels them differently. Most women have no or few menopausal symptoms, while some women have many moderate or severe symptoms. Research has shown that women's experience of menopause can be related to many things, including genetics, diet, life style, and social and cultural attitudes toward older women.

The clearest signs of the start of menopause are irregular periods (when periods come closer together or further apart), and when blood flow becomes lighter or heavier. There may be other physical and mental changes such as vasomotor hot flushes and vaginal symptoms. The physical and psychological symptoms related to menopause are detailed in Chapter 44.

Death rates for menopausal women have declined dramatically during the past several decades. Although previously, the leading cause of death for women was heart disease, cancer is now the major cause, and heart disease is the leading cause of death in women 65 years of age and older. The decline in heart-related mortality is attributed to changes in life style including smoking cessation, exercise, lowering of cholesterol levels, and controlling hypertensive disorders.

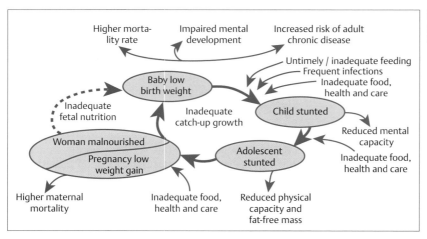

Fig. 1.4 The potential consequences of poor nutrition for pregnant women and their offspring.

Breast Cancer and Hormone Replacement Therapy

Women 65 years or older account for about half of all new breast cancer cases, and the chances of developing the disease increase with age. About 70% of women diagnosed with breast cancer each year are over age 50 years, and almost half are age 65 and older. Other risk factors include:

- previous cancer in one breast
- late menopause (after age 55)
- starting menstruation early in life (before age 12)
- having a first child after age 30
- never having had children
- having used hormone replacement therapy

Besides age, hormone replacement therapy (HRT) has been found to significantly contribute to the risk of breast cancer. HRT often is given to postmenopausal women who have severe symptoms.

However, evidence suggests that the longer a woman is exposed to female hormones (either made by the body, taken as a drug, or delivered by a patch), the more likely she is to develop breast cancer. Thus, the longer a woman is on HRT, the greater her chances may be of being diagnosed with breast cancer.

In 2002, the Women's Health Initiative study revealed an increase in breast cancer, heart attacks, and stroke in older women given conventional HRT. This resulted in a significant decline in HRT prescriptions.

HRT is particularly contraindicated in women who have already been diagnosed with the disease. A recent large-scale clinical trial conducted in Sweden[**] found that breast cancer survivors who took HRT to relieve menopausal symptoms had more than three times as many breast cancer recurrences as survivors who did not take HRT. Results from a longer period of follow-up confirmed the link between HRT and an increased risk of breast cancer recurrence.

The United States Food and Drug Administration has since recommended that women discuss with their doctors whether the benefits of taking estrogen and progestin outweigh the risks. The FDA added that, if used, the hormones should be taken "at the lowest doses for the shortest duration to reach treatment goals."

It is particularly important for all menopausal women to get regular mammograms because menopause has effects on breast tissue that are greater than the effects of age. In order to prevent breast cancer, most menopausal women receive mammograms every year, as recommended by their doctors.

HRT not only increases a woman's risk of developing breast cancer, but also it makes detection of any breast cancer harder, should it occur. It has been demonstrated that use of postmenopausal HRT increases breast density (**Fig. 1.5**). Thus, benign mammographic findings, primarily cysts, in women undergoing HRT result in an increased use of diagnostic mammography and sonography.

** Holmberg L, Anderson H; HABITS steering and data monitoring committees. HABITS (hormonal replacement therapy after breast cancer--is it safe?), a randomised comparison: trial stopped. Lancet. 2004 Feb 7;363(9407):453-5.

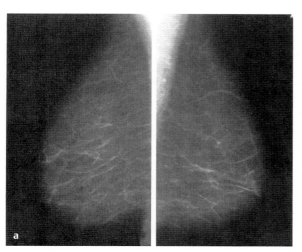 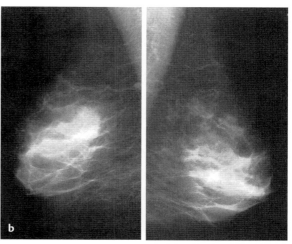

Fig. 1.5 a, b   A woman's mammogram before (**a**) and after 2 years of hormone replacement therapy (**b**) showing much denser breast tissue after therapy. From: Hashimoto B, Bauermeister D. Breast Imaging: A Correlative Atlas. New York: Thieme; 2003.

Heart Disease

Before menopause, women have less risk of cardiovascular disease (CVD) than do men. However, as women age, their risk of heart disease and stroke begins to rise. CVD is the most common cause of death in postmenopausal women. Owing to a greater female life expectancy, women who develop CVD tend to be older or elderly, and are therefore more likely to suffer from co-morbidities such as diabetes and hypertension.

It is beyond the scope of this chapter to discuss the management approach to CVD in postmenopausal women. This would typically be done in conjunction with a cardiologist. However, disease prevention, pharmacotherapy, percutaneous intervention, surgical revascularization, and cardiac rehabilitation are all viable approaches, depending on the condition of the patient.

Urinary Incontinence

Some women develop bladder control problems, or urinary incontinence, after menopause. Urinary incontinence can be slightly bothersome or totally debilitating. Incontinent women may lose a few drops of urine while exercising. Others may feel a strong, sudden urge to urinate just before losing a large amount of urine. Many women experience both symptoms. For some women,

the risk of public embarrassment keeps them from enjoying many activities with their family and friends. Urine loss can also occur during sexual activity and cause tremendous emotional distress. **Figure 1.6** presents a management scheme for urinary incontinence, depending on whether it is the result of stress or urge symptoms.

Osteoporosis

During menopause, estrogen levels in a woman's body drop rapidly, significantly impacting bone health. Estrogen keeps the osteoclasts in check, allowing the osteoblasts to build more bone. Unless the estrogen that is lost is being replaced, a woman's bones can become thin and brittle quite rapidly. This condition is known as osteoporosis.

The definitive method for diagnosing osteoporosis is a bone density scan. Bone density is measured on a point scale, called a T-score. Normal bone density has a T-score of 0 to 1. If a woman's T score is between 1 and 2.5, she has a high likelihood of being diagnosed with osteopenia, a milder form of osteoporosis. If her T-score is less than 2.5, osteoporosis is diagnosed.

Osteoporosis treatment can be quite effective, especially when taken quickly after diagnosis. A variety of new treatments for osteoporosis have also been introduced into the market. **Figure 1.7** presents a scheme for

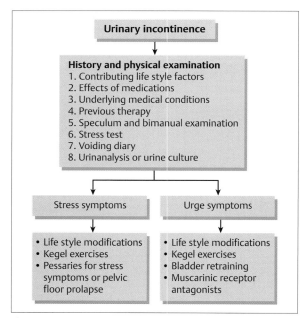

Fig. 1.6 Management scheme for urinary incontinence symptoms. Adapted with permission from O'Neil B, Gilmour D. Approach to Urinary Incontinence in Women. Diagnosis and Management by Family Physicians. Can Fam Physician 2003; 49:611–618

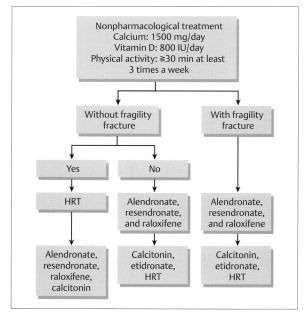

Fig. 1.7 Nonpharmacological versus pharmacological management of osteoporosis based on differential diagnosis. *HRT, hormone replacement therapy.*

the optimal management of osteoporosis, which depends on whether or not a fragility fracture is diagnosed.

Key Points

- OB/GYN care includes the entire spectrum of a woman's life and life style, not just pregnancy and childbirth.
- There is an ongoing controversy about whether young girls should be vaccinated against the human papilloma virus. Physicians need to be aware of these controversies and discuss them in a frank and open manner with parents of young girls.
- OB/GYN physicians should anticipate that overweight girls are more likely to show signs of early puberty, and take obesity and racial status into account when deciding how to manage early-maturing girls.
- Clinicians caring for young women must be able to recognize and help them reduce any risk-taking and other unhealthy behaviors, such as smoking or unprotected sexual intercourse, and discuss contraceptives when appropriate to protect them from unplanned pregnancy.
- OB/GYN physicians should be aware and alert to a number of endocrine and autoimmune disorders, such as thyroid disease, that are more common to pregnancy.
- OB/GYN physicians should be well-versed in the conservative management of uterine fibroids, which often grow rapidly during pregnancy but regress following delivery. After the onset of menopause, fibroids generally regress as well.
- Postpartum depression strikes 1–2 out of 10 pregnant women. OB/GYN physicians need to be keenly aware of the symptoms of postpartum depression and take immediate steps to prevent unnecessary risk to the mother and her newborn baby.
- Adequate nutrition is especially critical for pregnant women because inadequate nutrition wreaks havoc not only on their own health, but also on the health of their babies.

- Although menopause is not considered a classic medical problem, disease, or illness, OB/GYN physicians should be aware that many women have a difficult time adjusting to it because of the changes in hormone levels.
- Hormone replacement therapy presents a serious breast cancer risk, and such risks must be discussed with a patient in great detail before she considers whether to use it to address serious menopausal symptoms.
- Heart disease and urinary incontinence are two conditions that are exacerbated in menopausal women. OB/GYN physicians need to be aware of this increased risk and competent to take appropriate management steps, which have been clearly established.

Further Reading

Holmberg L, Iversen OE, Rudenstam CM, et al; HABITS Study Group. Increased risk of recurrence after hormone replacement therapy in breast cancer survivors. *J Natl Cancer Inst* 2008;100(7):475–482

Holmberg L, Anderson H; HABITS steering and data monitoring committees. HABITS (hormonal replacement therapy after breast cancer—is it safe?), a randomised comparison: trial stopped. *Lancet* 2004;363(9407):453–455

Menopause and Hormones. Available at: http://www.fda.gov/womens/menopause/pdfFiles/FSeng.pdf. Accessed October 31, 2009.

Rossouw JE, Anderson GL, Prentice RL, et al; Writing Group for the Women's Health Initiative Investigators. Risks and benefits of estrogen plus progestin in healthy postmenopausal women: principal results From the Women's Health Initiative randomized controlled trial. *JAMA* 2002;288(3):321–333

2 OB/GYN Examinations and Evaluations

Avi Harlev, Eyal Sheiner, and Arnon Wiznitzer

Achieving the right diagnosis and suggesting the proper treatment is a process that is greatly dependent upon the confidence the patient has in her caregiver. This process begins with an open, patient–physician dialogue, in which the patient feels comfortable relaying all relevant medical information to enable her physician to make the best medical decision.

Since intimate details are to be discussed, a private and quiet environment is required to allow the patient to relax and not only share enough details for her physician to understand her medical condition, but also voice her concerns and expectations. After a thorough medical history is taken, the next steps involve a physical examination as well as the appropriate imaging procedures and laboratory tests, depending on the setting (i.e., ambulatory care, outpatient, or in-patient hospitalization).

In addition to the history, this chapter focuses primarily on the gynecologic physical examination. Complete examination of the breast, abdomen, and pelvis are the core, vital elements of the gynecologic examination. The remainder of the examination depends upon the patient's specific symptoms and complaints. For example, a thyroid gland examination should be performed for infertile women or women with menstrual disorders. Additionally, patients using hormonal therapy should be examined for any hypercoagulability event, such as deep vein thrombosis (DVT). Thus, the examining physician must be flexible about the questionnaires and specific tests that will be administered, and stay attuned to the patient's specific verbal and other cues in order to guide this process.

Definitions

Ascites: This is an accumulation of fluid in the peritoneal cavity. Although most commonly due to cirrhosis and severe liver disease, its presence can portend other significant medical problems. Diagnosis of the cause is usually with blood tests, an ultrasound scan of the abdomen and direct removal of the fluid by needle or paracentesis (which may also be therapeutic). Treatment may be with medication (diuretics), paracentesis, or other treatments directed at the cause.

Auscultation: This is a technical term for listening to the internal sounds of the body, usually using a stethoscope. Based on the Latin verb *auscultare* "to listen," auscultation is performed for the purposes of examining the circulatory system and respiratory system (heart sounds and breath sounds), as well as the gastrointestinal system (bowel sounds).

Ectopic pregnancy: This is a complication of pregnancy, in which the fertilized ovum is implanted in any tissue other than the uterine wall. Most ectopic pregnancies occur in the fallopian tube (so-called **tubal pregnancies**), but implantation can also occur in the cervix, ovaries, and abdomen.

Endometriosis: This is a common health problem in women. The condition gets its name from the word endometrium, which is the tissue that lines the uterus (womb). In women with this problem, tissue that looks and acts like the lining of the uterus grows outside of the uterus, in other areas. These areas can be called growths, tumors, implants, lesions, or nodules.

Menarche: This term refers to a girl's first menstrual period, or first menstrual bleeding (see below). From both a social and medical perspective, it is often considered the central event of female puberty, as it signals the possibility of fertility. Timing of menarche is influenced by both genetic and environmental factors, especially nutritional status. The average age of menarche has declined over the last century, but the magnitude of the decline and the factors responsible remain subjects of contention.

Menstruation: This term refers to a woman's monthly bleeding cycle, also called a period. Menstruation is part of the menstrual cycle, which prepares a woman's body for pregnancy each month. A cycle is counted from the first day of one period to the first day of the next period. The average menstrual cycle is 28 days long. Cycles can range anywhere from 21 to 35 days in adults and from 21 to 45 days in young teenagers.

Müllerian duct anomaly: This is a congenital anatomical abnormality of the female internal genitalia due to nondevelopment or nonfusion of the muüllerian ducts or a failure of reabsorption of the uterine septum. Müllerian duct anomalies are common, occurring in 1–15% of women. However, clinically significant congenital uterine abnormalities are rare, with a reported incidence of between 0.1 and 0.5%.

Myoma: This is a kind of tumor, of which there are of two types: the leiomyoma may occur in the skin or gut, but the common form is the uterine fibroid; rhabdomyoma is a rare tumor of muscles, which occurs in childhood and often becomes malignant.

Palpation: This technique is used as part of a physical examination, in which an object is felt (usually with the hands of a health care practitioner) to determine its size, shape, firmness, or location. Palpation should not be confused with palpitation, which is an awareness of the beating of the heart.

Thrombophilia: This term describes the propensity to develop thrombosis (blood clots) due to an abnormality in the system of coagulation. Most women with a thrombophilia have healthy pregnancies. However, pregnant women with a thrombophilia may be more likely than other pregnant women to develop a venous thromboembolism or other pregnancy complications related to circulatory problems.

History

Chief Complaint

The chief complaint is a condensed summary of the reason the patient is seeking medical care. This information is typically condensed into a single sentence containing the following information:

- name
- age
- familial status
- residency
- the main medical issue that brings her to the physician

For example: Mrs. R. T., married +2, living in New York City, admitted due to postmenopausal bleeding for the last 2 days.

Present Illness

The present illness is typically recorded and described in significantly more detail. The physician should begin with open questions, allowing the patient to speak freely about her main complaint, asking only short questions such as "When did it start?"

In order to complete the history, the physician should follow up with more direct questions, including asking more details about every symptom mentioned by the patient. This part of the conversation will help the physician to strengthen the differential diagnosis of the patient.

Gynecologic History

In taking a gynecologic history, the physician should ask about the patient's menstruation in great detail including:

- Age at menarche
- Regularity of her menstruation
- Date of her last menstrual period (LMP)
- Duration of her menstruation
- Length of her menstrual cycle (in days)

This information can be summarized in the formula: 5/28 (meaning 5 days of bleeding every 28 days).

The physician also should inquire about any pain experienced during menstruation (dysmenorrhea), as well as its severity, duration, and all other factors concerning general pain (**Table 2.1**).

Table 2.1 Menstrual history questionnaire

Menarche—age at first menstruation
Frequency, regularity, and duration of menstrual periods
Date of the last menstrual period
Current history of heavy, intermenstrual or postcoital bleeding
Current dysmenorrhea
History of menstrual irregularity
History of heavy or intermenstrual bleeding
History of dysmenorrhea
In postmenopausal women, further investigation:
Age at last menses
History of hormone replacement therapy
Current or past vasomotor symptoms, or mood swings
History of any postmenopausal bleeding

Table 2.2 Obstetric history questionnaire

History of any pregnancies:
Date of delivery
Gestational age at delivery
Mode of delivery (vaginal, operative, or cesarean delivery)
Maternal complications, such as hypertension, diabetes, or thrombophilia
Fetal complications, such as growth restriction, anomalies, or stillbirth
Delivery complications
Neonatal and current health of children
History of miscarriages—gestational age of the miscarriage, information from further investigation
Pregnancy terminations—gestational age and cause
Ectopic pregnancies—how were they treated
History of assisted reproduction in any pregnancy

Obstetric History

Taking a complete obstetric history (**Table 2.2**) is important at any age, since it may provide important clues about the general health of the patient. For example, any history of late abortions or stillbirths could raise a suspicion of thrombophilia, which is important before prescribing oral contraceptives.

The obstetric history includes the number of:
- pregnancies
- normal deliveries
- spontaneous abortions and the gestational week in which they occurred
- induced abortions
- ectopic pregnancies
- cesarean deliveries

Sexual History

When the physician inquires about sexual history, the patient also should be asked about her family planning practices and whether she uses, or has previously used, contraceptives. She also should be asked about the types of contraceptives used.

A significant detail in the sexual history-taking is ascertaining whether the patient experiences pain during intercourse (dispareunia). It is important to know if the pain is new or if it arises only during deep penetration. The patient also should be asked about bleeding during intercourse.

Other important questions to be asked during this phase of the history-taking include the general health condition of the patient, regularly taken medications, previous surgical procedures (especially any abdominal procedures), allergies to drugs or food, and whether there are significant diseases in the family history (e.g., heart disease, metabolic disorder, thrombophilic disease or events, cancer).

Physical Examination

The physical examination, particularly the pelvic examination, can sometimes evoke anxiety and fear in the patient. Therefore, a few preventive measures are recommended to reduce these unwanted feelings, including:
- having a preliminary discussion about the examination, emphasizing its importance and how crucial it is in the evaluation process
- educating the patient in advance about each next step in the examination process, thus allowing her to feel in control, which might lead to better cooperation
- encouraging the patient to immediately report any pain or discomfort during the examination
- strictly maintaining the patient's privacy. Her body should be completely covered except for the examined body part

Abdominal Examination

The abdominal examination should be performed when the patient is in a supine position. The head should be somewhat elevated by a pillow, and her legs should be bent with a slight flexion of the knees and thighs. Assuming this position will relax her abdominal muscles and facilitate the examination, which is composed of inspection, looking for skin rash or color change, signs of enlarged organs, ascites, etc.

Auscultation precedes palpation. Note bowel sounds, frequency and quality in all four abdominal quadrants (**Fig. 2.1**). Systematic palpation is performed in order to locate any abdominal mass, hepatomegaly or splenomegaly, and the configuration of the spleen and liver. The examiner should palpate the adnexal area and look for any mass or signs of pain. Palpation is performed superficially at first and then more deeply.

If the patient complains of any localized abdominal pain, the painful region should be palpated last. Note peritoneal signs and any local tenderness. Perform percussion to measure the dimensions of the liver and spleen, bladder, and ovaries, and to assess the severity of ascites, if present.

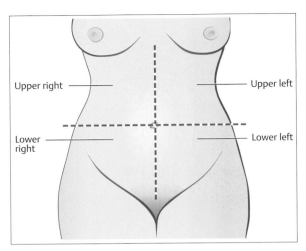

Fig. 2.1 During the physical examination, auscultation is performed on all four abdominal quadrants prior to palpation.

Pelvic Examination

The pelvic examination is performed when the woman lies on her back with her hips and knees bent, and her buttocks moved to the edge of the examining table. This position is called lithotomy (see **Fig. 2.2**). As noted earlier, the patient should be told in advance of every step being made in order to enable her to relax her muscles as much as possible.

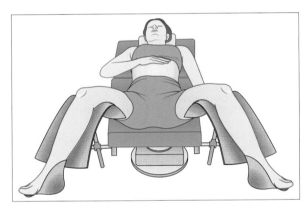

Fig. 2.2 The proper position for a lithotomy examination.

External Genitalia Inspection

The pelvic examination begins with inspection of the external genitalia. The physician should inspect the skin for discoloration, lesions of any kind (condylomata, herpes, etc.), edema or swelling, and wounds. Separation of the labia major and the skin folds around the clitoris allows inspection of the labia minor, clitoris, urethral myatus, vaginal outlet, and the hymen. The inspection may identify evidence of hormonal problems, cancer, infections, or sexual abuse.

Palpation enables detection of enlarged glands, such as in Bartholin abscess. Sebaceous cysts, if present, can be felt as well. If a Skene gland disease is suspected, the urethra should be milked for any excretion through the anterior vaginal wall. Any excretion should be cultured and viewed with a microscope. While separating the labias,

ask the patient to increase her intra-abdominal pressure, so that you can detect any pelvic organ prolapse and urinary stress incontinence.

Speculum Examination

The speculum examination typically precedes the digital vaginal examination. The speculum is a metal or plastic device that spreads the vaginal walls, thus enabling the examiner to view the inner part of the vagina and the cervix (**Fig. 2.3**).

The speculum enables examination of the vagina for signs of bleeding or any kind of discharge, which might hint of problems such as infectious diseases (bacterial vaginosis, trichomoniasis, etc.). Likewise, the mucosa should be inspected for any lesion (inflammatory, neoplastic, traumatic, etc.). The size and type of the speculum should be selected by the physician.

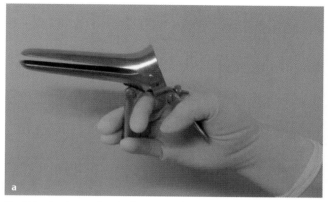

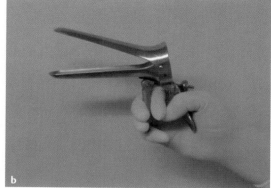

Fig. 2.3a, b   A speculum in the open and closed positions.

Inspect the cervix carefully looking for any signs of discharge as well as inflammation or cancer. A swab, brush, or spatula may be used to obtain a sample for culturing and Pap smear (see below). Bleeding from the cervix, except for menstruation, mandates further evaluation to exclude neoplasia.

Bimanual Examination

After removing the speculum the examiner usually inserts two fingers into the vagina, examining the strength of the vaginal wall, looking for any edematous or tender areas of the vagina. The other hand is placed on the lower abdominal wall (**Fig. 2.4**). The uterus can be palpated and assessed for its size, position, presence of tumors, consistency, mobility, or any tenderness. Subsequently, the cervix is palpated for size, position, mobility, and tenderness.

All four fornices should be evaluated. With the fingers in the right lateral fornix and the other hand on the right lower quadrant, outline the right adnexa (ovary and tube). Perform the same procedure on the other adnexa as well. Usually, normal adnexas are not palpable. Thus, any tenderness or adnexal mass should be further evaluated.

Fig. 2.4   Diagram showing the proper technique for the bimanual examination.

Rectovaginal Examination

With the index finger in the vagina, lubricate the middle finger and insert it into the rectum (**Fig. 2.5**). Palpate the posterior wall of the vagina for masses or irregularities. Raising the cervix will allow you to palpate the uterosacral ligaments. Nodules in the rectovaginal wall or along the uterosacral ligaments are potential indicators of endometriosis.

Laboratory Evaluations

Papanicolaou (Pap) Test

The Pap test, as a screening tool for cervical cancer, has helped to achieve a significant reduction in the incidence and mortality from cervical cancer during the last decades. The sensitivity of the test, according to the US

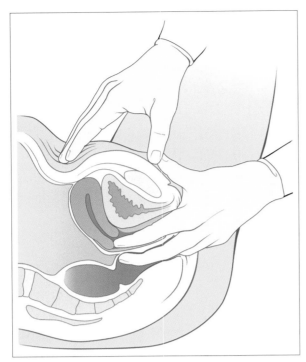

Fig. 2.5 Diagram showing the proper technique for the rectovaginal examination.

Agency for Healthcare Research and Quality, is 51%. This section provides an overview of the Pap test. Chapter 6 contains a significantly more detailed discussion of this powerful screening tool.

In the Pap smear, cervical cells are collected and inspected under a microscope. When collecting the sample the patient lies in the lithotomy position (see **Fig. 2.2**). A speculum is placed in the vagina, exposing the cervix. The speculum should be lubricated only with water, and the patient should not be menstruating.

The cell sample is collected with an endocervical brush used in combination with a plastic spatula inserted into the cervix canal and rotated 360° to scrape cells from the squamocolumnar junction. In the conventional method, the sample is spread on a glass slide, fixed with a spray and sent to the laboratory.

The second method is to insert the sample into a liquid-based medium, which is then sent to the laboratory. This method is considered more accurate, since 80–90% of the sampled cells are transferred to the medium as compared to 10–20% cell transfer rate on the glass slide. The liquid-based medium also eliminates air drying and is associated with fewer unsatisfactory samples compared with the conventional glass slide method.

A third, but not commonly used, method is the Auto-Pap Screening System. This technology attempts to increase the sensitivity of the Pap smear by scanning the slides with a digital microscope and camera using ad-

vanced imaging techniques. Every slide is inspected for any abnormality. Any "suspect" slides undergo further evaluation by a cytopathologist. Although this technique has reduced the false-negative rate by 32%, it is not yet in widespread use.

Guidance for clinical management of the patient uses the Bethesda III System (2001) (see Chapter 6), which was developed as a uniform system of cytology that would provide clear clinical recommendations for patient management based on the results of the Pap test.

Laboratory Biopsies

A biopsy is a technique in which a tissue sample is removed for laboratory evaluation, usually via a microscopic inspection. A biopsy is usually taken when there is suspicion of a malignancy or a premalignant state.

Colposcopy

A uterine–cervix biopsy is usually taken during colposcopy. Colposcopy in most cases is performed after an abnormal Pap smear cytology or a lesion is found during the examination. The colposcope is a binocular microscope used for the direct visualization of the cervix enabling a view of the transformation zone which is the junction between the endocervix and exocervix epithelial cells (**Fig. 2.6**).

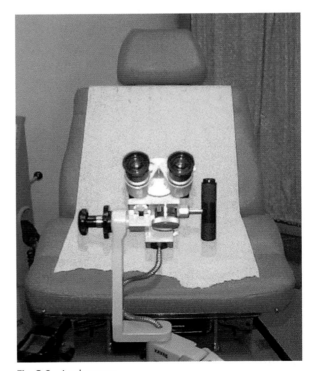

Fig. 2.6 A colposcope.

Using biopsy forceps, sample the suspected areas for any abnormality visualized under the colposcope. Usually, no anesthesia is required for cervical biopsy, which can cause a sharp pinch feeling or a cramp in some cases. Nonsteroidal anti-inflammatory drugs can be administered 30 minutes prior to the biopsy to reduce any discomfort.

If a colposcope is not available, take a biopsy from every quadrant of the squamocolumnar junction at the 12, 3, 6, and 9 o'clock positions. In these cases, use the **Schiller test**, which relies an iodine-based substance called Lugol solution to paint the cervix. Normal tissue stains brown, while tissue suspicious for cancer does not stain and appears pale compared to the surrounding tissue. Obtain a sample from any unpainted area suspected for premalignancy or malignancy.

Vulva and Vagina

A biopsy of a suspected vulvar or vaginal lesion requires the use of local anesthesia. The biopsy can be taken using a scalpel knife or a skin punch. Direct pressure over the biopsy area is usually effective to stop the bleeding. Sutures are rarely needed.

Endocervical Curettage

Endocervical curettage is a procedure performed when a cervical or endometrial malignancy is suspected. A sharp curette is inserted into the cervical canal to obtain a tissue sample (**Figs. 2.7 and 2.8**). This procedure is usually performed during colposcopy. A cervical biopsy is usually taken as well. The sample is sent for examination by a pathologist.

Endometrial Biopsy

An endometrial biopsy is an important test for diagnosing cases of irregular uterine bleeding, suspected endometrial carcinoma, or during an infertility or amenorrhea work-up. An endometrial sample can be collected using a flexible device such as Pipelle (**Fig. 2.9a**). Using a speculum to view the cervix, the device is inserted into the uterus and scratched over the uterine wall. Pulling the inner part of the device guides the endometrial sample into the cannula (**Fig. 2.9b**).

Dilation and Curettage

Dilation and curettage (D&C) is a method used either to evacuate the uterus when an incomplete abortion or a dead fetus is diagnosed, or to obtain a tissue sample from the endometrium. The procedure can be performed under sedation or general anesthesia, though a cervical block is optional. A D&C is not commonly used for biopsy these days, as the Pipelle test generally gives sufficient information.

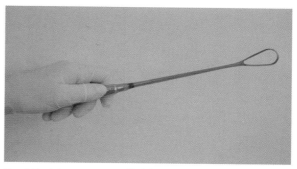

Fig. 2.7 A large curette, called the Bumm curette, which is used for curettage after termination of an advanced gestational age pregnancy.

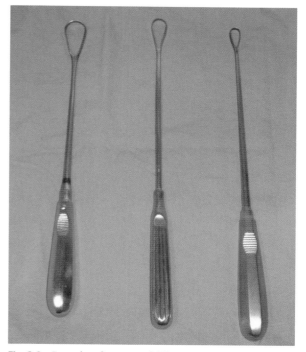

Fig. 2.8 Examples of curettes of different sizes.

Diagnostic Imaging Procedures

Hysterosalpingography

Hysterosalpingography is a radiograph of the uterus and fallopian tubes that involves the injection of dye through the cervix (**Fig. 2.10**). It is performed to assess the tubal patency and to find abnormalities in the uterine cavity, usually as part of infertility work-up. In addition to tubal patency, this test can also detect a uterine filling defect,

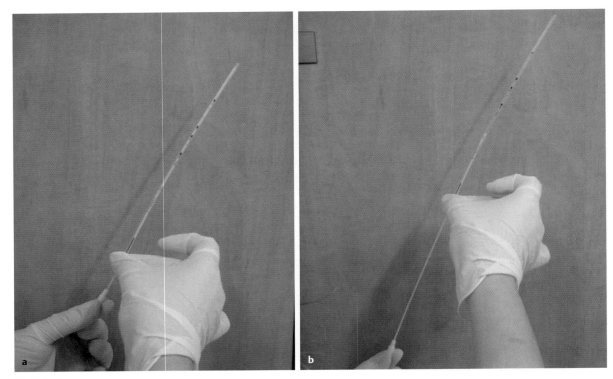

Fig. 2.9a, b
a The plastic Pipelle cannula.
b Pulling the inner device to guides the biopsy material into the cannula.

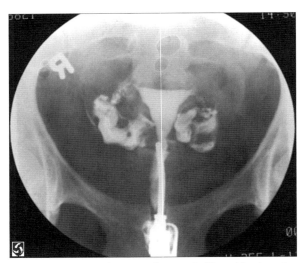

Fig. 2.10   A hysterosalpingography is a valuable tool for detecting any blockages in the fallopian tubes as well as abnormalities of the uterine cavity.

which can be an indication of myomas, polyps, or müllerian duct anomalies, all of which require further evaluation.

A hysterosalpingography typically is performed in the follicular phase of the menstrual cycle. The contrast ma-

terial can be any oil-based dye with good resolution of tubal architecture and a high postprocedure pregnancy rate. The main disadvantage of using an oil-based dye is the risk for lipid embolism caused by dye extravasation or lipid granuloma formation. The other option for a contrast material is a water-soluble dye. After a radiopaque dye is injected, radiographs are taken and the uterus and tubes outline is demonstrated.

Ultrasonography

An ultrasonographic test uses sound waves reflected from anatomical structures to produce three-dimensional images. Depending on the organ density, a different echo is returned from the organ to the wave source. This differentiation enables the machine to create an image of different shades of gray.

Ultrasonography is considered a safe and painless method. It allows for measuring the uterus size and endometrium, demonstrating and defining myomas, observing early pregnancy in the uterus or in ectopic places, and diagnosing of an abnormal molar pregnancy.

Furthermore, ultrasonography can be used to measure the ovaries, diagnose cysts, and differentiate them as simple or complex, and to detect any other pelvic masses.

Indeed, ultrasonography is considered more sensitive in the diagnosis of pelvic masses than computed tomography, and is widely used for such diagnoses.

Using Doppler ultrasound studies, an ovarian or pelvic mass is further evaluated, raising or decreasing the suspicion of malignancy. Free fluid in the pelvis is an important aspect when evaluating ectopic pregnancy, hemorrhagic corpus luteum, and ascites in ovarian malignancy or ovarian hyperstimulation syndrome (Evidence Box 2.1).

Hysteroscopy

A hysteroscope is a fiberoptic device that enables the direct visualization of the uterine cavity. The procedure is performed under sedation and paracervical block, or under anesthesia. During the procedure, the uterus is inflated with fluid (e.g., saline, dextran), and the hysteroscope is inserted through the cervix into the uterine cavity (**Fig. 2.11**).

Hysteroscopy can be carried out as a diagnostic test or a therapeutic procedure, in which uterine septa can be resected, an endometrial polyp can be removed, a submucos myoma can be resected, or the endometrium can be ablated. Complications of hysteroscopy mainly involve perforation, bleeding, or infection.

Hysteroscopy is sometimes used in conjunction with other procedures, such as curettage, in the evaluation of abnormal vaginal bleeding evaluation or laparoscopy (see below) during an infertility work-up.

Laparoscopy

Laparoscopy is a procedure in which the abdominal and pelvic cavities are viewed directly by a fiberoptic device: the laparoscope. Under general anesthesia, the laparoscope is inserted through a small incision in the umbilical area. The abdominal cavity is inflated with carbon dioxide in order to lift the abdominal wall and enable a good view of the organs.

In some cases, laparoscopy is used for diagnostic purposes, such as in diagnosing the cause of chronic pelvic or abdominal pain, evaluating the cause of infertility, or for taking a biopsy. In other cases, laparoscopy is used in surgery, such as for removing an ovarian cyst or an ectopic pregnancy. It also is used for tubal sterilization and even laparoscopic hysterectomy. When a surgical procedure is performed, additional tools are inserted to the abdomen through extra-abdominal incisions. Common complications of laparoscopy include bladder, urethra or bowel injury, and bleeding.

Key Points

- The chief complaint is a condensed summary of the reasons why the patient is seeking medical care, and includes name, age, familial status, residency, and the main medical issue for which care is sought.
- To complete the history, the physician should follow up with more direct questions, asking for more details about every symptom mentioned by the patient.
- A gynecologic history involves asking the patient a number of detailed questions regarding her age of menarche, menstrual regularity, last menstrual period, duration of menstruation, and length of her menstrual cycle
- A complete obstetric history may provide important clues about the general health of the patient.
- A sexual history is important to learn about a patient's family planning and contraceptive practices as well as information regarding symptoms experienced during intercourse such as bleeding, dyspareunia etc., which provide important clues for a diagnosis.
- The physical examination, particularly the pelvic examination, can sometimes evoke anxiety and fear in the patient, and a few, relatively simple preventive measures can reduce these feelings.

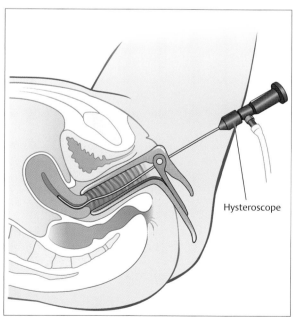

Hysteroscope

Fig. 2.11 The hysteroscope is typically used by doctors to diagnose and treat uterine polyps.

Evidence Box 2.1

A comparative study of different imaging methods has shown that ultrasonography, computed tomography, and magnetic resonance imaging are equally efficacious at diagnosing and staging ovarian cancer.

Kurtz et al. evaluated potential masses in 280 women suspected to have ovarian cancer using Doppler ultrasonography (US), computed tomography (CT), and magnetic resonance imaging (MRI). They also used conventional US, CT, and MRI to stage spread. All three modalities had high accuracy (0.91) for the overall diagnosis of malignancy. In the ovaries, the accuracy of MRI (0.91) was higher than that of CT and significantly higher than that of Doppler US (0.78). In the extra-ovarian pelvis and in the abdomen, conventional US, CT, and MRI had similar accuracies (0.87–0.95). In differentiation of disease confined to the pelvis from abdominal spread, the specificity of conventional US (96%) was higher than that of CT and significantly higher than that of MRI (88%), whereas the sensitivities of MR imaging (98%) and CT (92%) were significantly higher than that of conventional US (75%). The researchers concluded that although MRI is superior to Doppler US and CT in diagnosing malignant ovarian masses, there is little variation among conventional US, CT, and MR imaging as regards staging.

Kurtz AB, Tsimikas JV, Tempany CM, et al. Diagnosis and staging of ovarian cancer: comparative values of Doppler and conventional US, CT, and MR imaging correlated with surgery and histopathologic analysis—report of the Radiology Diagnostic Oncology Group. Radiology 1999 Jul;212(1):19–27.

Further Reading

American College of Obstetricians and Gynecologists. ACOG Committee Opinion. Primary and preventive care: periodic assessments. *Obstet Gynecol* 2003;102(5 Pt 1):1117–1124

Practice Bulletin ACOG; ACOG Committee on Practice Bulletins. ACOG Practice Bulletin: clinical management guidelines for obstetrician-gynecologists. Number 45, August 2003. Cervical cytology screening (replaces committee opinion 152, March 1995). *Obstet Gynecol* 2003;102(2):417–427

Berek JS, ed. Berek and Novak's Gynecology. 14th ed. Philadelphia, Pa: Lippincott Williams & Wilkins; 2007

Bickley LS, ed. Bates' Guide to Physical Examination and History Taking. 7th ed. Rochester, NY: Lippincott Williams & Wilkins; 1999

Frye CA, Weisberg RB. Increasing the incidence of routine pelvic examinations: behavioral medicine's contribution. *Women Health* 1994;21(1):33–55

Kurtz AB, Tsimikas JV, Tempany CM, et al. Diagnosis and staging of ovarian cancer: comparative values of Doppler and conventional US, CT, and MR imaging correlated with surgery and histopathologic analysis—report of the Radiology Diagnostic Oncology Group. *Radiology* 1999;212(1):19–27

3 Embryology of the Female Reproductive System

Shimrit Yaniv Sakem

This chapter describes the normal development of the female reproductive system as well as the defects that sometimes occur in the female reproductive tract during embryogenesis.

Definitions

Agenesis: This term refers to failure of an organ to develop during embryonic growth and development. Many forms of agenesis are referred to by individual names, depending on the organ affected.

Canalization: The production of a canal structure.

External genitalia: These are comprised of the labia majora, labia minora, mons veneris (mons pubis) clitoris, vulvar vestibule and urethral meatus, and glandular structures opening to the vaginal vestibule.

Hemivagina: This is a rare urogenital malformation characterized by a transverse vaginal septum.

Internal genitalia: The internal genitalia include the uterus, cervix, ovaries, and fallopian tubes.

Müllerian duct: The internal female sex duct, which forms on each side of a female embryo to connect the peritoneal cavity with the outside of the embryo.

Genital Embryogenesis

Embryogenesis of the genital tract occurs at 8 weeks of gestation. The external genitalia are derived from the genital tubercle (**Fig. 3.1**). The labial structures are of ectodermal origin; the urethra vaginal introitus and vulvar vestibule are derived from uroepethelial endoderm. Thus, the upper two-thirds are of müllerian origin, and the lower third is of urogenital sinus origin.

The internal genitalia originate from the genital ridge. The embryologic ovaries migrate caudaly to the true pelvis. The primordial follicles remain dormant until adolescence. The müllerian ducts migrate caudally to form the fallopian tubes and fuse in the midline to create the uterus. A vertical midline septum is present until the end of the first trimester (**Fig. 3.2**), at which time it is reabsorbed. Failure of lateral fusion or of the septal reabsorption will result in what is referred to as müllerian duct anomalies (**Fig. 3.3**).

Malformations of the external genitalia vary from vaginal agenesis, as can be found in Mayer–Rokitansky–Kuster–Hauser syndrome, through to failure of vaginal canalization. Failure of canalization might manifest as imperforated hymen, requiring further evaluation for transverse or lateral axis defects resulting in obstructed hemivagina or nonsignificant septa, which is found in up to 1 in 80 000 women.

The incidence of uterine anomalies is between 1 in 100 and 1 in 1000 women. Clinical presentation might be primary amenorrhea, dysmenorrhea, a symptomatic pelvic mass; and more commonly, infertility, repeat abortions, and preterm labor. The most common uterine malformations are listed in **Table 3.1**.

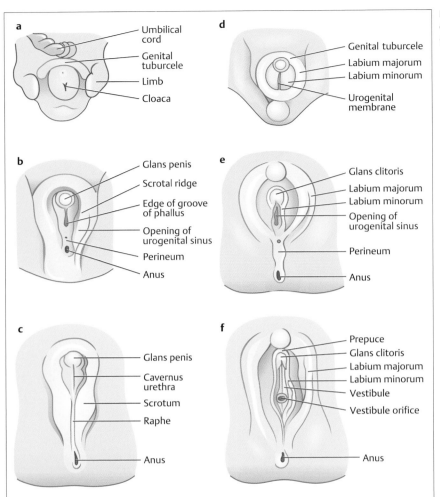

Fig. 3.1 Differentiation to male (**a**, **c**, **e**) and female (**b**, **d**, **f**) external genitalia.

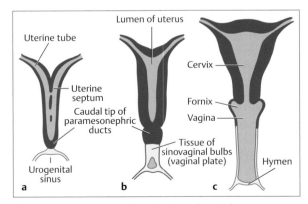

Fig. 3.2 Embryogenesis of female internal genitalia.

Table 3.1 Common müllerian abnormalities

Organ	Abnormality
Ovary	Duplication of ovary; secondary ovarian rests; para-ovarian cysts (wolffian remnants)
Tube	Congenital absence; paratubal cyst (hydatid of Morgagni); hydrosalpinx—accumulation of serous fluid in the fallopian tube, often an end-result of pyosalpinx
Vagina	Agenesis; transverse or longitudinal septum; para-vaginal (Gartner duct) cyst; hydrocolpos—accumulation of mucus or nonsanguineous fluid in the vagina; hemihematometra—atretic segment of vagina with menstrual fluid accumulation
Uterus	Didelphic uterus—two cervices, each associated with one uterine horn; bicornuate uterus—one cervix associated with two uterine horns; unicornuate uterus—result of failure of one müllerian duct to descend

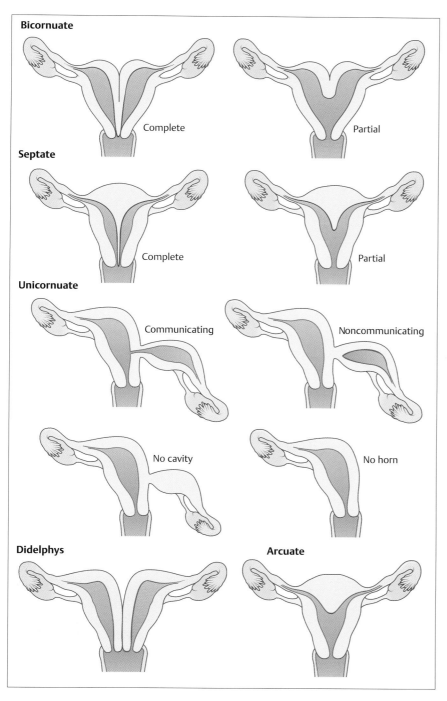

Bicornuate

Complete

Partial

Septate

Complete

Partial

Unicornuate

Communicating

Noncommunicating

No cavity

No horn

Didelphys

Arcuate

Fig. 3.3 Types of müllerian uterine anomalies.

Anatomy

External Genitalia

The external genitalia are comprised of the labia majora, labia minora, mons veneris (mons pubis) clitoris, vulvar vestibule and urethral meatus, and glandular structures opening to the vaginal vestibule (**Fig. 3.4**). These structures vary between individuals in morphology and hair distribution. Beneath these structures lie the fascial and muscular layers of the perineum.

The muscles of the external genitalia consist of the deep and superficial transverse perineal muscles, the ischiocavernosus muscles that cover the crura of the clitoris, and the bulbocavernosus muscles lying on either side of the vagina covering the vestibular bulbs.

The layers of the external genitalia as detailed are of clinical importance while performing an episiotomy—an incision of the pudenda and the covering perineum made during the second stage of labor—as illustrated in **Fig. 3.5**.

The Uterus

The uterus is a midline, pear-shaped pelvic organ situated between the bladder anteriorly and the rectum posteriorly. It is covered posteriorly by serosa or peritoneum, covering also the upper anterior side, while the lower anterior side is connected with the posterior side of the bladder via a loose layer of connective tissue. The size of the uterus varies greatly. At reproductive stage it is about $8 \times 6 \times 4$ cm, and much smaller during childhood and postmenopause. It is of course much larger during pregnancy.

The uterus may be divided to two main areas: the broad triangular body and the narrow cylindrical cervix as illustrated in **Fig. 3.6**. The fallopian tubes emerge at the superior poll of the uterus at the cornea, defining the fundus. The endometrium is a fine mucosal layer that lines the uterus and varies in thickness and histology, according to age and menstrual phase.

The thick myometrium is a deeper layer of smooth muscle united by connective tissue. The structure is not even, and the greatest muscular mass is found in the fundi and diminishes gradually to comprise only about 10% of the cervical mass. This is of great importance when considering uterine contractile ability. Blood supply is by the uterine artery, a branch of the anterior portion of the internal iliac.

The uterus is suspended from the pelvic walls by various ligaments (**Fig. 3.7**). The broad ligaments are wing-shaped structures extending from both lateral portions of the uterus. The broad ligaments give rise at their upper portion to the mesosalpinx to which the fallopian tubes are connected, and to the suspensory ligament of the ovary where ovarian vessels pass through. At its lower portion, the broad ligament gives rise to the cardinal ligament which fuses with connective tissue adjacent to the cervix. The round ligaments extend from the lateral part of the uterus downward through the broad ligament to the upper portion of the labia majora. The uterosacral ligaments suspend the uterus in the height of the supravaginal portion of the cervix.

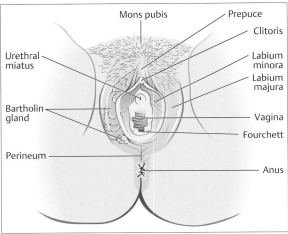

Fig. 3.4 Female external genitalia.

Labels: Mons pubis, Prepuce, Clitoris, Urethral miatus, Labium minora, Labium majura, Bartholin gland, Vagina, Fourchett, Perineum, Anus

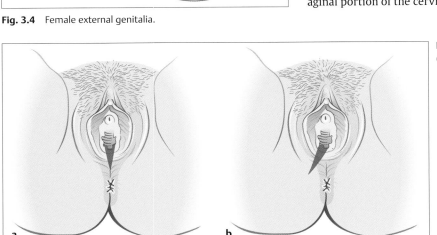

Fig. 3.5 Medial (**a**) and lateral (**b**) episiotomy.

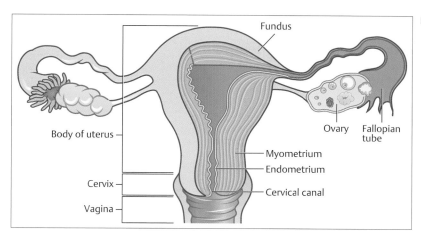

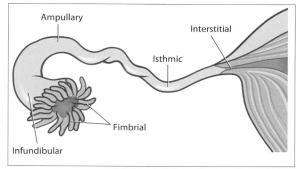

Fundus

Body of uterus

Cervix

Vagina

Ovary   Fallopian tube

Myometrium

Endometrium

Cervical canal

Fig. 3.6   The uterus.

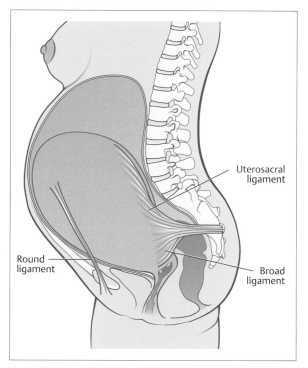

Uterosacral ligament

Round ligament

Broad ligament

Fig. 3.7   Uterine ligaments at term pregnancy.

Ampullary

Interstitial

Isthmic

Fimbrial

Infundibular

Fig. 3.8   Regions of the fallopian tube.

The Ovaries

The ovaries are almond-shaped, white silvery organs, varying in size according to the age and ovulatory stage of the woman. They are situated in the upper part of the pelvic cavity, on either side of the uterus. Blood supply to the ovaries is via the ovarian arteries arising directly from the aorta.

The Bony Pelvis

The pelvis is composed of four bones: the sacrum, coccyx, and two innominate bones. The innominate bones are formed by the fusion of the ilium, ischium, and pubis.

There are three diameters described at the level of the pelvic inlet: anteroposterior, transverse, and oblique. The obstetrically important anteroposterior diameter is the shortest distance between the promontory of the sacrum and the symphysis pubis, and measures normally 10 cm or more.

The anteroposterior diameter of the pelvic inlet has been identified as the *true conjugate.* The shortest distance

Fallopian Tubes

The fallopian tubes, less commonly known as the oviducts, are cylindrical structures 8–14 cm in length. They may be divided into four anatomical regions (**Fig. 3.8**). The **interstitial** portion is embedded in the uterine wall, the **isthmus** is the narrow part opening to the wide **ampulla**, and the **infundibulum** is the funnel-shaped extremity ending in the fimbria. The tubes are lined with ciliated cells participating in the peristalsis found in the tube. Blood supply is from branches of the uterine artery and anastomosis with the ovarian vessels.

between the promontory of the sacrum and the symphysis pubis is the *obstetric conjugate*, which is the shortest anteroposterior diameter through which the head must pass when descending through the pelvic inlet.

The obstetric conjugate cannot be measured directly digitally. For clinical purposes, the obstetric conjugate is estimated indirectly by subtracting 1.5–2 cm from the diagonal conjugate. The latter is determined by measuring the distance from the lower margin of the symphysis to the promontory of the sacrum.

Key Points

- Embryogenesis of the female genital tract occurs at 8 weeks of gestation.
- The incidence of uterine anomalies is between 1 in 100 and 1 in 1000 women. Clinical presentation might be primary amenorrhea, dysmenorrhea, a symptomatic pelvic mass, and more commonly, infertility, repeat abortions, and preterm labor.
- The external genitalia are comprised of the labia majora, labia minora, mons veneris (mons pubis), clitoris, vulvar vestibule and urethral meatus, and glandular structures opening to the vaginal vestibule.
- The uterus is a midline pear-shaped pelvic organ situated between the bladder anteriorly and the rectum posteriorly.
- The fallopian tubes, less commonly known as the oviducts, are cylindrical structures 8–14 cm in length.
- The ovaries are almond-shaped silvery-white organs, varying in size according to the age and ovulatory stage of the woman.
- The pelvis is composed of four bones: the sacrum, coccyx, and two innominate bones.

Further Reading

Cunningham FG, Leveno KJ, Bloom SL, et al, eds.ds. Williams Obstetrics. 22nd ed. New York: McGraw-Hill Medical; 2005.

Edmonds DK. Congenital malformations of the genital tract. *Obstet Gynecol Clin North Am* 2000;27(1):49–62

Folch M, Pigem I, Konje JC. Müllerian agenesis: etiology, diagnosis, and management. *Obstet Gynecol Surv* 2000; 55(10):644–649

Nelson Textbook of Pediatrics. 18th ed. New York: Elsevier/ WB Saunders, 2007.

Stelling J, Gray M, Davis A, van Lingen B, Reindollar R. Müllerian agenesis: an update. *Obstet Gynecol* 1997;90(6):1024–1025

Spence JE. Vaginal and uterine anomalies in the pediatric and adolescent patient. *J Pediatr Adolesc Gynecol* 1998;11(1): 3–11

Townsend CM, Beauchamp RD, Evers BM, Mattox KL. Sabiston Textbook of Surgery. 18th ed. St. Louis, Mo: Elsevier/WB Saunders; 2007.

4 The Menstrual Cycle and Fertilization

Arnon Wiznitzer

Menarche is often considered to be the central event of female puberty. The age of onset of menarche is variable, and ranges between 9.1 and 17.7 years with a mean of almost 13 years. The events that initiate puberty are still unknown. However, adrenal steroids and melatonin are probable initiators of these events. Maturation at puberty probably involves changes in the hypothalamus that are independent of ovarian steroids.

An orderly sequence of events follows the maturational changes in the hypothalamus, which includes an increased secretion and response to gonadotropin-releasing hormone (GnRH). This, in turn, leads to an increased production and secretion of gonadotropins, which are responsible for follicular growth and development in the ovary and increased sex steroid levels. This series of events leads finally to the monthly cycle of hormone production and simultaneous proliferation of the uterine lining to prepare for possible fertilization of the ovum and implantation of the embryo—a process known as the "menstrual cycle."

To facilitate understanding in this chapter, discussion of the menstrual cycle is divided between cyclic changes that occur in ovary and the uterus. There is also a brief discussion of the process of fertilization.

Definitions

Amenorrhea: The absence of menstrual bleeding is known as amenorrhea.

Follicular atresia: This is the process by which a primary follicle or a tertiary follicle stops growing, leading to disappearance (apoptosis) of its follicle cells and the oocyte, or egg, they contain. Such a follicle is called an atretic follicle.

Gamete: This term refers to a mature sexual reproductive cell having a single set of unpaired chromosomes.

Gametocyte: This describes an immature animal or plant cell that develops into a gamete by meiosis.

Hypophysis: This is a term for the pituitary gland. The anterior lobe is sometimes identified as the adenohypophysis and the posterior lobe as the neurohypophysis.

Menarche: The time in a girl's life when menstruation first begins is known as menarche. During the menarche period, menstruation may be irregular and unpredictable. Mood, weight, activity level, and growth rate may fluctuate with the hormone levels. This term is often used synonymously with female puberty.

Menses: This refers to the monthly flow of blood from the genital tract of a woman.

Menorrhea: This term describes the normal discharge of the menses.

Oocyte: A female gametocyte that develops into an ovum after two meiotic divisions is known as an oocyte.

Oogonia: This term describes a descendant of a primordial germ cell that gives rise to oocytes.

Pubarche: This is a term for the beginning of puberty marked by the first appearance of pubic hair in the genital region.

Puberty: This is the process of physical changes by which a child's body becomes capable of reproduction. Puberty is initiated by hormone signals from the brain to the gonads (the ovaries and testes). In response, the gonads produce a variety of hormones that stimulate the growth, function, or transformation of brain, bones, muscle, skin, breasts, and reproductive organs.

Thelarche: The start of breast development in a woman at the beginning of puberty is known as thelarche.

The Menstrual Cycle

The menstrual cycle can be divided into three phases:
1. Follicular phase
2. Ovulation
3. Luteal phase

Follicular Phase

Follicular development is a dynamic process designed to allow the monthly recruitment of a cohort of follicles, and the selection of one dominant follicle that will release a single mature oocyte each month.

In humans, the average length of the follicular phase ranges from 10 to 14 days (**Fig. 4.1**), and variability in this length is responsible for most of the variation in total cycle length. The follicular phase initiates at the first day of the menses. At this time the levels of gonadal steroids are low, and with the demise of the corpus luteum follicle-stimulating hormone (FSH) levels begin to rise recruiting a cohort of follicles.

In response to FSH, the follicles initiate the secretion of estrogen, which increases through the follicular phase and is responsible for endometrial growth. The rise in estrogen exerts a negative feedback on FSH at the hypophysis (pituitary gland) level.

In addition, the growing follicles produce inhibin B, which also suppresses FSH secretion by the pituitary.

Conversely, the rise in estrogen levels at the beginning of the cycle produces a negative effect on the secretion of luteinizing hormone (LH), but late in the follicular phase LH levels increase dramatically.

During the follicular phase, hormonal feedback promotes the orderly development of a single dominant follicle, which is destined to ovulate from a period of initial growth of a primordial follicle through the stages of the preantral, antral, and preovulatory follicular growth (**Fig. 4.2**).

This phase corresponds to the proliferative phase in the uterus, in which there is building of the endometrial lining. In the middle of the follicular phase of menstrual cycle, after growth of a follicle has been achieved, local concentrations of prostaglandins and proteolytic enzymes induce the extrusion of the oocyte through the follicular wall, and ovulation occurs.

After ovulation, the menstrual cycle enters the luteal phase, the ruptured follicle becomes the corpus luteum and secretion of both progesterone and estrogen provide the adequate environment for the fertilized oocyte to implant in the endometrium. This phase corresponds to the secretory phase in the uterus.

If fertilization occurs, the secretion of human chorionic gonadotropin (HCG) by the embryo rescues the corpus luteum, allowing the continued secretion of progesterone and estrogen to sustain the pregnancy. If fertilization does not occur, the corpus luteum dies, which causes a drop in progesterone and estrogen levels and eventual shedding of the endometrium (menses).

Ovarian Follicular Development

Most oogonia are lost during fetal development, and the remaining follicles are recruited during the reproductive years until menopause occurs, in which the oocyte reserve is depleted.

During fetal development, the oogonia are arrested at the diplotene stage of the prophase in the first meiosis, the germ-cell process of reduction division. At this stage, a single layer of 8 to 10 granulosa cells surrounds the oogonia to form the primordial follicle. Those oogonia that fail to be properly surrounded by granulosa cells undergo atresia.

When the developing oogonia begin to enter the meiotic prophase I, they are known as primary follicles (**Fig. 4.3**), or oocytes, and remain arrested in this phase, until the time of ovulation, by a probable stasis mechanism involving an oocyte maturation inhibitor (OMI) produced by granulosa cells.

It is believed that the inhibitory action of this substance is achieved via gap junctions connecting the oocyte to its surrounding granulosa cells. When the LH surge at midcycle occurs, the gap junctions are disrupted, and the connection between the oocyte and granulosa cells is interrupted, allowing meiosis I to resume.

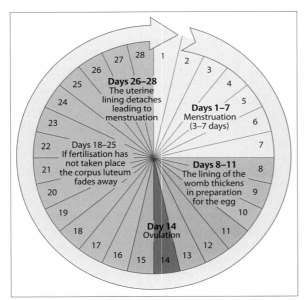

Fig. 4.1 A diagram of the menstrual cycle. The follicular phase constitutes the period beginning with menstruation and ending at ovulation, which is approximately 14 days in most women.

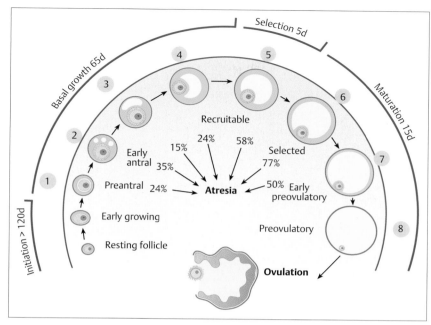

Fig. 4.2 Folliculogenesis and the classes of growing follicles in the human ovary. The early stages of folliculogenesis proceed very slowly, and it has been estimated that in humans the process can take more than 300 days. Even in the preantral stage (class 1), many growing follicles fail to survive, and degenerate through a process termed follicular atresia. Growing follicles enter class 2 usually in the late luteal phase, class 3 between late luteal and early follicular phases, class 4 during late follicular phase, and become recruitable class 5 follicles during late luteal phase.

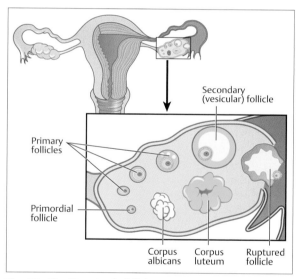

Fig. 4.3 The life cycle of a follicle.

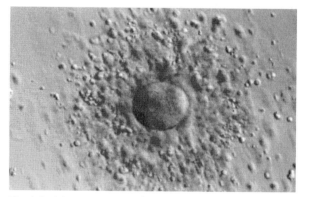

Fig. 4.4 A human oocyte with surrounding granulosa cells, after aspiration.

Primordial Follicles

In each cycle there is growth of a cohort of oocytes. The initial recruitment and growth of the primordial follicles is independent of gonadotropin and affects a cohort over several months. The factor(s) responsible for the recruitment in each cycle is unknown. After initial recruitment, control of follicular growth and differentiation shifts from gonadotropin-independent to gonadotropin-dependent growth, presumably by FSH. The action of FSH promotes growth of the oocyte and expansion of the granulosa cells (**Fig. 4.4**) from a single layer to a multilayer of cuboidal cells.

Preantral Follicle

Driven by the stimulus of FSH, the zona pellucid, a glycoprotein-rich substance, is formed, which separates the oocyte from the surrounding granulosa cells. Simultaneously with the proliferation of granulosa cells, there is proliferation of theca cells in the stroma bordering the granulosa. Both granulosa and theca cells function synergistically to produce estrogen, which is then secreted into the circulation. One of the follicles attains dominance over the rest of the cohort, which undergo atresia.

The mechanism for selection of the dominant follicle is still not clear, but follicular development can be explained by the "two-cell, two-gonadotropin theory," which states that during follicle development, steroid hormone synthesis takes place in a compartmentalized

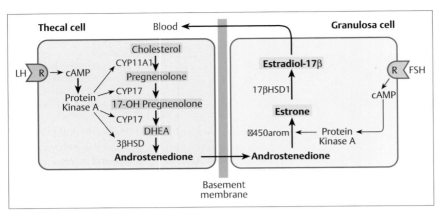

Fig. 4.5 Schematic diagram of the two-cell theory. DHAE, dehydroepiandrosterone; R, receptor; HSD, hydroxysteroid dehydrogenase; P450arom, androgen aromatase; CYP, cytochrome P450 enzyme; LH, luteinizing hormone; FSH, follicle-stimulating hormone; cAMP, cyclic AMP.

manner (**Fig. 4.5**). According to the two-cell theory, estrogen is produced in the granulosa cell by aromatization of androgens; the activity of the enzyme (aromatase) that catalyzes this reaction is enhanced by FSH stimulation of specific receptors on these cells.

Androgens, in turn, are synthesized by theca cells primarily in response to stimulation by LH. The androgens produced in theca cells, which have most of the LH receptors at this early stage of the menstrual cycle, are transferred to the granulosa cells and are aromatized into estrogens. This, in turn, contributes to the continuous growth of the follicle and to a positive feedback on FSH. Positive feedback on FSH further stimulates estrogen production by inducing FSH receptor synthesis and expression.

Androgens have two different regulatory roles in follicular development. At low concentrations, they stimulate aromatase activity via specific receptors in granulosa cells in the early preantral follicle. However, at higher levels, androgens are converted enzymatically by 5α-reductase to forms that cannot be aromatized, thus creating an androgenic environment in the follicle that inhibits the expression of FSH receptors and aromatase activity. This androgenic environment eventually results in follicle atresia.

When the peripheral estrogen level rises, it exerts a negative feedback on the pituitary that decreases circulating FSH levels. In addition, the ovary produces inhibin B, which further decreases FSH production. The resulting decrease in FSH level can only be survived by those follicles with the greatest number of FSH receptors.

This process ends when a single dominant follicle emerges, while the remaining follicles from the cohort suffer atresia (**Fig. 4.6**) due to decreasing FSH support, which interrupts granulosa proliferation and function, promotes a conversion to an androgenic microenvironment, and induces irreversible atretic changes.

During the cycle, sex steroids are not the only gonadotropin regulators of follicular development and ovulation initiation. At the level of the pituitary gland, there are two related granulosa cell-derived peptides that play opposing roles: inhibin A and inhibin B. Inhibin B is se-

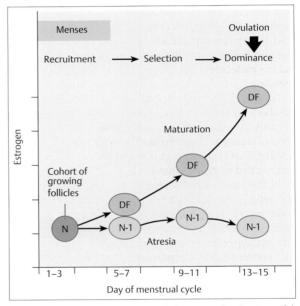

Fig. 4.6 The follicle that eventually becomes the dominant follicle (DF) is the one which is best at continuing to develop, grow, and produce estrogen, and by this process is able to strengthen its advantage against other follicles (N–1) by outcompeting them for follicle-stimulating hormone.

creted primarily in the follicular phase and is stimulated by FSH, whereas inhibin A is mainly active in the luteal phase. Both forms of inhibin act to inhibit FSH synthesis and release. A second peptide, activin, stimulates FSH release from the pituitary and potentiates its action in the ovary.

A third important peptide involved in follicular development is follistatin, which inhibits FSH synthesis, secretion, and response to GnRH. Follistatin is believed to work by binding to activin and decreasing its activity. It is expressed by granulosa cells in response to FSH and activin.

In addition to these peptides, there are many other intra-ovarian regulators known to play an important role in promoting the normal ovulatory process. Some of these include insulinlike growth factor 1(ILGF-1), epidermal growth factor (EGF)/transforming growth factor (TGF)-α, TGF-β₁, β-fibroblast growth factor (FGF), interleukin-1, tissue necrosis factor-α, oocyte maturation inhibitor, and renin–angiotensin.

Preovulatory Follicle

When the dominant follicle reaches it maximal growth, it is characterized by a fluid-filled antrum composed of plasma and granulosa cell secretions (**Fig. 4.7**). At this point granulosa cells surround the oocyte and maintain their connection to it via gap junctions. This group of cells that surrounds the oocyte also is known as the *cumulus oophorus*. The granulosa cells depend upon these specialized gap junctions that communicate with the oocyte for the purpose of metabolic exchange, the transport of signalling molecules, and the inhibition and stimulation of meiosis.

As the rising levels of estrogen exert their negative feedback on FHS secretion, they also enhance LH release. For this to occur, however, a high and sustained serum level of estrogen of 200 pg/mL for more than 48 hours is needed. This typically occurs when the dominant follicle has reached at least 15 mm in diameter.

At the same time, LH receptors on the granulosa cells are induced by local estrogen and FSH interactions. This positive feedback is responsible for the midcycle LH surge, with exposure to high levels of LH that result in three specific responses by the dominant follicle:
1. Luteinization of the granulosa cells
2. Production of progesterone
3. Initiation of the ovulation process

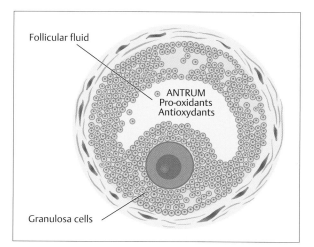

Fig. 4.7 The follicular fluid consists of a pro-antioxidant and an antioxidant-rich solution of secretions from plasma and granulosa cells.

In general, ovulation will occur in a single, mature, dominant follicle in every cycle, 10–12 hours after the LH peak, or 34–36 hours after the initial LH surge

In the follicles that fail to achieve maturity and undergo atresia, the theca cells return to their origin as a component of stromal tissue, retaining their ability to respond to LH with androgen production. Thus, the increase in stromal tissue in the late follicular phase is associated with a rise in androgen levels in the peripheral plasma at midcycle, which is believed to play a role in enhancing the process of atresia, stimulating libido, and increasing sexual activity at the time most likely to achieve pregnancy.

Ovulation

Ovulation occurs approximately 10–12 hours after the LH peak and 24–36 hours after peak estradiol level is attained. The onset of the LH surge appears to be the most reliable indicator of impending ovulation, occurring 34–36 hours prior to follicle rupture (see Evidence Box 4.1).

The rise in progesterone levels at this stage increases the distensibility of the follicle wall, which helps to explain the rapid increase in follicular fluid volume prior to ovulation that is unaccompanied by any significant change in intrafollicular pressure. After selection of the dominant follicle takes place with distention of the antrum caused by the increment of antral fluid, there is compression of the granulosa against the limiting membrane separating the avascular granulosa and the luteinized, vascularized theca interna.

The thinning of the thecal layer over the surface with the creation of an avascular area causes the ovarian capsule to weaken and finally rupture with extrusion of the oocyte in its cumulus. This process is more than a mere elevation of intrafollicular pressure. Rather, it involves multiple complex processes in order to attain oocyte maturation.

Apparently, there is the need for a preovulatory surge in prostaglandin synthesis within the follicle, caused by the LH surge, which is thought to increase the concentration and activity of local proteases. These proteases are responsible for weakening the follicular wall by disrupting the collagenous layer and causing the loss of intercellular gap junction integrity fibers. Also in the follicle, an inflammatory-like response is promoted by angiogenesis and hyperemia.

Moreover, the LH surge is responsible for luteinization of granulosa cells, expansion of the cumulus, and resumption of meiosis in the oocyte, which is not completed until after the sperm has entered the oocyte and the second polar body is extruded. The latter is caused by LH-induced cyclic AMP activity that overcomes the local inhibitory action of OMI and luteinization inhibitor.

Ovulation is the result of proteolytic digestion of the follicular apex, a site called the stigma. Prostaglandins may also contract smooth muscle cells that have been identified in the ovary, thereby aiding in the extrusion of the oocyte and cumulus cell.

With the LH surge, levels of progesterone in the follicle continue to rise up to the time of ovulation. The progressive rise in progesterone may act as a negative feedback to terminate the LH surge (**Fig. 4.8**), although the exact mechanism responsible for the end of the LH surge is unknown.

Luteal Phase

Shortly before ovulation, the ruptured follicle continues to suffer profound alterations in cellular organization. The granulosa cells hypertrophy markedly during the first 3 days after ovulation, and capillaries begin to penetrate into the granulosa layer reaching the central cavity, gradually filling in the cystic, sometimes hemorrhagic, cavity of the early corpus luteum.

In addition, granulosa cells become markedly luteinized by the incorporation of lipid-rich vacuoles within their fully vascularized cytoplasm. Angiogenesis is an important feature of the luteinization process, and is a response to LH mediated by growth factors produced in luteinized granulosa cells, such as vascular endothelial growth factor. The theca cells of the corpus luteum become less prominent. As a result, a new yellow body is formed that is dependent on the small, but important, quantities of LH available in the luteal phase, which in turn stimulates the production of estradiol and progesterone. The secretion of progesterone and estradiol during the luteal phase is episodic, and the changes correlate closely with LH pulses.

Indeed, normal luteal function requires optimal preovulatory follicular development with adequate levels of FSH and estradiol. Moreover, the successful conversion of the avascular granulosa of the follicular phase to the vascularized luteal tissue (corpus luteum) is responsible for the adequate transport of cholesterol by low-density lipoprotein (LDL), which serves as substrate for the production of progesterone. Thus, the capacity of the corpus luteum to produce steroids (primarily progesterone) is dependent on continued LH secretion (**Fig. 4.9**).

Luteal cells are both large and small. The former are believed to be derived from granulosa cells. The small cells, which are greater in number, are believed to derive from thecal cells. Most of the steroidogenesis takes place in the large cells, although it is the small cells that contain LH and HCG receptors. Intercellular communication through gap junctions is mediated the passage of regulating factors from small to large cells.

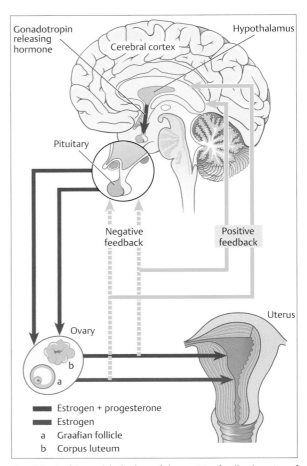

Fig. 4.8 In this model, the loss of the positive feedback action of estradiol, the increasing negative feedback of progesterone, or a depletion in pituitary LH content due to downregulation of gonadotropin-releasing hormone (GnRH) receptors, are responsible for the abrupt end of the luteinizing hormone (LH) surge.

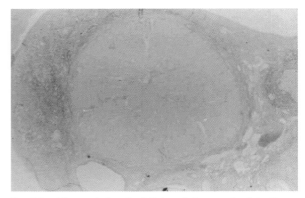

Fig. 4.9 After ovulation the follicle cells form a glandular tissue, called the corpus luteum, which secretes progesterone.

Besides the luteal cells, endothelial cells, leukocytes, and fibroblasts are responsible for the secretion of non-steroidal products during the luteal phase, including cytokines, interleukin-1b, and tissue necrosis factor-α, and are an directly involved in angiogenesis, steroidogenesis, and luteolysis.

By day 8 or 9 after ovulation, peak vascularization is reached, which is accompanied by peak levels of progesterone and estradiol in the blood. New follicular growth is suppressed by progesterone and low levels of gonadotropins as a result of negative feedback by estrogen, progesterone, and inhibin A.

The average life of the corpus luteum is 14 days unless a new source of stimulation becomes available. If successful implantation occurs, HCG secreted by the embryo becomes the LH-like stimulus for the continued secretion of estradiol and progesterone by the corpus luteum. If no stimulus becomes available, the corpus luteum rapidly ages, losing its vascularity and lipid content, and a scar tissue is formed. As the levels of estrogen and progesterone drop, menstrual bleeding ensues.

During the last days of the luteal phase of the cycle, hormonal changes responsible for the transition from the luteal phase to a new follicular phase include changes in the secretion of GnRH, FSH, LH, estradiol, progesterone, and inhibins. There is also a selective increase in FSH that begins approximately 2 days before the onset of menses, caused by a decrease in estrogen, progesterone, and inhibin, and a change in GnRH pulsatile secretion brought about by the process of luteolysis.

Fertilization

Fertilization involves fusion of gametes to produce a new organism of the same species. In humans and other animals, the process involves a sequence of events that begins with the contact of a sperm cell with an egg cell (ovum) and ends with the fusion of their two pronuclei (each containing 23 chromosomes) to form a new diploid cell, called a *zygote*. Fertilization normally occurs in the *ampulla* region of the fallopian tube 12–24 hours after ovulation (**Fig. 4.10**).

To reach the ovum, however, sperm must travel through the vagina and the cervix, through the uterus, and then up the fallopian tube. Smooth muscle contractions in the fallopian tube as well as ciliary activity (the waving of hairlike structures) of the tube's lining are both important in the transport of sperm up to the ovum, into and then down, the fallopian tube.

Although tens, or even hundreds, of millions of sperm are ejaculated, many fewer will actually reach the ovum. Those sperm that do survive the trip must get through follicle cells and zona pellucid covering the ovum (**Fig 4.11**) and finally contact and bind to the ovum's membrane by means of specialized structures in the head of the sperm cell.

When a sperm does get into the ovum, then the ovum membrane changes to prevent additional sperm from entering. The lone sperm cell that enters into the egg is also changing, and its specialized structures dissolve.

The haploid nuclei of both the sperm and the egg are now called male and female pronuclei. Both swell, as their densely packed DNA loosens prior to replication. They then migrate toward the center of the ovum, where their nuclear membranes disintegrate. The chromosomes contributed by the sperm and the ovum then pair up, an event called syngamy.

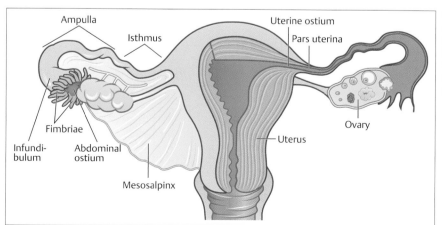

Fig. 4.10 Schematic diagram showing, among other structures, the infundibulum, ampulla, and isthmus regions of the oviduct and the regions where oocyte cumulus complexes and preimplantation embryos can be found.

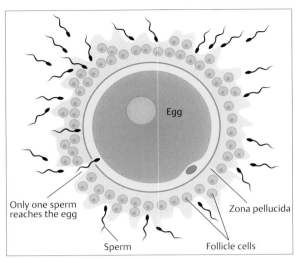

Fig. 4.11 Once sperm reach the ovum, they face even more obstacles in their attempts to fertilize the ovum. Once one sperm does enter, the ovum makes it difficult for others to follow suit.

In this integration, the diploid chromosome number (46) is restored, and a new complete genome comes into being. The result of syngamy is a zygote, or fertilized egg, which is already entering the first stage of its first mitotic division and beginning cleavage. If all goes well, the zygote will eventually mature into a fully formed human being.

After fertilization occurs, the zygote remains in the fallopian tube for about 72 hours and undergoes several cellular divisions. At around 72 hours, the zona pellucida fragments and falls away, and the dividing zygote, or blastocyst, enters the uterine cavity for an additional 60–72 hours. During this time, the central cavity begins to form, and a defined cell mass, called a trophoblast, is formed on one side of the blastocyst by the time implantation occurs.

The trophoblast cells, which will eventually form the placenta, burrow into the stroma of the endometrium to form a syncytiotrophoblast, which then invaginates and projects into the endometrium of the uterine wall. During placental development, these protrusions become surrounded by lacunae (cavernous spaces) filled with maternal blood. Primitive amniotic and chorionic cavities begin to form, and a germ disk is recognizable soon after implantation.

Key Points

- The menstrual cycle is monthly cycle of hormone production and simultaneous proliferation of the uterine lining to prepare for possible fertilization of the ovum and implantation of the embryo.
- In humans, the average length of the follicular phase ranges from 10 to 14 days, and variability in this length is responsible for most variation in total cycle length. The follicular phase initiates at the first day of the menses.
- The onset of the luteal hormone surge appears to be the most reliable indicator of impending ovulation.
- Normal luteal function requires optimal preovulatory follicular development with adequate levels of follicle-stimulating hormone and estradiol.
- Fertilization involves a sequence of events that begins with the contact of a sperm cell with an egg cell (ovum), and ends with the fusion of their two pronuclei to form a *zygote*.

Evidence Box 4.1

Testing of luteinizing hormone levels in urine using a home based assay kit is reliable and highly predictive of the timing of ovulation.

Miller and Soules assessed the predictive value of monitoring urine luteinizing hormone (LH) levels at home using a rapid, colorimetric enzyme immunoassay test once every evening among 26 normal women with no history of infertility. Each woman also were given sonographs and serum LH tests two times per day The time of the peak serum LH measurement was considered to be the surge. Ovulation was determined using sonographic criteria with confirmation by normal luteal-phase progesterone levels (3 ng/mL or greater). All 26 cycles examined were ovulatory, based on sonographic and progesterone level criteria, and the test had a positive predictive value for follicular collapse within 24 or 48 hours after positive urine LH testing of 73% and 92%, respectively. Based on these results, the investigators concluded that urine LH testing every evening is a highly reliable method of predicting ovulation within the next 48 hours.

Miller PB, Soules MR. The usefulness of a urinary LH kit for ovulation prediction during menstrual cycles of normal women. Obstet Gynecol 1996 Jan;87(1):13–17.

Further Reading

Adams JM, Taylor AE, Schoenfeld DA, Crowley WF Jr, Hall JE. The midcycle gonadotropin surge in normal women occurs in the face of an unchanging gonadotropin-releasing hormone pulse frequency. *J Clin Endocrinol Metab* 1994;79(3):858–864

Cahill DJ, Wardle PG, Harlow CR, Hull MGR. Onset of the preovulatory luteinizing hormone surge: diurnal timing and critical follicular prerequisites. *Fertil Steril* 1998;70(1):56–59

Filicori M, Butler JP, Crowley WF Jr. Neuroendocrine regulation of the corpus luteum in the human. Evidence for pulsatile progesterone secretion. *J Clin Invest* 1984;73(6):1638–1647

Filicori M, Santoro N, Merriam GR, Crowley WF Jr. Characterization of the physiological pattern of episodic gonadotropin secretion throughout the human menstrual cycle. *J Clin Endocrinol Metab* 1986;62(6):1136–1144

Gordts S, Campo R, Rombauts L, Brosens I. Endoscopic visualization of the process of fimbrial ovum retrieval in the human. *Hum Reprod* 1998;13(6):1425–1428

Hall JE, Schoenfeld DA, Martin KA, Crowley WF Jr. Hypothalamic gonadotropin-releasing hormone secretion and follicle-stimulating hormone dynamics during the luteal-follicular transition. *J Clin Endocrinol Metab* 1992;74(3):600–607

Lockwood GM, Muttukrishna S, Ledger WL. Inhibins and activins in human ovulation, conception and pregnancy. *Hum Reprod Update* 1998;4(3):284–295

McLachlan RI, Cohen NL, Vale WW, et al. The importance of luteinizing hormone in the control of inhibin and progesterone secretion by the human corpus luteum. *J Clin Endocrinol Metab* 1989;68(6):1078–1085

Maruncic M, Casper RF. The effect of luteal phase estrogen antagonism on luteinizing hormone pulsatility and luteal function in women. *J Clin Endocrinol Metab* 1987;64(1):148–152

Miller PB, Soules MR. The usefulness of a urinary LH kit for ovulation prediction during menstrual cycles of normal women. *Obstet Gynecol* 1996;87(1):13–17

Pauerstein CJ, Eddy CA, Croxatto HD, Hess R, Siler-Khodr TM, Croxatto HB. Temporal relationships of estrogen, progesterone, and luteinizing hormone levels to ovulation in women and infrahuman primates. *Am J Obstet Gynecol* 1978;130(8):876–886

Retamales I, Carrasco I, Troncoso JL, Las Heras J, Devoto L, Vega M. Morpho-functional study of human luteal cell subpopulations. *Hum Reprod* 1994;9(4):591–596

Roseff SJ, Bangah ML, Kettel LM, et al. Dynamic changes in circulating inhibin levels during the luteal-follicular transition of the human menstrual cycle. *J Clin Endocrinol Metab* 1989;69(5):1033–1039

Tedeschi C, Hazum E, Kokia E, Ricciarelli E, Adashi EY, Payne DW. Endothelin-1 as a luteinization inhibitor: inhibition of rat granulosa cell progesterone accumulation via selective modulation of key steroidogenic steps affecting both progesterone formation and degradation. *Endocrinology* 1992;131(5):2476–2478

Urban RJ, Veldhuis JD, Dufau ML. Estrogen regulates the gonadotropin-releasing hormone-stimulated secretion of biologically active luteinizing hormone. *J Clin Endocrinol Metab* 1991;72(3):660–668

Xiao S, Robertson DM, Findlay JK. Effects of activin and follicle-stimulating hormone (FSH)-suppressing protein/follistatin on FSH receptors and differentiation of cultured rat granulosa cells. *Endocrinology* 1992;131(3):1009–1016

5 Genetics and Genomic Applications in OB/GYN Practice

Arie Koifman and Arnon Wiznitzer

The fundamentals of classic genetics were established by Gregor Johann Mendel (1822–1884), who elucidated the process of single-gene inheritance. Traditionally, "Mendelian" genetics was thus studied through relatively rare, single-gene diseases. However, a steadily growing body of evidence has suggested that multiple genes are involved in the vast majority of medical abnormalities. In fact, if neoplastic diseases are included, up to 90% of the general population will be affected during their lifetime by a disease with a multigene component.

Traditionally, clinical geneticists have dealt with three main areas: 1) the diagnosis and management of pediatric patient abnormalities (including dysmorphology, chromosomal abnormalities, mendelian disorders, and other rare diseases); 2) prenatal genetic diagnosis and prenatal counseling; and 3) adult genetics (mainly the genetics of cancer). However, with recent advances in clinical knowledge—based on the enormous achievements in molecular genetics, genomics, and many other related disciplines—the field of clinical genetics is expanding rapidly. Furthermore, clinical geneticists must interact with an increasing diversity of other medical specialties, making a basic understanding of genetic and genomic concepts an essential tool for routine clinical practice.

Definitions

Autosome: This term refers to any paired chromosome that is alike in the cell of males and females, as distinguished from the two sex chromosomes X and Y. Humans have 22 pairs of autosomes.

Cell nucleus: This is a membrane-enclosed structure found in most eukaryotic cells that contains most of the cell's genetic material, which is organized as multiple, long, linear DNA molecules incomplexes with a large variety of proteins, such as histones, to form chromosomes.

The genes within these chromosomes are the cell's nuclear genome. The function of the nucleus is to maintain the integrity of these genes and to control the activities of the cell by regulating gene expression.

Conceptus: This refers to all structures that develop from the zygote, both embryonic and extra-embryonic. It includes the embryo as well as the embryonic part of the placenta and its associated membranes: amnion, chorionic (gestational sac), and yolk sac.

Chromosomes: These are the organized structures composed of DNA and proteins that are found in cells. A chromosome is a singular piece of DNA, which contains many genes, regulatory elements and other nucleotide sequences. Chromosomes also contain DNA-bound proteins, which serve to package the DNA and control its functions.

Cytoplasm: This gelatinous, semitransparent fluid fills much of the volume of a cell. Eukaryotic cells contain organelles, such as mitochondria, that are filled with liquid which is kept separate from the cytoplasm by cell membranes.

DNA: Deoxyribonucleic acid (DNA) is a complex molecule that contains the genetic instructions used in the development and functioning of all known living organisms and some viruses. The main role of DNA molecules is the long-term storage of information so that cells can make copies of themselves.

Gamete: This describes a cell that fuses with another cell (gamete) during fertilization (conception) in organisms that reproduce sexually. In species that produce two morphologically distinct types of gametes, and in which each individual produces only one type, a female is any individual that produces the larger type of gamete—called an ovum (or egg)—and a male produces the smaller tadpole-like type—called a sperm.

Gene: The functional and physical unit of heredity that passes from parent to offspring is called a gene. Genes are pieces of DNA, and most genes contain the information for making a specific protein.

Gene expression: This is the process by which inheritable information from a gene, such as its DNA sequence, is converted into a functional gene product, such as a protein or ribonucleic acid (RNA).

Genome: The complete package of genetic material of a living organism, organized in chromosomes, is known as the genome. A complete copy of the genome is found in most cells.

Genotype: This defines the genetic constitution of a cell, an organism, or an individual.

Haploid: This term refers to a set of chromosomes containing only one member of each chromosome pair. Human sperm and egg are haploid and have 23 chromosomes compared to a somatic cell, which is diploid and has 46.

Karyotype: This is a pictorial representation of the chromosomes in a cell, which is used to check for abnormalities. A karyotype is created by staining the chromosomes with dye and photographing them through a microscope. The photograph is then cut up and rearranged so that the chromosomes are lined up into corresponding pairs.

Mosaicism: This term describes the presence of two populations of cells with different genotypes in one individual, who has developed from a single fertilized egg.

Pedigree: A pedigree is a diagram of family relationships that uses symbols to represent people and lines to represent genetic relationships. These diagrams make it easier to visualize relationships within families, particularly large extended families. Pedigree analyses are often used to determine the mode of inheritance (dominant, recessive, etc.) of genetic diseases.

Phenotype: This term refers to any observable characteristic of an organism, such as its shape, development, biochemical or physiological properties, or behavior. Phenotypes are influenced by a combination of genetic and environmental factors.

Sex chromosome: In females, the sex chromosomes are the XX chromosomes. Males have one X chromosome and one Y chromosome. The presence of the Y chromosome is decisive for unleashing the developmental program that leads to a baby boy.

Translocation: This is a process by which chromosomes break and the fragments rejoin to other chromosomes, resulting in chromosomal abnormalities.

Impact of Genetics and Genomics on OB/GYN Practice

Genetics has a profound impact on all different fields of OB/GYN patient care. Obstetricians must deal with genetic issues on a daily basis, such as in counseling women before pregnancy on how to prevent neural tube defects (NTDs), during pregnancy regarding screening tests for aneuploidy, ultrasonographic findings, and after pregnancy for risk assessment of future pregnancies Similarly, gynecologists routinely face genetic issues when seeking the etiology of recurrent miscarriages, the management of hydatidiform moles, and so on. Clinicians practicing reproductive medicine also deal with genetics in their daily medical practice, such as in managing infertility, delineating the etiology of infertility (e.g., chromosomal abnormalities, Turner syndrome, Klinefelter syndrome) as well as in preimplantation genetic diagnoses during in vitro fertilization.

Basic Concepts of Genetics

A basic knowledge of mitosis and meiosis is essential for the understanding genetics. The two processes are described briefly below.

Mitosis is the process by which all the chromosomes in the nucleus duplicate themselves in order to generate two, identical, daughter nuclei. It is generally followed immediately by cytokinesis, which divides the nuclei, cytoplasm, organelles, and cell membrane into two daughter cells, each with the genetic equivalent of the parent cell (**Fig. 5.1**).

Meiosis is a process of reduction division in which the number of chromosomes per cell is cut in half. In humans, meiosis always results in the formation of gametes and is essential for sexual reproduction. During meiosis, the genome of a diploid germ cell undergoes DNA replication followed by two rounds of division, resulting in four haploid cells. Each of these cells contains one complete set of chromosomes, or half of the genetic content of the original cell. Because the chromosomes of each parent undergo genetic recombination between homologous chromosomes during meiosis (**Fig. 5.2**), each gamete, will have a unique genetic blueprint encoded in its DNA.

The genetic information in cells is arranged in several structural levels, from the basic DNA sequence to the chromosomes which are visible by light microscopy after staining.

Basic chromosome structure consists of a short arm (p), long arm (q), and a centromere in between (**Fig. 5.3**).

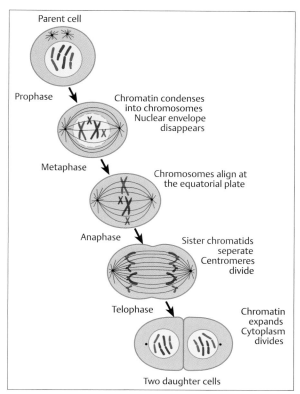

Fig. 5.1 Mitosis consists of four distinct phases—prophase, meta-phase, anaphase, and telophase—which result in the production of two genetically identical daughter cells.

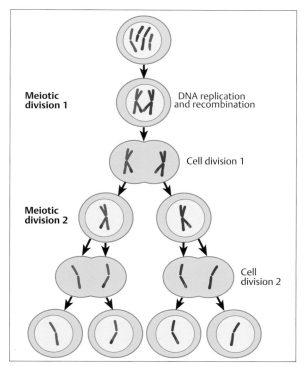

Fig. 5.2 The process of meiosis in humans involves the halving of a cell's chromosomes to form gametes for sexual reproduction.

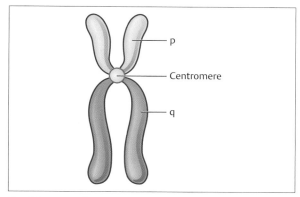

Fig. 5.3 General structure of a chromosome showing the short arm (p), long arm (q) and the centromere which divides the two.

In 1985, a standard nomenclature for chromosomes was developed and named the International System for Human Cytogenetic Nomenclature (ISCN). In this ISCN nomenclature, each arm of a chromosome is divided into one to four major regions, depending on chromosomal length; each band, positively or negatively stained, is given a number, which rises as the distance from the centromere increases.

Chromosomes are grouped according to their size and the location of the centromere. Of a special interest are the acrocentric chromosomes (chromosomes 13, 14, 15, 21, 22), in which the short arm (p) is absent and there exists only a stalk in its place containing satellite DNA (i.e., highly repetitive, noncoding sequence). Translocations involving these chromosomes are called "robertsonian translocations" and are important in inheritance mechanism of chromosomal rearrangements (see below).

Types and Mechanisms of Genetic Abnormalities

There are several types of common genetic abnormalities, each resulting from a different mechanism. These include numerical abnormalities.

Numerical Abnormalities

Numerical abnormalities can be divided into two main categories: 1) aneuploidy—meaning a loss or addition of one (or in very rare occasions two) chromosome(s); and 2) polyploidy—meaning an addition of one or more set of chromosomes.

Aneuploidies

The diseases in this group are quite common, and are well recognized and described. The aneuploidy group can be categorized into trisomies (meaning that cells have an extra copy of one of the chromosomes giving them three copies overall instead of two) and monosomies (a missing copy of one of the chromosomes). Trisomies can occur for each of the autosomes (i.e., chromosomes 1–22) or for each of the sex chromosomes (X or Y). All monosomies of autosomes are lethal and result in death before birth or immediately afterward.

The only monosomy compatible with life is Turner syndrome, in which women are missing an X chromosome (see below). A normal female karyotype is labeled 46,XX; individuals with Turner syndrome are 45,X. In Turner syndrome, female sexual characteristics are present but generally underdeveloped (see below).

The main reason 45,X females are able to survive the loss of one of an X chromosomes in each cell is that one of the two X chromosomes in each somatic cell of a female is typically inactivated early in the life of the embryo. This inactivated X chromosome is referred to as the "Barr body." Recent genetic studies have demonstrated that although not all genes on the Barr body are inactivated, most are. Thus, X chromosome abnormalities are relatively benign compared with autosomal chromosomal abnormalities. An exception to this "rule of thumb" is the case of autosome/sex chromosome translocations, in which the translocated chromosome stays activated.

Polyploidies

Trisomy 21 (Down syndrome): Individuals who have all or part of an extra copy of chromosome 21 (i.e., trisomy 21) have significant physical and mental developmental problems. The condition is widely known as Down Syndrome. It is named after John Langdon Down, the British doctor who first described the syndrome in 1866.

The overall incidence of Down syndrome among live births is about 1 in 800, but there is a marked variability depending on maternal age (**Fig. 5.4**). The vast majority (95%) of trisomy 21 is derived from an extra whole chromosome 21, which in most cases is due to maternal non-disjunction during meiosis. Other etiologies includes mainly "robertsonian" translocations (see below) between two acrocentric chromosomes and mosaicism (when two different cell types are present in a person).

The Down syndrome phenotype includes marked hypotonia (low muscle tone), a protruding tongue, a small head with flattened occiput (back of the head), flat nasal bridge, and epicanthal folds with up-slanting palpebral fissures (separation between upper and lower eyelids) (**Fig. 5.5**). There is frequently loose skin at the nape of the neck, short fingers, a single palmar crease, and absence or hypoplasia of the middle phalanx, causing clinodactyly (inward curving) of the fifth finger, and the "sandal toe" gap.

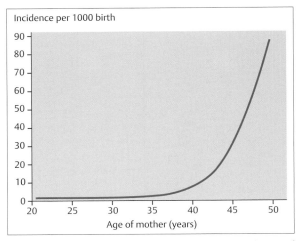

Incidence per 1000 birth

Age of mother (years)

Fig. 5.4   The incidence of Down syndrome increases as the age of the mother increases and is nearly 10% by age 50 years.

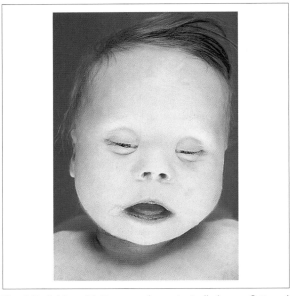

Fig. 5.5   Babies with Down syndrome typically have a flattened nasal bridge and protruding tongue, among many other facial and physical abnormalities. From: Riede UN, Werner M. Color Atlas of Pathology. Stuttgart: Thieme; 2004.

Associated major abnormalities include heart defects (particularly endocardial cushion defects) in 30–40% of cases and gastrointestinal malformations. These children also have a high incidence of neonatal or childhood leukemia and thyroid disease. The intelligence quotient (IQ) ranges from 25 to 50, with a few individuals testing higher. Most affected children have social skills averaging 3–4 years ahead of their mental age. Life expectancy is decreased because of heart disease and susceptibility to acute leukemia. Most affected persons survive to adulthood, but the aging process seems to be accelerated, with death often occurring in the fifth or sixth decade.

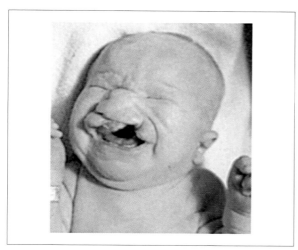

Fig. 5.6 A child with trisomy 13 showing the characteristic cleft lip. Passarge E. Color Atlas of Genetics, 3rd ed. Stuttgart: Thieme; 2007.

Trisomy 13 (Patau syndrome): Trisomies of chromosome 13 occur in about 1 in every 10 000 live births; about 80 % of cases are complete trisomy 13 (i.e., they have a full extra chromosome). There is an increased risk of this condition with advanced maternal age.

Characteristic symptoms in babies with trisomy 13 include midline anomalies, such as gross anatomical defects of the brain, especially holoprosencephaly; cleft lip and palate (**Fig. 5.6**), microphthalmi, colobomas (fissures) of the iris, and retinal dysplasia. Additionally, the supraorbital ridges (bony ridges above the eye) are shallow and the palpebral fissures usually are slanted. The ears are abnormally shaped and usually low-set. Deafness also is common.

Infants with trisomy 13 tend to be small for gestational age. Simian crease, polydactyly, and hyperconvex narrow fingernails are common. About 80 % of cases have severe congenital cardiovascular anomalies and dextrocardia (i.e, the heart is situated on the right side of the body) is common. Other midline defects include scalp defects and dermal sinuses. Loose folds of skin are often present over the posterior aspect of the neck. The genitalia are frequently abnormal in both sexes; cryptorchidism and an abnormal scrotum occur in the male, and a bicornuate uterus occurs in the female. Apneic spells in early infancy are frequent. Mental retardation is severe. Most patients (70 %) do not survive more than 6 months, and less than 10 % survive longer than 1 year.

Trisomy 18 (Edwards syndrome): Trisomy 18 occurs in 1 in every 6000 live births. More than 95 % of affected children have complete trisomy 18. Advanced maternal age increases the risk. The incidence is significantly higher in girls (75 % vs. 25 % for boys).

Newborns with trisomy 18 are markedly small for their gestational age, with hypotonia and severe hypopla-

sia of skeletal muscle and subcutaneous fat. Their crying is weak, and they have a decreased response to sounds. The orbital ridges are hypoplastic, the palpebral fissures short, and the mouth and jaw small—all of which give the face a pinched appearance (**Fig. 5.7**).

Microcephaly, prominent occiput, low-set malformed ears, and a short sternum are common. A peculiar clenched fist with the index finger overlapping the third and fourth fingers usually occurs. The distal crease on the fifth finger is absent, and there is a low-arch dermal ridge pattern on the fingertips. The fingernails are hypoplastic, and the big toe is shortened and frequently dorsiflexed. Clubfeet and rocker-bottom feet are common. Severe congenital heart disease and anomalies of lungs, diaphragm, abdominal wall, kidneys, and ureters also are common, as are hernias and/or diastasis recti, cryptorchidism, and redundant skinfolds (particularly over the posterior aspect of the neck). Association with single umbilical artery is present. Survival for more than a few months is rare; less than 10 % of such individuals are still alive at 1 year of age. Those who do survive have marked developmental delay and disability.

47,XXY (Klinefelter syndrome): Klinefelter syndrome is a sex chromosome abnormality that occurs in about 1 in 800–1000 of male live births. It involves the inheritance of two or more X chromosomes and one Y (i.e., 47,XXY), resulting in a male with female physical features. The extra X chromosome is maternal in origin in 60 % of cases.

Affected persons tend to be tall, with disproportionately long arms and legs (**Fig. 5.8**). They often have small, firm testes, and up to 30 % develop gynecomastia. Puberty usually occurs at the normal age, but often facial hair growth is light. There is a predisposition for learning

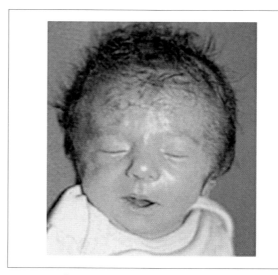

Fig. 5.7 A baby with trisomy 18 displaying the characteristic pinched face. From Passarge E. Color Atlas of Genetics, 3rd ed. Stuttgart: Thieme; 2007.

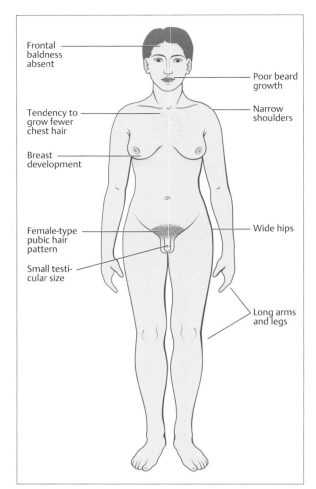

Frontal
baldness
absent

Poor beard
growth

Narrow
shoulders

Tendency to
grow fewer
chest hair

Breast
development

Female-type
pubic hair
pattern

Small testi-
cular size

Wide hips

Long arms
and legs

Fig. 5.8   Individuals with Klinefelter syndrome often appear male but have many female features due to their inheritance of multiple X chromosomes and a single Y chromosome.

difficulties, and many have deficits in verbal IQ, auditory processing, and reading.

However, there is a great variation in clinical symptoms. Many 47,XXY males are normal in appearance and intellect and are diagnosed in the course of an infertility work-up (probably all 47,XXY males are sterile) or in cytogenetic surveys of normal populations.

Testicular development varies from hyalinized nonfunctional tubules to some production of spermatozoa. Mosaicism occurs in 15 % of cases. Some affected persons have three, four, or even five X chromosomes along with the Y. In general, as the number of X chromosomes increases, the severity of mental retardation and of malformations also increases.

47,XXX (triple X syndrome): Triple X syndrome (47,XXX) occurs in about 1 in every 2000 apparently normal females. Physical abnormalities are rare. However, sterility and menstrual irregularity sometimes occur. Affected persons may have a mildly impaired intellect with IQ

scores averaging just below 90 when compared with siblings. Advanced maternal age increases risk, and the extra X chromosome is usually maternally derived.

Monosomies

45,X (monosomy X, Turner syndrome): Turner syndrome occurs in about 1 in every 4000 female live births and 1 in every 5000 live-born neonates. It is the most common aneuploidy in naturally aborting fetuses and accounts for 20 % of chromosomally abnormal first-trimester abortions. It is the only monosomy compatible with life.

There are three distinct phenotypes seen with 45,X. Ninety nine percent of conceptuses are so abnormal that they abort in the first trimester. In the majority of the remainder, cystic hygromas may be detected and may be accompanied by hydrops and fetal demise.

The third, least common phenotype comprises most live-born individuals, who may have only minor problems. Features of this last group include short stature, broad chest with widely spaced nipples (**Fig. 5.9**), congenital lymphedema with puffy fingers and toes, low hairline with webbed posterior neck, and minor bone and cartilage abnormalities. From 30 % to 50 % of cases have a major cardiac malformation, usually aortic coarctation or bicuspid aortic valves.

Intelligence is generally in the normal range; however, 45,X females frequently have visual–spatial organization deficits and difficulty with nonverbal problem-solving and with interpretation of subtle social cues. More than 90 % of cases also have ovarian dysgenesis and require life-long hormone replacement therapy beginning just before adolescence.

The variety of phenotypic appearance in girls with Turner syndrome can be explained by the significant rate of mosaicism that occurs. Live-born infants will typically have karyotypes such as 45,X/46,XX or 45,X/46,XY. If ultimately the majority of cells are 45,X, that individual will have the Turner phenotype, but modified by the presence of the other cell populations . The missing X chromosome does not appear to be lost randomly because the maternal X is retained in 80 % of surviving cases.

Polyploidy: Polyploidy occurs when at least one whole *set* of haploid chromosomes are added to the chromosomal milieu. Usually polyploidy will result in miscarriage. Up to 66 % of triploidy cases (e.g., 69,XXX/XXY/XYY) result from fertilization of one egg by two sperm. Other causes of triploidy involve a failure of one of the meiotic divisions, resulting in a diploid chromosomal complement in either the egg or, more frequently, the sperm.

The phenotype of the individual is dependent on the origin of the extra set of chromosomes. A *partial hydatidiform mole* with abnormal fetal structures is the result of an extra set of parternal chromosomes. In cases of polyploidy of maternal origin, a fetus and placenta develop, but the

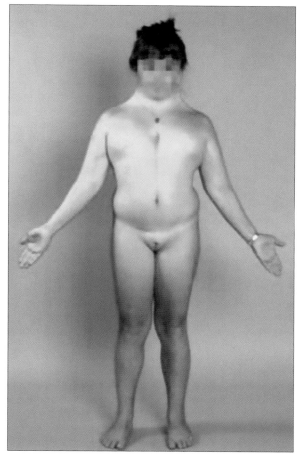

Fig. 5.9 A young girl with Turner Syndrome displaying the characteristic short stature, broad chest, and widely spaced nipples. Reproduced by kind permission of Professor P.E. Mullis, Inselspital, Bern, Switzerland.

fetus is severely growth-restricted which, in some cases, will result in sacral teratoma in the fetus. Triploid fetuses of either kind are frequently dysmorphic. If a woman had a triploid pregnancy with a fetus that survived past the first trimester, the risk of a future recurrence is 1–1.5%.

Tetraploidy always results in 92,XXXX or 92,XXYY, indicating a postzygotic failure to complete an early cleavage division. The recurrence risk for tetraploidy is minimal.

Structural Chromosomal Abnormalities

Several mechanisms are involved in structural abnormalities in chromosomes. These include deletions (when a part of chromosome is missing), duplications (a part is added), translocations (replacement of parts of two different chromosomes), and inversions (breakage and fusion of a piece of a chromosome in a different orientation from that which normally occurs).

Deletions

Deletions occur mainly during pairing of homologous chromosomes in meiosis and usually arise from an abnormal alignment mechanism. There are some common, well-described syndromes arising from chromosomal deletions. For instance, deletions on the short arm of chromosome 4 (4p) give rise to Wolf–Hirschhorn syndrome, which is characterized by intrauterine growth restriction, hypotonia, dysmorphism, severe mental deficiency, polydactyly, cutis aplasia, and severe seizures.

Duplications

Duplications occur when part of a chromosome is added in a repetitive manner. Duplications usually do not cause a phenotypic abnormality. A large proportion of all duplications are inherited from a parent with balanced translocations (see below) or inversions.

Inversions

Inversions result from two breaks on the same chromosome, just before the breaks are repaired. Inversions result in no gain or loss of genetic material. However, the break points can disrupt the integrity of coding genes, leading to a phenotypic abnormality. Two main types of inversions are possible: *pericentric* and *paracentric.*

Pericentric inversions occur when the break points are on different sides of the centromere, whereas *paracentric inversions* occur when the breaks occur on the same side of the centromere. It is important to differentiate one from the other, because they result in different types of gamete and increase the risk of offspring inheriting unbalanced genetic material. Pericentric inversions cause problems in chromosomal alignment during meiosis, so that the carrier of an inversion is at a high risk of producing abnormal gametes and thus abnormal offspring. Paracentric inversions, on the other hand, produce either balanced gametes or gametes that are so abnormal that they cannot produce a viable conceptus.

Each type of inversion should be considered individually regarding recurrence risk. Empirically, if the ascertainment is the result of an abnormal stillbirth or abnormal live birth, the recurrence risk is 5–10%. If found coincidentally (i.e., when a chromosomal analysis is done for another reason) the recurrence risk is 1–3%.

Translocations

Translocations occur when there is a break and exchange of chromosomal segments between two chromosomes. Translocations can be further defined as *reciprocal* or *robertsonian.*

Reciprical translocations involve the exchange of chromosomal segments between two different chromosomes. Thus, two break points and two fusion points are present on each chromosome. Usually, no chromosomal material is gained or lost in a carrier, making it a balanced translocation.

The transposition of chromosomal segments, however, can cause abnormalities due to repositioning of specific genes. In most cases, the function of the gene is not compromised, and the balanced carrier is phenotypically normal (although, up to 6.5% can be phenotypically abnormal).

On the other hand, carriers of a balanced translocation can produce unbalanced gametes that result in abnormal offspring. The unbalanced offspring will carry a partial monosomy and a partial trisomy of the involved chromosomes, usually leading to a phenotypic abnormality. Again, recurrence risk is dependent on whether the abnormality was found after the birth of a phenotypically abnormal baby or as a coincidental finding, and ranges from 5–30% to 5%, respectively.

Robertsonian translocations occur when there is a fusion of the whole q arm of two acrocentric chromosomes and the loss of the p arm in those same chromosomes (**Fig. 5.10**). Since the p arm in acrocentric chromosomes contains virtually a completely noncoding DNA, a carrier of such a translocation will have 45 chromosomes but with no gain or loss of genetic material. Carriers of robertsonian translocation are normal and considered to be carriers of a balanced translocation.

The segregations of the translocated chromosomes give rise to either balanced or unbalanced gametes, which can lead to a phenotypically affected individual. Among robertsonian translocations, translocation of chromosomes 13,14, and 21 are common as well. As discussed above, the translocation t(14:21) accounts for up to 5% of all Down syndrome cases. A diagnosis of a translocation as the etiology of a trisomy has a crucial impact on counseling for the patient and for calculating parents' risks for future genetic problems when deciding to have more children.

Isochromosomes and Ring chromosomes

Isochromosomes

Isochromosomes occur when either a p or a q arm of a chromosome is duplicated and all genetic material from the other arm is lost. The result is two identical arms on each side of the centromere. When occurring between two acrocentric chromosomes, a "robertsonian-like" genotype is found. However, unlike in true robertsonian translocations, only abnormal unbalanced gametes can be made.

Isochromosomes may be important in imprinting disorders (see below), trisomies (e.g., patients with Down syndrome because of isochromosome 21q will have a risk of 100% for an offspring inheriting the syndrome), or in cases of sex chromosome abnormalities. Up to 15% of Turner syndrome patients with clinical symptoms have an isochromosome Xq genotype meaning they have a monosomy of Xp.

Ring Chromosomes

Ring chromosomes are the result of deletions from both ends of a chromosome. When the ends fuse, they form a ringlike structure (**Fig. 5.11**). The phenotype of the carrier of a ring chromosome depends on which regions of the chromosome are deleted. Chromosomal alignment during meiosis is altered in patients with a ring chromosome

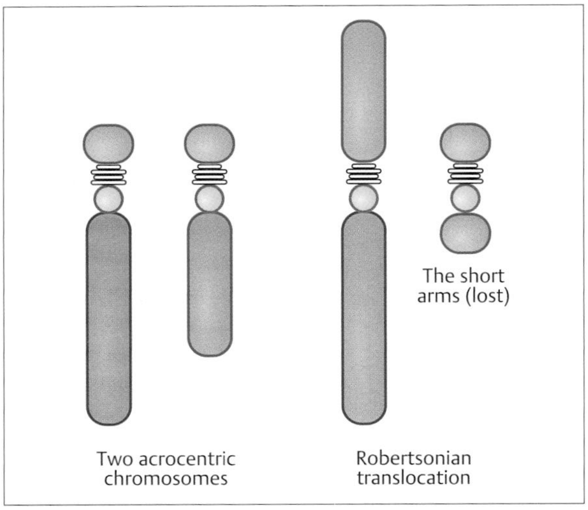

Fig. 5.10 A robertsonian translocation is a fusion between the centromeres of two chromosomes with loss of the short arms, forming a chromosome with two long arms, one derived from each chromosome.

The short arms (lost)

Two acrocentric chromosomes

Robertsonian translocation

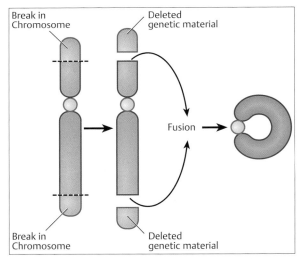

Break in Chromosome

Deleted genetic material

Fusion

Break in Chromosome

Deleted genetic material

Fig. 5.11 Carriers of ring chromosomes have variable phenotypes depending on which regions of the chromosome are deleted.

mutation leading to abnormal gametes. Most ring chromosomes are de novo but inherited forms are present as well. In cases of inherited ring chromosome, it is always maternal in origin, possibly because a ring chromosome defect compromises spermatogenesis.

Mendelian Disorders

Gregor Mendel first observed inheritance patterns of certain traits in pea plants and demonstrated that they obeyed simple statistical rules. From his observations, Mendel defined the concept of a basic unit of heredity, which he named an "allele." Today, the term allele is used synonymously with the term gene. In mendelian inheritance patterns, a single gene is responsible for a single trait. The following briefly reviews the basic principles of mendelian inheritance patterns.

Autosomal Dominant Disorders

An autosomal dominant disorder is present when only one copy of an abnormal allele of a gene leads to a specific phenotypic appearance or disorder. In those disorders, an affected person has an affected parent. Unaffected children of an affected parent can have unaffected children and grandchildren. Males and females are equally likely to be affected, and the risk for occurrence among children of an affected person is 50%.

Not all carriers of an autosomal dominant disease will present with the same phenotype, however. When the same disease has a range of appearances, it is considered to have variable expression. Another term often used in describing autosomal dominant diseases is *penetrance*, which is an all-or-nothing phenomenon. For example, an adult-onset genetic disease is considered to have no penetrance if the carrier dies before expressing the disease. In pedigrees where autosomal dominant inheritance is suspected and there is no sign of the disease in some generations, the genetic mutation is believed to have only partial penetrance. *Anticipation* is another phenomenon seen with autosomal dominant inheritance. It is defined as a disease that is expressed in a more severe manner and at an earlier age in each successive generation.

Autosomal Recessive Disorders

Autosomal recessive disorders are the result of mutations in two copies of the same allele. When only one allele is affected, the person is considered to be a heterozygotic carrier of the disease. If an affected offspring with a recessive condition is diagnosed, both parents must be carriers of the mutation. Males and females are equally likely to be affected. Many rare genetic diseases, such as cystic fibrosis, are autosomal recessive and, in many cases, the parents of the offspring are closely related (i.e., the result of a consanguious marriage or relationship).

X-linked Disorders

When the mutated gene is located on one of the sex chromosome (X or Y) it is considered to be X-linked or Y-linked. Because the Y chromosome carries a relatively small number of genes, Y-linked diseases extremely rare. Thus, most known sex-linked diseases are X-linked and are usually recessive.

X-linked dominant disorders affect females predominantly because they tend to be lethal in male offspring, who have only one X chromosome.

Mitochondrial Inheritance Disorders

In the mitochondrion of each cell in the body, there is a small circular chromosome that encodes only a few proteins, various RNAs, and several enzymes. Mitochondrial disease arise from deletions, duplications, or mutations in mitochondrial DNA. Since mitochondria are derived exclusively from the ovum, mitochondrial disorders are maternally inherited.

Polygenic and Multifactorial Inheritance Disorders

Polygenic traits are defined as more than one gene causing a disorder. *Multifactorial* traits are determined by multiple genes and environmental factors. Many inherited human traits are multifactorial or polygenic.

Congenital anomalies caused by such inheritance are recognized by their tendency to recur in families, rather than according to a classic mendelian inheritance pattern. For example, neural tube defects (NTDs) and cardiac anomalies are polygenic and multifactorial. Because these conditions are multifactorial, they can sometimes be prevented. This concept was proven unequivocally when folic acid was added to the diet of women prior to and during pregnancy and NTDs were prevented in their offspring.

Non-mendelian Inheritance and Disorders

Unstable DNA Disorders

Most regions of DNA in chromosomes are extremely stable. However, there are several regions prone to breakage. These are usually in *trinucleotide repeat* sites, which tend to get expanded during DNA replication, leading to chromosomal instability. The genes affected by the instability may be altered and lead to dysfunction. Those regions can be transmitted from parent to child. Trinucleotide repeat disorders generally show genetic anticipation, that is, their severity increases with each successive generation that inherits them.

Fragile X syndrome: The fragile X syndrome is a type of unstable DNA disorder and is the most common cause of *familial* mental retardation. It accounts for 5–8% of all cases of mental retardation in males and females. The incidence of the full fragile X syndrome is generally 1 in every 1000 males and 1 in every 2000 females.

The fragile X mutation is a region of unstable DNA on the X chromosome located at Xq27 (i.e., the long arm of chromosome X) where there is a region of CGG triplet repeats. As previously noted, these triplet repeats tend to expand in each successive generation. When the number of triplet repeats reaches a critical size, the normal gene is inactivated and the protein product it encodes (FMR-1) is not produced. The exact function of FMR-1 is not completely known, but it is believed to work in localized expression of mRNA. The FMR-1 gene is highly conserved in all species and is most active in brain and testes.

When the repeat number of DNA triplets is between 2 and 49, individuals are usually phenotypically normal. However, those carrying from 50 to 199 repeats are considered to have a pre-mutation, which will lead eventually to fragile X syndrome in successive generations. Those with more than 230 repeats have the full mutation and are usually affected. Even individuals carrying the pre-mutation, who are considered "not affected," are prone to mild cognitive and behavioral deficits, premature ovarian failure, and a neurodegenerative disorder that affects older adults.

The number of repeats usually remains stable when the gene is transmitted from the father. When a mother carries the pre-mutation, however, the triplet repeat can expand during meiosis. Thus, if a woman carries a pre-mutation that increases in size as she transmits it to her offspring, it is possible for her child to manifest fragile X syndrome. Eighty percent of males and 50–70% of females carrying the full mutation are mentally handicapped. Males are moderately to severely affected and may show attention-deficit/hyperactivity disorder, autistic behavior, and speech and language problems. Phenotypic variability is found in up to 10–20% of individuals with the full mutation.

Genomic Imprinting and Uniparental Disomy

The expression of genes is tightly regulated. One of the more important mechanisms of gene expression is *genomic imprinting*. Genomic imprinting is an *epigenetic* mechanism (meaning that there is a change in expression of genes without altering the actual DNA sequence).

Genomic imprinting relates to a different expression of genetic information depending on whether it has been inherited from the father or mother. A classic example of a disorder regulated by genomic imprinting is the 15q11-13 deletion. If the deletion is paternally inherited, the person will develop Prader–Willi syndrome, which is manifested in obesity and hyperphagia, short stature, small hands, feet, and external genitalia and mild mental retardation. However, if the same deletion is inherited maternally, the individual will develop Angelman syndrome, which is characterized by normal stature and weight but with severe neurologic deficits, including mental retardation, speech impairment, seizure disorder, ataxia, and jerky arm movements.

Uniparental disomy occurs when two chromosomes of a pair are inherited from only one parent. Imprinting effects may be seen because genetic information from the other parent is absent. In addition, if the same chromosome is duplicated and that chromosome carries a mutated allele for an autosomal recessive disorder, the individual will express the disorder even though only one parent is a carrier.

Diagnosis and Management

Prenatal Genetic Screening

Because genetic defects can be so devastating, a substantial effort must be put into diagnosing genetic disorders during pregnancy. Because of its relatively high incidence, much of this effort will be put into screening for aneuploidy.

Aneuploidy Screening Tests

Aneuploidy screening tests are traditionally done during the second trimester by measuring several markers in blood serum, including total beta human chorionic gonadotropin (β-HCG), alpha fetoprotein (αFP), and unconjugated estriol (E3). By combining these assays with the age-related risk of the patient, these screening tests can detect up to 70% of trisomy 21 cases. In an attempt to detect aneuploidy (mainly trisomy 21) earlier, several strategies have been developed, most of them employing combined testing strategies.

First trimester screening: First-trimester screening (FTS) combines measurements of a nuchal translucency by ultrasound scan (see below), serum levels of free β-HCG, and pregnancy associated plasma protein A (PAPP-A) to estimate the risk of a fetus with Down syndrome. The results of these tests, which are typically done on the same day, adjust for the woman's age and give a numerical estimate of the chance of Down syndrome.

These tests are usually done between 11 and 13 weeks' gestation, and the results are categorized as either "screen-positive" or "screen-negative." If the risk for Down syndrome is greater than 1/350, a further diagnostic test is suggested. The test will also indicate a screen-positive for trisomy 18 and 13. The cutoff value for those disorders is 1/100. The detection rate is estimated at 80% with a 5.5% false-negative rate. The false-positive rate with FTS is higher at 4–5% than the 2–3% with integrated prenatal screening (see below).

Integrated prenatal screening: Integrated prenatal screening (IPS) is the most accurate and widely accepted combined screening test for Down syndrome during the first and second trimesters. This screening test combines measurements from a nuchal translucency ultrasound scan and two blood tests to estimate the chances of having a baby with Down syndrome. In addition, unlike FTS for Down syndrome, the IPS also determines if there is an increased chance of NTDs.

The ultrasound exam and initial blood test for β-HCG and PAPP-A are done at 11–13 weeks' gestation. The second set of blood tests (αFP, unconjugated E3, and inhibin A) are done between 15 and 18 weeks' gestation. This fully integrated battery of tests can be used to calculate the total risk of having an affected fetus. The detection rate for Down syndrome is 85% with a false-positive rate of 0.9%. The advantages of IPS include a lower false-positive rate compared with FTS and the added ability to screen for NTDs (see Evidence Box 5.1).

Nuchal translucency utrasound scan: Nuchal translucency (NT) ultrasonography measures the fluid at the back of a baby's neck between 11 and 14 weeks of pregnancy. An increased NT in the first trimester is associated with fetal Down syndrome. Research has demonstrated that an NT of at least 3 mm between 10 and 13 weeks' gestation is present in 86.1% of fetal trisomies but in only 4.5% of chromosomally normal fetuses. Studies have demonstrated that an NT of 3 mm or greater is associated with a 12-fold increase in fetal aneuploidy and is independent of maternal age.

Women who are pregnant with twins or triplets will not require a blood test, as current guidelines do not recommend using blood tests to screen for Down syndrome (or trisomy 13/18). Thus, the best screening for a multiple pregnancy is the use of each NT measurement, as it is unique to each baby. Chapter 18 contains a detailed discussion of screening methods used in multiple pregnancy situations.

Diagnostic tests for fetal aneuploidy: Most prenatal diagnostic testing is aimed at diagnosing chromosomal numerical abnormalities. Indication for such testing in pregnant women includes an advanced maternal age, other abnormal screening test results, and any abnormal ultrasound findings. The different methods of obtaining and analyzing the sample are discussed below.

Invasive Testing Methods

Chorionic villus sampling: Routinely performed between 10 and 12 weeks' gestation, chorionic villus sampling (CVS) allows an earlier detection of abnormalities and a safer pregnancy termination, if indicated. During the procedure, approximately 25 mg of villi are aspirated from the chorion frondosum (the fetal portion of the placenta), transvaginally. Results can be obtained within 24–48 hours.

CVS is a relatively safe procedure and the spontaneous abortion rate is less than 0.5% to 1%. However, there is an increased association of limb defects when the procedure is performed earlier than 10 weeks of gestation. Confined placental mosaicism (i.e., more than one cell line is present in the sample from the placenta) is present in up to 2% of all cases of CVS, even though the associated fetus is usually normal.

This placental mosaicism is caused by nondisjunction during early mitotic divisions in one or more cells destined to become the placenta or from partial "correction" of a trisomy resulting from a meiotic error, with the extra chromosome lost from all cells destined to become the fetus, but retained in some cells destined to become the placenta. CVS findings should be confirmed by examining cultured mesenchymal cells, as they are more reliably derived from the fetus.

Amniocentesis: Amniocentesis is the most common genetic screening procedure and is routinely performed at 15–17 weeks' gestation. On some occasions, early amniocentesis at 12–14 weeks is performed to expedite results, although less amniotic fluid can be obtained during this time period. Early amniocentesis also carries a greater risk of spontaneous abortion or fetal injury.

Fetal blood sampling: Fetal blood can be collected directly from the umbilical cord. To do this, a percutaneous needle is inserted into the uterine cavity and directed by ultrasound imaging to the umbilical artery (**Fig. 5.12**). Indications for the procedure includes late second-trimester abnormalities detected by ultrasound exam or inconclusive results of cytogenetic analysis derived from amniocentesis.

Noninvasive Screening Methods

Fetal blood extraction from maternal circulation: Fetal nucleated red blood cells may be present in the maternal blood as early as 10 weeks' gestation. Thus, sampling maternal blood allows for first-trimester diagnosis of fetal aneuploidy . However, aggressive purifying techniques are needed to accomplish this, since the concentration

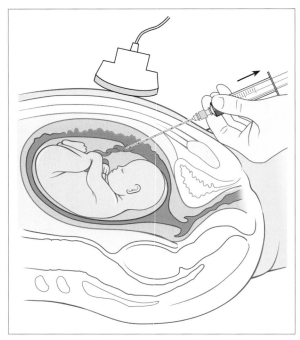

Fig. 5.12 The proper method for obtaining a sample of fetal blood involves carefully inserting a percutaneous needle through the cervical cavity and into the umbilical artery, using ultrasound imaging to guide the needle.

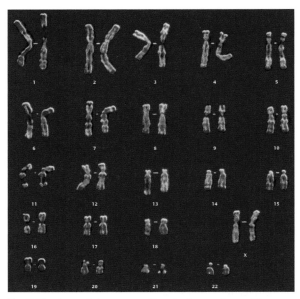

Fig. 5.13 A sample karyogram. Karyotyping can be used for many purposes but is most often used to study chromosomal aberrations, such as translocations or ring chromosomes.

of fetal blood cells is extremely low in maternal blood. Polymerase chain reaction (PCR) technology (see below) is usually used for this type of diagnosis. Detection rate are reportedly as high as 97 % with a false-positive rate of 13 %.

Fetal cells in the cervix: Fetal cells recovered from the cervix have been used in prenatal diagnosis, but the quality of cells collected has limited the use of this technique.

Free fetal DNA in maternal blood: Free fetal DNA in maternal plasma can be detected as early as the fifth week of gestation. This could theoretically be used as a noninvasive method for prenatal diagnosis. High detection rates have been reported with X-linked disorders and for gender determination. This technique also can help in fetal genotyping in cases of suspected Rhesus incompatibility between mother and baby (see Chapter 17).

Laboratory Techniques Used in Prenatal Genetic Diagnosis

Karyotyping

Karyotyping is used to detect chromosomal abnormalities. This assay involves culturing cells in the laboratory with phytohemagglutinin to stimulate cell division.

Colchicine is then added to arrest mitosis during metaphase, when each chromosome has replicated into two chromatids attached at the centromere. The cells, which are spread onto microscope slides, are then stained. Computer imaging is used to produce a visual display of the chromosomes. The chromosomes are depicted (by rearranging a microphotograph) in a standard format, known as a *karyogram* or *idiogram*, in pairs which are ordered by size and position of centromere for chromosomes of the same size (**Fig. 5.13**). Chromosome staining is performed by G (Giemsa) or Q (fluorescent) banding techniques. Additional staining procedures and techniques for extending chromosome length have greatly increased the precision of cytogenetic diagnosis

Fluorescence in situ Hybridization

The technique of fluorescence in situ hybridization (FISH) provides a rapid method for determining ploidy of select chromosomes or confirming the presence or absence of a specific gene or large DNA sequence. It involves fixing cells and labeling them with a fluorescent compound. A chromosome or gene probe is then allowed to hybridize to the fixed chromosomes. Each probe is complementary to a unique area of the chromosome or gene being investigated, thus preventing cross-reaction with other chromosomes. A fluorescent signal, visible by microscopy (**Fig. 5.14**), is produced when the chromosome or gene of interest is present. The number of signals indicates the number of chromosomes or genes of that type in the cell being analyzed.

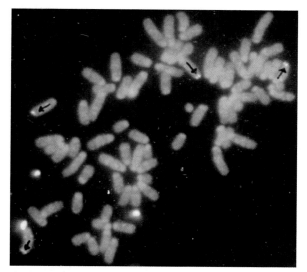

Fig. 5.14 Fluorescence in situ hybridization (FISH) is limited to detecting chromosome duplications, deletions, and rearrangements.

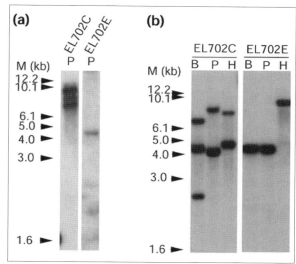

Fig. 5.15 A Southern blot showing bands that correspond to DNA fragments of different sizes and molecular weight.

This technique is limited to detecting chromosome duplications, deletions, and rearrangements. Thus, FISH is used when ploidy status would change clinical management and there is limited time for conducting cytogenetic analyses. A full karyotype should be performed along with all FISH analyses to confirm the ploidy status and to rule out structural chromosomal alterations.

Polymerase Chain Reaction

This technique enables the rapid synthesis of large amounts of a specific DNA sequences or entire genes. Either the entire gene sequence or the sequences at the beginning and end of the gene must be known, however.

PCR involves repeating three steps over and over again:

1. Denaturing double-stranded DNA by heating
2. Adding of oligonucleotide primers corresponding to the target sequence on each separate DNA strand
3. Adding of a mixture of nucleotides and heat-stable DNA polymerase to elongate the primer DNA sequence

The procedure is repeated with exponential amplification of the DNA segment. Different DNA probes are used for different genes or suspected diseases but can be used for sex determination and even for the detection of numerical chromosomal abnormalities.

Southern Blotting

Southern blotting involves cutting chromosomal DNA into large fragments with enzymes that cleave the DNA at specific sites, separating these large fragments by a special type of electrophoresis, and "annealing" the DNA frag-

ments to cDNA probes (a laboratory-made copy of RNA corresponding to a known sequence of a gene or DNA region). The result is a series of bands on a gel that can be visualized by a number of methods and allow for detection of a number of type of genetic mutations (**Fig. 5.15**). The basic principles of Southern blotting also can be applied to RNA, in which case it is called Northern blotting, and to proteins—Western blotting.

DNA Microarray Chips

DNA microarray chips are a high-throughput technology used in molecular biology and in medicine. A chip consists of an arrayed series of thousands of microscopic spots of DNA oligonucleotides, called features, which each contain a very small amounts of a specific DNA sequence. These can be a short sections of a gene or other DNA element that are used as probes to hybridize a cDNA or cRNA sample (called target) under high-stringency conditions. Probe–target hybridization is usually detected and quantified by fluorescence-based detection of fluorophore-labeled target to determine relative abundance of nucleic acid sequences in the target (**Fig. 5.16**). There are not only different microarray applications, but also differences in the fabrication and workings of the microarrays, which result in differences in accuracy, efficiency, and cost. Their greatest use is in detecting mutations or genetic variations in large numbers of genes simultaneously or for determining how active a gene or genetic sequence is in a particular type of cell. Although not widely available in clinics, the use of DNA microarrays in biomedical research for detecting genetic imbalances or imperfections is growing exponentially.

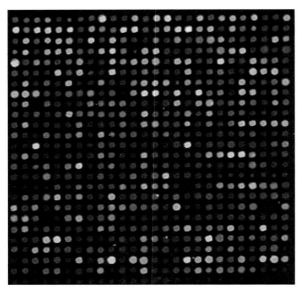

Fig. 5.16 A DNA microarray chip. Each spot corresponds to a different gene, and the color corresponds to the intensity of the gene's expression in the cell.

Key Points

- Genetics has a profound impact on all different fields of OB/GYN patient care, including counseling preventing neural tube defects before pregnancy, screening for genetic abnormalities during pregnancy, and assessing the risk of certain conditions for future pregnancies.
- There are several types of common genetic abnormalities found in pregnancy, each resulting from a different mechanism and leading to a different complication.
- Genetic defects can be so devastating that a substantial effort must be put into diagnosing genetic disorders during pregnancy.
- Because of its relatively high incidence, much of this effort will be put into screening for aneuploidy. Indeed, most prenatal diagnostic testing is aimed at diagnosing chromosomal numerical abnormalities.

Evidence Box 5.1

Ultrasound combined with serum screening for multiple genetic markers has a 90 % sensitivity for Down syndrome.

Benn et al. evaluated the efficacy of a combined measurement of second-trimester maternal serum analytes and continuous ultrasound measurements of nuchal fold thickness and proximal long-bone length in detecting Down syndrome. In all, they reviewed ultrasound measurements of nuchal fold, femur length, and humerus length for 72 second-trimester Down syndrome fetuses and 7063 unaffected fetuses. Overall efficacy of ultrasound screening alone, the quad test (αFP, HCG, E3 and inhibin A), and the combination of the ultrasound and quad tests were compared using a 1/270 second-trimester risk cutoff applied to 1999 US births.

Using ultrasound, there was a sensitivity of 79.9 % and false-positive rate of 6.7 % and positive predictive value: 1 in 42. The quad test had a sensitivity of 81.5 % and false-positive rate of 6.9 % (positive predictive value: 1 in 42). The combination of the quad test with nuchal fold and long bone measurements achieved a 90 % sensitivity and a 3.1 % false-positive rate (positive predictive value: 1 in 18). The investigators concluded that the combined modality was substantially more effective than either serum screening or ultrasound alone, and its efficacy is comparable to that reported for combined first and second trimester (integrated) screening.

Benn PA, Kaminsky LM, Ying J, Borgida AF, Egan JF. Combined second-trimester biochemical and ultrasound screening for Down syndrome. Obstet Gynecol 2002 Dec;100(6):1168–1176.

Further Reading

Al-Mufti R, Hambley H, Farzaneh F, Nicolaides KH. Investigation of maternal blood enriched for fetal cells: role in screening and diagnosis of fetal trisomies. *Am J Med Genet* 1999;85(1):66–75

Baty BJ, Blackburn BL, Carey JC. Natural history of trisomy 18 and trisomy 13: I. Growth, physical assessment, medical histories, survival, and recurrence risk. *Am J Med Genet* 1994;49(2):175–188

Benn PA, Kaminsky LM, Ying J, Borgida AF, Egan JF. Combined second-trimester biochemical and ultrasound screening for Down syndrome. *Obstet Gynecol* 2002;100(6):1168–1176

Bronshtein M, Rottem S, Yoffe N, Blumenfeld Z. First-trimester and early second-trimester diagnosis of nuchal cystic hygroma by transvaginal sonography: diverse prognosis of the septated from the nonseptated lesion. *Am J Obstet Gynecol* 1989;161(1):78–82

Cockwell A, MacKenzie M, Youings S, Jacobs PA. A cytogenetic and molecular study of a series of 45,X fetuses and their parents. *J Med Genet* 1991;28(3):151–155

de Vries BB, Mohkamsing S, van den Ouweland AM, et al; The Collaborative Fragile X Study Group. Screening for the fragile X syndrome among the mentally retarded: a clinical study. *J Med Genet* 1999;36(6):467–470

Gardner RJM, Sutherland JR. Chromosome Abnormalities and Genetic Counseling. Oxford Monographs on Medical Genetics No. 29. New York: Oxford University Press; 2003

Lyon MF. X-chromosome inactivation as a system of gene dosage compensation to regulate gene expression. *Prog Nucleic Acid Res Mol Biol* 1989;36:119–130

Malone FD, Canick JA, Ball RH, et al; First- and Second-Trimester Evaluation of Risk (FASTER) Research Consortium. First-trimester or second-trimester screening, or both, for Down's syndrome. *N Engl J Med* 2005;353(19):2001–2011

Migeon BR, Luo S, Stasiowski BA, et al. Deficient transcription of XIST from tiny ring X chromosomes in females with severe phenotypes. *Proc Natl Acad Sci U S A* 1993;90(24):12025–12029

Nicolaides KH, Brizot ML, Snijders RJ. Fetal nuchal translucency: ultrasound screening for fetal trisomy in the first trimester of pregnancy. *Br J Obstet Gynaecol* 1994;101(9):782–786

Roizen NJ, Patterson D. Down's syndrome. *Lancet* 2003;361(9365):1281–1289

Rousseau F, Rouillard P, Morel ML, Khandjian EW, Morgan K. Prevalence of carriers of premutation-size alleles of the FMRI gene—and implications for the population genetics of the fragile X syndrome. *Am J Hum Genet* 1995;57(5):1006–1018

Saenger P. Turner's syndrome. *N Engl J Med* 1996;335(23):1749–1754

Sybert VP, McCauley E. Turner's syndrome. *N Engl J Med* 2004;351(12):1227–1238

Wald NJ, Watt HC, Hackshaw AK. Integrated screening for Down's syndrome on the basis of tests performed during the first and second trimesters. *N Engl J Med* 1999;341(7):461–467

Zoll B, Wolf J, Lensing-Hebben D, Pruggmayer M, Thorpe B. Trisomy 13 (Patau syndrome) with an 11-year survival. *Clin Genet* 1993;43(1):46–50

6 Pap Smear and Human Papilloma Virus Testing

Benjamin Piura and Ruthy Shaco-Levy

After breast cancer, cervical cancer is the second most common malignancy diagnosed in women worldwide. Approximately 500 000 new cases of cervical cancer are diagnosed each year, and nearly 250 000 women die of this disease each year worldwide.

Cervical cancer is the most common malignancy encountered in women in developing countries. The majority of these cases occur in countries with limited or no effective screening programs using the Papanicolaou (Pap) smear test[1] for detecting cervical cellular abnormalities, which places women at a greater risk for developing cervical cancer. In the United States, Finland, Sweden, Iceland, and other developed countries where Pap smear screening is widely used, rates of cervical cancer have noticeably dropped up to 50% over the past 20–30 years (see Evidence Box 6.1).

However, health disparities prevent more lives from being saved with Pap smear screening, even in developed countries. Indeed, despite the test's widespread availability in the United States, for example, more than 10 000 new cases of cervical cancer are diagnosed each year, and almost 4000 women die each year unnecessarily from this preventable disease. About 50% of women with cervical cancer in the United States did not have a Pap smear test in the preceding 3 years, and an additional 10% had not been screened in the past 5 years.

Nevertheless, more than 50 million Pap smears are performed each year in the United States alone, and 7% (3.5 million) of these give abnormal test results. It has been estimated that women who never had a Pap smear have a 3.5% risk of developing cervical cancer, whereas the risk is reduced to 0.8% with Pap smear screening. Since infection with human papilloma virus (HPV) has been found in almost all cervical cancers, testing for the presence of high-risk HPV types in cervical samples has now become a part of routine clinical work-up in women with equivocal Pap smear test results.

Pap Smear Terminology

There are a number of outdated terminologies regarding Pap smear results (**Table 6.1**). The lack of a common terminology initially resulted in widespread confusion about what really constitutes an abnormal test result. This confusion necessitated further action. In December 1988, a National Cancer Institute workshop held in Bethesda, Maryland, provided for the first time a consensus, now known as the Bethesda System, on how to properly read Pap smears. The result was initial guidelines designed to decrease the variability among laboratories reporting the results.

The three most important contributions of this Bethesda System were:

1. Establishing a special category of abnormal squamous cells of undetermined significance (ASCUS)
2. Organizing the four grades of atypical squamous cells (mild, moderate, severe, and carcinoma in situ) of the old classifications into two distinctive groups: low-

---

[1] In 1928, George Papanicolaou began sampling vaginal cells, speculating that the presence of any atypical cells might predict the development of cervical cancer. It was only in 1943 when he and Herbert Traut published a monograph on the topic that the Papanicolaou (Pap) smear became the standard cervical cancer screening test. In 1947, Ayers introduced a specially designed wooden spatula (Ayer spatula) for the direct collection of cells from the uterine cervix.

Table 6.1 Historical Pap smear terminology

Papanicolaou	United States	United Kingdom
Normal	Normal	Normal
Inflammatory	Inflammatory	Inflammatory
Atypical cells	Mild atypia Moderate atypia	Mild dyskariosis Moderate dyskariosis
Carcinoma in situ	Severe atypia	Severe dyskariosis
Carcinoma	Carcinoma	Carcinoma

grade squamous intra-epithelial lesion (LSIL) (**Fig. 6.4**), and high-grade squamous intra-epithelial lesion (HSIL) (**Fig. 6.5**). LSIL (previously referred to as "mild atypia") is compatible with grade 1 cervical intraepithelial neoplasia (CIN 1) and HSIL (encompassing "moderate atypia," "severe atypia," and "carcinoma in situ") is compatible with grade 2 or 3 cervical intra-epithelial neoplasia (CIN 2, 3) and carcinoma in situ (CIS)

3. Establishing a new category of abnormal glandular cells of undetermined significance (AGCUS)

Key Terminology Changes in the 2001 Bethesda System

The Bethesda System was revised in 1991 and 2001. The 2001 Bethesda System (**Table 6.2**) reflects the most current knowledge about the biology of Pap test abnormalities and addresses new screening technologies such as the liquid-based, thin-layer Pap smear and HPV testing. It recommends dividing the category of atypical squamous cells (ASCs) into two subcategories: a) atypical squamous cells of undetermined significance (ASCUS), and b) atypical squamous cells that cannot exclude high-grade intra-epithelial lesion (ASC-H).

Overall, among all women with ASC, the risk of developing invasive cancer is low (0.1–0.2%). Nevertheless, the prevalence of CIN 2, 3 confirmed by biopsy among women with ASC is 7–12%, whereas the prevalence of CIN 2, 3 confirmed by biopsy among women with ASC-H ranges from 26% to 68%. Rates of high-risk HPV DNA positivity are 40–51% among women with ASCUS, whereas they are 74–88% among women with ASC-H. Consequently, ASC-H should be considered to represent equivocal HSIL and a productive HPV infection. Thus, the performance of HPV testing allows for clear statements regarding the meaning of an ASC interpretation.

The 2001 revisions to the Bethesda System also eliminated the category of AGCUS (atypical glandular cells of undetermined significance) and identified three subcategories of atypical glandular cells (AGCs):

- AGC not otherwise specified
- AGC favoring neoplasia
- adenocarcinoma in situ (AIS)

Table 6.2 The 2001 Bethesda System

Specimen adequacy	
Satisfactory for evaluation (8000–12 000 well-visualized squamous cells for conventional smears and 5000 squamous cells for liquid-based preparations (*note presence/absence of endocervical/transformation zone component*—there should be at least 10 well-preserved endocervical or squamous metaplastic cells)	
Unsatisfactory for evaluation (specimens with >75% of epithelial cells obscured)	

Table 6.2 Continued

General categorization
Negative for intra-epithelial lesion or malignancy
Epithelial cell abnormality
Other
Interpretation/result
Negative for intra-epithelial lesion or malignancy

- **Organisms**
  - *Trichomonas vaginalis*
  - Fungal organisms morphologically consistent with *Candida* species
  - Shift in flora suggestive of bacterial vaginosis
  - Bacteria morphologically consistent with *Actinomyces* species
  - Cellular changes consistent with herpes simplex virus

- **Other non-neoplastic findings**
Reactive cellular changes associated with:
  - inflammation (includes typical repair)
  - radiation
  - intrauterine contraceptive device
Glandular cells status posthysterectomy
Atrophy

Epithelial cell abnormalities

- **Squamous cell**
  - Atypical squamous cells (ASC)
  - of undetermined significance (ASC-US)
  - cannot exclude HSIL (ASC-H) (*5–10% of ASC cases overall*)

- **Low-grade squamous intra-epithelial lesion (LSIL)** (generally a transient infection with HPV) encompassing: human papilloma virus/mild dysplasia/cervical intra-epithelial neoplasia (CIN) 1

- **High-grade squamous intra-epithelial lesion (HSIL)** (more often associated with HPV persistence and higher risk of progression) encompassing: moderate and severe dysplasia, carcinoma in situ; CIN 2 and CIN 3

- **Invasive squamous cell carcinoma**

- **Glandular cell**

- **Atypical glandular cells (AGC)** (*specify endocervical, endometrial, or glandular cells not otherwise specified*)

- **Atypical glandular cells (AGC)** (*specify endocervical, endometrial, or glandular cells not otherwise specified*)

- **Endocervical adenocarcinoma in situ (AIS)**

- **Invasive adenocarcinoma**

Other
Endometrial cells in a woman ≥40 years of age

Reproduced with permission from Salomon D et al. The 2001 Bethesda System: terminology for reporting results of cervical cytology. JAMA 2002; 287:2116.

Types of Pap Smear, Their Sensitivity, and Screening Guidelines

There are two main types of Pap smear: a conventional Pap smear, and liquid-based Pap smear.

Conventional Pap Smear

For a conventional Pap smear, the cell specimen on the collection instrument is spread across a glass slide and fixed to it by either spraying a fixative on the glass slide (**Fig. 6.1**) or placing it in a vial containing an ethanol fixative.

Ideally, samples for this type of a Pap smear should be obtained from three locations: (i) the endocervical canal (E), (ii) the exocervix (including the entire transformation zone) (C), and (iii) posterior vaginal pool (posterior fornix) (V). The samples can be smeared separately on three glass slides that are marked with the letters E, C, or V, respectively.

Some investigators, however, do not advocate collecting samples from the posterior vaginal pool. Nevertheless, for screening, all three samples can be smeared and mixed on one glass slide. The smear should be thick enough that it is not transparent.

Pap smears on a glass slide should be evaluated by a trained laboratory technician or cytopathologist, utilizing a regular light microscope (**Fig. 6.2**). In 1997, the US Food and Drug Administration (FDA) approved two systems for routine use as quality control (rescreening) devices. Although studies have shown that these systems can catch problems not detected on a microscopic evaluation of Pap smears, such technical triumphs have been overshadowed by conflicting opinions about their cost-effectiveness and accuracy among cytopathology professionals, clinicians, patients, and device manufacturers.

Liquid-Based, Thin-Layer (ThinPrep) Pap Smear

A ThinPrep Pap smear involves rinsing or dropping the collection instrument into a vial containing a liquid fixative (**Fig. 6.3**). The cells obtained are filtered, placed on a

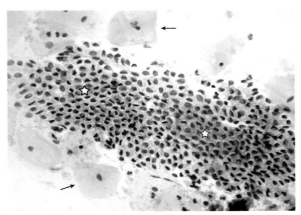

Fig. 6.2 The normal Pap smear. Benign superficial squamous cells (arrows) and endocervical cells (white stars) can be visualized by light microscopy.

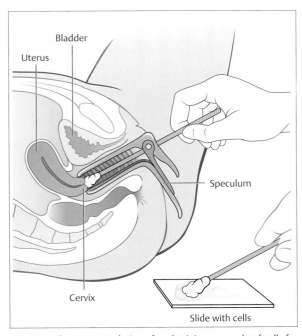

Fig. 6.1 The proper technique for obtaining a sample of cells for a Pap smear.

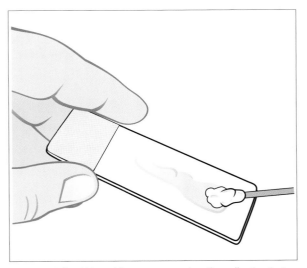

Fig. 6.3 A liquid-based Pap smear requires the collection instrument to be inserted into a vial containing a liquid fixative.

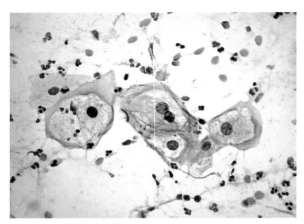

Fig. 6.4 Low-grade squamous intra-epithelial lesion characterized by perinuclear halo with peripheral thickening, binucleation, increased nuclear size and mild hyperchromasia.

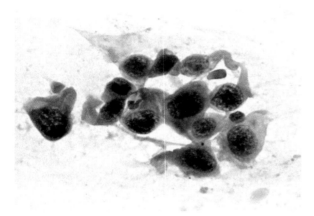

Fig. 6.5 High-grade squamous intra-epithelial lesion characterized by markedly increased nuclear to cytoplasm ratio and coarse chromatin.

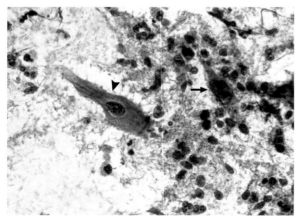

Fig. 6.6 Cytology of invasive squamous cell carcinoma. In addition to cells with features of high-grade squamous intra-epithelial lesion (arrow), spindle cells (arrowhead) may be identified in a background of necrotic debri.

slide and analyzed. Analysis usually includes initial computer screening followed by review by trained personnel. The ThinPrep Pap test screens for cervical cancer or precancerous changes.

ThinPrep technology may help detect up to 95% of high-grade lesions in the body, and is considered almost 100% accurate when combined with HPV testing for screening of cervical cancer.

Sensitivity and Specificity of Pap Smear Tests

Pap smear test sensitivity, specificity, and predictive value (negative and positive) are displayed in **Table 6.3**. A single conventional Pap smear test has a sensitivity to detect histological abnormality of 43–84% (mean, 62%) and specificity of 70–100% (mean, 89%). The single, liquid-based thin-layer cytology test has a sensitivity of 68–96% (mean, 81%) and specificity of 41–100% (mean, 78%). The repeat conventional Pap smear test has a sensitivity of 60–93% (mean, 75%) and specificity of 57–65% (mean, 62%).

There are two main contributors to false-negative readings on cervical cytology:

1. *Sampling error:* improper sample collection, poor transfer from collecting device to slide, poor fixation (air drying), and contamination with lubricant
2. *Laboratory error:* failure of identification of an abnormality, even though it is present on the smear

Because of the slow natural history of the disease, women who initially have a normal Pap smear test should have a repeat test approximately 1 year later. This will increase the sensitivity of the test to 75%. A third smear after an additional year will increase the sensitivity of the test to about 90%. Thus, the consensus recommendation is for women to have three consecutive annual Pap smears at the beginning and every 3 years thereafter, unless there is a reason to do otherwise.

Table 6.3 Sensitivity and specificity calculations

Histology of Pap smear	Abnormal	Normal	Total
Abnormal	TP	FP	TP + FP
Normal	FN	TN	TN + FN
Total	TP + FN	TN + FP	–

TP, true positive; FP, false positive; TN, true negative; FN, false negative.
Sensitivity = TP / TP + FN.
Specificity = TN / TN + FP.
Predictive value positive = TP / TP + FP.
Predictive value negative = TN/TN + FN.

Identification of cytologic abnormalities by means of the Pap test allows eradication of precursor lesions (CIN 2, 3), which could potentially evolve into invasive cancer (**Fig. 6.6**). Howell et al., for example, investigated the role of the new Pap test terminology in the detection of carcinoma in situ and invasive carcinoma in medically underserved Californian women. The results of their study are displayed in **Table 6.4**. Among HSIL Pap tests (N = 285), 40.7% had follow-up showing carcinoma in situ (CIS) and 3.9% invasive squamous cell carcinoma (SCC). Among SCC Pap tests (N = 28), 17.9% had follow-up results of CIS and 28.6% SCC. Of the 191 patients with CIS as a follow-up finding, the initial Pap smear showed: HSIL 60.7%, SCC 2.6%, LSIL 10.5%, ASC-US 13.6%, and negative or infection 9.9%. Of the 27 patients with SCC, the initial Pap test showed: HSIL 40.7%, SCC 29.6%, LSIL 7.4%, ASC-US 7.4%, and negative or infection 11.1%.

Screening Guidelines

American Cancer Society Screening Guidelines

The American Cancer Society recommends routine Pap screening based on a woman's age or medical status as follows.

1. *Age of screening initiation:* 3 years after onset of sexual activity, no later than age 21
2. *Screening frequency:* annually with conventional cytology or every 2 years with liquid-based cytology. After age 30, women with three consecutive normal Pap tests may be screened every 2–3 years
3. *Screening after hysterectomy:* no cytologic testing after total hysterectomy for benign conditions
4. *Discontinuation of screening:* after age 70
5. *Routine screening for high-risk HPV infection:* conventional or liquid-based cytology combined with test for DNA for high-risk HPV subtypes should be performed not more often than every 3 years

American Society of Colposcopy and Cervical Pathology Screening Guidelines

Following the 2001 Bethesda System, the American Society of Colposcopy and Cervical Pathology (ASCCP) sponsored two consensus conferences in 2001 and 2006, respectively, for establishing consensus guidelines for the management of women with abnormal cervical screening tests. These management guidelines are summarized in **Table 6.5**.

Table 6.4 The 2001 Bethesda System Pap test terminology in relation to the detection of carcinoma-in-situ and invasive carcinoma in medically underserved California women (Howell et al., 2004)

Pap screening result	Number of women	Carcinoma in situ	Invasive cancer
Negative	42 868 (81.9%)	14 (0.03%)	2 (0.004%)
Infection	5541 (10.6%)	5 (0.09%)	1 (0.02%)
ASCUS	1758 (3.4%)	26 (1.48%)	2 (0.11%)
LSIL	441 (0.8%)	20 (4.5%)	2 (0.45%)
HSIL	285 (0.5%)	116 (40.7%)	11 (3.86%)
Squamous cell carcinoma	28 (0.1%)	5 (17.86%)	8 (28.57%)
Other	435 (0.8%)	3 (0.69%)	1 (0.23%)
Unsatisfactory	983 (1.9%)	2 (0,2%)	0 (0.00%)
Total	52 339 (100.0%)	191 (0.36%)	27 (0.05%)

Reproduced with permission from Howell LP et al. Role of Pap test terminology and age in the detection of carcinoma in situ in medically underserved California women. Diagn Cytopathol 2004; 30(4):227–234.

Table 6.5 The 2006 American Society of Colposcopy and Cervical Pathology (ASCCP) consensus guidelines for the management of women with abnormal cervical screening tests

Pap smear result	Management
ASCUS	HPV testing, Repeat Pap smear, Colposcopy and biopsy
ASC-H	Colposcopy and biopsy
LSIL	Colposcopy and biopsy
HSIL	Colposcopy and biopsy, endocervical curettage, Further treatment with LEEP (LLETZ), cryotherapy, LASER therapy, conization, or hysterectomy
AGC	Colposcopy and biopsy, endocervical curettage

HPV, human papilloma virus; LEEP, loop electrosurgical excision procedure; LLETZ, large loop excision of transformation zone; LASER, light augmentation of stimulated emission of radiation. For Pap smear terminology, see text. Reproduced with permission of Elsevier from Wright TC et al. 2006 Consensus guidelines for the management of women with abnormal cervical cancer screening tests. AJOG 2007; 197:346–355.

Human Papilloma Virus DNA Testing

In 2003, the FDA approved the use of HPV DNA testing as an adjunct to cervical cytology screening in women aged 30 years and older. HPV DNA testing should be restricted to the known 13 high-risk (oncogenic) HPV types: 16, 18, 31, 33, 35, 39, 45, 51, 52, 56, 58, 59, and 66.

HPV DNA testing is performed using commercially available, highly sensitive molecular methods to detect high-risk types of HPV (the Hybrid Capture II HPV DNA Assay). The sensitivity (TP/TP + FN; for notation key, see **Table 6.3**) of HPV DNA testing for the detection of biopsy-confirmed CIN 2, 3 in women with ASC is 0.83 to 0.96 and is higher than the sensitivity of 0.7 to 0.85 attributed to a single repeat cervical cytological test (conventional or liquid-based).

The negative predictive value (TN/TN + FN) of DNA testing for high-risk types of HPV is generally reported to be 0.98 or greater. For comparison, a colposcopy in women with ASC to distinguish normal cervical tissue from abnormal tissue has a sensitivity of 0.96 and a specificity (TN/TN + FP) of 0.48 (high rate of false-positive). Between 31% and 60% of all women with ASC will have high-risk types of HPV identified, but the proportion with high-risk HPV decreases with increasing age.

Sensitivity using a combination of HPV testing and cytology is significantly higher than that of either test alone, with negative predictive value of 99–100%. The frequency of combined cytology and HPV testing should not be more than every 3 years, provided that both tests are negative. HPV testing should differentiate patients with SILs from those with reactive conditions. A positive HPV test will therefore prompt colposcopy more quickly than might otherwise happen if the patient were followed up with serial repeat Pap tests.

Management

Currently, there are three possible approaches to managing women with ASCUS:

1. Perform two repeated cytological examinations at 6 and 12 months.
2. Test for HPV.
3. Administer a single colposcopic examination.

Although all three management approaches are acceptable for managing women with ASCUS, "reflex" HPV testing is preferred. Reflex testing refers to testing either the original liquid-based cytology residual specimen or a separate sample co-collected at the time of the initial screening visit for HPV testing. All women with ASCUS who test positive for HPV DNA should be referred immediately for colposcopic evaluation and biopsy.

Management options for women who are positive for high-risk types of HPV, but who do not have biopsy-confirmed CIN, include follow-up with a repeat Pap test at 6 and 12 months. Patients should be referred back to colposcopy if a result of ASCUS or greater is obtained. All HPV DNA-positive women should be referred back for HPV-DNA testing and colposcopy. Women with ASCUS who test negative for high-risk HPV DNA can be followed up with a repeat Pap test at 12 months.

The management of women with ASC-H and LSIL is identical; all should be referred immediately for colposcopy and biopsy. If biopsy fails to confirm CIN, acceptable management options include follow-up with repeat smear screening at 6 and 12 months. Women with HSIL should be referred immediately for colposcopically directed biopsy and endocervical curettage.

If a CIN 2, 3 or a more advanced lesion is confirmed, further treatment options include loop electrosurgical conization, laser conization, cold-knife conization, or hysterectomy. Recent studies have found that a single colposcopic examination identifies CIN 2,3 or cancer in 53–66% of women with HSIL cytologic results and that CIN 2,3 or cancer is diagnosed in 84–97% of women evaluated using a loop electrosurgical excision. Approximately 2% of women with HSIL have invasive cancer.

Women younger than 35 years of age with AGC (except atypical endometrial cells) should be referred immediately for colposcopically directed biopsy with endocervical curettage, HPV DNA testing, and endometrial sampling. Women with atypical endometrial cells should be referred for endometrial and endocervical sampling. If there is no endometrial pathology, they should be referred for colposcopy.

Key Points

- After breast cancer, cervical cancer is the second most common malignancy diagnosed in women worldwide, and is the most common malignancy encountered in women in developing countries with limited or no effective screening programs.
- Human papilloma virus (HPV) infection has been found in almost all cervical cancers. Thus, testing for HPV in cervical samples has now become a part of routine clinical work-up in women with equivocal Pap smear test results.
- The American Cancer Society recommends that all women receive a Pap smear test 3 years after onset of sexual activity and no later than age 21 years.
- Women who initially have a normal Pap smear should have a repeat test approximately 1 year later.
- HPV DNA testing is a useful adjunct to cervical cytology screening in women aged 30 years and older.

Further Reading

The 1988 Bethesda System for reporting cervical/vaginal cytologic diagnoses. Developed and approved at the National Cancer Institute Workshop, Bethesda, Maryland, U.S.A., December 12-13, 1988. *Acta Cytol* 1989;33(5):567–574

Apgar BS, Brotzman G. Management of cervical cytologic abnormalities. *Am Fam Physician* 2004;70(10):1905–1916

Apgar BS, Zoschnick L, Wright TC Jr. The 2001 Bethesda System terminology. *Am Fam Physician* 2003;68(10):1992–1998

Cangiarella JF, Chhieng DC. Atypical glandular cells—an update. *Diagn Cytopathol* 2003;29(5):271–279

Emerson RE, Puzanov A, Brunnemer C, Younger C, Cramer H. Long-term follow-up of women with atypical squamous cells of undetermined significance (ASCUS). *Diagn Cytopathol* 2002;27(3):153–157

Hatch KD, Hacker NF. Intraepithelial disease of the cervix, vagina, and vulva. In: Berek JS, Adashi EY, Hillard PA, eds. Novak's Gynecology. 12th ed. Baltimore, Md: Williams & Wilkins; 2000:447–486.

Howell LP, Tabnak F, Tudury AJ, Stoodt G. Role of Pap Test terminology and age in the detection of carcinoma invasive and carcinoma in situ in medically underserved California women. *Diagn Cytopathol* 2004;30(4):227–234

Hughes AA, Glazner J, Barton P, Shlay JC. A cost-effectiveness analysis of four management strategies in the determination and follow-up of atypical squamous cells of undetermined significance. *Diagn Cytopathol* 2005;32(2):125–132

Koong SL, Yen AM, Chen TH. Efficacy and cost-effectiveness of nationwide cervical cancer screening in Taiwan. *J Med Screen* 2006;13(Suppl 1):S44–S47

Rowe LR, Aldeen W, Bentz JS. Prevalence and typing of HPV DNA by hybrid capture II in women with ASCUS, ASC-H, LSIL, and AGC on ThinPrep Pap tests. *Diagn Cytopathol* 2004;30(6):426–432

Solomon D, Davey D, Kurman R, et al; Forum Group Members; Bethesda 2001 Workshop. The 2001 Bethesda System: terminology for reporting results of cervical cytology. *JAMA* 2002;287(16):2114–2119

Stoler MH. New Bethesda terminology and evidence-based management guidelines for cervical cytology findings. *JAMA* 2002;287(16):2140–2141

Wright TC, Cox JT, Massad LS, Twiggs LB, Wilkinson EJ; for the 2001 ASCCP-Sponsored Consensus Conference. 2001 consensus guidelines for the management of women with cervical cytology abnormalities. *JAMA* 2002;287:2120–2129

Wright TC Jr, Massad LS, Dunton CJ, Spitzer M, Wilkinson EJ, Solomon D; 2006 ASCCP-Sponsored Consensus Conference. 2006 consensus guidelines for the management of women with abnormal cervical screening tests. *J Low Genit Tract Dis* 2007;11(4):201–222

7 Genetic Screening and Obstetric Procedures

Aria Koifman and Arnon Wiznitzer

Maternal age of 35 years and over is the single most important risk factor for having a child with trisomy 21 (Down syndrome). In the past decade, amniocentesis and chorionic villous sampling (CVS) were introduced as methods of diagnosing Down syndrome for women who would be over the age of 35 years at time of delivery.

Since both of these diagnostic techniques, which will be discussed later in this chapter, are quite invasive, noninvasive screening test were developed in the early 1980s and have since evolved. Today, several noninvasive screening strategies are available to clinicians. This chapter, which supplements Chapter 5, discusses the relative advantages and disadvantages of these common screening tests and their applications in common clinical practice.

Definitions

α-Fetoprotein: This is a major plasma protein, which is produced by the yolk sac and the liver during fetal life.

Aneuploidy: This term refers to an abnormal number of chromosomes. Syndromes caused by an extra or missing chromosome are among the most widely recognized genetic disorders in humans.

Dimeric inhibin A: This is a glycoprotein of placental origin, similar to human chorionic gonadotropin. Levels of this glycoprotein in maternal serum remain relatively constant through the 15th to 18th weeks of pregnancy. Maternal serum levels of dimeric inhibin A are twice as high in pregnancies affected by Down syndrome than in unaffected pregnancies.

Human chorionic gonadotropin: This glycoprotein hormone is produced in pregnancy, by the developing embryo soon after conception and later by the placenta. Its role is to prevent the disintegration of the corpus luteum of the ovary and thereby maintain progesterone production that is critical for the maintenance of a healthy pregnancy in humans.

Nuchal translucency: This term is used to describe the area at the back of the neck (nuchal region) of the developing baby as assessed by ultrasound scanning. Measurement of the nuchal translucency is performed in the first trimester (between 11 weeks and 13 weeks, 6 days). Measurements of greater than 3.0 mm may warrant further investigation.

Pregnancy associated plasma protein A: This is a large, zinc-binding protein that acts as an enzyme, specifically a metallopeptidase. Women with low blood levels of this protein at 8–14 weeks of gestation have an increased risk of intrauterine growth restriction, trisomy 21, premature delivery, pre-eclampsia, and stillbirth.

Trisomy: This is a form of aneuploidy with the presence of three copies, instead of the normal two, of a particular chromosome. Down syndrome, in which affected individuals have an extra copy of chromosome 21, is called trisomy 21.

Unconjugted estriol: Estriol is a steroid hormone derived from cholesterol and is the major estrogen produced during pregnancy. It is only produced in significant amounts during pregnancy as it is made by the fetal liver and the placenta.

Screening Strategies

Although current screening strategies offer high sensitivity and specificity rates, patients should be informed that a screening test provides an individual risk assessment but is not diagnostic for chromosomal abnormalities. The main disadvantage of screening tests is that not all affected fetuses will be detected.

A screen is considered positive when a value for one or more of the screened disorders falls above a designated risk cutoff. A risk cutoff might be chosen based upon the desired detection rate, false-positive rate, or a combination of both. The results in the screening tests are expressed (aside from their proper measuring units for each marker) in multiples of the median (MoM). Each marker result, including both biochemistry and nuchal translucency measurements, can be expressed in MoM. This allows for direct comparison of results between laboratories.

Historically, a biochemical marker in maternal serum, combined with maternal age, has been the main screening method. As ultrasound imaging became a common practice in obstetrics, it was only natural to use it in aneuploidy screening. Combination of the methods is the basis for current screening strategies. In cases identified as "screen positive," proper counseling should be provided in order to deliver the information in a clear and accurate manner.

First Trimester Screening

Nuchal Translucency

One early study reported that increased nuchal translucency (NT), which can be visualized by ultrasound scanning at 11–14 weeks of gestation (**Fig. 7.1**), is associated with trisomy 21. Unfortunately, the detection rate, which was validated by several studies, was only 65–71%, with a false-positive rate of about 5–8%. Only with large-scale studies, when the option of using NT in a quantitative manner (i.e., with MoM) became available, could NT be combined with biochemical markers to improve detection rates for trisomy 21.

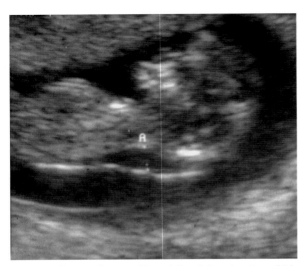

Fig. 7.1 Ultrasound scan at 11 weeks' gestation showing a thickened nuchal translucency (A) of 3.5 mm.

NT has proven to be useful not only in aneuploidy screening, but also for fetal cardiac malformations, diaphragmatic hernia, and some rare single-gene disorders as well. An NT value above the 95th percentile warrants a detailed ultrasonographic anatomy scan, and in many centers even fetal echocardiography is employed in such cases.

Biochemical Markers

The most widely studied markers in the first trimester of pregnancy are free beta human chorionic gonadotropin (β-HCG), total β-HCG, and pregnancy associated plasma protein A (PAPP-A). Of these, β-HCG has been found to be useful in both the first and second trimesters and provides predictive information concerning pregnancy outcomes. The level of PAPP-A, a glycoprotein produced by the trophoblast, is reduced in Down syndrome and trisomy 18. This marker is only useful as a quantitative screen in the first trimester. Regarding detection rates, first-trimester biochemical markers alone are not superior to the second-trimester triple test (see below). However, as previously mentioned, PAPP-A in combination with NT provides detection rates of 82–87%.

Around 10% of circulating estriol (E3) in the maternal compartment remains in the unconjugated form. Decreased levels of uconjugated estriol (uE3) have been seen in pregnancies affected with Down syndrome in the second trimester of pregnancy. Low levels of midtrimester uE3, alone or in association with other midtrimester markers, has been associated with adverse pregnancy outcomes.

Second Trimester Screening Tests

Triple Test

Alpha fetoprotein (αFP) was the first biochemical marker to be associated with a birth defect, when it was discovered that high levels of αFP in maternal serum were associated with neural tube defects (NTDs). Later reports described low levels of maternal serum αFP (MS αFP) as being associated with trisomonies 21 and 18. Eventually, it was shown that adding β-HCG and E3 testing to an assay for αFP (i.e., the triple test) could significantly increase the sensitivity of detecting trisomy 21 (see Evidence Box 7.1).

Quad Test

In order to improve the detection rate for trisomy 21, an assay for measuring blood levels of dimeric inhibin A was added to the triple test. The detection rate of the quad test has increased to approximately 80%, with a false-positive rate of 5%.

Common Screening Strategies

The following provides an overview of the common genetic screening strategies in use around the world.

First Trimester Screening

- NT alone: detection rate of 65–70%. Rarely used as a sole screening method
- Combined test: NT + Free β-HCG and PAPP-A; detection rates of 82–87%. Can be used as a sole method or part of the integrated testing

Second Trimester Screening

- Triple marker: MS αFP, uE3, total β-HCG; detection rates of about 70%. Still used extensively as the sole screening method for trisomy 21, especially wherever NT measurement is difficult to obtain
- Quad marker: MS αFP, uE3, total β-HCG, inhibin A; detection rates reach about 81%. Currently not a very commonly used method of screening

Combined First and Second Trimester (Integrated) Screening

- Integrated screen: NT and PAPP-A are done in the first trimester (results are not reported), then β-HCG, uE3, MS αFP, and inhibin A are done in the second trimester. The risk for trisomy 21 is reported after all results are available. Detection rates reach 95%, with a false-negative rate of 5%
- Integrated serum screen: this is similar to integrated screen without the NT measurement. Serum-only integrated screening has been tested in clinical practice and shown to have a Down syndrome detection rate of 79–87%. However, 13% of first-trimester samples were not usable because of dating errors, resulting in this segment of the the population receiving quad marker test results only. **Figures 7.2 and 7.3** show a comparison of a first trimester prenatal screening protocol with second trimester integrated screening and the benefits and limitations of each

Patients undergoing integrated screening usually get their results only when the test is completed, meaning not until the second trimester. This has created some concerns among medical ethicists and patient advocacy groups, because they believe that not conducting a risk estimate in the first trimester of pregnancy could prevent women from acting upon the results, thus carrying a pregnancy that may be problematic.

Some studies have indicated that holding-back test results from the patient until the second trimester increases maternal anxiety and promotes lack of bonding to the pregnancy until the test results are known. Such concerns led recently to the development of two additional strategies regarding integrated testing: (i) stepwise sequential testing, and (ii) contingent sequential testing, which are discussed in detail below.

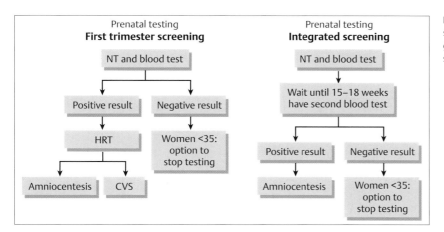

Fig. 7.2 Flowchart of first trimester screening versus second trimester integrated screening. CVS, chorionic villus sampling; NT, nuchal translucency.

	First trimester screening	Integrated screening
Down syndrome detection rate	85%	94%
Trisomy 18 detection rate	80%	90%
Spina bifida detection rate	No detection	80%
Results and diagnosis available	First trimester	Second trimester

Fig. 7.3 Comparative benefits and limitations of fist trimester only screening versus integrated second trimester screening. *A blood test can be done between 16 and 18 weeks of pregnancy.

Stepwise sequential testing: First trimester (i.e., NT and free β-HCG assays) screening is initiated, reported, and a risk is calculated. If the risk is very high from the first-trimester analysis, diagnostic testing is discussed, and no further serum screening is performed. First-trimester risk assessments that are less than 1 in 270 are considered "low risk" and do not require further evaluation and testing. Approximately 95% of pregnant women tested will have a "low risk" result. Since this is a screening test, there is still a small chance that the fetus may be affected, even when the screening test is negative.

For this low-risk population, the first-trimester result is discussed. If the physician elects to continue with screening, a quad test is typically performed at 15–20 weeks of gestation. Results are analyzed in conjunction with the first-trimester screen results, and a single-risk estimate is calculated. In order to calculate risk in the first trimester as well as in the integrated test, a β-HCG value is collected in both the first and second trimesters.

Contingent sequential testing: The initial steps in contingent sequential testing are the same as in stepwise sequential screening. If the risk is high, the patient is offered further diagnostic testing. However, in contrast to stepwise sequential testing, contingent sequential testing requires further delineation of low-risk versus intermediate-risk individuals. Patients in the low-risk group are advised that no further risk testing is needed. However, they can undergo further diagnostic testing, if they elect to do so. Patients in the intermediate-risk group undergo automatic second trimester serum testing, are given an integrated risk assessment, and counseled accordingly.

Some factors are known to influence the serum screening results, including exact dating (i.e., early dating ultrasound exam is preferred), maternal weight (both height and low body mass index affect results and a proper calculation adjustment is needed), ethnic origin, and insulin-dependent diabetes mellitus status.

Diagnostic Testing

Chorionic Villus Sampling

Chorionic villus sampling (CVS), which is discussed in detail in Chapter 5, utilizes either a catheter or needle to obtain a biopsy containing a small sample of the fluid that surrounds the fetus. This fluid contains placental cells that are derived from the same fertilized egg as the fetus and are shed primarily from the fetal skin, bladder, gastrointestinal tract, and amnion.

Typically, CVS is done at 10–12 weeks' gestation, and amniocentesis is done at 15–18 weeks' gestation. In the United States, the current standard of care in obstetric practice is to offer either CVS or amniocentesis to women who will be equal to or greater than 35 years of age when they give birth, because these women are at increased risk for giving birth to infants with Down syndrome and certain other types of aneuploidy. Karyotyping of cells obtained by either amniocentesis or CVS is the standard and definitive means of diagnosing aneuploidy in fetuses (**Fig. 7.4**).

The risk that a woman will give birth to an infant with Down syndrome increases with age. For example, for women of 35 years of age, the risk is 1 per 385 births (0.3%), whereas for women of 45 years of age, the risk is 1 per 30 births (3%). The background risk for major birth defects (with or without chromosomal abnormalities) for women of all ages is approximately 3%.

Confined placental mosaicism (i.e., a discrepancy between the chromosomal make-up of the cells in the placenta and the cells in the baby) is present in up to 2% of all CVS, even though the associated fetus is usually normal. This placental mosaicism is caused by a "nondisjunction" during early mitotic divisions in one or more cells destined to become the placenta or from partial "correction" of a trisomy resulting from a meiotic error (see Chapter 5). This correction results in a chromosome being lost from all cells destined to become the fetus but retained in some cells destined to become the placenta. CVS findings should be confirmed by analyses of cultured mesenchymal cells, as they are more reliably derived from the fetus.

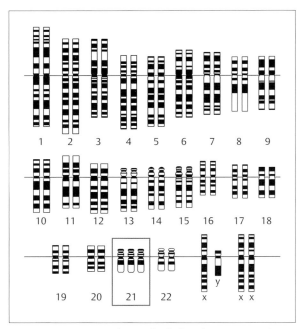

Fig. 7.4   Karyotype of an individual with trisomy 21 (Down syndrome).

Amniocentesis

Amniocentesis is the most common procedure performed during pregnancy. It is routinely performed at 15–17 weeks' of gestation. On some occasions, early amniocentesis at 12–14 weeks is performed to expedite results, although less fluid is obtained at this time. Early amniocentesis also carries a greater risk of spontaneous abortion or fetal injury but provides important diagnostic results at an earlier stage of pregnancy.

Fetal Blood Sampling

Fetal blood can be collected directly from the umbilical cord. A percutaneous needle is inserted to the uterine cavity and directed by ultrasound imaging to the umbilical artery (see Chapter 5, Fig. 5.12). Indications for this procedure include late second-trimester abnormalities detected by ultrasound exam or inconclusive results of cytogenetic analysis derived from amniocentesis.

Screening for Neural Tube Defects

When introduced, second trimester maternal serum screening was directed to detecting neural tube defects. With detection rates of 75–80%, MS αFP determination is still a good screening tool for NTDs, especially when ultrasonography is unavailable. It is recommended that all pregnant women should have an MS αFP test for NTDs. However, high-resolution ultrasonography is currently the most useful method for diagnosing NTDs. The sensitivity of ultrasound imaging for the detection of NTDs has been reported to be as high as 94–100%. It has been suggested that ultrasonography will soon replace MS αFP determination as the predominant screening tool for NTDs.

Key Points

- Maternal age of 35 years and over is the single most important risk factor for having a child with trisomy 21 (Down syndrome).
- Because early testing for Down syndrome, such as amniocentesis and chorionic villi sampling, are quite invasive and carry significant risks for mother and infant, several noninvasive screening strategies have been developed and are available to clinicians.
- Nuchal translucency (i.e, the thickness of the area at the back of the neck of the developing baby, which can be visualized by ultrasound scanning at 11–14 weeks of gestation) is strongly associated with trisomy 21.
- Human chorionic gonadotropin (β-HCG) has been found to be useful as a biochemical marker in both the first and second

trimester for providing predictive information concerning pregnancy outcomes.
- The serum level of pregnancy associated plasma protein A, a glycoprotein produced by the trophoblast, is reduced in Down syndrome and trisomy 18. This marker is only useful as a quantitative screen in the first trimester.
- Decreased levels of uconjugated estriol in the second trimester have been seen in pregnancies affected with Down syndrome.
- Combining measures of nuchal translucency with assays for biochemical markers has significantly improved the diagnosis of aneuploidies and other developmental abnormalities.
- The detection rate of the quad test, the most sensitive screening test available, is approximately 80%, with a false-positive rate of 5%.

Evidence Box 7.1

The triple test combined with maternal age can detect two-thirds of fetuses with trisomy 21.

Wald and Watt introduced the first multiple marker screening test for trisomy 21 (Down syndrome) in the second trimester (15–20 weeks). They then conducted a study to investigate the effect of parity on the six serum markers used in screening for Down syndrome. Of the six markers, only human chorionic gonadotropin (HCG) levels were affected by parity; HCG levels decreased by 3.1% per previous birth (95% confidence interval, 2.2% to 4.0%); there was no significant relationship between the number of previous abortions and HCG level after adjustment for the number of previous births. The effect of previous births on HCG was not due to maternal age.

Overall, they demonstrated that combining determinations of maternal serum α-fetoprotein, maternal serum β-HCG, maternal serum unconjugated estriol, and maternal age could detect 65–69% of fetuses with trisomy 21, with only a 5% false-positive rate. Numerous later studies have validated this initial finding.

Wald NJ, Watt HC. Serum markers for Down's syndrome in relation to number of previous births and maternal age. Prenat Diagn 1996;16:699–703.

Further Reading

Chervenak FA, McCullough LB, Chasen ST. Clinical implications of the ethics of informed consent for first-trimester risk assessment for trisomy 21. *Semin Perinatol* 2005;29(4):277–279

Haddow JE, Palomaki GE, Knight GJ, Williams J, Miller WA, Johnson A. Screening of maternal serum for fetal Down's syndrome in the first trimester. *N Engl J Med* 1998;338(14):955–961

Knight GJ, Palomaki GE, Neveux LM, et al. Integrated serum screening for Down syndrome in primary obstetric practice. *Prenat Diagn* 2005;25(12):1162–1167

Malone FD, Canick JA, Ball RH, et al; First- and Second-Trimester Evaluation of Risk (FASTER) Research Consortium. First-trimester or second-trimester screening, or both, for Down's syndrome. *N Engl J Med* 2005;353(19):2001–2011

Merkatz IR, Nitowsky HM, Macri JN, Johnson WE. An association between low maternal serum alpha-fetoprotein and fetal chromosomal abnormalities. *Am J Obstet Gynecol* 1984;148(7):886–894

Nicolaides KH, Azar G, Byrne D, Mansur C, Marks K. Fetal nuchal translucency: ultrasound screening for chromosomal defects in first trimester of pregnancy. *BMJ* 1992;304(6831):867–869

Norton ME. Genetic screening and counseling. *Curr Opin Obstet Gynecol* 2008;20(2):157–163

Summers AM, Farrell SA, Huang T, Meier C, Wyatt PR. Maternal serum screening in Ontario using the triple marker test. *J Med Screen* 2003;10(3):107–111

Wald NJ, Rodeck C, Hackshaw AK, Walters J, Chitty L, Mackinson AM. First and second trimester antenatal screening for Down's syndrome: the results of the Serum, Urine and Ultrasound Screening Study (SURUSS). *J Med Screen* 2003;10(2):56–104

Wald NJ, Watt HC. Serum markers for Down's syndrome in relation to number of previous births and maternal age. *Prenat Diagn* 1996;16(8):699–703

Wapner R, Thom E, Simpson JL, et al; First Trimester Maternal Serum Biochemistry and Fetal Nuchal Translucency Screening (BUN) Study Group. First-trimester screening for trisomies 21 and 18. *N Engl J Med* 2003;349(15):1405–1413

Part II Obstetrics

Section I   Normal Obstetrics

8 Maternal–Fetal Physiology

Natalia P. Zeff and Gustavo F. Leguizamón

During pregnancy, extensive physiologic changes occur in both the mother and her developing fetus. Physiological activity increases markedly in most pregnant women, and an understanding of these normal physiological changes is necessary in order to provide adequate care. Furthermore, physicians caring for pregnant women must have a basic knowledge of embryology and fetoplacental physiology.

Maternal Physiology

Carbohydrate Metabolism

Early pregnancy can be viewed as an anabolic state, with increased peripheral utilization of glucose and fasting hypoglycemia. Therefore, energy is stored in this early stage to meet future fetal demands in late pregnancy. The second half of pregnancy is characterized by a significant increase in insulin resistance and, consequently, postprandial hyperglycemia.

Two common symptoms/findings presented by pregnant women can be explained by the following physiologic changes.
1. *Tendency to interprandial hypoglycemia.* This occurs because the fetus continues to draw glucose from the maternal bloodstream across the placenta, even during periods of fasting.
2. *Gestational diabetes.* Progressive tissue resistance to insulin, secondary to increased levels of various diabetogenic hormones, leads to increased pancreatic production of insulin—up to 30% higher in pregnant women in the third trimester than in nonpregnant women. Therefore, women not able to cope with these demands, or those presenting other complications that increase insulin resistance (e.g., obesity), are susceptible to develop gestational diabetes.

Hyperglycemia also is associated with significant fetal complications. Since glucose readily crosses the placenta by facilitated diffusion, abnormal values in the maternal compartment are immediately followed by abnormal fetal glycemic levels. Therefore achieving euglycemia during pregnancy is of utmost importance (see Evidence Box 8.1).

Cardiovascular System

Pregnancy affects all of the components of the mother's cardiovascular system, including cardiac volume and output as well as blood volume and red blood cell count (**Fig. 8.1**). Changes in cardiac function begin in the first trimester of pregnancy. There is an initial increase in cardiac output due to reduced systemic vascular resistance, and an increase in heart rate, which continues to increase and remains elevated during the remainder of pregnancy.

At just about mid-pregnancy, arterial blood pressure decreases to a nadir and rises thereafter until term, but

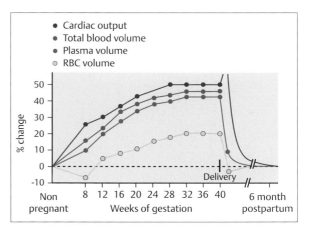

Fig. 8.1 Beginning in the first trimester, many changes occur in a pregnant woman's cardiovascular and hematologic system to compensate for the need to supply additional blood and nutrients to her growing body and the fetus.

even then, it is still 21% lower than nonpregnant values. This overall decrease in maternal blood pressure is a result of the decreased systemic vascular resistance due to the smooth muscle-relaxing effects of the elevated progesterone levels.

Respiratory Tract

The diaphragm rises by about 4 cm during pregnancy, causing a reduction in the lung residual volume. The increased ventilation observed during pregnancy is secondary to increased tidal volume (TV) with no change in the respiratory rate (RR). This is caused by a direct effect of progesterone on the CNS respiratory center. Functional residual capacity (FRC) is defined as the volume remaining in the lungs after a forced expiration. The increase in TV observed occurs at expense of the FRC. The VC does not change (**Fig. 8.2**).

Minute ventilation is defined as tidal volume (TV) × respiratory rate (RR). The increase observed in minute ventilation is responsible for the physiologic fall of the P_{ACO_2} and the P_{ACO_2}. This fall facilitates the transfer of CO_2 from the fetus to the mother and results in respiratory alkalosis observed under physiological conditions in pregnancy.

Spirometric measurements and peak expiratory flow rates are not altered in pregnancy, suggesting that airway function remains stable. However, despite pulmonary function not being altered during pregnancy, diseases of the respiratory tract may be more serious. Indeed, pregnancy increases the woman's risk of a number of non-infectious respiratory diseases, including asthma, aspiration pneumonia, venous air embolism, adult respiratory distress syndrome, pulmonary embolism, and deep venous thrombosis. These conditions often have unique manifestations in pregnant women.

Renal Function

During pregnancy, the kidneys enlarge significantly, owing to an increase in their vasculature, interstitial volume, and urinary dead space (, dilation of the renal pelvis, calyces, and ureters) and reach their maximal size by mid-pregnancy.

There is a corresponding marked increase in renal plasma flow as well as the rate of glomerular filtration, which are reflected by a significant increase in creatinine clearance, from approximately 120 mL/min in the non-pregnant state to approximately 150–200 mL/min during pregnancy.

Glucose excretion increases in pregnancy as well and glycosuria may occur. About 90% of pregnant women with normal blood glucose levels excrete 1–10 g of glucose per day. No increase in proteinuria is found in normal pregnancies.

Pregnancy-Related Changes in Placental Structure and Physiology

Although the placenta acts as an anatomical barrier between the mother and the fetus, it has important metabolic, endocrine, immunological, and nutritional properties.

Placental development is initiated by blastocyst implantation. Ten days after conception two different

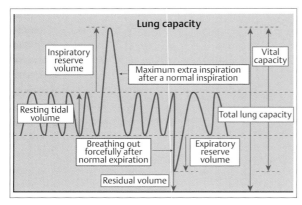

Fig. 8.2 Lung capacity is the total volume of the lung (i.e., the volume of air in the lungs after maximum inspiration). It is calculated by adding the inspiratory reserve volume to the tidal volume plus expiratory reserve volume and the residual volume (IRV + TV + ERV + RV). The increase in oxygen requirement caused by pregnancy is accommodated by an increase in tidal volume without an increase in respiratory rate.

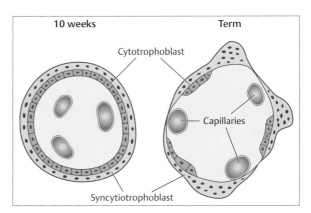

Fig. 8.3 The trophoblast, which develops during the first week to 10 days following implantation, consists of an inner layer of rapid proliferating cells known as the cytotrophoblast and an outer layer of multinucleated cells known as the syncytiotrophoblast. By term, the capillaries have migrated toward the syncytiotrophoblast, and the cytotrophoblast has degenerated leaving a thin barrier between maternal and fetal blood.

cell layers can be observed in the invading trophoblast (**Fig. 8.3**):

- *the inner layer* composed of individual and rapidly proliferating cells, the cytotrophoblast, and
- *the outer layer*, which is thick and comprises a continuous mass of cell plasma containing multiple nuclei with indistinct cell borders the syncytiotrophoblast

Three different compartments can be identified in the maternal–fetal interaction:

1. *Fetal circulation.* Blood coming from the umbilical arteries enters the villus and is subsequently drained back to the fetus by the umbilical veins.
2. *Maternal circulation.* Blood coming from the uterine spiral arteries (maternal) enters the intervillous space and is subsequently drained by the endometrial veins.
3. *Intervillous space.* Maternal blood drains into this space, which is in early pregnancy a barrier between maternal and fetal blood constituted by the capillary endothelium, cytotrophoblast, and syncytiotrophoblast. As pregnancy progresses, the capillaries migrate toward the syncytiotrophoblast, and the cytotrophoblast degenerates leaving a thin barrier between maternal and fetal blood.

Certain villi extend from the "chorionic plate" to the decidua, serving as "anchoring villi" (**Fig. 8.4**). However, most of them end fully in the intervillous space without

reaching the decidua. As the placenta matures, the villi branch and form finer subdivisions with small villi.

Each of the main stem villi and their ramifications constitute a placental cotyledon. This structure allows maternal–fetal interaction without significant contact between maternal and fetal blood. The main placental functions are gas exchange, passing nutrients from mother to fetus, passive immunity, and endocrine regulation.

Fetal Physiology

An understanding of fetal and neonatal physiology is critical in order to provide proper care for these infants. It is particularly needed if one is going to perform interventions via the umbilical cord or within the intrauterine environment. Fortunately, recent advances in fetoscopy, Doppler ultrasonography, and umbilical cord blood sampling have made the detection and treatment of fetal disorders significantly more manageable.

Fetal Circulation

Beginning about 25 days after conception, the circulatory system of the fetus becomes fully functional, and well-oxygenated blood from the placenta enters the fetus through the umbilical vein.

1. The umbilical vein gives off branches to the left lobe of the liver, which assumes the major role in blood formation at about 10 weeks postconception, and then continues as the ductus venosus. Subsequently, a major right branch is given off which joins the portal vein supplying the right hepatic lobe.
2. On the left side, the left hepatic vein fuses with the well-oxygenated ductus venosus and flows into the inferior vena cava to reach the left atrium by crossing through the foramen ovale. Therefore, blood with the highest oxygen content reaches the left ventricle. Then, via the aorta and carotid circulation, this blood supplies the brain and upper body.
3. It is worth mentioning that left hepatic lobe is supplied almost exclusively by umbilical venous blood (>95%). In contrast, the right lobe receives both umbilical venous blood (60%) and portal venous blood (30%). Therefore, while the left hepatic lobe is perfused with blood which has an oxygen saturation of 80–85%, the right lobe is perfused by a mixture of umbilical and portal venous blood, with a much lower oxygen saturation (35%).
4. Blood from the right hepatic vein and the inferior vena cava join to form a stream directed through the

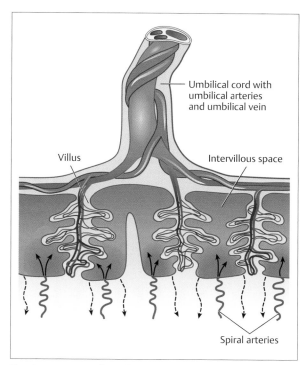

Umbilical cord with umbilical arteries and umbilical vein

Villus

Intervillous space

Spiral arteries

Fig. 8.4 Certain villi in the intervillous space extend from the "chorionic plate" to the decidua, serving as "anchoring villi."

tricuspid valve to the right ventricle. Therefore, right ventricular output is directed through the ductus arteriosus to the descending aorta. Since the pulmonary vascular resistance is high and the mean pulmonary artery pressures are higher than aortic pressures, the flow is mainly directed toward the ductus arteriosus, leaving the pulmonary circulation with 5–10% of the ventricular output.

Amniotic Fluid

During the early stages of pregnancy, the mechanism of formation of amniotic fluid is an active transport of solute (probably sodium or chloride) by the amnion into the amniotic space, with water moving passively down the chemical potential gradient.

During the second half of gestation, other important pathways come into play. The excretion of fetal urine and the swallowing of amniotic fluid by the fetus are the two major mechanisms for the formation and clearance, respectively, of amniotic fluid. The fetal lungs also contribute to the production of amniotic fluid, secreting 300–400 ml per day near term. There is also a transmembranous pathway, which consists of movement of water and solutes between amniotic fluid and maternal blood. Finally, fluid may be secreted by the fetal oral–nasal cavities. Amniotic fluid circulates with a turnover time of approximately one to two days.

Endocrinology

The thyroid gland and the pancreas are the first endocrine glands to become fully functional in the fetus and can be producing thyroxine and insulin as early as 4 weeks and 12 weeks postconception, respectively. Maternal insulin does not reach the fetus in physiological quantities, so the fetus must supply whatever is needed to metabolize glucose for energy. Therefore, the availability of insulin is the rate-limiting process controlling fetal growth and development.

The normal B cells of the fetus respond poorly to hyperglycemia unless the stimulus is constant. Thus, maternal diabetes may cause hyperplasia of fetal B cells, so that larger quantities of insulin can be manufactured. Many believe that this is why some infants of diabetic mothers grow so large or show evidence of hyperinsulinism when born.

The fetal adrenal gland consists mainly of a fetal zone, which disappears about six months after birth, and a cortex, and is an extremely active organ that produces large quantities of steroid hormones (**Fig. 8.5**). Research suggests that the steadily increasing activity of the fetal zone triggers the initiation of labor, and premature atrophy of the fetal adrenal gland leads to markedly prolonged labor. The fetal adrenal gland also is an important source of catecholamines, which respond when stress is placed on the fetal myocardium.

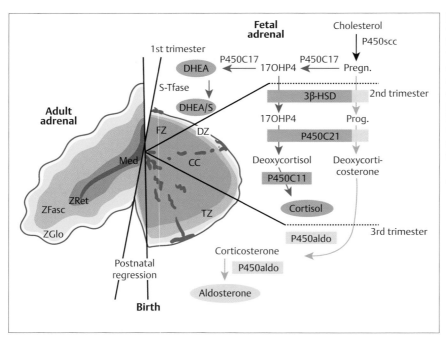

Fig. 8.5 This schematic representation is divided into portions showing the fetal adrenal gland (right) at the first, second and third trimesters of pregnancy, and the adult adrenal gland (left). DHEA: Dehydroepiandrosterone; DHEA/S: Dehydroepiandrosterone sulfate; 3β-HSD: 3β-hydroxysteroid dehydrogenase; P450C21: Steroidogenic enzyme cytochrome P450C21; P450C11: Steroidogenic enzyme cytochrome P450C11; P450aldo: P450 aldosterone synthase.

Key Points

- During pregnancy, physiological activity increases markedly in most pregnant women, and an understanding of these normal physiological changes is necessary in order to provide adequate care.
- In early pregnancy, there is an increased peripheral utilization of glucose and fasting hypoglycemia, and energy is stored to meet future fetal demands in late pregnancy.
- Pregnancy affects all of the components of the cardiovascular system, including cardiac volume and output as well as blood volume and red blood cell count.
- Pregnancy increases women's risk of a number of noninfectious respiratory diseases, which often have unique manifestations in pregnant women.
- During pregnancy, the kidneys enlarge significantly, and there is a corresponding marked increase in renal plasma flow as well as in the rate of glomerular filtration.
- Recent advances in fetoscopy, Doppler ultrasonography, and umbilical cord blood sampling have made the detection and treatment of fetal disorders significantly more feasible.

Evidence Box 8.1

Maternal glucose levels below those diagnostic for diabetes are associated with increased birth weight and increased cord-blood serum C-peptide levels.

The HAPO Cooperative Study Research Group analyzed the outcomes of 75-g oral glucose-tolerance testing at 24–32 weeks of gestation among a total of 25 505 pregnant women at 15 centers in nine countries. Data remained blinded if the fasting plasma glucose level was 105 mg/dL (5.8 mmol/L) or less, and the 2-hour plasma glucose level was 200 mg/dL (11.1 mmol/L) or less. The primary outcomes of the study were birth weight above the 90th percentile for gestational age, primary cesarean delivery, clinically diagnosed neonatal hypoglycemia, and cord-blood serum C-peptide level above the 90th percentile. For the 23 316 participants, there were no obvious thresholds at which risks increased. However, significant associations were observed for maternal glucose levels below those diagnostic of diabetes, with increased birth weight and increased cord-blood serum C-peptide levels.

HAPO Study Cooperative Research Group, et al. Hyperglycemia and adverse pregnancy outcomes. N Engl J Med 2008 May 8;358(19):1991–2002.

Further Reading

Reece EA, Hobbins JC, eds. Clinical Obstetrics: the Fetus and Mother. 3rd ed. Malden, Mass: Blackwell Synergy Publishing; 2007

Creasy RK, Resnik R, Iams JD, eds. Maternal–Fetal Medicine: Principles and Practice. 5th ed. Philadelphia, Pa: WB Saunders; 2004

Gabbe SG, Niebyl JR, Simpson JL, eds. Obstetrics—Normal and Problem Pregnancies. 4th ed. New York: Churchill Livingstone; 2002

9 Preconception and Antepartum Care

Gustavo F. Leguizamón

Preconception and antepartum care are excellent examples of effective primary prevention. Because more than 50% of pregnancies in the United States are unplanned, health care providers should advise every woman in her reproductive years to seek preconception care and counseling. This chapter offers an overview of the key components of effective preconception and antepartum care, and refers the reader to other chapters for more detailed descriptions of specific approaches and procedures.

Definitions

Preconception care: Preconception care is a set of interventions that identify and modify biomedical, behavioral, and social risks to a woman's health prior to her conceiving a child. It includes both prevention and management, emphasizing health issues that require action before conception, or very early in pregnancy, for maximal impact. The target population for preconception care is women of reproductive age, although men are also targeted by several components of preconception care.

Antepartum care: The antepartum period refers to events occurring or existing after conception and before birth. This is also known as the "prenatal" period. So, antepartum care has the dual goals of ensuring a healthy baby and a healthy mother. Antepartum care includes the evaluation of the health status of both mother and fetus, estimation of the gestational age of the baby, identification of the patient at risk for complications, anticipation of problems before they occur (and prevention, if possible), and patient education and communication.

Preconception Care

Primary prevention consists of intervening before pathological changes have begun, to prevent the occurrence of disease. Preconception care is an excellent example of how primary prevention methods and the identification/modification of risk factors can markedly improve pregnancy outcomes, particularly for women with chronic diseases such as diabetes, hypothyroidism, and substance abuse issues.

Because more than 50% of the pregnancies in the United States are unplanned, health care providers should advise every woman in her reproductive years to seek preconception care and counseling. Indeed, an overwhelming amount of evidence suggests the best time to evaluate, counsel, and potentially treat specific conditions affecting pregnancy is *before* conception.

There are four critical areas for determining risks and implementing interventions during the preconception period:
1. History and physical examination
2. Serology to evaluate mostly infectious diseases
3. Management of chronic disease
4. Preconception supplementation

History

The most relevant variables to determine are maternal age and life-style factors as well as the presence of previously existing conditions, such as infections or chronic disease. How these factors impact preconception care is described below.

Maternal Age

Extremes of reproductive years are of special concern. The pregnant teenager is at increased risk for sexually transmitted diseases, and requires special attention paid to issues such as nutrition and emotional support. Mothers older than 35 years present an increased risk for chromosomal abnormalities, such as Down syndrome, which lead to a significant increase in the risk for spontaneous abortion as well as major congenital anomalies.

Timely education would most likely increase the opportunity to prevent teenage pregnancy and help women to make decisions regarding the age of conception. Finally, advanced paternal age is associated with increased genetic risk to the fetus and is considered when the father is older than 55 years.

Life-Style Factors

Tobacco: Smoking is a well-known, modifiable risk factor. It has been associated with increase risk for spontaneous abortion, prematurity, intrauterine growth restriction (IUGR), premature rupture of membranes (PROM), abruptio placentae, and placenta previa. Of significant clinical importance is the fact that smoking discontinuation before or during early pregnancy reduces these tobacco-associated risks.

Alcohol: Drinking alcohol has been clearly identified as a risk factor for adverse pregnancy outcome. There is also strong evidence that harm can occur early in gestation, even before the patient is aware of her pregnancy.

The so-called "fetal alcohol syndrome" (FAS) is defined by the presence at least one of the following signs:
- growth restriction either before or after birth
- facial anomalies
- central nervous system dysfunction

When these findings are associated with maternal alcohol consumption during pregnancy, the diagnosis is confirmed. In addition to growth and neurological deficits, children with FAS tend to have distinctive facial anomalies (**Fig. 9.1**), making it particularly difficult for them to adjust socially. Thus, it is truly a devastating condition for a child, and would-be mothers should be made fully aware of the potential consequences of drinking alcohol on the developing fetus.

When taking the medical history, four specific questions, which are often referred to as TACE (Tolerance, Annoyed, Cut down, and Eye opener), will help to identify women at risk for alcohol-related fetal complications (**Table 9.1**).

Since alcohol-related fetal complications can be completely prevented by stopping alcohol consumption before conception, all women seeking preconception care should be advised to do so.

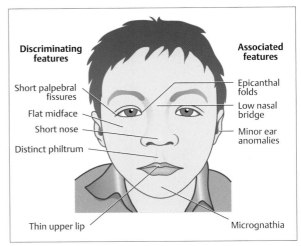

Fig. 9.1 Facial anomalies in young children are among the discriminating characteristics of fetal alcohol syndrome.

Table 9.1 Common questions used to screen for alcohol abuse. A positive answer for tolerance adds 2 points, while a positive answer to the other questions adds 1 point

T (tolerance)	How many drinks does it take to make you feel high (can you hold?)
A (annoyed)	Have people annoyed you by criticizing your drinking?
C (cut down)	Have you felt you ought to cut down on your drinking?
E (eye opener)	Have you ever had to drink first thing in the morning to steady your nerves or to get rid of a hangover?

Source: Sokol RJ, Martier SS, Ager JW: The TACE questions. Practical prenatal detection of risk-drinking. Am J Obstet Gynecol 1989;160:863.

Prescription drugs: Millions of women of childbearing age receive prescriptions for potentially teratogenic class D and X medications each year (**Table 9.2**). The most often prescribed potentially teratogenic prescription drugs are anxiolytics, anticonvulsants, statins, and certain antibiotics. Therefore, physicians should ascertain whether a woman is taking any of them in early gestation. Because the indications for clinical use, as well as the risk of an adverse birth outcome, vary significantly among medications classified as class D or X, it is important for clinicians to counsel women about potential risks and benefits as well as about planning the timing of conception.

Table 9.2 Volume of prescriptions for potentially teratogenic (US Food and Drug Administration class D or X) medications to women of childbearing age, by medication

Medication class	Annual prescriptions for class D or X* drugs, in millions (95% CI)	Proportion of prescriptions for class D or X* drugs
Anxiolytics	4.06 (3.88–4.23)	35%
Alprazolam	1.46	
Clonazepam	0.99	
Lorazepam	0.76	
Diazepam	0.69	
Temazepam	0.12	
Chlordiazepoxide	0.03	
Anticonvulsants	1.42 (1.33–1.51)	12%
Divalproex sodium	0.71	
Carbamazepine	0.44	
Phenytoin	0.18	
Valproate	0.05	
Phenobarbital	0.04	
Primidone	0.01	
Antibiotics	1.38 (1.29–1.47)	12%
Doxycycline	0.90	
Tetracycline	0.38	
Tobramycin	0.10	
Statins	0.76 (0.69–0.83)	6%
Atorvastatin	0.45	
Pravastatin	0.16	
Simvastatin	0.11	
Fluvastatin	0.02	
Lovastatin	0.01	
Isotretinoin	0.54 (0.49–0.59)	5%
Methotrexate	0.40 (0.35–0.45)	3%
Lithium	0.40 (0.35–0.45)	3%
Warfarin	0.21 (0.18–0.24)	2%
Others	1.67 (1.57–1.77)	14%
Total	11.7 (11.3–12.1)	100% †

CI, confidence interval.
*Potentially teratogenic class D or X medications.
†Proportions listed do not total 100% as a result of rounding.

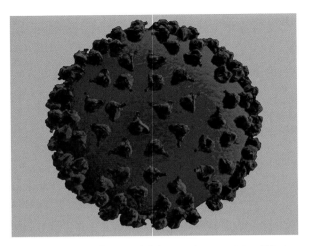

Fig. 9.2 Human immunodeficiency virus particle. HIV has emerged as one of the leading infectious agents threatening young mothers and their newborns around the world. Effective preconception can significantly reduce the chance that a mother will pass the virus to her newborn.

Serological Evaluations

Hepatitis B Virus

Infectious diseases can have a serious impact on newborns and their families. Congenital rubella syndrome, for example, can provoke deafness, ocular problems, and defects in the cardiac and central nervous systems. Serologic screening with immunoglobulin G (IgG) antibodies in the preconception period is mandatory, since vaccination provides protective seropositivity and prevents congenital rubella syndrome.

If a patient is considered to be at risk, screening for hepatitis B virus (HBV) should be performed. When the patient is susceptible vaccination should be indicated. Preventing HBV infection in women of childbearing age eliminates the risk of vertical transmission as well as potential long-term sequelae.

Human Immunodeficiency Virus

AIDS is another infectious disease with potentially serious implications for mothers and their newborns. Medical intervention during pregnancy has led to a significant decrease in vertical transmission of human immunodeficiency virus (HIV), the agent that causes AIDS (**Fig. 9.2**). Decreasing maternal viral load and choosing the appropriate mode of delivery can potentially decrease the transmission rate to as low as 4%. Identifying HIV-infected women in the preconception period allows timely antiretroviral treatment as well as counseling to the prospective parents.

Syphilis

Vertical transmission of syphilis has been well documented, and it is known to occur with a frequency ranging from 10% to 50% according to the stage of maternal infection. Manifestations such as IUGR, fetal death, preterm labor and delivery, and physical manifestations of congenital syphilis are well known. Furthermore, if HIV infection is also present, syphilis accelerates its progression in the mother. Screening for this condition, thus, should be considered. If an infection is detected, it should be treated preconceptionally to improve perinatal outcome.

At this time, serologic status for toxoplasmosis may also be evaluated. A positive IgG test can can indicate a lack of risk. On the other hand, women who screen negative should be advised to avoid ingestion of raw meat as well as to avoid contact with wild felines.

Chronic Disease Detection and Management

Certain chronic maternal diseases, such as hypothyroidism, diabetes, and epilepsy can have a significant impact on perinatal outcome. During the preconception period efforts should be made to assess the presence of these conditions and to bring them under control before any pregnancy is considered.

Hypothyroidism

Untreated or undertreated hypothyroidism has been associated with an excess risk of spontaneous abortion, as well as IUGR and fetal death. It has been suggested that normal maternal thyroid function is required for the development of the fetal nervous system. Although universal screening is not currently recommended, an effort should be made to identify patients who have a history or physical examination that is suggestive of hypothyroidism during the preconception period. These findings should be followed by serologic determination of thyroid-stimulating hormone (TSH) level which, if high, should be treated accordingly before conception.

Diabetes

Early sustained maternal hyperglycemia, such as when diabetes mellitus complicates pregnancy, is associated with increased risk of spontaneous abortion and congenital malformations. Furthermore, certain stages of maternal disease can be worsened by pregnancy itself. Women suffering from diabetes should be counseled and educated regarding strategies to optimize perinatal outcome. They also need to be made aware of the potential impact of pregnancy on the natural course of diabetes.

The following recommendations are associated with an improved maternal and perinatal outcome.

- Hemoglobin (Hb) A1c values should not exceed 1% of the normal value.
- While achieving the desired HbA1c value, diabetic women should be educated regarding:
  - proper contraception methods
  - glucose self-monitoring and the use of insulin
  - identification and management of hypoglycemia
- Regular physical activity should be included in the life style.
- Establish fluent communication with the health team.
- Physical examination should determine the presence of hypertension, orthostatic hypotension, retinopathy (especially proliferative), and coronary heart disease.
- Initial lab tests should include: monthly HbA1c until an acceptable value is achieved, renal function (serum creatinine, creatinine clearance and 24-hour protein excretion), and TSH level.
- Daily folic acid supplementation should be indicated from the preconception period and throughout the first trimester (see below).

Epilepsy

Epileptic women taking anticonvulsants have almost double the risk for having children with congenital malformations compared with women in the general population (5% versus 2–3%, respectively). Common anomalies observed are cleft lip with or without cleft palate, cardiac, and neural tube defects. Furthermore, children born to epileptic women have increased incidence of epilepsy later in life.

The etiology of this increased risk of malformations is still unresolved, since women with epilepsy and no treatment also have increased risk for fetal anomalies. So, an attempt to achieve seizure control should be performed with the lowest effective doses and the least number of drugs.

Preconception Supplementation

Folic acid supplementation has been definitively shown to decrease the incidence of neural tube defects (NTDs) in both high-risk women and the general population (Evidence Box 9.1). The following recommendations should be followed for an effective intervention:

- Start supplementation 4 weeks before conception and continue throughout the first 3 months of pregnancy.
- Dose for women at high risk (e. g., previous child with NTD): 4 mg/day.
- Dose for the general population: 0.4 mg/day.

Summary

There are a number of important issues for the physician to address during the preconception visit, including maternal age, addictions (alcohol, smoking, illicit drugs), chronic diseases (diabetes, epilepsy, hypothyroidism), and infectious diseases (syphilis, HIV, Hepatitis B, rubella).

Table 9.3 provides a summary of the standard recommended interventions to be used in preconception care according to well-defined clinical scenarios.

Table 9.3 Summary of the recommended interventions according to defined clinical scenarios

Clinical scenario	Intervention
Nutritional	Folic acid supplementation
Advanced maternal/ paternal age	Counseling
Alcohol/tobacco	Education/discontinuation
Rubella negative IgG	Vaccination. Avoid pregnancy for 1 month
Toxoplasmosis negative IgG	Education to avoid exposure
HIV positive	Education/treatment/decrease viral load
Syphilis	Treat before conception
Diabetes	Education/glycemic control
Hypothyroidism	Levotiroxin targeted to normal TSH

Antepartum Care

Antepartum, or prenatal, care can occur with a pregnant woman who has already had preconception care and counseling, or it can arise from the first contact with the health care provider. In the latter scenario, the initial evaluation should be comprehensive and involve all the variables recommended above for preconception care.

All women who are pregnant need routine prenatal care. The following schedule of visits is generally recommended for women with uncomplicated pregnancies:

- every 4 weeks until 28 weeks of gestation
- every 2–3 weeks until 36 weeks of gestation
- weekly after 36 weeks of gestation
- 4–6 weeks postpartum

Initial Prenatal Visit

A general physical examination at the initial visit should include blood pressure, maternal weight, a Pap smear, and tests to identify risk factors for pregnancy complications. This is especially crucial for patients who did not have preconception care or education regarding taking medications or leading a healthy life style.

Immune status for infectious diseases with teratogenic or fetal infectious potential should be assessed at this visit. Chiefly, the presence of antibodies against syphilis, rubella, HIV, and hepatitis B should be determined. In some countries it is also recommended to determine cytomegalovirus, toxoplasmosis, and varicella immune status. Tests for hemoglobin and hematocrit, blood type and group should be carried out; and the presence of antibodies against red blood cell antigens should be determined by an indirect Coombs test (see Chapter 17).

Repeat Prenatal Visits

At every prenatal visit until delivery, every pregnant woman needs a physical examination including blood pressure and maternal weight. The obstetric part of the examination should include determination of fundal height and fetal heart tones after 12 weeks of gestation, as well as analyses for proteinuria and urinary tract infections.

Screening for Chromosomal Anomalies

The negative impact of chromosomal anomalies on perinatal outcome is well documented, and different methods are currently available to approach this issue. Ideally, all pregnant women should be offered noninvasive screening (e.g., ultrasonography) before 20 weeks of gestation, regardless of maternal age. Those women with a positive screening should be offered an invasive diagnostic test (e.g., amniocentesis).

The selection of the screening test depends on many factors including:
- gestational age at first prenatal visit
- number of fetuses
- test availability
- desire for early test results
- sensitivity and false positives
- obstetrical and family history

Those women who elect no screening or only first trimester screening should be offered neural tube defect (NTD) screening in the second trimester (16–20 weeks). This may include determination of second trimester maternal serum α-fetoprotein or ultrasonography. Details of screening protocols are given in Chapter 7.

Obstetric Ultrasonography

Ultrasound imaging is frequently used in pregnancy to follow fetal growth and development. An ultrasound scan performed at 16–18 weeks will allow appropriate dating and identification of fetal anomalies.

Glucose Screening

Between 24 and 28 weeks of gestation, screening for gestational diabetes is performed. There are different approaches available, including *universal* and *selective* screening. Universal glucose screening consists of screening every pregnant woman. Selective screening seeks to avoid the screening of low-risk women, defined according to the following criteria:
- younger than 25 years of age
- normal weight
- absence of history of abnormal glucose metabolism or poor obstetric outcome, and
- no first-degree relative with diabetes

Screening can be performed by the glucose challenge test, which consists of a 50 g oral glucose load followed by blood extraction after 1 hour. Normal blood glucose concentration is below 140 mg/dL. A positive screening test should be followed by a diagnostic test. The oral glucose tolerance test (OGTT) consists of 100 g of glucose given orally in at least 400 mL of water with blood glucose determinations at fasting, 1, 2, and 3 hours after the glucose load. Diagnosis of gestational diabetes requires that at least two of four blood glucose levels determined thereafter should exceed the upper limits of normal values.

Vaccinations/Prophylaxis

Rhesus Isoimmunization

Between 24 and 28 weeks of gestation, nonimmunized Rh-negative patients should receive D immunoglobulin (RhIg). Although cost-effectiveness of repeated anti-D (Rh) antibodies screening before RhIg administration is questionable, it is a reasonable practice.

Group B Streptococcus

Approximately 10–20% of pregnant women are colonized by group B Streptococcus (GBS). It is well known that in susceptible neonates this organism is able to cause significant disease. Therefore, screening for vaginal and rectal group B Streptococcus should be performed between 35 and 37 weeks of gestation for all pregnant women, with the exception of patients who have GBS bacteriuria during the current pregnancy, or had a previous infant with invasive GBS disease. When necessary, prophylaxis is administered during labor to susceptible individuals (see Chapter 23).

Other Vaccines

Immunizations with inactivated virus vaccines, toxoids, tetanus immunoglobulin, and bacterial vaccines are safe in pregnancy and they should be administered when indicated. Measles, mumps, and rubella viruses are not transmitted after immunization; therefore, children of pregnant women can safely receive such immunizations when indicated. Finally, influenza vaccination is an important element of prenatal care. Women who will be pregnant during the influenza season should be vaccinated. This intramuscular inactivated vaccine may be used in all three trimesters.

Nutritional Support and Weight Management

Recommended energy intake for healthy pregnant women is 2500 kcal/day, with 60 g of protein mainly obtained from meat, fish, poultry, and dairy products. In general, a well-balanced diet provides all the required nutrients, with the exception of iron. Therefore, 30 mg daily of ferrous iron supplements is recommended for pregnant women. For groups at significant risk, such as adolescents, a vitamin and mineral supplement should be indicated. Finally, strict vegetarians my need supplements of vitamin B_{12}.

Obstetricians have known for some time that obesity in women can cause serious pregnancy-related complications, such as hypertension, diabetes, and large birth-weight babies. Recently, evidence also has emerged that maternal obesity is a significant contributor to birth defects as well. Studies show that obese women and overweight women are at a much higher risk of having a child with a range of life-threatening birth defects compared with women of normal weight. Thus, proper weight maintenance during pregnancy is crucial the health of the mother and her fetus.

The recommended weight gain in pregnancy is 11.5–16 kg for women with adequate preconception weight. Underweight women can gain up to 18 kg, and obese patients should limit this increase to 7–11.5 kg. However, already-obese pregnant women should not be put on a dieting program to prevent complications, because low weight gain during pregnancy is associated with increased risk of perinatal complications. These women thus need additional monitoring to control high blood glucose levels and hypertension, as well as additional nutritional supplementation. For example, there is growing evidence that obese pregnant women need more than 400 mg of folate supplementation per day to prevent an elevated risk of NTDs in their offspring.

Summary

In addition to receiving a thorough physical examination and medical history at their initial prenatal visit to ascertain blood pressure and maternal weight, proteinuria, and any urinary tract infections, after 12 weeks of gestation all pregnant women should be given an obstetric examination that includes measuring fundal height and monitoring fetal heart tones. This should be performed at every visit until delivery.

Furthermore, pregnant women should be offered noninvasive screening before 20 weeks of gestation independently of maternal age. Those women with a positive screening should be offered an invasive diagnostic test. Neural tube defect (NTD) screening should be performed in the second trimester, either by maternal serum α-fetoprotein determination or by ultrasonography.

Between 24 and 28 weeks of gestation either universal or selective screening for gestational diabetes should be performed. Anti D (Rh) antibodies screening early in pregnancy should be performed and non immunized Rh negative patients should receive D mmunoglobulin (RhIg) between 24 and 28 weeks of gestation. Screening for vaginal and rectal group B Streptococcus (GBS) should be performed between 35 and 37 weeks of pregnancy for all pregnant women with the exception of patients with GBS bacteriuria during current pregnancy, or a previous infant with invasive GBS disease.

Folic acid supplementation decreases the incidence of neural tube defects (NTDs) in both high-risk patients and general population. Thus, folic acid supplementation should begin 4 weeks before conception and continue throughout the first 3 months of pregnancy.

Table 9.4 summarizes the standard prenatal screening tests and interventions and when they should be administered in the course of care.

Part II Obstetrics

Table 9.4 Standard routine prenatal care schedule and screening tests/interventions performed

		6–8 weeks	10–12 weeks	16–18 weeks	22 weeks
Screening		Risk profile	Weight	Weight	Weight
		Height/weight	Blood pressure	Blood pressure	Blood pressure
		OB H&P	Fetal heart rate	Fetal heart rate	Fundal height
		Blood pressure	Biochemical screening	Biochemical screening	Fetal heart rate
		Breast exam		OB ultrasonography	
		Pap smear		Fundal height	
		Hemoglobin/hematocrit			
		Rubella/varicella			
		HBV S Ag/RPR			
		HIV			
		ABO/Rh/Ab			
		Urine culture			
		Domestic abuse screening			
Immunization and chemo-prophylaxis		Nutritional supplements Td Booster			
		28 weeks	**32 weeks**	**36 weeks**	**38–41 weeks**
Screening		Blood pressure	Weight	Weight	Weight
		Hemoglobin/hematocrit	Blood pressure	Blood pressure	Blood pressure
		Fetal heart tones	Fetal heart tones	Fetal heart tones	Fundal height
		Fundal height	Fundal height	Fundal height	Fetal heart tones
		Ab screen		Group B Streptococcus culture	Cervix
		GDM screen			
Immunization and chemo-prophylaxis		RhoGAM (if indicated)			

RPR: rapid plasma reagin; RhoGAM: $Rh_0(D)$ immune globulin; GDM: Gestational diabetes mellitus.

Key Points

- More than 50% of pregnancies in the United States are unplanned. Thus, health care providers should advise every woman in her reproductive years to seek preconception care and counseling.
- The target population for preconception care is women of reproductive age, although men are also targeted by several components of preconception care.
- A general physical examination at the initial visit should include blood pressure, maternal weight, a Pap smear, and tests to identify risks factors for pregnancy complications.
- At every prenatal visit until delivery, every pregnant woman needs a physical examination, including blood pressure and maternal weight.
- Ideally, all pregnant women should be offered noninvasive screening (e. g., ultrasonography) before 20 weeks of gestation, regardless of maternal age. Those women with a positive screening should be offered an invasive diagnostic test (e. g., amniocentesis).

Evidence Box 9.1

Folic acid supplementation given to women before conception decreases recurrance of neural tube defects in their babies.

Upon discovering an unusually high neural tube defect (NTD) incidence rate of 27 out of 10 000 in a Texas border county, the Texas Department of Health initiated a folic acid intervention for prevention of recurrent NTDs in this predominantly Mexican-American population. Enrollees were provided folic acid at home visits at 3-month intervals throughout the project. Folic acid supplementation of 0.4 mg/day or more occurred during the last month preconception in 161 (83.4%) of the 193 pregnancies. No NTDs were detected in the 130 live births to women who received 0.4 mg/day supplementation nor were NTDs detected in the 23 supplemented women who experienced pregnancy loss. The authors concluded that supplementation was successful in preventing recurrent NTDs in Mexican-American women.

Felkner M, Suarez L, Hendricks K, Larsen R. Implementation and outcomes of recommended folic acid supplementation in Mexican-American women with prior neural tube defect-affected pregnancies Prev Med. 2005 Jun;40(6):867–871.

Further Reading

Carroli G, Villar J, Piaggio G, et al. WHO Antenatal Care Trial Research Group. WHO systematic review of randomised controlled trials of routine antenatal care. *Lancet* 2001;357(9268):1565–1570

Schrag S, Gorwitz R, Fultz-Butts K, Schuchat A Centers for Disease Control and Prevention (CDC). Prevention of perinatal group B streptococcal disease. Revised guidelines from CDC. *MMWR Recomm Rep* 2002;51(RR-11):1–22

Diabetes Care. Preconception care of women with diabetes. American Diabetes Association. Position Statement. Vol. 26, Suppl 1, Jan 2003

Felkner M, Suarez L, Hendricks K, Larsen R. Implementation and outcomes of recommended folic acid supplementation in Mexican-American women with prior neural tube defect-affected pregnancies. *Prev Med* 2005;40(6):867–871

Kent H, Johnson K, Curtis M, et al, eds. Proceedings of the Preconception Health and Health Care Clinical, Public Health, and Consumer Workgroup Meetings. CDC National Center on Birth Defects and Developmental Disabilities. June 27–28, 2006

Screening for fetal chromosomal abnormalities. ACOG Practice Bulletin, No. 77, Jan 2007:217–227

10 Intrapartum Care and Fetal Surveillance

Carolina Ghia, Luciana Prozzillo, and Gustavo F. Leguizamón

In the last 50 years different techniques have been developed to assess fetal health during labor. From intermittent auscultation to the most recent invasive techniques, the objective of these methods is to detect fetal stress early, so that complications, such as intrapartum fetal hypoxia leading to cognitive impairment, cerebral palsy, or even fetal death, can be prevented.

Persistent intrapartum hypoxia, which complicates about 1% of all labors, can lead to severe acidemia, which in turn may compromise those vital tissues requiring strict oxygen levels, such as in the renal, cardiovascular, and central nervous systems. The latter is the most vulnerable to oxygen deprivation and is, therefore, frequently involved in long-term sequelae.

Thus, an ideal method of intrapartum fetal surveillance should be able to differentiate between transient hypoxia without metabolic acidosis and pathologic hypoxia leading to acidosis and tissue damage. This is of utmost importance, since it allows accurate intervention and prevention of long-term sequelae without increasing unnecessary cesarean sections. In other words, it requires a method with a high degree of sensitivity and a low false-positive rate.

Since alterations in maternal blood pressure, heart rate, and uterine contractions have direct effects on fetal oxygenation, maternal vital signs should be monitored during labor, especially in the event of a non-reassuring fetal pattern.

Fetal heart rate and its variations is a good parameter of fetal response to labor events. In particular, knowledge of normal and abnormal patterns will allow both detection of fetal distress and accurate intervention. Other methods of measuring metabolic status, such as fetal blood sampling, pulse oximetry, and lactate measurement, have been developed in order to complement fetal assessment. These methods are discussed in detail in this chapter.

Definitions

Acceleration: This describes a short-term rise in fetal heart rate of greater than 15 beats per minute (bpm) that lasts for more than 15 seconds.

Acidemia: This condition arises from increased hydrogen content in the blood.

Acidosis: This term describes a state of increased hydrogen content in the tissues.

Respiratory acidosis: The accumulation of CO_2 leads to respiratory acidosis. When the umbilical cord is compressed, CO_2 rapidly accumulates in the fetal blood.

Metabolic acidosis: During the peak of uterine contraction, intramyometrial pressure exceeds uterine arterial pressure and therefore, the blood flow decreases, leaving the fetus in a transient state of hypoperfusion. In the event of basal inadequate oxygen delivery to the fetus, this transitory lack of perfusion leads to fetal hypoxia, which can result in metabolic acidosis.

Asphyxia: This is a state of hypoxia with metabolic acidosis.

Deceleration: This describes a fall in the fetal heart rate of greater than 15 bpm that lasts for more than 15 seconds (but less than 10 minutes).

Hypoxemia: This condition occurs following decreased oxygen concentration in the blood.

Hypoxia: This term describes decreased oxygen concentration in the tissues.

Fetal Heart Rate: Normal and Pathologic Patterns

The normal fetal heart rate at term varies between 110 and 160 bpm. This is measured by a cardiotachometer during intrapartum fetal monitoring and is defined as the baseline heart rate, which is much higher in the second trimester and declines thereafter with increasing gestational age. This decline in baseline heart rate is a good indicator of development of the vagal tone.

A heart rate above 160 bpm that persists for more than 10 minutes (a shorter period could represent a transient acceleration) is referred to as tachycardia. Among the most frequent causes of tachycardia are maternal fever (as seen in chorioamnionitis), the use of drugs that elevate heart rate (e.g., ritodrine), fetal anemia, and fetal arrhythmias. However, if tachycardia is persistent, it can also indicate fetal hypoxia.

A heart rate of less than 110 bpm that persists for more than 10 minutes (as distinct from transient deceleration) is known as bradycardia. Some fetuses have normal baselines of 100–105 bpm. However, in most cases, it indicates some metabolic alteration (e.g., maternal hypothermia or hypoglycemia), use of drugs that diminish heart rate (e.g., magnesium sulfate), or cardiac abnormalities (e.g., heart block, umbilical cord occlusion).

Variability

The difference in heart rate from beat to beat, which is registered by a device known as a cardiotachometer as a trace moving over and under the baseline, is known as variability (**Fig. 10.1**). Normal variability ranges from 5 bpm to 25 bpm, and is an indicator of a well-functioning fetal brain. However, heart rate variability increases with gestational age, reaching a stable pattern at approximately 28 weeks of gestation. Variations between fetuses are also observed.

Decreased variability is defined as less than 5 bpm for longer than 80 minutes (**Fig. 10.2**). It may reflect different physiological conditions, including fetal sleep and prematurity, or may be secondary to drugs such as narcotics, barbiturates, tranquilizers, phenotiazines, and general anesthetics. Among the pathologic causes of decreased heart rate variability are maternal hypoglycemia, reduced fetal oxygenation and acidosis, major anomalies of the fetal central nervous system, chorioamnionitis, and fetal heart block.

Transient Accelerations

Heart rate accelerations are usually a response to fetal movement or external stimulations, such as uterine contractions (**Fig. 10.3**). Their spontaneous presence indicates absence of hypoxia, especially in the context of normal baseline and variability. The presence of provoked accelerations, even in a context of non-reassuring fetal heart rate, rules out a pH lower than 7.20 on scalp sampling.

The absence of accelerations should be interpreted in the context of other variables. In general, if the fetal heart rate pattern is non-reassuring with no accelerations, approximately half of such fetuses will be acidotic. On the other hand, the lack of accelerations in an otherwise reassuring pattern is generally not associated with an increased fetal risk of hypoxia.

Transient Decelerations

Decelerations are classified in three groups, according to their location regarding uterine contractions:
- *Early decelerations.* These coincide with uterine contractions and appear as vagal reactions in response to fetal head compression during the final stages of labor and they are not associated with fetal hypoxia, however. The drop in fetal heart rate appears as a

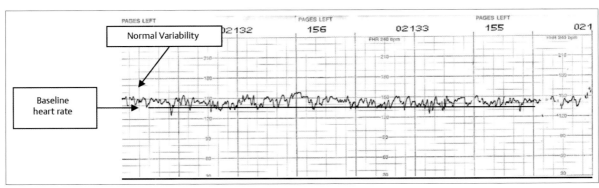

Fig. 10.1   Fetal heart rate variability that changes with gestational age is an indicator of a well-functioning fetal brain.

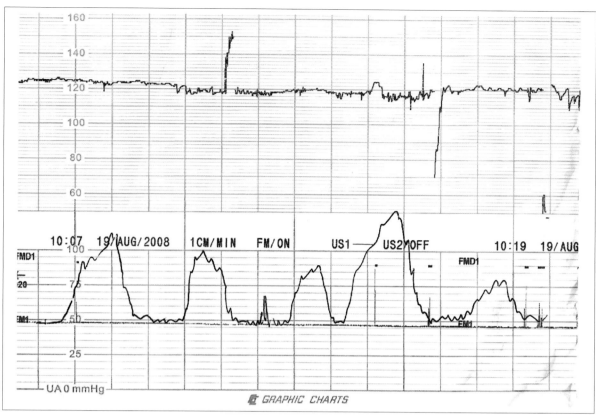

Fig. 10.2 Decreases in fetal heart rate variability (as indicated by the changes in peak size) may reflect aberrant physiologic conditions that may harm the fetus.

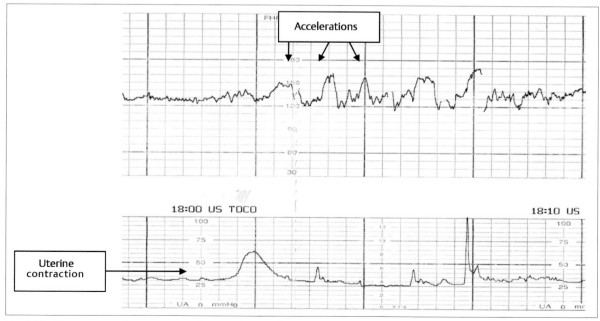

Fig. 10.3 The presence of accelerations, which can be provoked by uterine contractions, can rule out problems such as hypoxia and acidosis.

V-shaped pattern coinciding with the uterine contraction, and does not persist beyond it. They create a "mirror" image of the contraction in the monitor trace, with their nadir in coincidence with the peak of the contraction.

- *Variable decelerations.* These are the most common type of deceleration during labor. They are called "variable" because of the lack of a particular relation with contractions, and the absence of a consistent pattern (**Fig. 10.4**). These decelerations usually are not associated with fetal hypoxia. They are caused by fetal heart rate changes in response to blood pressure alterations, which are frequently due to cord compression. When the cord vein is compressed, CO_2 accumulates in fetal blood; this can produce respiratory acidosis. If compression continues, oxygen delivery becomes insufficient; producing metabolic acidosis, turning the situation into mixed acidosis.

Variable decelerations can be further classified according to their severity:
- *Mild decelerations.* These have duration of less than 30 seconds regardless of the depth, or heart rate not below 80 bpm regardless of duration.
- *Moderate decelerations.* These fall below 80 bpm.
- *Severe decelerations.* These are decelerations that last for more than 60 seconds and fall to less than 70 bpm.
- *Late decelerations.* These generally appear within 30 seconds of a contraction; their nadir is delayed with respect to the peak of the contraction, usually descend no more than 40 bpm from the baseline, and last a variable amount of time beyond the contraction (**Fig. 10.5**). Late decelerations reflect transient periods of fetal hypoxia due to a diminished uterine–placental blood flow during a contraction. The severity of hypoxia cannot be predicted from the depth of the deceleration. The persistence in time of late

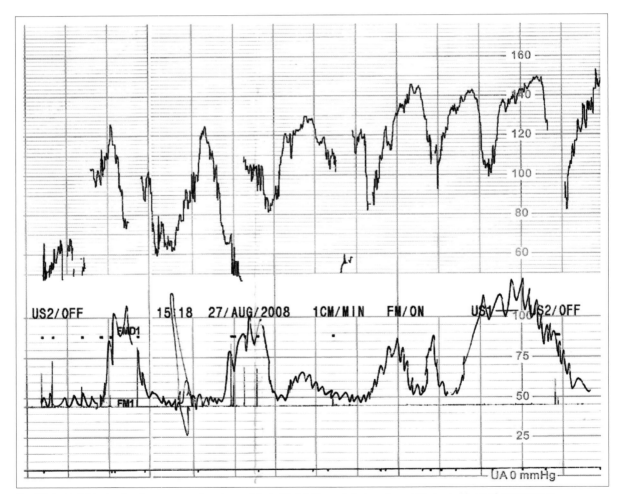

Fig. 10.4 Variable decelerations are usually not associated with fetal hypoxia but are frequently caused by cord compression.

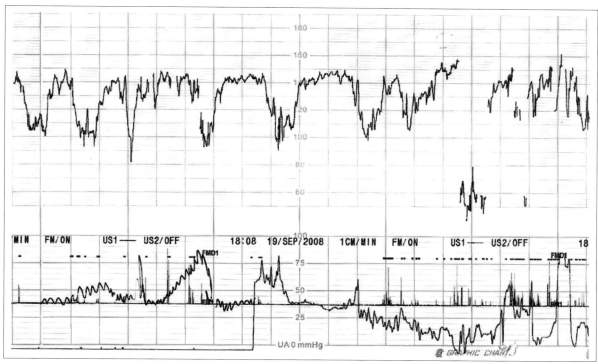

Fig. 10.4 (continued)

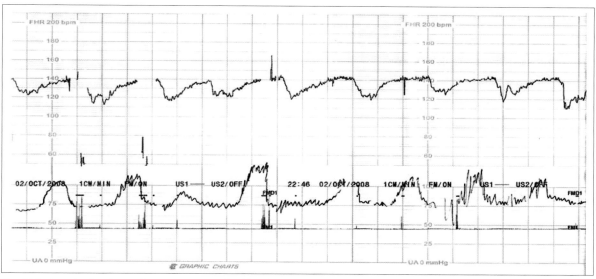

Fig. 10.5 Late decelerations reflect transient periods of fetal hypoxia during contractions.

decelerations gives a more reliable reason to suspect hypoxia and fetal metabolic acidosis.

A fetus whose placenta suffers from any pathologic condition is more likely to develop late decelerations in response to decreased oxygen exchange. This condition usually includes maternal hypertension or pre-eclampsia, maternal diabetes, or collagen vascular diseases.

Sinusoidal Pattern

A sinusoidal pattern is strongly associated with severe fetal anemia and hypoxia. Its characteristics include:
1. Stable baseline fetal heart rate of 120–160 bpm with regular sine-wave–like oscillations (**Fig. 10.6**)
2. Amplitude of 5 to 15 bpm

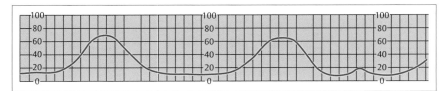

Fig. 10.6 A sinusoidal pattern, which is characterized by regular sine-wave–like oscillations with little variability and an absence of accelerations, is a potential indicator of fetal hypoxia and anemia.

3. Frequency of 2 to 5 cycles/min
4. Fixed or absent short-term variability
5. Oscillation of sine wave above and below the baseline
6. Absence of accelerations

Other Methods for Intrapartum Fetal Surveillance

Intermittent Auscultation

Intermittent auscultation was originally performed with the Pinard stethoscope (**Fig. 10.7**). In the 1950s it was replaced by Doppler sonographic technology, which has the advantage of easier localization of fetal heart tones as well as giving the patient the ability to hear her baby's heart beat, giving her more confidence in the labor process.

Fetal auscultation should be performed every 15 minutes and 5 minutes, respectively, in the first and second stage of labor. It then should be performed throughout labor as well as for 60 seconds following each contraction. In low-risk patients, the frequency should be at least every 30 minutes in the first stage and every 15 minutes in the second stage. Even with correct techniques, there are disadvantages to this method, including inaccurate information about late decelerations and the inability of registering baseline variability.

Although comparisons between continuous fetal heart rate monitoring (see below) and intermittent auscultation during labor in low-risk patients has failed to demonstrate benefits in neonatal outcomes, the number of personnel needed for the latter technique (one-to-one care is required) make it difficult to perform.

Continuous Electronic Fetal Heart Rate Monitoring

Although reactivity is often absent in intrapartum heart rate tracings, a healthy fetus usually tolerates labor well, showing normal variability and without severe persistent decelerations.

Continuous monitoring of fetal heart rate has several advantages over intermittent auscultation, including:
- requiring fewer personnel to administer
- the ability to obtain a printed strip, which allows comparisons of fetal responses during the progressive stages of labor
- being more accurate in diagnosing late decelerations
- producing reduced variability, and
- allowing for the simultaneous measurement of uterine contractions

This method has an excellent sensitivity in detecting fetal hypoxia during labor, but very poor specificity (Evidence Box 10.1). It employs a Doppler heart-rate detector that translates heart beats into dots in a paper strip which, joined together, form the line moving above and below the horizontal baseline, representing variability. A transducer is placed on the mother's abdomen upon the pro-

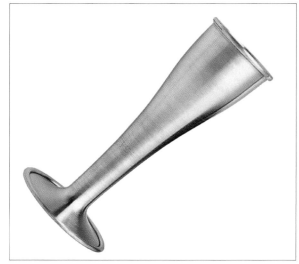

Fig. 10.7   An aluminum Pinard fetal stethoscope.

jection of the fetal shoulder. A tocodynamometer is also placed in the mother's abdomen, in the projection of the uterine fundus, to obtain simultaneous reading of uterine contractions.

Approximately one-half of fetuses that present with a non-reassuring pattern during labor (e.g., reduced variability, persistent decelerations progressing in severity, tachycardia, or bradycardia) are born with normal Apgar scores. If the patient's membranes are ruptured and there is difficulty in obtaining good recordings with external monitoring, an internal electrode can be applied to the fetal scalp for a more accurate tracing.

Fetal Metabolic Status Assessment

In order to improve the specificity of continuous monitoring for fetal hypoxia/acidemia and to prevent unnecessary operative interventions, invasive procedures have been developed to further evaluate non-reassuring patterns in the electronic heart-rate monitoring.

One such method is fetal pulse oximetry, whereby a specially adapted device is placed in contact with the fetus' cheek to provide information about fetal oxygenation during labor. Another method involves sampling fetal blood in order to measure pH, base deficit, and lactate as direct parameters of the fetal metabolic status. This involves obtaining samples by puncturing the fetal scalp. However, this method can only be used if the membranes are ruptured and the woman's a cervix is dilated at least 4–5 cm).

Fetal Scalp pH

This is the most accurate technique to diagnose fetal acidosis. It consists of taking a blood sample from the fetal scalp using a lancet and a capillary collection tube. During labor, normal pH is above 7.24. A pH value between 7.20 and 7.24 indicates pre-acidemia, and a pH lower than 7.20 indicates acidosis. Complementing electronic fetal monitoring with fetal scalp pH measurement should reduce cesarean rates for non-reassuring fetal status. However, the technique is rarely used. Measurement of base excess of umbilical artery is a great tool for differentiating respiratory from metabolic acidosis. Base excess below −12 mmol/L has a high correlation with increased risk of neonatal neurologic injury.

Fetal Pulse Oximetry

Fetal pulse oximetry is a tool that measures fetal arterial O_2 saturation using a sensor attached to the fetus' temple or cheek. Normal fetal O_2 saturation during labor is 40–70%. Values below 30% are strongly associated with pH under 7.20. The American College of Obstetricians and Gynecologists states that further studies confirming safety and efficacy are required before recommendation of this technology. To use it, the membranes must be ruptured and the cervix ought to be dilated 2 cm or more.

Meconium

Meconium is the normal content of the fetal gut. When the fetus is suffering from hypoxia, because of gut vasoconstriction, there can be passage of meconium to the amniotic fluid. Hypoxia also works as an important stimulus for fetal gasping, which can result in fetal aspiration of meconium. Thick meconium is frequently associated with oligohydramnios, which in turn is a sign of placental dysfunction. Nevertheless, with normal fetal heart rate, the presence of meconium does not always reflect fetal hypoxia.

Amnioinfusion

In variable decelerations caused by oligohydramnios, this technique can improve Apgar score and pH values and can also reduce the number of cesarean sections for non-reassuring fetal status. Amnioinfusion might reduce the cord compression that leads to hypoxia. It is also used in the presence of meconium to dilute it.

Interventions for Altered Heart Rate Patterns

Clinical Management

The following steps should be taken when an altered heart rate pattern is detected via continuous monitoring:
*   *Assess the mother's vital signs and uterine tone.* It is possible that fever, hypotension, hypertonic uterus, or tachysystolia may be causing fetal distress.

- *Place the mother in the left lateral position.* This action relieves uterine compression of the vena cava, allowing better blood flow.
- *Increase oxygen supply.* Administer oxygen to the mother via a nasal cannula or a mask to improve the mother's P_{O_2} and therefore placental O_2 exchange.
- *Increase intravenous hydration.* This helps to maximize uterine flow and perfusion and to correct a possible hypotension as a cause of the abnormal pattern.
- *Discontinue oxytocin infusion (if being administered).* This will improve placental perfusion as it decreases uterine contractions.
- *Initiate acoustic or scalp stimulation.* Fetuses who respond with increased heart rate upon stimulation have better outcomes than those who don't. Usually, fetal response to either acoustic or scalp stimulation reflects a lack of acidosis.

Operative Management

When a fetus is considered to be "at risk" due to a persistent non-reassuring pattern in continuous fetal monitoring, and back-up studies cannot offer reassurance, the physician must proceed with rapid delivery.

The choice between instrumental vaginal delivery and cesarean section will depend on the stage of labor, cervical dilatation, vertex station, and the estimated time for performing each procedure. Therefore, each case must be analyzed individually in order to achieve delivery in the least amount of time and without exposing the mother and fetus to unnecessary procedures.

Key Points

- The objective of the intrapartum fetal testing is to determine whether the fetus presents hypoxia and/or metabolic acidosis.
- If hypoxia is detected, attempts to reverse it by interventions such as hydration, discontinuation of oxytocin, oxygen supply, or fetal stimulation must be performed.
- If persistent non-reassuring results are observed in spite of such interventions, expedited delivery must be initiated.

Evidence Box 10.1

Careful interpretation of specific FHR patterns can be a useful screening test for fetal asphyxia. However, supplementary tests are required to identify the large number of false-positive patterns to avoid unnecessary intervention.

   Low et al. analyzed selected patterns of important fetal heart rate variables, during the last hour before delivery, for their predictive value for fetal asphyxia among a group of 71 term infants with umbilical artery base deficit >16 mmol/L, and a control group of 71 term infants with umbilical artery base deficit <8 mmol/L. The fetal heart rate variables associated with fetal asphyxia included absent and minimal baseline variability and late and prolonged decelerations. Fetal heart rate patterns with absent baseline variability were the most specific, but identified only 17% of the asphyxia group. The sensitivity of this test increased to 93% with the addition of less specific patterns. The estimated positive predictive value ranged from 18.1% to 2.6%, and the negative predictive value ranged from 98.3% to 99.5%. The investigators concluded that a narrow 1-hour window of fetal heart rate patterns, including minimal baseline variability and late or prolonged decelerations, can predict fetal asphyxial exposure before decompensation and newborn morbidity. Thus, with careful interpretation, predictive fetal heart rate patterns can be a useful screening test for fetal asphyxia. However, supplementary tests are required to confirm the diagnosis and to identify the large number of false-positive patterns to avoid unnecessary intervention.

   Low JA, Victory R, Derrick EJ. Predictive value of electronic fetal monitoring for intrapartum fetal asphyxia with metabolic acidosis. Obstet Gynecol 1999 Feb;93(2):285-91.

Further Reading

American College of Obstetricians and Gynecologists. Fetal Distress and Birth Asphyxia. ACOG Committee Opinion 1994, No 137, Washington, DC

American College of Obstetricians and Gynecologists. Fetal Heart Rate Monitoring, Interpretation and Management. ACOG Technical Bulletin 1995, No. 207, Washington, DC

Dildy G. Intrapartum assessment of the fetus: historical and evidence-based practice. Obstet Gynecol Clin 2005, Vol. 32, Issue 2.

National Institute of Child Health and Human Development Research Planning Workshop. Electronic fetal heart rate monitoring: research guidelines for interpretation. *Am J Obstet Gynecol* 1997;177(6):1385–1390

Gabbe SG, Niebyl JR, Simpson JL. Obstetrics—Normal and Problem Pregnancies. 5th ed. New York: Churchill Livingstone / Elsevier; 1997

Graham E. Intrapartum electronic fetal heart rate monitoring and the prevention of perinatal brain injury. ACOG 2006, Vol. 108, No.3, Part 1

Jibodu OA, Arulkumaran S. Intrapartum fetal surveillance. *Curr Opin Obstet Gynecol* 2000;12(2):123–127

Smith JF Jr, Onstad JH. Assessment of the fetus: intermittent auscultation, electronic fetal heart rate tracing, and fetal pulse oximetry. *Obstet Gynecol Clin North Am* 2005;32(2):245–254

11 Labor and Delivery

Vanina S. Fishkel and Gustavo F. Leguizamòn

This chapter reviews the determinants of human parturition, or labor. Labor is a physiologic process consisting in organized uterine contractions of adequate intensity, frequency, and duration to affect complete cervical dilatation and expulsion of the fetus, placenta, and fetal membranes through the birth canal.

Labor progresses from a state of uterine quiescence (latent phase) to a phase characterized by uterine contractions and cervical dilatation (active phase). Maternal structures (e.g., pelvis) and functions (e.g., uterine contractions) as well as fetal structures (e.g., presenting parts) and functions (e.g., fetal cardinal movements) are of utmost importance in the progression of labor.

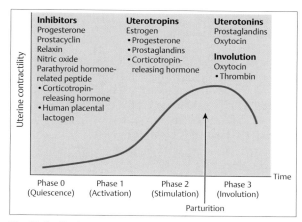

Fig. 11.1 Uterine activity in pregnancy. Adapted from Challis JRG, Gibb W: Control of Parturition. Prenatal and Neonatal Medicine 1996;1:283.

Labor Physiology

The physiology of term labor initiation is not fully elucidated, but during the past several decades significant information has been added to our understanding of this process.

Uterine activity can be classified as having four distinct phases (**Fig 11.1**):

- *Phase 0 (quiescence).* This Phase is characterized by uterine quiescence and the leading hormone is progesterone.
- *Phase 1 (activation).* In this Phase, receptors for oxytocin and prostaglandins are actively synthesized as well as an increased number of gap junctions, leading to a progressive increase in uterine sensitivity to different uterotonics. Estrogens play a pivotal role in this phase.
- *Phase 2 (stimulation).* Once the uterus has reached its potential to respond, oxytocin and prostaglandins stimulate contractions actively.
- *Phase 3 (involution).* After delivery, oxytocin leads to uterine contraction and bleeding decreases significantly.

Mechanics of Labor

Adequate interaction between the fetus' features and maternal pelvis allows vaginal delivery. Thus, maternal contractions to propel the fetus through the birth canal and the ability of the fetus to pass through the mother's pelvic bones are crucial to successful labor and birth.

Contractions

Uterine contractions are characterized by the following measurable parameters:

Amplitude or intensity: The ability of the external tocodynamometer or manual palpation to determine contraction intensity is limited and of no clinical value. Intensity can be measured more precisely by an intrauterine pressure catheter. This device is placed transcervically inside the uterine cavity after membrane rupture and above the fetal presenting part.

The Montevideo Unit attempts to measure objectively the intensity of the contraction. It is calculated by the average strength of contractions in millimeters of mercury multiplied by the number of contractions in 10 minutes. During the active phase of labor, 200–250 Montevideo Units are considered normal. Since an internal catheter is not routinely used in clinical practice, the ability to measure intensity of uterine contractions is limited.

Frequency: Laboring patients in the active phase usually contract 3–5 times in 10 minutes. The presence of more than 5 contractions in 10 minutes for a period of 20 minutes is abnormal and is defined as tachysystole. When an alteration in the fetal heart rate accompanies tachysystole it is called hyperstimulation.

Duration: The sensitivity to detect the uterine contractions varies with different methods. The highest sensitivity is observed with internal catheters followed by palpation and, finally, patient perception. External tocodynamometer determinations are biased by the sensitivity of the device as well as maternal body habit.

The Pelvis

Since the progression of labor and fetal descent are determined in part by the relationship of the fetal presenting part and the bony pelvis, the obstetrician must become familiar with the evaluation of the pelvic dimensions, which is traditionally determined by a pelvimeter (**Fig. 11.2**).

Overall, four different shapes of female bony pelvis have been described. Two of them with favorable characteristics for vaginal delivery (gynecoid, anthropoid), and two (android, platypelloid) more frequently associated with cephalopelvic disproportion (CPD).

The bony pelvis (**Fig. 11.3**) is composed of the sacrum, ilium, ischium, and pubis. The pelvic brim separates the false (greater) pelvis from the true (lesser) pelvis. The true pelvis is further divided into three sections: 1) the pelvic inlet, 2) midpelvis, and 3) pelvic outlet.

Pelvic Inlet

The following are the measurable parts of the pelvic inlet.

Diagonal conjugate: This is the distance from the sacral promontory to the inferior margin of the symphysis pubis. This measure can be obtained by vaginal examination.

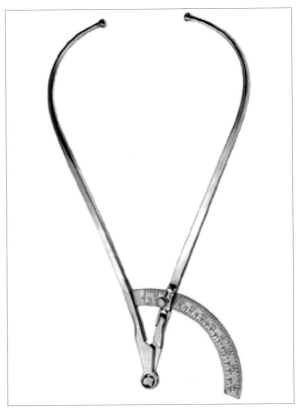

Fig. 11.2   A Martin pelvimeter.

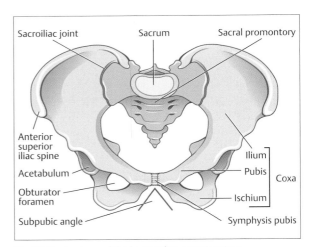

Fig. 11.3   Anatomy of the bony pelvis, anterior view.

True or obstetric conjugate: This is the distance from the sacral promontory to the superior margin of the symphysis pubis. It is the shortest diameter of the pelvic inlet. Values below 10 cm are frequently associated with CPD. Although this measure cannot be obtained by vaginal examination, it can be calculated by subtracting 2 cm from the diagonal conjugate.

Midpelvis

The interspinous diameter: This is the distance between the ischial spines. It is the shortest diameter and measures below 10 cm are associated with CPD.

Pelvic Outlet

Clinical examination allows evaluation of the pubic angle, prominence of the coccyx, and intertuberous diameter of the pelvic outlet.

The Fetus

Fetal characteristics are of utmost importance in the progression of labor. Important parameters include fetal size, lie, presentation, attitude, position, and station.

Fetal size: The impact of this measure in the progression of labor is relative to the maternal pelvis. However, macrosomic infants (>4500 g) need to be delivered by cesarean section significantly more often than normal birth weight babies.

Lie: This term refers to the relation between the fetal and maternal longitudinal axis. It can be longitudinal, transverse, or oblique. Longitudinal lie is required to achieve a successful vaginal delivery.

Presentation: This refers to the fetal part being offered to the pelvic inlet. It can be cephalic (vertex), breech, or compound (when multiple fetal parts are offered to the pelvic inlet). The presentation is further classified according to the main bony presenting part. For example, in a cephalic presentation, different degrees of fetal cervical flexion can offer different anatomical landmarks such as occiput (vertex), the chin (mentum), and the brow.

Attitude: This consists in the position of the head with regard to the fetal spine. The optimal attitude is with the head flexed and the chin against the chest, presenting the smallest possible head diameter to the pelvic inlet, or the suboccipitobregmatic diameter.

Position: In cephalic presentation the occiput is the anatomical reference, and its localization in relation to the maternal axis determines the fetal position. For example, if the occiput is localized anterior straight to the pubic arch, it is occiput anterior (OA), and if it is toward the mother's right, then it is right occiput anterior (ROA). **Figure 11.4** depicts the possible fetal positions in vertex presentation.

Station: This refers to the relation of the lowest bony fetal part to the ischial spines. It is a measure of descent of the fetus in labor and is classified according to the distance in centimeters from the plane of the ischial spines (**Fig. 11.5**).

Cardinal Movements of Labor

During labor, the fetus dynamically interacts with the rigid maternal bony pelvis to offer the best possible diameter to the pelvic path. Seven main movements are identified in the fetus (**Fig. 11.6**).

Engagement: This occurs when the widest diameter of the presenting part (biparietal diameter in cephalic or bitrocantheric diameter in breech presentation) reaches a plane below the pelvic inlet. In cephalic presentation as seen at vaginal examination, the presenting part is at 0 station and the fetus is engaged.

Descent: The descent of the presenting part is through the pelvic birth canal.

Flexion: To improve the ability to pass through the birth canal, flexion of the head (the chin lies against the chest) occurs. This allows presentation of the smallest diameter of the fetal head, the suboccipitobregmatic.

Internal rotation: Most frequently, the presenting head enters the pelvis in transverse position. By internal rotation the head turns to OA position (towards the pubis), offering the best diameter to the pelvic canal.

Extension: Once the fetal head reaches the introitus, it extends leaving the pubis symphysis at the base of the occiput. This facilitates the delivery of the fetal head.

External rotation: Once the fetal head is delivered it rotates back in line with the anatomical position of the fetal body.

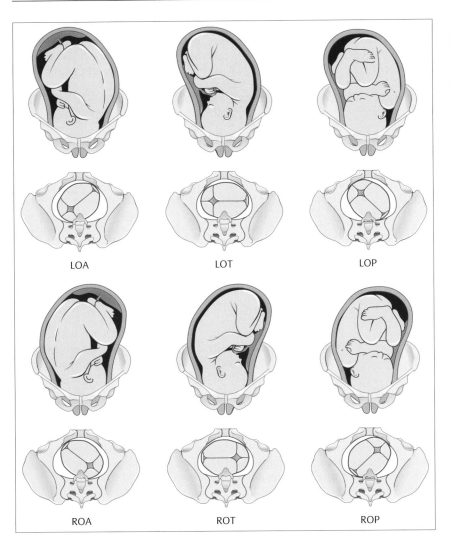

Fig. 11.4 Fetal presentation and position. LOA, left occiput anterior; LOT, left occiput transverse, LOP, left occiput posterior; ROA, right occiput anterior; ROT, right occiput transverse; ROP, right occiput posterior.

LOA

LOT

LOP

ROA

ROT

ROP

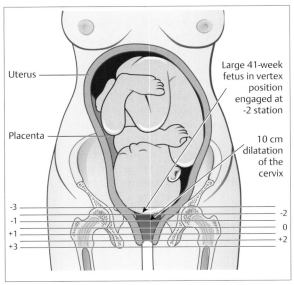

Uterus

Placenta

Large 41-week fetus in vertex position engaged at -2 station

10 cm dilatation of the cervix

-3
-1
+1
+3

-2
0
+2

Fig. 11.5 Fetal descent stations (birth presentation).

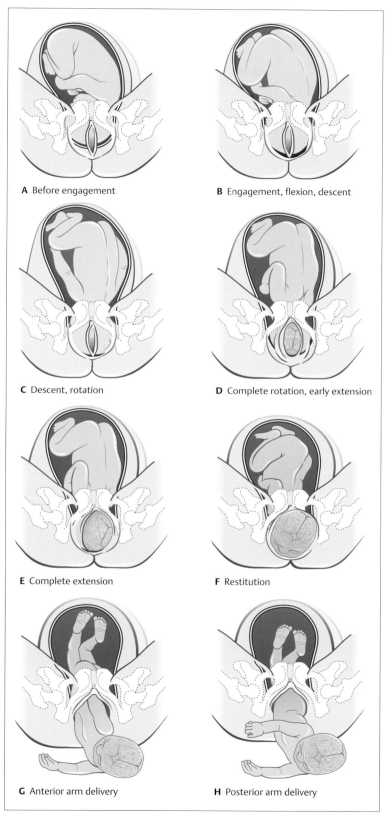

Fig. 11.6 Cardinal movements of labor.

A Before engagement

B Engagement, flexion, descent

C Descent, rotation

D Complete rotation, early extension

E Complete extension

F Restitution

G Anterior arm delivery

H Posterior arm delivery

Expulsion: This describes the delivery of the rest of the fetal body. The delivery of the anterior shoulder follows the same pattern of rotation as the delivery of the head.

Progress of Labor

Stages

The three stages of labor are:
- *First stage.* Extending from the onset of labor to full cervical dilatation
- *Second stage.* Extending from full cervical dilatation until fetal delivery
- *Third stage.* Extending from the delivery of the baby until the placenta is delivered

Phases

There are two phases of labor: latent and active.
- *Latent phase.* Extending from initiation of labor until active labor is achieved. The diagnosis of labor initiation is subjective, and usually refers to the presence of regular contractions.
- *Active phase.* Labor usually is considered active when there is 80% effacement and greater than 4 cm of cervical dilatation is achieved.

To objectively monitor the progress of labor and to identify patients that require further evaluation, it is practical to plot the progress of labor as a labor curve (**Fig. 11.7**). In general, the rate of dilation during the active phase is 1.2 cm and 1.5 cm per hour for nulliparous and multiparous women, respectively. The use of epidural analgesia appears to prolong these time periods. **Table 11.1** depicts mean and 95th percentile for duration of first and second stage of labor.

During labor, risk factors for a prolonged second stage, such as macrosomia or maternal diabetes, must be identified. Once the fetal head is crowning, the physician must control the delivery of the head. It is critical to protect the perineal region with the other hand to diminish the risk for tears.

Once the head is delivered, external rotation is permitted or gently assisted. At this point, look for the nuchal umbilical cord and, if present, reduce it. If it is tight and reduction is not feasible, perform clamping and section at this point, before delivery of the rest of fetal body. Currently, there is not robust evidence to support routine oropharynx aspiration. The anterior shoulder is then delivered by gentle downward traction. Subsequently, the delivery of the posterior shoulder is assisted by gentle upward traction. Again, protection of the maternal perineal region is important at this stage.

The placenta and membranes are delivered passively. Manual intervention is only considered after 30 minutes of expectant management. After delivery, examine the placenta and membranes for integrity, and document the number of cord vessels.

Table 11.1 Duration of second stage of labor (mean and 95th percentile)

Parameter	Mean	95th percentile
Nulliparas		
Latent labor	7.3–8.6 h	17–21 h
First stage	7.7–13.3 h	16.6–19.4 h
First stage epidural	10.2 h	19 h
Second stage	53–57 min	122–147 min
Second stage epidural	79 min	185 min
Multiparas		
Latent labor	4.1–5.3 h	12–14 h
First stage	5.7–7.5 h	12.5–13.7 h
First stage epidural	7.4 h	14.9 h
Second stage	17–19 min	57–61 min
Second stage epidural	45 min	131 min

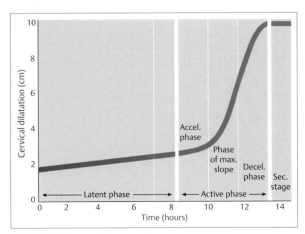

Fig. 11.7   A typical labor graph.

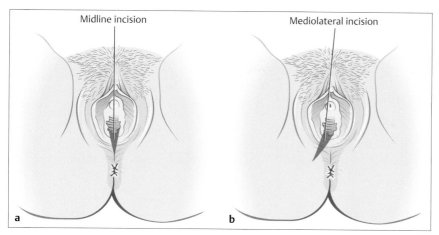

Midline incision   Mediolateral incision

a   b

Fig. 11.8 Options for an episiotomy incision.

Episiotomy

Episiotomy is an incision in the perineal region performed when the fetal head crowns. The objective of this intervention is to reduce the risk of perineal trauma. It could be median (vertical medial midincision from the vagina toward the anal sphincter) or mediolateral (at a 45° angle from the vagina) (**Fig. 11.8**).

Although it was previously believed that episiotomy could favor delivery and decrease perineal trauma, current studies have shown that midline episiotomy increases the risk of third and fourth degree tears. Therefore, episiotomy should not be used routinely (See Evidence Box 11.1) and must be reserved for special circumstances, such us the relief of shoulder dystocia.

Operative Vaginal Delivery

In selected cases operative delivery either by forceps or vacuum extraction, instrumentation is required.

Forceps Delivery

Three general classes of forceps exist:
- *Classic forceps.* These are designed for traction in vertex presentation, but are not designed for rotation of the fetal head. The most common forceps in this group are Tucker-McLane, Simpson, and Elliot.
- *Rotational forceps.* This is characterized by the lack of pelvic curvature (to avoid pelvic damage on rotation) and sliding lock (to facilitate the application on asynclitic presentations). The most common forceps in this group is Kielland.

- *Forceps to deliver the aftercoming head in breech presentation.* This forceps has a cephalic curve consisting of a reverse pelvic curve. When its application is required, the trunk of the baby is held horizontally and the forceps is applied from below (**Fig. 11.9**). This maneuver is feasible because of the inverse pelvic curve. This forceps is called Piper.

Vacuum Extraction

The vacuum extraction device consists of a stainless steel or a plastic cup attached to a handle grip and a tube that connects to a vacuum source. Fundamentals for application are the same for either vacuum extraction or forceps delivery and require:
- baby to be in an engaged vertex presentation
- cervix to be fully dilated
- membranes to be ruptured
- bladder to be drained
- adequate assessment of fetal position in relation to the maternal pelvis
- availability of maternal analgesia
- acquisition of informed consent
- operator to be trained in forceps delivery/vacuum extraction
- willingness to abandon the procedure if unsuccessful

Indications to consider operative vaginal delivery are also similar for both techniques and include a prolonged second stage. For, nulliparous women, indications for vaginal delivery include the lack of progression for 2 hours when no regional anesthesia is used, and for 3 hours if analgesia was applied. For multiparous women, indicators for vaginal delivery include lack of progression for 1 hour when no regional anesthesia is used, and for 2 hours if analgesia was applied.

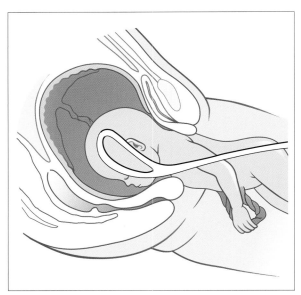

Fig. 11.9 The Piper forceps is applied to the fetal head from below. This is the preferred method of delivering the head of a breech baby.

Key Points

- Labor is a physiologic process consisting in the occurrence of organized uterine contractions of adequate intensity, frequency, and duration leading to complete cervical dilatation and expulsion of the fetus, placenta, and fetal membranes through the birth canal.
- Physiology of labor initiation involves different phases characterized by quiescence, activation, stimulation, and involution.
- Normal labor pattern consists in 3–5 contractions in 10 minutes. The presence of more than 5 contractions in 10 minutes for a period of 20 minutes is abnormal and is defined as tachysystole.
- The cardinal movements of labor are engagement, descent, flexion, internal rotation, extension, external rotation, and expulsion.
- Routine median episiotomy is associated with increased incidence of pelvic tears.

Evidence Box 11.1

Restrictive use of episiotomy leads to fewer complications than routine use.

Carroli and Mignini reviewed the scientific literature to determine the effects of restrictive use versus routine use of mediolateral and midline episiotomy. In reviewing eight randomized, controlled trials that included more than 5500 women, they found that compared with routine use, restrictive episiotomy resulted in less severe perineal trauma, less suturing, and fewer healing complications. There was no difference in severe vaginal/perineal trauma, dyspareunia, urinary incontinence, or several pain measures between the two groups. Restrictive episiotomy was, however, associated with more anterior perineal trauma. The authors concluded that restrictive episiotomy appears to have a number of benefits compared to policies based on routine episiotomy.
Carroli G, Mignini L. Episiotomy for vaginal birth. Cochrane Database Syst Rev 2009 Jan 21;(1):CD000081.

Further Reading

American College of Obstetricians and Gynecologists: Dystocia and augmentation of labor. ACOG Practice Bulletin No. 49, December 2003

American College of Obstetricians and Gynecologists: Episiotomy. ACOG Practice Bulletin No. 71, April 2006

Reece EA, Hobbins JC, eds. Clinical Obstetrics—the Fetus and Mother. 3rd ed. Malden, Mass: Blackwell Synergy Publishing, 2007

Gabbe SG, Niebyl JR, Simpson JL. Obstetrics: Normal and Problem Pregnancies. New York: Elsevier/Churchill Livingstone; 2007

12 Immediate and Postpartum Newborn Care

Julieta E. Irman and Gustavo F. Leguizamòn

The neonatal period comprises the four weeks following delivery. During this phase, the newborn must rapidly adjust to its extrauterine life. To survive and achieve normal development, it must make major physiologic changes, including increased respiratory gas exchange, switching from fetal to neonatal circulation, and taking over its own thermoregulation. This chapter addresses these major physiologic changes involved in the newborn's transition to its extrauterine life. It also offers the basics of medical interventions commonly used to assist newborns throughout this critical transition.

Definitions

Apgar score: The Apgar score provides an objective method of evaluating the physical condition of a newborn infant soon after delivery. The score takes into account the heart rate, respiratory effort, muscle tone, skin color, and responce to a catheter in the nostril. Each of these objective signs can receive 0, 1, or 2 points, and each test is performed at 1 minute and 5 minutes after delivery. A common mnemonic is APGAR: **A**ppearance, **P**ulse, **G**rimace, **A**ctivity and **R**espiration.

Hyperbilirubinemia: This term refers to excess bilirubin in the blood, usually characterized by jaundice or yellowing of the eyes.

Hyperthermia: Abnormally high body temperature that occurs when the body's metabolic heat production or environmental heat load exceeds the normal heat loss capacity (or when heat loss is impaired).

Hypothermia: A dangerous lowering of body-core temperature, caused by losing heat faster than it is produced by the body.

Postpartum: A term used to describe something that occurs after childbirth, usually involving the mother.

Tachypnea: This refers to an excessively rapid respiratory rate, defined as greater than 20 breaths per minute.

Transition: The transition period is referred to as 6–12 hours after birth, when the baby goes through physiological adaptation to extrauterine life.

Vaginal introitus: This is the anatomical term for the vaginal opening.

The Respiratory Transition

The alveoli of the fetus in utero are filled with fluid that must be cleared during the initial transitional period, so that the baby can breathe. In addition, to ensure effective pulmonary perfusion and to match perfusion to ventilation, the baby must be able to increase blood flow to the lungs.

During the last few weeks of pregnancy, there is a maturation and recruitment of sodium channels in the epithelial cells of the lungs in response to endogenous steroid and catecholamine surges that are triggered by the onset of labor. It is through these epithelial sodium channels that a significant part of the fluid in the fetus' lungs is purged. Liquid is also driven out of the fetus' lungs through the pulmonary epithelium into the vasculature as well as through the mechanical *squeeze* and Starling forces that occur during the process of labor and vaginal delivery.

Newborns sometimes have difficulty purging all the liquid from their lungs, particularly if they are late preterm babies. As a result, they may exhibit respiratory difficulties that require stabilization and immediate supportive therapy, such as supplemental oxygen and assisted ventilation. They are also at increased risk for associated morbidities.

Wang et al. estimated that nearly one-third of late preterm newborns exhibit respiratory difficulties. Neonates who are born by cesarean delivery before labor begins are at increased risk for respiratory distress, as are late preterm males compared with late preterm females. Hemodynamic instability caused by hypothermia or hypoglycemia may worsen the newborn's underlying respiratory distress.

Acute respiratory distress syndrome (RDS) is the most common respiratory condition experienced in newborns. The condition, which is characterized by severe difficulty in breathing and related complications, occurs primarily in neonates born between 34 and 36 weeks' gestation. It is the fourth leading cause of death for neonates in the United States (**Fig. 12.1**).

Late preterm infants also are at increased risk of having low Apgar scores, transient tachypnea of the newborn (TTN), persistent pulmonary hypertension, and respiratory failure. TTN and RDS are both common respiratory conditions in the late preterm newborn and are related to difficulty in clearing fluid from the lungs or a surfactant deficiency, or both. The protocols for managing a child in respiratory distress are covered later in this chapter.

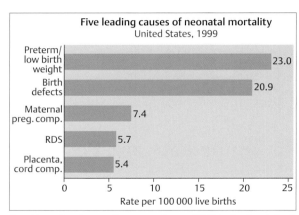

Fig. 12.1   Respiratory distress syndrome (RDS) is the fourth leading cause of death among neonates in the United States at approximately 6 per 100 000 live births. Adapted from the National Center for Health Statistics, 1999 period birth/infant death data; prepared by March of Dimes Perinatal Data Center, 2002

versing the right-to-left shunt and leading to the closure of the ductus arteriosus. Prostaglandins play a pivotal role in maintaining patency of the ductus arteriosus in utero and in its closure during early neonatal life.

The Circulatory Transition

As described in Chapter 9, there is a substantial difference between the circulation of a fetus and a neonate. In the womb, well oxygenated blood from the placenta is delivered to the fetus through the umbilical vein. The umbilical vein gives off branches to the left lobe of the liver and then continues as the ductus venosus (**Fig. 12.2**). The left hepatic vein fuses with the well oxygenated ductus venosus and flows into the inferior vena cava to reach the left atrium by crossing thorough the foramen ovale. Then, via the aorta and carotid circulation, this blood supplies the brain and upper body. The right ventricular output is directed through the ductus arteriosus to the descending aorta.

Since the pulmonary vascular resistance is high and the mean pulmonary artery pressures are higher than aortic pressures, the flow is mainly directed toward the ductus arteriosus, leaving the pulmonary circulation with 5–10% of the ventricular output. Finally, fetal blood returns to the placenta through the umbilical arteries.

However, when delivery occurs, clamping the umbilical cord provokes a sudden decrease in the amount of neonatal blood draining toward and away from the baby. This leads to a sudden increase pressure in the systemic circulation and a decrease in the right side circulation, re-

The Thermoregulatory Transition

Thermoregulation is a critical physiologic function that is closely related to the transition and survival of the infant. An understanding of transitional events and the physiologic adaptations that must be made is essential in helping the neonate to maintain its thermal stability. This section reviews neonatal thermal regulation, heat loss and gain, and infant thermoregulatory behavior. Measures to ensure thermal stability for the neonate are discussed later in this chapter.

Neonatal Thermoregulation

Babies are not as adaptable as adults to temperature change. A baby's body surface is about three times greater than an adult's, relative to the weight of the body. Babies can lose heat rapidly, as much as four times more quickly than adults. Premature and low birth weight babies usually have little body fat and may be too immature to regulate their own temperature, even in a warm environment. Even full-term and healthy newborns may not be able to maintain their body temperature if the environment is too cold.

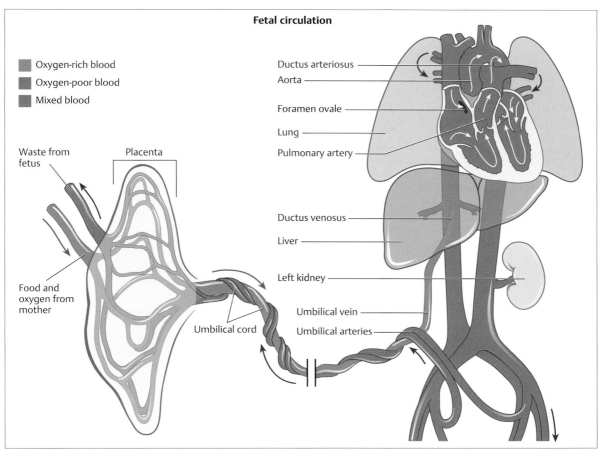

Fetal circulation

Oxygen-rich blood
Oxygen-poor blood
Mixed blood

Waste from fetus
Placenta
Food and oxygen from mother
Umbilical cord

Ductus arteriosus
Aorta
Foramen ovale
Lung
Pulmonary artery
Ductus venosus
Liver
Left kidney
Umbilical vein
Umbilical arteries

Fig. 12.2 The fetus receives all the necessary nutrition, oxygen, and life support from the mother's placenta via the blood vessels in the umbilical cord. Waste products and carbon dioxide from the fetus are sent back through the umbilical cord and placenta to the mother's circulation to be eliminated.

When babies are stressed by cold, they use energy and oxygen to generate warmth. If skin temperature drops just one degree from the ideal 36.5 °C (97.7 °F), a baby's oxygen use can increase by 10%. Keeping babies at optimal temperatures, neither too hot nor too cold, enables them to conserve energy and build up reserves. This is especially important when babies are sick or premature.

For optimal thermal stability the baby's temperature must be kept within the Thermal Neutral Zone (**Fig. 12.3**). Once stabilized within the Thermal Neutral Zone, the baby's energy expenditure and oxygen consumption are minimized, promoting optimal growth.

Thermoregulation is controlled by the hypothalamus, a region of the central nervous system responsible for certain metabolic process and other activities of the autonomic nervous system. Thermal stimuli from the skin and body's deep (central) thermal receptors provide information on body temperature to the hypothalamus (**Fig. 12.4**). It is in the hypothalamus that sensory information describing thermal status throughout the body is processed and compared against the temperature set

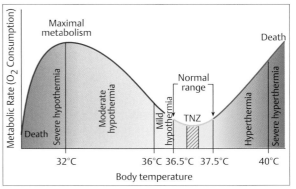

Fig. 12.3 Thermal stability is essential for every baby, especially those with limited metabolic capacity due to illness, prematurity, or low birth weight. Research has shown that the Thermal Neutral Zone for preterm babies less than 30 weeks old is less than 0.5 °C.

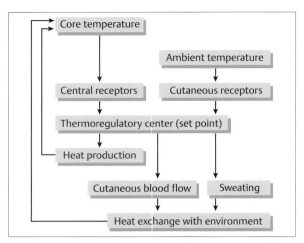

Fig. 12.4 Thermoregulation is mediated by a population of neurons in the hypothalamus that act to integrate the receptor information and compare it to the temperature set point (normal core temperature). Their output regulates the metabolic, cutaneous, vascular, and sudomotor (sweating) activity to control heat balance and, therefore, body temperature.

point. Just like a thermostat, the hypothalamus modifies body heat—and therefore body temperature—by altering metabolism, motor tone and activity, vasomotor activity, and sweating to produce either heat gain or loss.

Heat Loss and Gain

Neonates are especially prone to sudden heat loss or gain. The intrauterine temperature of 37.9° C (100.2 °F) fluctuates very little under normal circumstances. At birth, the transition from an intrauterine to extrauterine environment creates a significant thermal change that challenges the infant's thermoregulatory abilities. Because of differences in physiological function and small body size, neonates are particularly vulnerable to both underheating (hypothermia) and overheating (hyperthermia).

Neonates have higher metabolic rates than do children or adults. Metabolism reflects the overall energy needs supporting maintenance, repair, and growth. The higher metabolic rate is due not only to energy demands related to growth, but also to increased maintenance requirements related to the neonate's large body surface area and large surface-to-mass ratio.

Body heat generated by body mass (weight of metabolizing cells producing heat) is lost over the surface area. Therefore, the smaller the neonate, the greater the imbalance between its heat-producing ability (mass) and heat loss (surface area). The infant's relatively large surface area relative to body mass requires a higher caloric intake to support temperature balance.

Thermoregulatory Behaviors

Because of immature motor and cognitive abilities, the neonate has limited, but subtle, thermoregulatory behaviors. When cool, infants will increase flexion and motor activity. Warm infants will increase extension and may sleep or be lethargic. Irritability may be a sign that the infant is too warm or too cool, suggesting the need for intervention.

Newborn Management

Evaluation and Resuscitation

Approximately 10% of newborns require some type of respiratory assistance at birth, and about 1% need more complex measures to survive. Conversely, 90% of newborns undergo the transition into extrauterine life without difficulties and require little or no assistance to sustain spontaneous and regular breathing.

The following steps are needed immediately after delivery:
1. Dry the baby and place him or her under a radiant heat source to maintain body temperature; avoid letting the baby become hyperthermic.
2. Apply suction to the nose and oropharynx
3. Assess the baby's condition using an Apgar score, as defined above and detailed in **Table 12.1**. If the first cumulative score is less than 7, an additional valuation should be obtained every 5 minutes until at least 20 minutes after delivery.

Table 12.1 Apgar score

Sign	0	1	2
Heart rate	Absent	<100 bpm	>100 bpm
Respiratory effort	Apneic	Weak, irregular, gasping	Regular
Reflex	No response	Some response	Facial grimace, cough
Muscle tone	Flaccid	Some flexion	Good flexion: arms and legs
Color	Blue, pale	Body pink: hands and feet blue	Pink

4. If the heart rate is more than 100 beats per minute (bpm) and the baby is breathing, no further intervention is generally required.

5. If the heart rate is below 100 bpm and the baby is apneic or with inadequate respiratory effort, stimulate by rubbing the baby's back and apply an oxygen mask over the face.

6. If the baby does not respond to these initial measures, initiate bag and face mask ventilation with 100% oxygen immediately. If bagging is appropriate, chest expansions are observed and color as well as perfusion and heart rate should improve. The rate of bagging should not exceed 40–60 per minute.

7. If there is no response to appropriate bag and mask ventilation after approximately 40 seconds, endotracheal intubation must be performed.

8. If the heartbeat drops below 60 bpm, epinephrine is indicated.

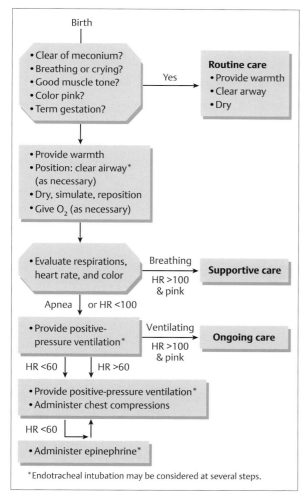

Fig. 12.5 Schematic for managing the respiratory needs of newborns.

Figure 12.5 depicts the conditions under which specific resuscitation interventions need to be initiated to achieve optimal outcome.

General Care

Once the baby is delivered, the mouth and nose must be cleared up. This is done by holding the baby face down to help drain the fluids from the mouth and nose. To prevent a significant shifting of blood away from the neonate, he or she must be held at the level of vaginal introitus. Meanwhile:

- Cover the baby with a sterile warm blanket and rub the head and back.
- Wait 30 seconds before clamping the cord. It is clamped and cut 4–5 cm from the baby's abdomen. Later, once the baby is stabilized, an umbilical clamp can be secured to the cord 1–2 cm distal from the abdominal wall and the excess cut off. If the baby is preterm or unstable, and catheterization of the umbilical vessels is likely, the cord can be clamped more distally, around 3 cm.
- Place the baby on a heated radiant warmer bed, dressed in a diaper, shorts, hat, and wrapped in a double blanket. Then transfer the baby to the mother.
- If the baby is vigorous, has good tone and color, let him or her rest on the mother's chest, while still drying the baby. In this way, mother–child bonding and feeding can be stimulated.

Identification and Security

Each country, state, city, and hospital has its own regulations regarding identification of the newborn. In the delivery room, footprinting, palmprinting of the infant, and fingerprinting of the mother can be taken. Both mother and infant should wear matching wrist and ankle ID bands.

Thermal Regulation

The newborn infant is highly dependent on environmental temperature. Thus, providing thermal support is a primary objective of newborn care. Indeed, without immediate thermal support, a newborn's body temperature can drop 4–5 °C during the first minute after birth.

Since neonates are particularly vulnerable to hypothermia, special attention should be given to their environmental support. It has been suggested that these very small infants should be incubated like eggs and that early in the postnatal period they may require air temperatures warmer than body core temperature.

Requirements for "thermoneutrality" are met when central and skin temperatures are within normal limits of 36.7–37.3 °C (98.1–99.1 °F) and stable, that is, changing less than 0.2–0.3 °C (0.36–0.54 °F) per hour. Smaller and less mature infants, particularly very preterm infants, are usually cared for in air-heated perspex incubators or in open cots, where they are placed under clear polyethylene blankets and there are overhead radiant heaters (**Fig. 12.6**). The air temperature of the incubator or the power of the overhead heater can be set to respond to changes in the temperature of the infant's abdominal wall to try to maintain the infant's temperature between 36.5 °C and 37 °C.

Closed incubators allow adjustment of the ambient humidity, and this further reduces heat and fluid evaporation. Consequently, incubator care is associated with less insensible water loss, and lower fluid requirements, than nursing infants in open cots under radiant heaters.

Both closed incubator and open cot care have other potential advantages and disadvantages. Environmental noise and light can be reduced with incubator care, and this may improve sleep patterns. Open cots, however, allow easy access for caregivers. Additionally, parents might find it easier to bond with their babies if they are nursed in an open cot rather than in a closed incubator. At present there are insufficient data to determine whether open cots or incubators confer more beneficial effects on important clinical outcomes.

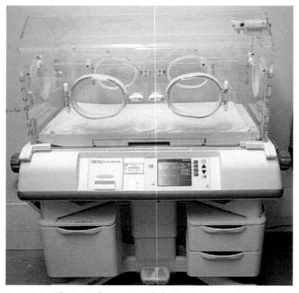

Fig. 12.6   The typical premature baby incubator consists of a clear Perspex chamber. In addition to temperature and humidity, oxygen levels also can be controlled.

Initial Physical Assessment and Prophylaxis

The initial physical assessment of the baby should be done every half an hour for at least 2 hours of stability, then every 8 hours. It includes:
- determining vital signs, heart rate, respiratory rate, and temperature
- measuring weight, length, and head circumference
- conducting a complete physical examination at least daily

If the baby stays in the hospital for an extended period, follow-up assessment includes:
- recording feeding volume, frequency, and behavior
- recording urine and stool output
- recording daily weight: check percentage of loss from birth weight
- cord and circumcision care

Eye Infection Prophylaxis

To prevent gonococcal and chlamydial ophthalmia in all children, 1% silver nitrate or 0.5% erythromycin is instilled into the conjunctival sac.

Vitamin K Prophylaxis

Newborns have low levels of active vitamin K-dependent clotting factors because in utero placental transport of vitamin K is poor, and no intestinal flora produce this vitamin. Therefore, 1 mg of vitamin K during the first hour of life is indicated to prevent hemorrhagic disease in the newborn.

Breast-feeding

The American College of Obstetricians and Gynecologists endorses breast-feeding as the "gold standard" for newborn feeding (see also Evidence Box 12.1) Among the main health benefits observed with breast-feeding are improved growth, less vulnerability to infections, less allergies, and lower incidence of childhood cancer or type I diabetes. Furthermore, maternal benefits have also been reported such as: faster postpartum weight loss, lower incidence of premenopausal breast cancer, as well as improved maternal–infant bonding.

The first day of breast-feeding is usually disorganized. Each time the baby feeds, however, it should take from 10 to 15 minutes on each breast, every 3 to 4 hours, adding up to 8–12 times per day. To be adequate, breast-feeding should occur at least eight times a day (24 hours) with a duration no shorter than 15 minutes each time.

Stooling

As many as 99% of newborns pass stool in the first day. At first, their stool will be dark brown or blackish. As feeding is established, the stool will be lighter, green, yellowish, or orange. Since neonates already present the gastrocolic reflex, they can stool every time they eat.

Voiding Micturition

Most babies void during the first 16 hours of life. Be alert, and closely monitor and evaluate any baby that hasn't done so by 24 hours.

Discharge Procedures

Before discharge, the mother must be instructed in the proper use of an approved safety car seat. She should also receive instructions on how to prevent burns, falls, aspiration, and harm by siblings and pets.

Home Routines and Visitors

Establishing home routines can be difficult, challenging, and exhausting because the mother may still be recovering from delivery and the newborn has no routines per se. The following are five basic steps for caring for the newborn at home.

1. **Bathing**: The baby should be bathed at least twice a week. However, avoid overbathing, which can dry the baby's skin.
2. **Clothing**: Dress the baby comfortably. In cold weather, the baby may need an extra layer of clothing in addition to a hat and a coat.
3. **Sunlight**: Avoid exposing the baby to direct sunlight for any significant length of time.
4. **Diaper changes**: Change the baby's diapers frequently to protect the skin from dermatitis. Use warm water with mild soap to clean stools and diaper wipes when not at home. Do not apply ointments unless the skin shows signs of dermatitis.
5. **Umbilical cord**: The umbilical cord clamp can be safely removed after 24 hours. Alcohol can be used to wipe the cord at least daily. It should be left outside the diaper to dry and mummify. A little bleeding is normal. It usually stops around 7 to 10 days.

Managing Neonatal Jaundice

Among term infants the problem most frequently encountered is neonatal hyperbilirubinemia. Under physiological conditions, the largest amount of bilirubin is the product of the normal red blood cell destruction. Heme is converted to bilirubin in the reticuloendothelial system. Unconjugated bilirubin reversibly binds to plasma protein reaching the liver, where it is conjugated with glucuronic acid to become water-soluble. Finally, it is secreted into the small intestine.

Most jaundice is benign and generally occurs in otherwise healthy infants. However, because of the potential toxicity of bilirubin, newborns must be monitored to identify severe hyperbilirubinemia and, in rare cases, acute bilirubin encephalopathy or kernicterus. This latter complication involves the deposition of bilirubin in specific parts of the brain, such as the basal ganglia, producing neuronal necrosis.

When bilirubinemia occurs it is usually observed at 7–10 days of life. It presents with lethargy, poor feeding, hypertonisity, and opisthotonos. Severe, lifelong sequelae occur in survivors. **Figure 12.7** depicts the risk of developing significant hyperbilirubinemia based on hour-specific bilirubin determinations.

Major risk factors for hyperbilirunemia include:
- blood group incompatibility with positive direct Coombs test
- presence of other hemolytic disease
- gestational age 35–36 weeks.
- jaundice observed during the first 24 hours of life
- previous sibling receiving phototherapy.
- cephalohematoma or extensive bruising
- exclusive breast-feeding, particularly if inadequate or more than 12% weight loss.
- east Asian race.

The American Academy of Pediatrics recommends that clinicians:
(1) perform a systematic assessment before discharge for the risk of severe hyperbilirubinemia;
(2) provide early and focused follow-up based on the risk assessment; and
(3) when indicated, treat newborns with phototherapy or exchange transfusion to prevent the development of severe hyperbilirubinemia and possible bilirubin encephalopathy.

The guidelines emphasize the importance of universal systematic assessment for the risk of severe hyperbilirubinemia, close follow-up, and prompt intervention.

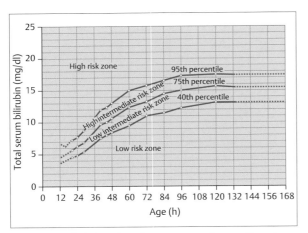

Fig. 12.7   Risk designation of term and near-term well newborns based on their hour-specific serum bilirubin values. The high-risk zone is designated by the 95th percentile track. The intermediate-risk zone is subdivided into upper and lower risk zones by the 75th percentile track. The low-risk zone has been electively and statistically defined by the 40th percentile track. (Dotted extensions are based on <300 total serum bilirubin values per epoch).

General Laboratory Evaluation

The recommended laboratory screening tests for the newborn include:

- Blood type and direct Coombs test in infants born to mothers with type O or Rhesus (Rh)-negative blood. Hemolytic disease due to Rh or major blood group incompatibility takes place when Rh negative mothers deliver an Rh-positive child, or type O mothers with type A/B children. Furthermore, every Rh-negative mother should receive immunoprophylaxis (see Chapter 6 for a more detailed discussion).
- a serologic test for syphilis
- hemoglobin and hematocrit
- urinalysis
- blood glucose test in infants with either symptoms or risk factors for hypoglycemia
- newborn metabolic screening: this test is mandatory for every infant

Key Points

- Most babies are able to perform the transition from intrauterine to extrauterine life without complications. A few will need assistance to decrease morbidity and mortality. Current protocols should be followed in these circumstances.
- Acute respiratory distress syndrome is the most common respiratory condition experienced by newborns. This condition, which is characterized by severe difficulty in breathing

and related complications, occurs primarily in neonates born between 34 and 36 weeks' gestation. Immediate assessment and appropriate intervention, particularly oxygen supplementation, can ameliorate this condition in most newborns.

- The American College of Obstetricians and Gynecologists endorses breast-feeding as the "gold standard." Infant breast-feeding improves growth, lessens vulnerability to infections, reduces the development of allergies, and lowers incidence of childhood cancer and type 1 diabetes.
- The newborn infant is highly dependent on environmental temperature. Indeed, without immediate thermal support, a newborn's body temperature can drop by 4–5 °C during the first minute after birth. Thus, providing thermal support is a primary objective of newborn care.
- Neonatal hyperbilirubinemia is the problem most frequently encountered among term infants. Because of the potential toxicity of bilirubin, newborns must be monitored to identify severe hyperbilirubinemia and acute bilirubin encephalopathy or kernicterus.

Evidence Box 12.1

Breast-feeding confers developmental and behavioral advantages to very low birth weight infants compared with those not given breast milk.

Vohr et al. analyzed the effects of breast milk on cognitive skills and behavior ratings of 1035 extremely low birth weight infants. Specifically, they assessed neonatal characteristics and morbidities, interim history, and neurodevelopmental and growth outcomes at 18 to 22 months' corrected age. Infants in the breast milk group were similar to those in the no breast milk group in every neonatal characteristic and morbidity, including number of days of hospitalization. Children in the breast milk group were more likely to have a Bayley Mental Development Index ≥85, higher mean Bayley Psychomotor Development Index, and higher Bayley Behavior Rating Scale percentile scores for orientation/engagement, motor regulation, and total score. There were no differences in the rates of moderate to severe cerebral palsy or blindness or hearing impairment between the two study groups. There were no differences in the mean weight (10.4 kg vs. 10.4 kg), mean length (80.5 cm vs. 80.5 cm), or mean head circumference (46.8 cm. vs. 46.6 cm) for the breast-milk and no-breast-milk groups, respectively, at 18 months. Multivariate analyses, adjusting for confounders, confirmed a significant independent association of breast milk on all four primary outcomes

Vohr BR, Poindexter BB, Dusick AM, et al. Beneficial effects of breast milk in the neonatal intensive care unit on the developmental outcome of extremely low birth weight infants at 18 months of age. Pediatrics 2006;118(1):e115–e123.

Further Reading

American Academy of Pediatrics. Work Group on Breastfeeding. Breastfeeding and the use of human milk. *Pediatrics* 1997;100(6):1035–1039

American Academy of Pediatrics Subcommittee on Hyperbilirubinemia. Management of hyperbilirubinemia in the newborn infant 35 or more weeks of gestation. *Pediatrics* 2004;114(1):297–316

American Heart Association and American Academy of Pediatrics: Neonatal resuscitation Textbook; 2006.

Hermansen CL, Lorah KN. Respiratory distress in the newborn. *Am Fam Physician* 2007;76(7):987–994

Thomas K. Thermoregulation in neonates. *Neonatal Netw* 1994;13(2):15–22

Wang ML, Dorer DJ, Fleming MP, Catlin EA. Clinical outcomes of near-term infants. *Pediatrics* 2004;114(2):372–376

Vohr BR, Poindexter BB, Dusick AM, et al; NICHD Neonatal Research Network. Beneficial effects of breast milk in the neonatal intensive care unit on the developmental outcome of extremely low birth weight infants at 18 months of age. *Pediatrics* 2006;118(1):e115–e123

Section II   Abnormal Obstetrics

13 Ectopic Pregnancies

Eyal Sheiner and Arnon Wiznitzer

Ectopic pregnancy (EP) is a major health problem for women of reproductive age and is the leading cause of pregnancy-related death during the first 20 weeks of pregnancy. EP accounts for about 9% of all pregnancy-related deaths, and its incidence is higher for non-White women. This disparity increases with age. Accurate diagnosis and treatment of EP significantly decreases the risk of death and optimizes subsequent fertility.

Definition

Ectopic pregnancy (EP) refers to implantation of a fertilized ovum outside the uterus. The most common site of EP implantation is the fallopian tubes, accounting for about 98% of all EP cases. The majority of EPs (79.6%) are implanted in the ampullary part of the fallopian tube, approximately 12.3% implant in the isthmus, 6.2% in the fimbria, and 1.9% in the interstitial part (**Fig. 13.1**). In rare cases implantation can occur in other ectopic sites including the ovary, uterine cervix (i.e., cervical pregnancy), and abdomen. Coexistent intrauterine and extrauterine pregnancies are referred to as heterotropic pregnancy.

Diagnosis

The most common symptoms of EP are abdominal or pelvic pain accompanied with vaginal bleeding. The best diagnosis is based on the positive visualization of an extrauterine pregnancy outside the uterus. However, this is not seen in all cases. About 90% of EPs may be visualized using transvaginal sonography within 5 weeks of the last menstrual period.

Another method of EP detection is to measure the level of human chorionic gonadotropin (HCG). When the HCG level exceeds the transvaginal discriminatory zone (1000–2000 mIU/mL), it suggests the absence of an intrauterine gestational sac, and EP. It also may also suggest a failed intrauterine pregnancy. However, the combination of positive HCG and transvaginal ultrasound scan has a positive predictive value of 95% for an EP. If an intrauterine pregnancy is detected, this tends to exclude a diagnosis of EP, because coexisting intrauterine and extrauterine pregnancies (heterotropic) following spontaneous cycles are rare, with an estimated incidence of 1 in 30000.

Prevalence

There has been a significant increase in the number of cases of EP in the past several decades in developed countries. In the United States, for example, a sixfold increase in the number of cases of EP was noted between 1970 and 1992. The rate varies between 6 and 30 per 1000 pregnancies. However, with in vitro fertilization (IVF) cycles, the rate can be as high as 4.5%.

Etiology and Pathophysiology

The most common initiators of EP are tubal obstruction and injury. Previous pelvic inflammatory disease, especially due to *Chlamydia trachomatis*, is the leading risk factor for ectopic pregnancy.

Other factors associated with an increased risk of EP include prior ectopic pregnancy, a history of infertility (and specifically IVF), cigarette smoking (which causes alterations in tubal motility and ciliary activity), prior tu-

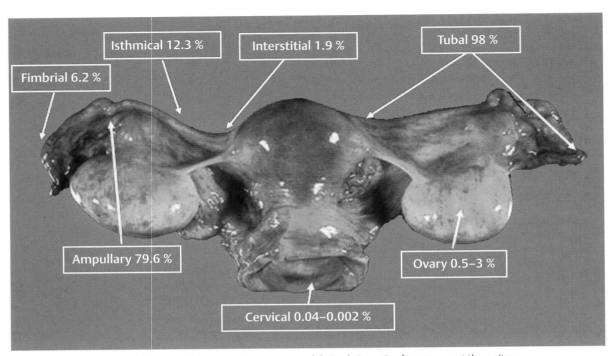

Fig. 13.1   Various locations where ectopic pregnancies can occur and their relative ratio of occurrence at those sites.

bal surgery, exposure to diethylstilbestrol (which alters fallopian tube morphology), non-White women, and advanced maternal age.

Women can be protected from developing an EP by intrauterine contraceptive devices (IUDs), progesterone-only contraceptives, and sterilization. Nevertheless, if a woman who has been sterilized or is a current user of an IUD or progesterone-only contraceptives becomes pregnant, her risk for an EP is increased 6 to 10-fold, since these methods of contraception provide greater protection against intrauterine pregnancies than EPs. **Table 13.1** summarizes risk factors for EP.

History

Physical Examination

The classic symptom triad of EP includes amenorrhea, irregular bleeding, and lower abdominal pain. The triad is present in only half of patients and most commonly when rupture has occurred.

The physical examination should include measurements of vital signs. Abdominal and pelvic tenderness, especially cervical motion tenderness, are common when rupture has occurred (and present in about 75% of pa-

Table 13.1 Risk factors for ectopic pregnancy

Risk factors	Predisposing conditions
Tubal obstruction and injury	Previous pelvic inflammatory disease, (especially *Chlamydia trachomatis*)
	Prior ectopic pregnancy
	A history of infertility (especially IVF)
	Prior tubal surgery, tubal ligation
	Diethylstilbestrol exposure
Non-White ethnicity	
Advanced maternal age	
Cigarette smoking	
Multiple partners	

tients). However, pelvic examination before rupture is usually nonspecific, and a palpable pelvic mass on bimanual examination is established in less than half of the cases. The accuracy of the initial clinical evaluation before rupture is less than 50% and additional tests are required in order to differentiate EP from early intrauterine pregnancy. Work-up includes first ruling out a normal intrauterine pregnancy.

Ultrasonography

The early sonographic appearance of a normal gestational sac is characterized by signs of a double decidual sac (i.e., two concentric echogenic rings separated by a hypoechogenic space) (**Fig. 13.2**). The presence of the characteristic double decidual sac is important in helping the physician diagnose an intrauterine pregnancy at a very early stage as well as to exclude EP.

However, an intrauterine pseudo-sac can be seen in some cases of EP, owing to intrauterine fluid or blood collection. A pseudo-sac is a uterine sac without a double decidual ring or a yolk sac.

Laboratory Assessment: β-HCG measurements

The first stage in the evaluation of women with a suspected EP is to determine whether the patient is pregnant. The enzyme immunoassay for HCG is positive in virtually all cases of EP. A "discriminatory cutoff of β-HCG" means the level at which a normal intrauterine pregnancy can reliably be visualized by ultrasound scanning. A viable intrauterine pregnancy should be seen by transvaginal sonography at HCG levels of about 1500 mIU/mL.

The level of HCG increases during gestation and reaches a peak of approximately 100 000 mIU/mL at 6–10 weeks. It then decreases and remains stable at approximately 20 000 mIU/mL. A 66% rise in the HCG level over a 48-hour period represents the lower limit of normal values for viable intrauterine pregnancy. Indeed, there is consensus that the predictable rise in serial β-HCG values is markedly different from the slow rise or plateau due to an EP.

Limitations of serial HCG testing include its inability to distinguish a failing intrauterine pregnancy from an ectopic pregnancy and the inherent 48-hour delay. Assays of serial HCG levels are typically required only when an initial ultrasound scan fails to detect either intrauterine or extrauterine pregnancy.

Serum Progesterone

The utility of measuring serum progesterone levels for diagnosing EP is still being debated. A baseline serum progesterone level of less than 20 nmol/L can be used to identify abnormal pregnancy (either intrauterine or extrauterine) with a positive predictive value of ≥95%.

Among pregnant patients with serum progesterone values of less than 5 nmol/L, 85% have spontaneous abortions, 0.16% have viable intrauterine pregnancies, and 14% have ectopic pregnancies. However, serum progesterone levels cannot distinguish ectopic pregnancy from spontaneous abortion. Thus, progesterone levels at defined times can be used to predict the immediate viability of a pregnancy, but cannot be used reliably to predict its location.

Dilatation and Curettage

When serial HCG values do not rise or fall appropriately, an abnormal gestation exists. When the pregnancy has been confirmed to be nonviable, a uterine dilation and curettage can be performed to obtain products of conception. It also can distinguish between an ectopic pregnancy and a miscarriage, when ultrasound scanning is not sufficient (**Fig. 13.3**).

Once tissue is obtained by curettage, it can be added to saline in order to investigate whether the sample floats. Visualization of villi in the tissue obtained indicates the occurrence of spontaneous intrauterine abortion. Because floating of the material is not 100% accurate, histological verification or serial HCG level measurement is needed.

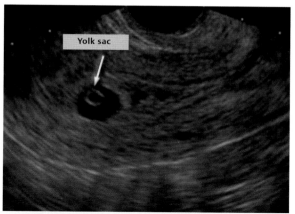

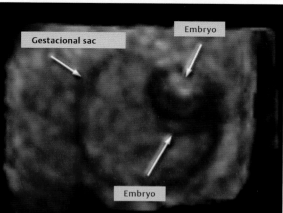

Fig. 13.2 Longitudinal ultrasound view of the uterus, gestational sac and yolk sac (top) and visualization of the embryo at the end of week 5 (bottom).

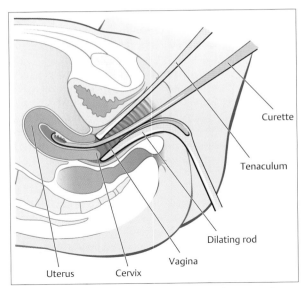

Fig. 13.3 For a dilation and curettage (D&C), the patient lies on her back, and a weighted retractor is placed in the vagina. A dilator is used to open the cervix, and a curette is used to scrape the inside of the uterus.

The absence of chorionic villi in the curettage specimen indicates the possibility of an EP.

Treatment Options

Less than 10% of patients with EP present with a surgical abdomen and signs of decreased blood volume (hypovolemia) and shock. Often, they present no diagnostic problem and require no specific intervention besides fluid and blood resuscitation, and immediate operation.

However, delayed hospital admission and treatment leads to maternal mortality. The majority of cases of EP can be treated medically (methotrexate), surgically (laparoscopy or laparotomy), or even by expectant management alone. The choice depends on the medical conditions, available resources, and the site of EP involved.

Surgical Treatment

Laparotomy Versus Laparoscopy

The standard operative procedure for the treatment of EP in the developed world is laparoscopy, which is a minimally invasive approach. Almost all tubal pregnancies in hemodynamically stable women can be removed laparoscopically, without the need for laparotomy. The excellent benefits of laparoscopic treatment include less blood loss, less analgesia, less postoperative pain, shorter recovery period, and decreased hospital costs.

Owing to lower perioperative and postoperative morbidity, lower cost and equivalent efficacy, laparoscopy is preferred to laparotomy for the treatment of EP. The only absolute contraindication for laparoscopy is shock or hemodynamic instability.

Salpingectomy, Salpingotomy, Salpingostomy, and Milking

The most commonly performed procedures are radical salpingectomy (removal of the affected tube), or salpingotomy (tubotomy that is closed) and salpingostomy (tubotomy that is left open). Salpingectomy is preferred in cases of ruptured ectopic pregnancy with uncontrolled bleeding, extensive tubal damage, recurrent EP in the same tube, and for sterilization. Salpingectomy for an unruptured EP is rarely performed. For a ruptured EP, linear salpingostomy, which preserves the tube, is the procedure of choice.

The EP is removed through a linear incision of 10–15 mm made into the tube on its antimesenteric border. The products will extrude from the incision and can be flushed out and evacuated. Both live birth rates and recurrent EP rates after a tubotomy were similar regardless of whether the incision was closed (salpingotomy) or left open to heal by secondary intension (salpingostomy). Laparoscopic salpingostomy is the preferred surgical procedure for an unruptured EP.

Manual expression or milking of the tube in order to effect a tubal abortion is possible only in cases of fimbrial pregnancy. The present consensus among tubal surgeons is that milking should be abandoned as it is associated with inordinately high recurrence of EPs, regardless of whether the procedure is performed by laparoscopy or laparotomy.

Medical Treatment with Methotrexate

Medical treatment with methotrexate has become a safe and effective treatment for EP. Methotrexate interferes with DNA synthesis, repair, and cellular replication.

Actively proliferating tissue such as the trophoblast cells of an EP are highly sensitive to these effects and become destabilized. More importantly, methotrexate does not subject patients to surgical intervention and possible associated complications. Thus, currently, methotrexate is considered the treatment of choice for EP.

Candidates for Medical Therapy

Hemodynamically stable patients without active bleeding or signs of hemoperitoneum are candidates for medical therapy. Also, these patients should be followed up for compliance because it requires careful use. Contraindications are summarized in **Table 13.2**. Absolute contraindications to medical therapy include breast-feeding, immunodeficiency, alcoholism, hepatic, pulmonary, renal or hematologic dysfunction, known sensitivity to methotrexate, blood dyscrasias, or peptic ulcer disease. Relative contraindications for methotrexate treatments include embryonic cardiac activity and gestational sac of 3.5 cm and above.

Because of its potential toxicity, patients receiving methotrexate should be followed-up cautiously and made aware of its potential side effects and signs of toxicity. During treatment, patients should be counseled to report promptly about signs and symptoms associated with tubal rupture, such as abdominal pain, dizziness, weakness, and syncope. Sexual intercourse, alcohol use, and nonsteroidal anti-inflammatory drugs as well as folic acid supplements, including prenatal vitamins consumption, are prohibited until serum HCG is undetectable.

It is clear that the main point for successful medical treatment is rigorous patient selection. Several orienting parameters aimed at choosing suitable patients should have already been assessed, such as the presence of fetal cardiac activity, size of the EP, initial levels of β-HCG and endometrial thickness.

Treatment Protocols

Typically, methotrexate is administered in a single dose, which is based on 50 mg/m^2 of body surface area, without the need for leucovorin rescue. Otherwise, methotrexate can be given using a multidose regimen of 1 mg/kg intramuscularly, alternating with 0.1 mg/kg of leucovorin intramuscularly for up to four daily doses of each drug. Both protocols have been demonstrated to have good success rates in the treatment of EP. The single-dose protocol is easier to administer and monitor, and results in fewer side effects. However, the single protocol is associated with a higher failure rate. Direct injection of methotrexate has lower efficacy than systemic administration and is not considered as a therapeutic alternative for EP.

Monitoring Efficacy of Therapy

The overall success rate of methotrexate treatments is 78–96%. Before treatment with methotrexate, blood analysis is required to establish baseline laboratory values for β-HCG levels and for renal, liver, and bone marrow functions. Blood type should be determined, since all patients with EP and who are Rh-negative require administration of Rh (D) immunoglobulin (50 μg).

For cost-effectiveness and convenience for the patient, outpatient observation is preferred. Patient monitoring continues until β-HCG levels are nondetectable. It usually takes a month or longer until HCG levels disappear from the plasma. With the single-dose treatment, levels of β-HCG generally increase during the first week subsequent to the treatment and peak at 4 days following injection.

If a response is observed and the fall in HCG level is above 15%, weekly serum HCG determinations should be measured until undetectable HCG levels are documented. Failure of the β-HCG level to decline requires that a second dose of methotrexate be administered. An additional dose of methotrexate may be given if β-HCG levels plateau or increase in one week. A persistent ectopic mass or hemoperitoneum may lead to a surgery.

Side Effects

Methotrexate has the potential for serious toxicity and, indeed, high doses can cause a number of serious side effects (see **Table 13.3**). Toxic effects usually are related to the amount and duration of therapy. Nevertheless, most side effects during regular treatment for EP are minor and self-limiting. They generally are restricted to an increase in hepatic transaminases, mild stomatitis, and gastrointestinal disturbances, including nausea and vomiting. Reproductive outcome after methotrexate treatment is basically favorable, and it seems that fertility depends more on the patients' previous medical history (i.e., a history of infertility) than on prior treatment for EP.

Table 13.2 Relative and absolute contraindications for methotrexate treatment

Absolute contraindications	Relative contraindications
Shock, hemodynamic instability	Embryonic cardiac activity
Known sensitivity to methotrexate	Gestational sac of 3.5 cm and above
Breast-feeding	
Immunodeficiency	
Alcoholism	
Hepatic, pulmonary, renal, or hematologic dysfunction	
Blood dyscrasias (bone-marrow hypoplasia, leukopenia, thrombocytopenia, significant anemia)	
Peptic ulcer disease	

Table 13.3 Potential side effects of methotrexate treatment

Adverse effect	Characteristics
Hepatotoxicity	Generally limited increase in hepatic transaminases
Stomatitis	Generally mild stomatitis, and gastrointestinal disturbance, nausea, vomiting.
Pulmonary fibrosis, pneomonitis	Severe neutropenia (rare)
Alopecia	
Photosensitivity	
Dizziness	
Bone marrow suppression (rare)	

Expectant Management

Some patients experience spontaneous resolution of their EP. In such patients an expectant management is optional in order to avoid unnecessary treatment. After clear demonstration that select cases of EP resolved without therapy, several studies of patients with EP have been conducted with consistently supportive results.

Candidates for successful expectant management must be asymptomatic, with an objective evidence of resolution (generally manifested by declining levels of HCG). In addition, they should be willing to accept the potential risks of tubal rupture and hemorrhage. Patients with early, small tubal gestations with lower (<200 mIU/mL) and falling HCG levels are the best candidates for expectant management.

Heterotropic Pregnancy

The occurrence of a heterotopic pregnancy (i.e., the coexistence of intrauterine and ectopic pregnancies) following spontaneous cycles is rare, with estimated incidence in the general population that varies between 1 in 4000 and 1 in 30000. Nevertheless, the incidence is increased to about 1 : 100 by the use of assisted reproductive techniques. It is particularly high among women undergoing ovulation induction with gonadotropins and among women undergoing IVF, since it has become standard practice to transfer at least two embryos with each IVF procedure.

Heterotropic pregnancy poses a diagnostic drawback. Serial HCG levels are not helpful due to the accompanying intrauterine pregnancy. Routine ultrasound scanning detects only half of the cases. This is because the intrauter-

ine pregnancy will be detected in the course of work-up, and the EP will be overlooked.

Also, in cases of nonviable intrauterine pregnancy, the presence of chorionic villi in the curettage specimen serves consistently to delay the correct diagnosis. Indeed, 50% of patients suffer from late diagnosis and arrive at the hospital after rupture.

There are no specific features to help the physician to make an accurate, early diagnosis of heterotopic pregnancy other than a general awareness for such a possibility. This is particularly important in cases of abdominal pain and tenderness accompanying normal intrauterine pregnancy, or following uterine curettage for a nonviable intrauterine pregnancy among patients who conceived following assisted reproductive techniques. Also, in cases of persistent or rising HCG levels following uterine curettage for a nonviable intrauterine pregnancy, the possibility of heterotopic pregnancy must be considered.

Treatment consists of removal of the EP by surgery and avoidance of intrauterine instrumentations, as well as systemic methotrexate treatment in cases where the pregnancy is desired (especially following assisted reproductive techniques). In hemodynamically unstable patients, an explorative laparotomy is necessary. Expectant management is problematic, since HCG levels cannot be monitored effectively due to the intrauterine pregnancy. On the other hand, the prognosis for the intrauterine pregnancy is excellent, and the majority are carried to term.

Nontubal Ectopic Pregnancy

In rare cases implantation can occur in other ectopic sites including the ovary, uterine cervix, and abdomen.

Interstitial (Cornual) Pregnancy

The interstitial part of the fallopian tube is the proximal portion that lies within the muscular wall of the uterus. Interstitial implantation of the blastocyst is the rarest form (1.9%) of *tubal* EP. Late diagnosis and treatment are the main contributing factors to the adverse outcome traditionally linked to these EP cases.

The traditional treatment of interstitial pregnancy has been hysterectomy or cornual resection by laparotomy. These patients tend to present later in gestation than other tubal pregnancies mainly because the myometrium (cornual part) is more distensible than the fallopian tube. However, progresses in diagnostic techniques lead toward conservative management with methotrexate, laparoscopic treatment including cornual resection, cornuostomy, salpingostomy, or salpingectomy, and even hysteroscopic removal (Evidence Box 13.1). Still, if uncontrolled hemorrhage occurs, hysterectomy might be the preferred treatment.

Abdominal Ectopic Pregnancy

Abdominal EP occurs in approximately 1 in 8000 births and represents 1.4% of EPs. The prognosis is generally poor with an estimated maternal mortality of 5.1 per 1000 cases. Several reports exist regarding abdominal pregnancies reaching near-term and viability. In such cases, the survival of the newborns is above 60%, although associated with a high rate of congenital anomalies. These include bone and joint deformities and central nervous system and skull anomalies, attributed to oligohydramnios.

Laparotomy is considered the treatment of choice for an abdominal EP with removal of the pregnancy with or without the placenta. However, alternative regimens have been used successfully and include the use of methotrexate or selective embolization of vessels feeding the placenta prior to definitive surgery and laparoscopic treatment.

Ovarian Pregnancy

Ovarian pregnancy is an infrequent variant of EP with an incidence of 0.5–3% of all EPs. It is likely, however, that the frequency is underestimated, since some of the suspected tubal pregnancies that are treated conservatively with methotrexate were, in fact, early ovarian pregnancies. Usually, the pathologist only retrospectively confirms such cases, since they often are mistakenly considered as ruptured corpus luteum. Recent improvements in ultrasonography and operative laparoscopy should lead to an earlier and a more accurate diagnosis of these pregnancies.

Clinical findings are similar to those encountered in tubal pregnancy. The major presenting symptom (in almost all patients) is abdominal pain. Oophorectomy was considered as the treatment of choice for ovarian pregnancies. Nevertheless, improvement in operative laparoscopic skills and instrumentation are leading to a more conservative approach. Laparoscopic wedge resection and ovarian cystectomy have become the preferred treatment. Successful treatment with methotrexate also has been reported, although immediate laparotomy is mandatory in patients with circulatory collapse.

Cervical Pregnancy

Cervical pregnancy results from implantation of the blastocyst within the cervical canal. Its incidence varies from 1 in 2400 to 1 in 50 000 pregnancies. Over the past 20 years, appropriate early diagnosis and treatment have dramatically reduced maternal mortality for this condition from 50% to less than 5%.

A close relationship has been found between cervical pregnancies and therapeutic abortions with sharp curettage (dilatation and curettage), previous cesarean sections, and IVF. Presenting symptoms include painless vaginal bleeding, although it may be accompanied by abdominal pain and urinary problems. On physical examination, the cervix is usually enlarged, global (barreled shaped), and distended. Occasionally, the external os is dilated.

Accurate diagnosis can be performed by transvaginal ultrasonography and magnetic resonance imaging, demonstrating an intracervical ectopic sac below a closed internal cervical os. Transvaginal demonstration of an intact part of the cervical canal between the endometrium and gestational sac is suggestive of cervical pregnancy.

Conservative medical (with systemic methotrexate) or surgical management of a cervical EP has been reported to be successful, obviating the need for surgical treatment, which entails a risk for hysterectomy. Dilation and evacuation followed by cervical tamponade has been successfully applied, specifically while using a Foley catheter tamponade. Methotrexate is the most commonly used chemotherapy for cervical pregnancies, with a success rate of about 80%. Other treatment regimens include arterial embolization, and even Shirodkar cerclage placement, in order to reduce bleeding. Still, in cases of massive and uncontrolled vaginal bleeding, abdominal hysterectomy is necessary.

Key Points

- Ectopic pregnancy (EP) is a major health problem for women of reproductive age and is the leading cause of pregnancy-related death during the first 20 weeks of pregnancy.
- The most common site of EP implantation (98% of cases) is the fallopian tubes.
- The most common initiator of EP is tubal obstruction and injury.
- The classic symptom triad of EP includes amenorrhea, irregular bleeding, and lower abdominal pain or tenderness.
- Abdominal and pelvic tenderness, especially cervical motion tenderness, are common when a rupture has occurred.

Evidence Box 13.1

The majority of cornual (interstitial) ectopic pregnancies can be effectively managed with laparoscopy.

Ng et al. retrospectively reviewed 53 cases of cornual ectopic pregnancy treated from 2001 to 2006 laparoscopically at the K. K. Women and Children's Hospital in Singapore. Fifty-two of the 56 cases were managed by laparoscopy, and one was converted to laparotomy. Laparoscopic wedge resection was carried out in 33 patients, cornuostomy in 13 patients, and salpingectomy in 7 patients. Nine patients received methotrexate injection after surgery because of persistently high serum β-HCG. Eighteen patients became pregnant, four had early miscarriages, and ten had pregnancies beyond 24 weeks' gestation. Five delivered vaginally, and three had cesarean section at term. Two patients traveled back to their native countries for delivery. There were no cases of uterine rupture or dehiscence reported. The investigators conclude that laparoscopic treatment of cornual pregnancy is safe and effective when carried out in an institution with a trained laparoscopist and adequate facilities.

Ng S, Hamontri S, Chua I, Chern B, Siow A. Laparoscopic management of 53 cases of cornual ectopic pregnancy. Fertil Steril 2009; 92 (2): 448–52

Further Reading

Al-Sunaidi M, Tulandi T. Surgical treatment of ectopic pregnancy. *Semin Reprod Med* 2007;25(2):117–122

Buster JE, Krotz S. Reproductive performance after ectopic pregnancy. *Semin Reprod Med* 2007;25(2):131–133

Cheong Y, Li TC. Controversies in the management of ectopic pregnancy. *Reprod Biomed Online* 2007;15(4):396–402

Hajenius PJ, Mol F, Mol BW, Bossuyt PM, Ankum WM, van der Veen F. Interventions for tubal ectopic pregnancy. *Cochrane Database Syst Rev* 2007; (1):CD000324

Menon S, Colins J, Barnhart KT. Establishing a human chorionic gonadotropin cutoff to guide methotrexate treatment of ectopic pregnancy: a systematic review. *Fertil Steril* 2007;87(3):481–484

Mukul LV, Teal SB. Current management of ectopic pregnancy. *Obstet Gynecol Clin North Am* 2007;34(3):403–419

Practice Committee of the American Society for Reproductive Medicine. Medical treatment of ectopic pregnancy. *Fertil Steril* 2006; 86(5, Suppl):S96–S102

Reece EA, Petrie RH, Sirmans MF, Finster M, Todd WD. Combined intrauterine and extrauterine gestations: a review. *Am J Obstet Gynecol* 1983;146(3):323–330

Tulandi T, Saleh A. Surgical management of ectopic pregnancy. *Clin Obstet Gynecol* 1999;42(1):31–38, quiz 55–56

Wiznitzer A, Sheiner E. Ectopic and heterotopic pregnancies. In: Reece EA, Hobbins JC, ed. Clinical Obstetrics: the Fetus and Mother. Malden, Mass: Blackwell Synergy Publishing; 2007, pp. 161–176

14 Spontaneous Abortion

Daniela Carusi

Many terms are used to describe spontaneous abortion, including miscarriage, chemical pregnancy, early pregnancy loss, embryonic or fetal demise, or blighted ovum. These refer to a pregnancy prior to 20 weeks of gestation that has ceased development, or has passed, or begun to pass, from the uterus. Though common, the event may be devastating to patients, and health care providers must be comfortable handling the woman's medical and psychological needs through this process.

Definitions

Chemical pregnancy: This is a pregnancy that is identified by a positive human chorionic gonadotropin (HCG) level, which is lost prior to 5 weeks' gestation. Clinical studies on miscarriage and recurrent pregnancy loss often do not include these common events.

Blighted ovum: Development of trophoblast and a gestational sac, but no evidence of embryonic development. This may also be called an *anembryonic gestation.* A sac that measures 16 mm or greater in diameter with no embryo is abnormal.

Missed abortion: A pregnancy is identified as "failed," but no tissue has passed and the cervix is closed.

Threatened abortion: The patient has vaginal bleeding, but the cervix is closed and the pregnancy otherwise appears viable. If a fetal heartbeat has been seen at 10 weeks' gestation, then these patients have a 98% probability of continuing the pregnancy without a loss.

Inevitable abortion: The patient has an open cervix, usually with bleeding and cramping, but the pregnancy has not passed and otherwise appears viable.

Incomplete abortion: The cervix has opened and some, but not all, pregnancy tissue has passed.

Completed abortion: A previously identified pregnancy has passed, the uterus has contracted down, bleeding has diminished, and the cervix has closed. HCG levels, if drawn, would fall to zero. If ultrasound scanning or pathological analyses were performed, there would be no evidence of pregnancy tissue.

Septic abortion: Pregnancy loss accompanied by uterine infection or endometritis. If not promptly treated, this can develop into pelvic inflammatory disease, sepsis, and death.

Molar pregnancy: This is a form of gestational trophoblastic disease marked by hydropic placental villi and abnormally high HCG levels. With a *complete mole*, there is no embryonic development and HCG levels may be dangerously high. With a *partial mole*, there may be development of a triploid fetus. Both types of molar pregnancy are nonviable.

Recurrent abortion: Also called *recurrent pregnancy loss (RPL)* or *habitual abortion*, this refers to three, sequential, pregnancy losses, usually with no history of a term delivery. Such an outcome is unlikely to occur by chance, and therefore evaluation for a medical problem in the parents is indicated. Some clinicians initiate a work-up after two miscarriages.

Incidence and Risk Factors

Spontaneous abortion is, unfortunately, a common event in early pregnancy: 15% of clinical pregnancies end in a spontaneous abortion, with an even higher proportion lost before 5 weeks' gestation. The vast majority (80%) of miscarriages occur before 12 weeks' gestation, while the risk of miscarriage after 16 weeks is less than 1%.

There is a strong relationship between maternal age and risk of miscarriage. While the risk of miscarriage is 9% for a 20–24-year-old, that risk increases to 15% for a 30–34-year-old and 51% for a 40–44-year-old. Advancing age of the father may contribute as well, but to a much lesser extent.

While most miscarriages are sporadic events, a history of miscarriages, particularly multiple miscarriages, increases the risk of having another. In one study, the miscarriage risk was 5% for women who had never had a prior miscarriage, 20% for those with one prior miscarriage, and 43% for those with three prior losses.

Miscarriage risk has also been associated with cigarette smoking, cocaine use, high levels of caffeine intake, and extremes of body mass index.

Etiology

In most cases of first trimester miscarriage, no specific cause is identified. A formal evaluation is generally not performed after one or two first-trimester losses. However, a more thorough work-up is performed if a woman has had recurrent pregnancy losses or one second-trimester spontaneous abortion.

Chromosomal Abnormalities

Aneuploidy (an abnormal number of chromosomes) is the most common cause of first trimester miscarriage. This is usually due to random nondisjunction during egg development, and the risk increases with maternal age. Genetic or chromosomal abnormalities can also develop as the embryo develops and cells rapidly divide. Trisomy 16 is the most common aneuploidy found in early pregnancy losses. Sex chromosome abnormalities and the trisomies 21, 13, and 18 are less common, but more likely to survive beyond the first trimester (**Fig. 14.1**).

Structural Problems

A physical defect in the cavity of the uterus may contribute to miscarriage. These include uterine fibroids, a septum (**Fig. 14.2**), scar tissue, or possibly a large polyp. While this could contribute to any pregnancy loss, it should be particularly considered with second trimester or recurrent losses.

Cervical insufficiency or incompetence refers to a second trimester condition in which the cervix inappropriately opens without labor. The cause of this condition is poorly understood.

Thrombosis

Blood clots forming in the placenta or uterus may lead to loss of the fetus. This is an unusual circumstance, but may occur in patients who carry a thrombophilia. This may be inherited (e.g., factor V Leiden mutation or prothrombin gene mutation) or acquired (e.g., antiphospholipid antibodies).

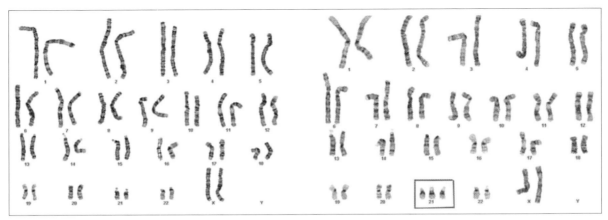

Fig. 14.1 Normal female karyotype (left), and karyotype of a female fetus with trisomy 21 (three copies of chromosome 21, boxed in red).

Placental Complications

Placental bleeding increases the risk of miscarriage. In the first trimester this is usually identified as a subchorionic hematoma, while in the second trimester the placenta may abrupt (prematurely separate). However, hematomas are frequently seen on early ultrasound scans, and do not imply that the pregnancy will be lost. In rare cases, placental insufficiency in the second trimester may lead to oligohydramnios, growth restriction, and fetal demise.

Infection

Certain viruses and bacteria may infect the placenta and fetus, leading to fetal demise in the second trimester. The infection may pass from the mother's blood stream or it may cross directly from the vagina. Rarely, the patient may develop a severe uterine infection, also called a septic abortion, which can be fatal if not promptly treated.

Endocrine Disorders

Miscarriage has been linked to uncorrected thyroid disease, diabetes, and hyperprolactinemia. Patients with the polycystic ovarian syndrome also have a higher rate of miscarriage than the general population. In a few women the corpus luteum produces insufficient progesterone, a condition known as luteal phase insufficiency. This is marked by a short luteal phase and recurrent chemical pregnancies, and usually requires an endometrial biopsy for diagnosis.

Fetal Abnormalities

Severe congenital abnormalities may lead to fetal demise in the second trimester.

Exposures

Medications, environmental exposures, and basic radiologic studies are highly unlikely to produce miscarriage. More extreme exposures, such as treatment with chemotherapeutic agents, high-dose radiation (such as for cancer treatment or thyroid irradiation), or prostaglandins can result in pregnancy loss.

Procedures

The risk of spontaneous loss is increased following chorionic villus sampling or amniocentesis. The risk of loss is slightly increased after nonuterine surgery performed under general anesthesia. Patients who undergo removal of the corpus luteum (owing to rupture, torsion, or hemorrhage) must have progesterone replacement prior to 9–10 weeks' gestation in order to avoid spontaneous loss.

Diagnosis

Diagnosis of a spontaneous abortion usually involves a combination of history, physical examination, ultrasonography, and laboratory tests, though not all of these may be required. While a history and physical examination are always used, the choice of other studies depends on the gestational age of the pregnancy.

By history, the patient often reports vaginal bleeding or spotting, which may be accompanied by menstrual-like cramps. With passage of the pregnancy, the bleeding may be heavy and the cramping quite severe. At times the patient may have no symptoms, and the miscarriage is identified incidentally when she has a routine ultrasound scan. A pregnancy loss may be marked by a loss of the usual pregnancy symptoms (nausea, breast tender-

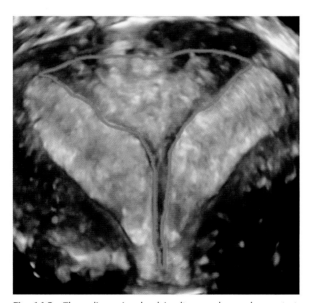

Fig. 14.2 Three-dimensional pelvic ultrasound scan demonstrating a complete uterine septum. The fibrous septum is outlined in blue.

ness, fatigue), but absence of such symptoms should not prompt concern on its own.

Physical examination should include an abdominal exam, speculum exam of the vagina, and bimanual pelvic exam. Findings may include a tender uterus, bleeding from the cervical os, or a dilated cervix. With a missed or completed abortion, the physical examination may be completely normal.

The health care provider must confirm that the patient is (or was) pregnant. This is generally accomplished with urine or serum HCG testing. If tissue is obtained—either by having the patient bring passed tissue to the provider or removing it from the cervix or vagina—pregnancy can be verified when chorionic villi or fetal parts are identified.

Prior to the fifth week of gestation, or a quantitative HCG level of 2000 mIU/mL, the pregnancy cannot be seen on ultrasound imaging. In this early stage, an abnormal pregnancy is diagnosed when the HCG level falls, or fails to rise by 50% over a 48-hour period. It is very important to confirm that the pregnancy is not ectopic (extra-uterine), as this can lead to a life-threatening emergency. Once the abnormal pregnancy is identified, the uterus is either evacuated to confirm that the tissue was in the uterus, or the HCG level is followed to zero.

At approximately 5 weeks' gestation, or an HCG level of 2000 mIU/mL, the gestational sac is usually visible on transvaginal ultrasonography (TVUS). Beyond this point, a miscarriage may be diagnosed using the following ultrasound criteria:

- The HCG level has reached 2000 mIU/mL or more and no sac is visible on high-quality TVUS (some will use a cutoff value of 4000 mIU/mL to account for a possible twin pregnancy).
- There is a large, empty sac (16–20 mm in dimension) with no embryo.
- The embryo has reached 6 mm or more, but has no heartbeat.
- A previously seen heartbeat is now absent.
- There is no growth of the pregnancy over 1 week or more.

Treatment

First Trimester

After a first trimester miscarriage, patients have three treatment options: medical management, surgical management with dilation and curettage (D&C), or expectant management with spontaneous pregnancy passage.

Traditionally, all miscarriages were treated with D&C of the uterus. Women are usually given intravenous seda-

tion or narcotics as well as a local paracervical block for the procedure. The cervix is then opened with rigid dilators, and a suction curette is passed into the uterus. The products of conception are then evacuated with suction. This is a very safe procedure, with small risks of heavy bleeding, infection, or uterine perforation. However, some patients prefer to avoid a surgical procedure and pass the products of conception on their own; recent studies show that this can be a safe option (Evidence Box 14.1).

Not all miscarriages will pass without intervention. When managed expectantly, rates of spontaneous passage are 50–60% within 2 weeks and 65–75% within 6 weeks. For this reason, women who want to avoid a surgical procedure may choose to induce miscarriage with misoprostol. The patient places 800 mcg of misoprostol into the vagina, and within 24–48 hours the uterus should contract and the gestational sac should pass. A second dose can be used if this does not occur. This method is 80–85% successful, and significantly more effective than expectant management. It produces more bleeding than D&C, but infection risk is no different than with surgical treatment or expectant management.

Patients with incomplete abortion have the same treatment options, though there is less evidence that medical management in this case is any better than expectant management. Patients who present with hemorrhage or infection need to undergo prompt treatment with D&C, and, in the latter case, intravenous antibiotics.

Second Trimester

Expectant management is generally not offered with second trimester pregnancy losses, and treatment (medical or surgical) takes place within a medical facility. This helps to ensure complete evacuation of the pregnancy, and allows for active management of heavy bleeding.

In the setting of a second-trimester fetal demise, misoprostol may be used to induce uterine contractions and expulsion of the pregnancy. Doses of 400–600 mcg are given vaginally every 6–12 hours until the pregnancy is expelled. Intravenous narcotics or epidural anesthesia (for larger pregnancies) is usually required for analgesia.

Cervical dilation and evacuation of the pregnancy is technically more challenging in the second trimester, and usually requires a health care professional with specialized training. If the cervix has not spontaneously dilated, laminaria tents are placed within the cervix one to two days before the procedure to allow wide dilation. The procedure is performed under intravenous conscious sedation or general anesthesia.

Post-Treatment Evaluation and Counseling

First Trimester

Following D&C or spontaneous passage of the gestational sac and fetus, patients will have moderate to light bleeding for up to 14 days. More prolonged bleeding, heavy bleeding, infection, or failure of menses to return suggests that some trophoblast is left behind. This may be treated with D&C or, in a very stable patient, with prolonged expectant management or misoprostol. HCG levels should fall quickly after a completed miscarriage, and a slow decline or persistently elevated levels after three or more weeks suggest retained tissue. However, a negative HCG level does not confirm that all of the tissue has passed. Rising or high levels may suggest trophoblastic disease or retained viable tissue.

No additional work-up is indicated after one or two first trimester miscarriages. These patients should be reassured that they did not cause their own miscarriage, and that the next pregnancy is very likely to proceed normally. Though the prognosis is good, these patients may be devastated by their pregnancy loss, and sensitivity and possible grief counseling are in order.

Recurrent First Trimester Losses

Following three or more sequential losses, work-up for an underlying cause is indicated. If possible, the pregnancy tissue from the most recent loss should be sent for chromosome analysis. Both parents should have their own karyotypes checked for balanced translocations. The uterus should be evaluated for structural defects, usually with hysterosalpingogram (HSG), hysteroscopy, or sonohysterography. The woman should have her blood tested for thyroid-stimulating hormone (TSH) and prolactin levels, and those at risk for diabetes should be screened for this disorder.

The woman should also be tested for antiphospholipid antibody syndrome (APAS) by checking levels of anticardiolipin antibodies and for the presence of the lupus anticoagulant. This disorder may also be diagnosed in the presence of a false-positive rapid plasma reagin (RPR) or anti-beta-2 glycoprotein antibodies. Patients diagnosed with APAS may be treated with heparin and aspirin for future pregnancy attempts, which appears to reduce the risk of miscarriage recurrence.

Inherited thrombophilias have been epidemiologically linked to recurrent miscarriage; however, there is no evidence that treating these patients with aspirin or heparin will decrease the risk of future losses. Thus screening for these thrombophilias after first trimester miscarriages is somewhat controversial.

Second Trimester Pregnancy Loss

Further work-up is indicated after any second trimester pregnancy loss. This should proceed in a stepwise fashion:

1. The fetal and placental tissue should be sent for a pathological analysis. The placenta may show signs of thrombosis or infection, and the fetus may have congenital anomalies or signs of a genetic syndrome.
2. The fetal and placental chromosomes should be analyzed.
3. Four to six weeks after the loss, the uterus can be evaluated for structural abnormalities, as with recurrent first trimester losses.
4. If the patient showed signs of infection, she should have bacterial blood cultures and antibody titers sent for analysis. The latter includes screening for cytomegalovirus, toxoplasmosis, parvovirus, and syphilis. Testing for herpes simplex virus or varicella may be guided by the clinical picture. If possible, the amniotic fluid and placenta should be tested for infection as well.
5. If the placental tissue showed signs of thrombosis or infarction, the patient can be tested for thrombophilias. This may also be done if no other explanation exists for the miscarriage. The link between thrombophilia and pregnancy loss is stronger in the second trimester than in the first, and there is some evidence that anticoagulant treatment will reduce the risk of recurrent loss.
6. If no other cause has been found, the parents' chromosomes may be analyzed for rearrangements.

If a likely cause is found, the other tests are usually not necessary. The order of the tests may be guided by the patient's history. For example, if there is a family history of blood clots or birth defects, these items may be evaluated right away.

Cervical incompetence is usually obvious at the time of miscarriage, as the patient presents with painless dilatation of her cervix. These women may choose to have a cerclage placed around the cervix in future pregnancies, or have the cervix watched closely with ultrasound imaging.

Often no cause is found for either recurrent early losses or a second trimester loss. This is understandably difficult for the patients involved, but they should still be encouraged that future normal pregnancies are possible. These patients should be followed closely with ultrasound scanning in the future, so that abnormalities can be detected early. Generally there is no proven treatment to offer these patients; however, one meta-analysis suggests that progesterone supplementation may benefit patients with two or more early miscarriages. Much more high-quality research is needed in this area.

Key Points

- Spontaneous abortion, also known as miscarriage, refers to a pregnancy that spontaneously ceases to progress before the embryo or fetus reaches viability. In practice this corresponds to about 20 weeks' gestation or 500 gm fetal weight.
- Spontaneous abortion occurs in about 10–20 % of clinically recognized pregnancies.
- Most women with a spontaneous abortion present with vaginal bleeding.
- Risk factors include advanced maternal age, smoking and a previous spontaneous abortion.
- Most spontaneous abortions are due to chromosomal or structural anomalies of the embryo and fetus.
- Ultrasonography of the pelvis is the most useful test in the evaluation of women suspected of having a spontaneous abortion.
- Spontaneous abortions can be managed expectantly, or with misoprostol to induce uterine contractions and expulsion of the pregnancy tissue or with surgical suction curettage.
- If a woman with an spontaneous abortion has a concomitant uterine infection, she should receive broad-spectrum antibiotics followed by surgical suction curettage in order to prevent sepsis.
- If a woman with a spontaneous abortion is bleeding heavily, she should have surgical suction curettage.

"unplanned" procedure for retained products of conception were higher in the expectant and medical groups than in the surgical group.

For those with incomplete spontaneous abortion, rates of D&C were even lower for the expectant and medical management groups, at 25 % and 29 %, respectively. Furthermore, those in the medical management groups had no increased risk of a delayed procedure for retained products of conception when compared to those in the surgical group.

In the medical management arm, this trial stands out in its use of mifepristone for patients with missed abortion, and its performance of D&C if there was no response to medication within eight hours. In a separate study, Zhang et al showed that by using misoprostol alone, repeating the dose if there were no initial response, and giving patients 8 days to pass the gestational sac, 84 % of patients with medical management could avoid D&C.

Trinder J, Brocklehurst P, Porter R, et al. Management of miscarriage: expectant, medical, or surgical? Results of randomised controlled trial (miscarriage treatment [MIST] trial). BMJ 2006;332(7552):1235–1240.

Zhang J, Gilles JM, Barnhart Kurt, et al. A comparison of medical management with misoprostol and surgical management for early pregnancy failure. N Engl J Med 2005;353(8):761–769.

Evidence Box 14.1

Expectant and medical management are appropriate treatment options for early spontaneous abortion.

Traditionally, spontaneous abortion was always treated with dilation of the cervix and evacuation of the uterus. However, this surgical procedure requires analgesia and carries small risks of uterine perforation. Some patients prefer to avoid a surgical procedure, and recent evidence shows that it can be safe for them to pass their pregnancies without a surgical intervention.

The MIST trial randomized 1200 women with a first trimester spontaneous abortion to suction curettage, medical management, or expectant management. They included women with missed abortion (either an empty gestational sac or embryonic/fetal demise) or incomplete abortion, as long as there were no signs of hemorrhage or infection. Their primary outcome measure was gynecologic infection within 14 days of study entry, while the secondary outcomes included success of the treatment (no unplanned uterine curettage within eight weeks of follow-up), side effects, and complications.

This trial found that the rates of infection were similarly low (approximately 3 %) with surgical, medical, and expectant management (see **Table 14.1**). For those with a missed abortion or early demise, 50 % in the expectant management arm were able to avoid any dilation and curettage (D&C), while 62 % in the medical management arm avoided a procedure. On the other hand, the rates of a later,

Table 14.1 Outcomes of various management approaches in missed and incomplete abortion

Outcome	Surgical management	Expectant management	Medical management
Missed abortion	N = 310	N = 306	N = 308
Infection	13 (4 %)	12 (4 %)	9 (3 %)
Any D&C	278 (90 %)	**154 (50 %)**	**116 (38 %)**
Unplanned D&C	20 (6 %)	**154 (50 %)**	**16 (15 %)**
Incomplete abortion	N = 92	N = 92	N = 90
Infection	3 (3 %)	2 (2 %)	3 (3 %)
Any D&C	78 (85 %)	**23 (25 %)**	**26 (29 %)**
Unplanned D&C	2 (2 %)	**23 (25 %)**	**6 (7 %)**

Source: Adapted from Trinder et al. BMJ 2006;332(7552):1235–1240. Items in bold face are significantly different from the surgical management arm.

Further Reading

Bagratee JS, Khullar V, Regan L, Moodley J, Kagoro H. A randomized controlled trial comparing medical and expectant management of first trimester miscarriage. *Hum Reprod* 2004;19(2):266–271

Barnhart KT, Bader T, Huang X, Frederick MM, Timbers KA, Zhang JJ. Hormone pattern after misoprostol administration for a nonviable first-trimester gestation. *Fertil Steril* 2004;81(4):1099–1105

Barnhart KT, Simhan H, Kamelle SA. Diagnostic accuracy of ultrasound above and below the beta-hCG discriminatory zone. *Obstet Gynecol* 1999;94(4):583–587

Cnattingius S, Signorello LB, Annerén G, et al. Caffeine intake and the risk of first-trimester spontaneous abortion. *N Engl J Med* 2000;343(25):1839–1845

Empson M, Lassere M, Craig J, Scott J. Prevention of recurrent miscarriage for women with antiphospholipid antibody or lupus anticoagulant. Cochrane Database of Systematic Reviews 2007 Issue 4

Goldhaber MK, Fireman BH. Re: "Estimates of the annual number of clinically recognized pregnancies in the United States, 1981-1991". [comment] *Am J Epidemiol* 2000;152(3):287–289

Haas DM, Ramsey PS. Progestogen for preventing miscarriage [Systematic Review] *Cochrane Database Syst Rev* 2009; 3:CD003511

Henriksen TB, Hjollund NH, Jensen TK, et al. Alcohol consumption at the time of conception and spontaneous abortion. *Am J Epidemiol* 2004;160(7):661–667

Kaandorp S, Di Nisio, Goddijn M et al. Aspirin or anticoagulants for treating recurrent miscarriage on women without antiphospholipid syndrome [Systematic Review] *Cochrane Database of Systematic Rev* 2009; 3:CD004734

Knudsen UB, Hansen V, Juul S, Secher NJ. Prognosis of a new pregnancy following previous spontaneous abortions. *Eur J Obstet Gynecol Reprod Biol* 1991;39(1):31–36

Luise C, Jermy K, Collons WP, Bourne TH. Expectant management of incomplete, spontaneous first-trimester miscarriage: outcome according to initial ultrasound criteria and value of follow-up visits. *Ultrasound Obstet Gynecol* 2002;19(6):580–582

Metwally M, Ong KJ, Ledger WL, Li TC. Does high body mass index increase the risk of miscarriage after spontaneous and assisted conception? A meta-analysis of the evidence. *Fertil Steril* 2008;90(3):714–726

Ness RB, Grisso JA, Hirschinger N, et al. Cocaine and tobacco use and the risk of spontaneous abortion. *N Engl J Med* 1999;340(5):333–339

Regan L, Braude PR, Trembath PL. Influence of past reproductive performance on risk of spontaneous abortion. *BMJ* 1989;299(6698):541–545

Rey E, Kahn SR, David M, Shrier I. Thrombophilic disorders and fetal loss: a meta-analysis. *Lancet* 2003;361(9361):901–908

Tabor A, Philip J, Madsen M, Bang J, Obel EB, Nørgaard-Pedersen B. Randomised controlled trial of genetic amniocentesis in 4606 low-risk women. *Lancet* 1986;1(8493):1287–1293

Trinder J, Brocklehurst P, Porter R, Read M, Vyas S, Smith L. Management of miscarriage: expectant, medical, or surgical? Results of randomised controlled trial (miscarriage treatment (MIST) trial). *BMJ* 2006;332(7552):1235–1240

Weiss JL, Malone FD, Vidaver J, et al; FASTER Consortium. Threatened abortion: A risk factor for poor pregnancy outcome, a population-based screening study. *Am J Obstet Gynecol* 2004;190(3):745–750

Zhang J, Gilles JM, Barnhart K, Creinin MD, Westhoff C, Frederick MM; National Institute of Child Health Human Development (NICHD) Management of Early Pregnancy Failure Trial. A comparison of medical management with misoprostol and surgical management for early pregnancy failure. *N Engl J Med* 2005;353(8):761–769

15 Pathological Labor and Delivery

Adi Y. Weintraub, Fernanda Press, and Arnon Wiznitzer

In order for labor and delivery to occur, uterine quiescence, which is the norm throughout pregnancy, is disrupted. Labor and delivery begin when regular uterine contractions activate and continue to the delivery of the fetus and the placenta. For a successful delivery, the fetus should be lying longitudinally, the presenting part is usually vertex, and there are effective contractions and an adequate relation between maternal pelvis and the passenger (i.e., the fetus). These conditions are termed the three "P's" for:

- passenger—the fetus
- pelvis—the maternal pelvis and birth canal
- power—the effectiveness of uterine contractions

An abnormal labor is defined as labor dystocia (see Definitions below) and refers to any deviation from the norm. The causes of abnormal labor may include maternal pathologic conditions (related or unrelated to gestation), fetal abnormalities, or problems in the relationship between both. This chapter will focus on pathologies in the timing of labor, most notably *preterm labor*, and problems that occur during labor and delivery, or *abnormal labor*.

Preterm Labor

Definitions

Cervical insufficiency: Also called *incompetent cervix*, this is a condition where the cervix begins to dilate during pregnancy (without contractions) before the fetus is ready to be born, such as in the second trimester. Depending on the point in pregnancy at which this occurs, cervical insufficiency can lead to miscarriage, stillbirth, or preterm delivery. Cervical insufficiency tends to be a recurring problem.

Cervical ripening: Refers to a change in the cervix with respect to its readiness to become softer, more flexible, more distensible, and shorter during the final weeks of pregnancy. These cervical changes can also be chemically induced (i.e., induced labor).

Contractility: This property relates to the ability of the uterus to shrink or contract.

Cervicovaginal secretions: Secretions that contain cytokines of maternal origin, inflammatory cells, and proteolytic enzymes, which act to protect the intra-amniotic compartment from infectious agents that may ascend along the birth canal.

Dystocia: A slow or difficult labor or delivery caused by an obstruction or constriction of the birth passage or the abnormal shape, size, position, or condition of the fetus.

Low birth weight neonates: Infants who weigh less than 2500 g at birth are regarded as low birth weight neonates. Those born with weights of 1500 g or less are considered *very low birth weight neonates*, and those who weigh less than 1000 g are defined as *extremely low birth weight neonates*.

Preterm birth: A human birth that occurs before 37 completed weeks of gestation (less than 259 days) is called preterm birth (PTB). A *very preterm birth* is typically defined as one of less than 32–34 weeks' gestation, and an *extremely preterm birth* is one that occurs at less than 28 weeks' gestation. Infants born prematurely at 34–36 weeks' gestation are referred to as "near-term" infants.

Preterm Labor: Labor that begins after 20 weeks, when the fetus is considered viable and before the 37th week, when the fetus is considered full-term, is referred to as preterm labor (PTL).

Diagnosis

The use of transvaginal cervical ultrasonography and assays to detect fetal fibronectin (fFN) in cervicovaginal secretions has greatly improved the diagnosis of *preterm labors* that have a likelihood of leading to PTBs. The value of these tests is that, if they are negative, they can help the physician avoid unnecessarily hospitalizing or transferring a woman who is experiencing false PTL. Other biomarkers have been found to have some association with the timing of birth but are not routinely used to predict PTB in women with symptoms of PTL.

Epidemiology and Prevalence

PTL that eventually leads to preterm delivery affects approximately 5–7% of live births in developed countries. Significantly higher rates are found in developing countries. Prematurity due to PTL is one of the leading causes of infant mortality and accounts for approximately 28% of neonatal mortality worldwide. Around 45–50% of PTBs are idiopathic, or spontaneous; 30% are related to premature rupture of membranes (PROM) (see Chapter 20); and another 15–20% are attributed to medically induced or elective preterm deliveries for maternal or fetal indications.

The percentage of preterm and low birth weight deliveries has been increasing steadily since the mid-1980s. The preterm delivery rate has been reported to be 11% in the United States, between 5% and 7% in Europe, and approximately 6.5% in Canada.

In the United States, there has been a 20% rise in the overall proportion of PTBs since 1990. However, due to better management of this condition, infant mortality rates in the United States have declined during this same period (**Fig. 15.1**).

The major reason for the increase in PTBs is a higher rate of multiple gestation. The shift toward earlier delivery that is observed among singletons is even more profound among multiples. Between 1990 and 2005, the percentage of twins delivered preterm has risen from 48% to 60% with large increases seen among twins born both at less than 34 weeks, and at 34–36 weeks. A marked trend to shorter pregnancies is also observed among triplets.

Additional contributors to the increase in the rate of PTBs include changes in obstetrical management (e.g., expanded use of ultrasound imaging and induction of labor for abnormal findings), patient demographic factors (e.g., more women giving birth at advanced maternal ages), and patient behavioral characteristics (**Fig. 15.2**).

Income level also has been implicated in the rate of PTBs. Researchers, for example, studied the trends in PTBs, low weight births, and intrauterine growth restriction rates in southern Brazil from 1982 to 2004. During

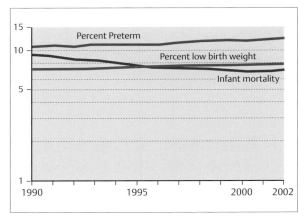

Fig. 15.1 Infant mortality rate per 1000 preterm births, and low birth weight per 100 live births. Rates are plotted on a log scale. Preterm is defined as less than 37 completed weeks of gestation and low birth weight as less than 2500 g. Reproduced from the National Vital Statistics System, National Center for Health Statistics, Centers for Disease Control and Prevention.

this time, they found a slight increase in the prevalence of low weight births from 9% to 10%. Intrauterine growth restriction decreased from 14.8% in 1982 to 12% in 2004, whereas PTBs more than doubled from 6.3% in 1982 to 14.7% in 2004. This dramatic increase in PTBs was only partially explained by pregnancy interruptions due either to caesarean sections or to labor inductions. When the investigators looked at other factors, they found that PTB rates more than doubled between 1982 and 2004 from 5.7% to 13.5% among higher income families (**Fig. 15.3**).

Etiology and Pathophysiology of Preterm Birth

Birth weight and gestational age are the two most important predictors of an infant's subsequent health and survival. Infants born too small or too soon or who weigh 2500 g or more have an increased risk of death or short-term and long-term disability than normal sized and weight infants born at term.

There is a remarkable relationship between gestational age and infant mortality. Infant mortality falls exponentially until term. Because of their much greater risk of death, infants born at the lowest gestational ages have a large impact on overall infant mortality. For example, in the United States only 0.8% of births occurred at less than 28 weeks' gestation, but they accounted for nearly half (46.4%) of all infant deaths in the United States in 2005.

The morbidity associated with prematurity is equally concerning. Disability occurs in 60% of survivors of birth at 26 weeks and in 30% of those born at 31 weeks. The morbidity and mortality rates of near-term infants approach those of term infants, but are still higher. In one

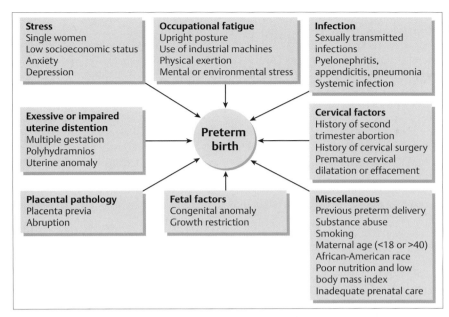

Fig. 15.2 Risk factors for preterm birth.

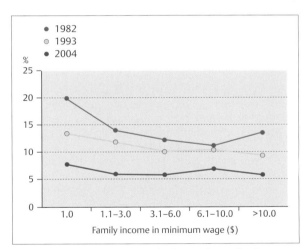

Fig. 15.3 Prevalence of preterm birth according to family income. Pelotas, southern Brazil, 1982, 1993, and 2004.

study, mortality rates at 34, 35, and 36 weeks of gestation were 0.11, 0.15, and 0.05%, respectively, compared with 0.02% at 39 weeks.

Preterm delivery is associated with immediate and long-term neonatal complications. Immediate neonatal complications include ventilator-treated respiratory distress, transient tachypnea, grade 1 or 2 intraventricular hemorrhage, sepsis work-ups, culture-proven sepsis, and hyperbilirubinemia. Intubation in the delivery room often is required to manage respiratory distress. Long-term morbidity for the child may include cerebral palsy, neurodevelopmental delay, chronic lung disease, and visual impairment.

Greater uncertainty exists in the assessment of gestational age than in the assessment of birth weight (see Chapter 27, Posterm Pregnancy). Therefore, perinatal outcomes are often reported in terms of birth weight rather than gestational age, even though gestational age is a more predictive parameter. It should be noted that not all infants of low birth weight are premature; some are born at term but are small for gestational age, while others are both premature and appropriate for gestational age.

Among preterm deliveries, approximately 80% occur spontaneously due to premature rupture of the membranes (PROM). Other reasons for spontaneous PTB include:

- pre-eclampsia/eclampsia (12% of cases)
- bleeding during pregnancy (6–9% of cases)
- fetal growth restriction (2–4% of cases)

Many risk factors have been associated with PTB (see **Fig. 15.2**). Approximately 10–30% are related to multiple gestations and other reasons, such as cervical insufficiency. Additionally, 20% are the result of iatrogenic intervention due to maternal or fetal indications.

Clinical and laboratory evidence suggest a final common pathway leading to PTL and delivery, which may result from a number of different pathogenic processes. **Table 15.1** presents pathological processes that are associated with preterm parturition.

Intrauterine Infection/Inflammation

Intrauterine infection or inflammation is the most important process leading to PTB. It is the only factor for which causality has been directly established. Laboratory and clinical data show a link between spontaneous PTB and both systemic and ascending genital tract infections. Both clinical and subclinical chorioamnionitis are much more common in preterm than term deliveries, and may account for 50% of PTBs before 30 weeks' gestation.

Intrauterine infection is involved in 25–40% of preterm deliveries. Finding bacterial particles in the sterile amniotic fluid is always abnormal. One study found a positive amniotic fluid culture in 13% of women with PTL. When the process progressed to preterm delivery, the rate of positive cultures was 22%. When labor started with PROM, the rate was found to be 32% and as high as 75% during active labor in this group. A high rate of positive cultures was found in women with cervical insufficiency, those with a short cervix, and those with twins and PTL as well (**Table 15.2**).

The final common pathway for triggering PTB is a maternal or fetal inflammatory response to infection in the amnion, chorion, or decidua. This response is characterized by the presence of activated neutrophils and macrophages that induce proinflammatory mediators, including interleukins (ILs) 1, 6, and 8; tumor necrosis factor-alpha (TNF-α); granulocyte colony-stimulating factor (G-CSF); and matrix metalloproteinases.

In addition to inducing an inflammatory response, bacteria may also have a direct role in the pathogenesis of PTB. Some organisms (e.g., Pseudomonas, Staphylococcus, Streptococcus, Bacteroides, and Enterobacter) are capable of producing proteases, collagenases, and elastases that can degrade the fetal membrane. Bacteria also produce phospholipase A2 (which leads to prostaglandin synthesis) and endotoxin, a substance that stimulates uterine contractions and can cause PTL. The presence of bacteria, without an inflammatory response, does not always lead to an adverse outcome.

Uterine Ischemia

Maternal and fetal vascular lesions are second only to inflammatory lesions as a factor in PTB. Such lesions are the most common pathological features in the placenta of women with PTB. Maternal lesions observed in the placenta of patients with a spontaneous PTB include failure of physiological transformation of the myometrial segment of the spiral arteries, atherosis, thrombosis of the spiral arteries (a form of decidual vasculopathy), and a combination of these lesions. Fetal lesions may include a decrease in the number of arterioles in the villi and fetal arterial thrombosis. Uteroplacental ischemia could be the cause of PTL in women with placental vascular lesions.

The precise mechanisms responsible for the onset of PTB in women with uteroplacental ischemia have not been determined. Some of these proposed mechanisms include a role for the following:

- *The renin–angiotensin system:* Fetal membranes are rich in functional renin–angiotensin system, and uterine ischemia increases the production of uterine rennin.
- *Angiotensin II:* Myometrial contractility can be induced directly by angiotensin II or through the release of prostaglandins.
- *Thrombin:* When uteroplacental ischemia is severe enough to lead to decidual necrosis and hemorrhage, thrombin may activate the common pathway of parturition. Also, fetal vascular lesions (i.e., abnormal development due to defective angiogenesis or fetal thrombosis) may lead to fetal compromise and PTL.

Uterine Overdistension

Women with müllerian duct abnormalities, polyhydramnios, and multiple pregnancies are at increased risk for spontaneous PTL and PTB. Intra-amniotic pressure remains relatively constant throughout gestation despite the growth of the fetus and placenta. This has been attributed to progressive myometrial relaxation caused by

Table 15.1 Pathological processes that have been implicated in preterm parturition syndrome

Intrauterine infection/inflammation
Uterine ischemia
Uterine overdistension
Abnormal allograft reaction
Allergy
Cervical insufficiency
Hormonal disorders (progesterone related and corticotropin-releasing factor related)

Table 15.2 Positive amniotic fluid culture in women with preterm delivery

Positive amniotic fluid culture	Percentage
Preterm labor	13
Progression to preterm delivery	22
Initial pPROM	32
Active labor in women with pPROM during active labor	75
Women with cervical insufficiency	51
Women with a shortened cervix (<25 mm by TVS)	9
Preterm labor in twins	12

pPROM, preterm premature rupture of membranes;
TVS, transvaginal sonography.

the effects of progesterone and endogenous myometrial relaxants such as nitric oxide. Stretching can, however, induce increased myometrial contractility, prostaglandin release, expression of gap junction protein or connexin-43, and increased oxytocin receptor expression in the myometrium of pregnant and nonpregnant women.

Progesterone inhibits the gene expression of a protein that is associated with stretch-induced contraction. The effect of stretch increases in late gestation. It is at its maximum level during labor as a result of the relative reduction in uterine growth compared with fetal growth, as well as due to declining circulating and/or local concentrations of progesterone. Not only may stretch induce increased myometrial contractility, it may also modify the contractile response through "mechanoelectrical feedback" similar to that seen in the heart. The chorioamniotic membranes are distended by 40% at 25–29 weeks of gestation, 60% at 30–34 weeks of gestation, and 70% at term.

Mechanical forces associated with uterine overdistension may result in activation of mechanisms leading to membrane rupture. In women with multiple gestations, premature cervical ripening is seen as well as certain müllerian duct anomalies (e.g., incompetent cervix in diethylstilbestrol-exposed daughters).

Abnormal Allograft Reaction

The fetoplacental unit is considered nature's most successful "graft." Reproductive immunologists have suggested that abnormalities in the recognition and adaptation to a set of foreign antigens (fetal) may be responsible for recurrent pregnancy loss, intrauterine growth restriction, and pre-eclampsia.

It has been observed that some women in PTL, without demonstrable infection, have elevated concentrations of the IL-2-soluble receptor. Also seen is an inverse pattern in IL-2 and IFN-gamma production in peripheral blood between weeks 20 and 30 in preterm delivery compared with patients delivering at term. Elevated plasma concentrations of the IL-2 receptor are an early sign of rejection in women with renal transplants.

The complement system is a group of proteins that are activated during an inflammatory response triggered by foreign invaders. It plays a central role in the first line of defense against invading pathogens, and its activation involves the release of potent pro-inflammatory mediators (C3a, C4a and C5a). Recent studies support the hypothesis that some components of the innate limb of the immune response may have a role in the development of PTL.

Allergy

Another potential mechanism for PTL and PTB is an immunologically mediated phenomenon induced by an allergic mechanism. There is some evidence that an allergylike immune response (type I hypersensitivity) is associated with PTL. However, this finding remains controversial.

Cervical Insufficiency

Although cervical insufficiency is traditionally considered a cause of midtrimester miscarriage, a wide spectrum of related diseases probably exists. This spectrum includes recurrent pregnancy loss in the midtrimester, some forms of PTL (presenting with bulging membranes in the absence of significant uterine contractility or rupture of membranes), and probably precipitous labor at term.

Cervical disease may be the result of:
- a congenital disorder (e.g., a hypoplastic cervix or diethylstilbestrol exposure in utero)
- surgical trauma (e.g., from conization resulting in substantial loss of connective tissue), or
- traumatic damage to the structural integrity of the cervix (e.g., repeated cervical dilation associated with termination of pregnancy)

Some cases of cervical insufficiency in the mid-trimester may be caused not by a primary cervical disease leading to premature ripening but by another pathological process, such as infection. Intrauterine infections have been found in nearly 50% of women with a clinical presentation consistent with acute cervical insufficiency.

Hormonal Disorders

Premature activation of the hypothalamic–pituitary–adrenal (HPA) axis can initiate PTB. Indeed, major maternal physical or psychological stress, which can activate the maternal HPA axis, has been associated with a higher rate of preterm delivery. HPA activation is thought to cause PTB via the increased release of corticotropin-releasing hormone (CRH), which appears to program the "placental clock." Another mechanism by which HPA activation could cause PTB is by increased fetal pituitary adrenocorticotropic hormone (ACTH) secretion, which stimulates the production of placental estrogenic compounds and may activate the myometrium and initiate labor.

Corticotropin-releasing hormone: CRH, which is released by the hypothalamus, plays a role in both term and PTB. However, during pregnancy it is also secreted by the placenta, chorionic trophoblasts, amnion, and decidual cells. CRH stimulates the secretion of ACTH from the pituitary, which then promotes the release of cortisol from the adrenal. In the maternal HPA axis, cortisol inhibits hypothalamic CRH and pituitary ACTH release, creating a negative feedback loop. In contrast, cortisol stimulates CRH release in the decidua-trophoblast-membranes compartment.

CRH, in turn, further drives maternal and fetal HPA activation, establishing a potent positive feedback loop.

One of the tissues targeted by CRH is the myometrial smooth muscle, which expresses an excess of specific CRH receptors. This finding suggests that CRH plays a role in preparing the myometrial microenvironment for the onset of labor and, possibly, in the regulation of active contractility during labor as well. CRH also targets other gestational tissues, including the placenta, fetal membranes, and fetal adrenals. Thus, CRH appears to regulate at least several distinct physiological functions, ranging from control of vascular tone to adrenal steroidogenesis and prostaglandin synthesis and activity.

Increased maternal plasma CRH levels are characteristic of some gestational diseases. Women with chronic hypertension and pre-eclampsia have high CRH levels. In addition, intrauterine growth retardation is associated with activation of the HPA axis, which is accompanied by increases in fetal plasma concentrations of ACTH, cortisol, and CRH.

Midgestational plasma CRH levels are higher in women delivering preterm (Evidence Box 15.1). If the sequence of events outlined above occurs too early in gestation, PTL and PTB may result. Although CRH levels may be a promising tool for predicting PTB, at present there are no clinical testing schemes available that use serum CRH concentrations to identify patients likely to deliver prematurely.

Estrogens: Estrogens produced by the placenta play a pivotal role in the endocrine control of pregnancy and induce many of the key changes involved in parturition. Activation of the fetal HPA axis leads to PTB through a pathway involving estrogens. Fetal pituitary ACTH secretion stimulates adrenal synthesis of dehydroepiandrosterone sulfate (DHEA-S), which is converted to 16-hydroxy-DHEA-S in the fetal liver.

Placental CRH also can augment fetal adrenal DHEA production directly. The placenta converts these androgen precursors to estrone (E1), estradiol (E2), and estriol (E3). These three hormones, in turn, activate the myometrium by increasing gap junction formation, oxytocin receptors, prostaglandin activity, and enzymes responsible for muscle contraction (myosin light chain kinase, calmodulin). Moreover, functional progesterone withdrawal leads to increasing concentrations of the myometrial estrogen receptor, further enhancing estrogen-induced myometrial activation.

Progesterone: Progesterone is central to pregnancy maintenance by specifically promoting myometrial quiescence, downregulating gap junction formation, inhibiting cervical ripening, and decreasing the production of chemokines (i.e., IL-8) by the chorioamniotic membranes, which is thought to be a key to decidual/membrane activation. Progesterone is considered important for pregnancy maintenance in humans because inhibition of progesterone action could result in parturition. In many species, a fall in maternal serum progesterone concentration (progesterone withdrawal) occurs prior to spontaneous parturition. The mechanisms that suppress progesterone's function to allow labor and delivery are still uncertain.

History

PTL is one of the most common reasons for hospitalization of pregnant women. Identifying women with preterm contractions who eventually will deliver preterm is challenging. That is why accurate diagnosis of PTL often requires a complete medical history, a comprehensive physical examination, and the appropriate laboratory and imaging tests.

As previously described, there are a numerous risk factors for PTL. The most common risk factors for PTL are listed in **Table 15.3**.

Chief Complaints

The most common signs and symptoms of early PTL include:
- menstrual-like cramping
- constant low back ache
- mild uterine contractions at infrequent and/or irregular intervals
- bloody show

However, these are nonspecific complaints that are common in women who achieve normal term deliveries. Uterine contractions, for example, are a normal finding at all stages of pregnancy, thereby adding to the challenge of distinguishing true from false labor. The frequency of contractions often increases with gestational age, the number of fetuses, and at night. A threshold contraction frequency that will effectively predict women who will deliver prematurely has not been identified.

Therefore, the diagnosis of PTL is generally based upon clinical criteria, such as regular painful uterine contractions accompanied by cervical dilatation and/or effacement. Specific criteria, which were initially developed to select subjects in research settings, include persistent uterine contractions (four every 20 minutes or eight every 60 minutes) with documented cervical change or cervical effacement of at least 80%, or cervical dilatation greater than 2 cm.

Table 15.3 Risk factors for preterm labor

Previous preterm delivery
Low socioeconomic status
Non-White race
Maternal age <18 years or >40 years
Preterm premature rupture of the membranes
Multiple gestation
Maternal history of one or more spontaneous second-trimester abortions
Maternal complications (medical or obstetric)
– maternal behaviors
– smoking
– illicit drug use
– alcohol use
– lack of prenatal care
Uterine causes
– myomata (particularly submucosal or subplacental)
– uterine septum
– bicornuate uterus
– cervical incompetence
– exposure to diethylstilbestrol
– over-distended uterus (multiple pregnancy, polyhydramnion)
Infectious causes
– chorioamnionitis
– bacterial vaginosis
– asymptomatic bacteriuria
– acute pyelonephritis
– cervical/vaginal colonization
– peridontal disease
Fetal causes
– intrauterine fetal death
– intrauterine growth retardation
– congenital anomalies
Abnormal placentation
– presence of a retained intrauterine device

Physical Examination

Examine the uterus to assess firmness, tenderness, fetal size, and fetal position. Perform a sterile speculum exam to rule out ruptured membranes, to visually examine the vagina and cervix, and to obtain specimens for laboratory testing.

You should also perform a digital examination to assess cervical dilation and effacement after placenta previa and PROM have been excluded (by history and physical, laboratory, and ultrasound examinations, as indicated).

Digital cervical examination has limited reproducibility between examiners, especially when changes are not prominent. Thus, some pregnancy care centers rely on transvaginal sonography (TVS) to confirm the diagnosis. TVS measurement of the cervical length (CL) is a more sensitive indicator of a patient's risk for PTB than cervical dilatation. CL is predictive of PTB in all populations studied, including asymptomatic women with prior cone biopsy, müllerian anomalies, or multiple dilatations and evacuations.

CL is measured by determining the distance between the internal os and external os. A short cervix has been variously defined as a CL less than 2.0 cm, 2.5 cm, or 3.0 cm. CL is typically taken between 16 and 32 weeks of gestation, with decreasing length associated with an increasing risk of delivery.

A CL below the 10th percentile (25 mm) is consistently associated with an increased risk of spontaneous PTB. Since most women with cervical shortening do not deliver preterm, TVS measurement of CL to screen pregnant women for PTB risk is not recommended. Rather, CL should be measured only in women deemed to at high risk of recurrent PTB, since the test is more predictive in this population. A suggested algorithm for the diagnosis and management of women with PTL by sonographic measurement of CL is presented in **Fig. 15.4**.

Laboratory Tests

A number of biologic markers in serum, amniotic fluid, and cervical secretions have been evaluated for their potential to predict PTD. However, the most clinically useful biochemical marker that can be used to differentiate women who are at high risk for impending PTD from those who are not is the level of fetal fibronectin (fFN) in the cervicovaginal secretions.

An extracellular matrix glycoprotein, fFN is localized at the maternal–fetal interface of the amniotic membranes, between the chorion and deciduas. Under normal conditions, fFN is found at very low levels in cervicovaginal secretions. Levels greater than 50 ng/mL beyond 22 weeks of gestation have been associated with an increased risk of spontaneous PTB.

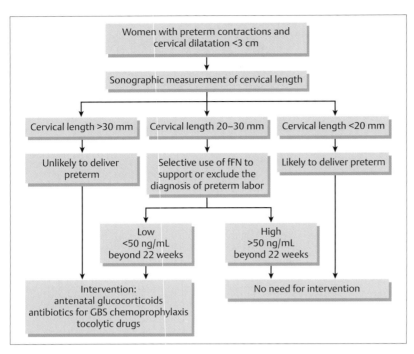

Fig. 15.4 Algorithm for the diagnosis and management of women with preterm labor by sonographic measurement of cervical length.

In symptomatic patients, the presence of high levels of fFN in the cervicovaginal secretions is associated with an increased risk for delivery within 7 days. The high negative predictive value of fFN enables the attending physician to take a more judicious and less invasive approach in these patients.

Although fFN is commonly used to help in the management of women with symptoms of PTL, there is currently not enough evidence to recommend its use as a screening tool. Some authors suggest sonographic measurement of CL in women with preterm contractions and cervical dilatation less than 3 cm. Women with CL over 30 mm are unlikely to deliver preterm, while preterm delivery is likely if the CL is less than 20 mm. In women with CL 20–30 mm, selective use of fFN to support or exclude the diagnosis of PTL is suggested.

Management

Hospitalization of women diagnosed with PTL at less than 34 weeks' gestation is recommended in order to initiate interventions. Such interventions can be primary (directed to all women), secondary (aimed at eliminating or reducing existing risks), or tertiary (intended to improve outcomes for preterm infants). Most efforts so far have been tertiary interventions, such as treatment with antenatal corticosteroids, tocolytic agents, and antibiotics.

Antenatal glucocorticoids: In the mid-1990s, the US National Institutes of Health assembled a Consensus Development Conference on the effect of corticosteroids used for fetal maturation on perinatal outcomes. The consensus panel concluded that antenatal corticosteroid therapy for fetal maturation reduces mortality, respiratory distress syndrome, and intraventricular hemorrhage in preterm infants. They stated that these benefits extend to a broad range of gestational ages (24–34 weeks) and are not limited by gender or race. Although the beneficial effects of corticosteroids are greatest more than 24 hours after beginning the treatment, a duration of treatment of less than 24 hours may also improve outcomes. The benefits of antenatal corticosteroids are additive to those derived from surfactant therapy. In the presence of preterm premature rupture of the membranes, antenatal corticosteroid therapy reduces the frequency of respiratory distress syndrome, intraventricular hemorrhage, and neonatal death, although to a lesser extent than with intact membranes. The consensus panel noted that data from trials in children who where followed for up to 12 years indicate that antenatal corticosteroid therapy does not adversely affect physical growth or psychomotor development.

Antibiotics for group B Streptococcus chemoprophylaxis: Group B Streptococcus (GBS) is an encapsulated, Gram-positive coccus that colonizes the gastrointestinal and genital tracts of 10–30% of pregnant women. Although GBS colonization usually remains asymptomatic in these women, maternal transmission to neonates is the most common cause of bacterial infection in young infants.

Vertical transmission primarily occurs after the onset of labor or rupture of the fetal membranes. The Centers for Disease Control and Prevention (CDC), and others, have published guidelines for prevention of neonatal GBS disease. In general, these guidelines involve intrapartum parenteral antibiotic prophylaxis of women with recent positive GBS cultures or risk factors for GBS colonization.

Screening for GBS colonization is usually performed at 35–37 weeks' gestation to maximize accordance between antepartum culture results and maternal GBS status at delivery. Thus, the colonization status of women who present with threatened preterm delivery is not generally known. If unknown, GBS cultures are obtained at the time of presentation, and then intrapartum antibiotic prophylaxis is administered until culture results are available.

Women with positive GBS cultures are treated with penicillin until the threat of impending delivery is over. The usual course of treatment is 48 hours, during which time antenatal glucocorticoids and/or tocolytic drugs may also be given. Patients who are discharged without having delivered should receive antibiotic prophylaxis when in labor. If the cultures are negative after 48 hours, penicillin can be discontinued. A GBS culture should be repeated in 4 weeks if the patient has not delivered, because GBS colonization can be intermittent.

Tocolytic therapy: Tocolytic therapy for an acute episode of PTL often eliminates contractions temporarily but does not remove the underlying stimulus that initiated the process of parturition or reverse changes in the uterus. The main goal of treating PTL is to delay delivery by at least 48 hours so that glucocorticoids given to the mother can achieve their maximum effect. An additional goal is to provide time for safe transport of the mother to a facility that can provide appropriate care for the premature neonate, if needed. Tocolytic therapy could also achieve prolongation of pregnancy when there are underlying, self-limited conditions that can induce labor, such as pyelonephritis or abdominal surgery, and are unlikely to cause recurrent PTL.

A variety of agents are used to inhibit acute PTL. These labor-inhibiting agents do so either by generating or altering of intracellular messengers, or by inhibiting the synthesis or blocking the action of a known myometrial stimulants. Drugs affecting intracellular messengers include ß-adrenergic receptor agonists, agents that generate nitric oxide (nitric oxide donors), magnesium sulfate, and calcium channel blockers. Drugs blocking the synthesis or action of known myometrial stimulants include prostaglandin synthesis inhibitors and oxytocin antagonists. The mechanisms of action of tocolytic agents are presented in **Table 15.4**. Maternal and fetal/neonatal side effects and contraindications for the use of tocolytic agents are presented in **Table 15.5**.

Table 15.4 The mechanisms of action of tocolytic drugs

Agent or class	Mechanisms of action
ß-adrenergic receptor agonists	• Bind with beta-2 adrenergic receptors and increase intracellular adenyl cyclase, activation of protein kinase, and phosphorylation of intracellular proteins
	• A drop in intracellular free-calcium occurs and interferes with the activity of myosin light-chain kinase and causes inhibition of the interaction between actin and myosin
Magnesium sulfate	• Competes with calcium at the level of the plasma membrane voltage-gated channels
	• Hyperpolarizes the plasma membrane and inhibits myosin light-chain kinase activity by competing with intracellular calcium at this site
Calcium channel blockers	• Directly block the influx of calcium ions through the cell membrane
	• Inhibit release of intracellular calcium from the sarcoplasmic reticulum and increase calcium efflux from the cell
	• Inhibit calcium-dependent myosin light-chain kinase phosphorylation
Nitric oxide (NO) donors	• Nitric oxide synthase synthesizes NO by oxidation of L-arginine to L-citrulline, which then diffuses from the generator cell
	• Couples NO formation with the synthesis of cyclic guanosine 3′, 5′-monophosphate (cGMP) in target cells
	• The increase in cGMP content in smooth muscle cells activates myosin light chain kinases
Cyclooxygenase inhibitors	• Cyclooxygenase (COX, or prostaglandin synthase) is responsible for conversion of arachidonic acid to prostaglandins
	• Prostaglandins enhance the formation of myometrial gap junctions and increase available intracellular calcium by raising transmembrane influx and sarcolemmal release of calcium
	• COX inhibitors decrease prostaglandin production by either general inhibition of COX or specific inhibition of COX-2
Oxytocin receptor antagonists	• Compete with oxytocin for binding to oxytocin receptors in the myometrium and decidua, thus preventing the increase in intracellular free calcium
	• More effective at later gestational ages, since oxytocin receptor concentration and uterine responsiveness to oxytocin increase with advancing gestation

Table 15.5 Maternal and fetal side effects and contraindications for tocolytic drugs

Agent or class	Drugs affecting intracellular messengers				Drugs blocking the synthesis or action of known myometrial stimulants	
	ß-adrenergic receptor agonists	Magnesium sulfate	Calcium channel blockers	Nitric oxide donors	Cyclooxygenase inhibitors	Oxytocin receptor antagonists
Maternal side effects	Tachycardia	Flushing	Dizziness	Dizziness	Nausea	Hypersensitivity
	Hypotension	Diaphoresis	Flushing	Flushing	Esophageal reflux	Injection-site reactions
	Tremor	Nausea	Hypotension	Hypotension	Gastritis and emesis	
	Palpitations	Magnesium toxicity (loss of deep-tendon reflexes, respiratory paralysis, cardiac arrest)	Elevation of hepatic aminotransferase levels		Platelet dysfunction (rarely significant)	
	Shortness of breath	Adverse effects when combined with calcium channel blockers	Adverse effects when combined with magnesium sulfate			
	Chest discomfort					
	Pulmonary edema					
	Hypokalemia					
	Hyperglycemia					
Fetal or neonatal side effects	Tachycardia	Possible perinatal mortality (conflicting data)			In utero closure of ductus arteriosus (when used for >48 hours)	*An increased rate of fetal or infant death
					Oligohydramnios (when used for >48 hours)	
					Patent ductus arteriosus in neonate (conflicting data)	
Contraindications	Tachycardia-sensitive maternal cardiac disease	Myasthenia gravis	Hypotension	Hypotension	Platelet dysfunction or bleeding disorder	None
	Poorly controlled diabetes mellitus		Preload-dependent cardiac lesions (eg, aortic insufficiency)	Preload-dependent cardiac lesions (eg, aortic insufficiency)	Hepatic or renal dysfunction	
					Gastrointestinal or ulcerative disease	
					Asthma	

*For atosiban (may be due to the lower gestational age of infants in the atosiban group).

Managing Asymptomatic Women at High Risk of Preterm Birth

Women with risk factors for PTB are sometimes followed with serial CL measurements. A CL ≥35 mm is generally considered normal and reassuring. A reverse relation exists between CL and risk of PTB. However, some centers manage asymptomatic patients at high risk of PTB similarly to symptomatic patients, but with a higher CL threshold for intervention.

Although symptomatic patients are divided into three groups according to their CL (>30 mm—low risk for PTB; 20–30 mm—intermediate risk for PTB; and <20 mm—high risk for PTB). In asymptomatic patients the CL threshold is higher (>35 mm—low risk for PTB, 25–35 mm—intermediate risk for PTB; and <25 mm—high risk for PTB). This minimizes overtreatment of high-risk asymptomatic patients and undertreatment of symptomatic patients. Surveillance with serial CL measurements may be initiated at 22 weeks. Early aggressive treatment of bacterial vaginosis in high risk patients may reduce PROM and PTB.

Key Points

- Preterm birth (PTB) refers to a birth that occurs before 37 completed weeks of gestation.
- Preterm labor (PTL) leading to preterm delivery affects approximately 5-7 % of live births in developed countries, but significantly higher rates are noted in developing countries.
- Prematurity due to PTB, is one of the leading causes of infant mortality and accounts for approximately 28 % of neonatal mortality worldwide. Most PTBs are spontaneous.
- The diagnosis of PTL is based on the presence of regular painful uterine contractions accompanied by cervical dilatation and effacement.
- Ultrasound measurement of cervical length and cervicovaginal fetal fibronectin level can help to confirm or exclude the diagnosis of PTL.
- Management of women with PTL includes administration of tocolytic drugs, antibiotic treatment given to women with positive urine culture results, antibiotic treatment for group B Streptococcus chemoprophylaxis (if indicated).
- Antenatal glucocorticoids can reduce neonatal morbidity and mortality associated with prematurity.

Abnormal Labor

Definitions

Abnormal labor: Traditional definitions of abnormal labor are presented in **Table 15.6**.

Arrest disorder: Arrest disorders include secondary arrest of dilation (no progress in cervical dilation in more than 2 hours), arrest of descent (fetal head does not descend for more than 1 hour in primiparous and more than 0.5 hour in multiparous), and failure of descent (no descent).

Labor: The presence of sufficient intensity, frequency, and duration of uterine contractions that brings about demonstrable effacement and dilation of the cervix. The definition and significance of the latent phase of labor is controversial, but it is agreed that women in labor enter the active phase when cervical dilatation is 3–4 cm. The active phase of labor includes both an increased rate of cervical dilation and the descent of the presenting fetal part.

Table 15.6 Traditional definitions of abnormal labor

| Stage of labor | Labor abnormality | |
	Protracted	Arrested
Latent phase		
Nulliparous	>20 hours	
Multiparous	>14 hours	
First stage		
Nulliparous	<1 cm per hour dilatation	≥2 hours of active labor without cervical change
Multiparous	<1.2–1.5 cm per hour dilatation	≥2 hours of active labor without cervical change
Second stage		
Nulliparous	With no regional anesthesia: >2 hours duration or <1 cm per hour descent	No descent after 1 hour of pushing
	With regional anesthesia: >3 hours duration	
Multiparous	With no regional anesthesia: >1 hour duration or <1.2 cm per hour descent	No descent after 1 hour of pushing
	With regional anesthesia: 2 hours duration	

Labor augmentation: The stimulation of uterine contractions when spontaneous contractions have failed to result in progressive cervical dilation or descent of the presenting fetal part. Augmentation should be considered if the frequency of contractions is less than three contractions in 10 minutes or the intensity of contractions is less than 200 Montevideo units as measured with an intrauterine pressure catheter, or both.

Protraction disorder: Protraction and arrest disorders occur in both the first and second stages of labor. The incidence is about 15% in either stage. A labor abnormality is the most common indication for primary cesarean delivery (CD). Approximately 70% of CDs are due to lack of progress in labor.

Diagnosis

Normal progress in labor was initially defined by Friedman in the 1950s based on data from labors of several hundred women. Labor abnormalities are characterized as protraction or arrest disorders. To follow labor most birth centers use a graph called a partogram, which plots cervical dilatation and station across time.

In the first stage of labor, a slow progression rate of cervical dilation on a partogram is suggestive of a protraction disorder. An arrest disorder can be diagnosed when the cervix ceases to dilate after reaching 4 cm dilatation despite adequate uterine contractions (i.e., more than three contractions in 10 minutes or greater than 200 Montevideo units for more than 2 hours).

In the second stage of labor, protracted labor is defined as a second stage longer than 2 hours in nulliparous women (3 hours when regional analgesia is used), and longer than 1 hour in multiparous women (2 hours when regional analgesia is used). An arrest of descent can be diagnosed after 1 hour if there is no descent, despite good maternal pushing efforts.

Prevalence and Epidemiology

Protraction and arrest disorders occur in both the first and second stages of labor. The incidence is about 15% in either stage.

Etiology and Pathophysiology

Abnormal labor can be the result of one or more abnormalities of the cervix, uterus, maternal pelvis, or fetus. Interestingly, it has been shown that a genetic component accounts for 28% of the susceptibility to dystocia. Risk factors for abnormal labor are shown in the **Table 15.7**.

Several factors are associated with longer duration of the second stage, including epidural analgesia, occiputoposterior position, longer first stage of labor, nulliparity, short maternal stature, birth weight, and high station at complete cervical dilatation. The following discusses in more detail the most common causes of abnormal labor.

Hypocontractile Uterine Activity

Hypocontractile uterine activity, which is commonly quantified as uterine contraction pressures less than 200 Montevideo units, is the most common cause of protraction or arrest disorders in the first stage of labor. Its name refers to uterine activity that is not strong enough or not coordinated properly to dilate the cervix and push out the fetus. It occurs in 3–8% of parturients.

Neuraxial Anesthesia

The potential impact of neuraxial anesthesia on uterine activity, fetal malposition, and ultimately arrest disorders, and its possible role in the increasing rates of cesarean deliveries has been widely addressed in research.

Table 15.7 Risk factors for abnormal labor

Older maternal age
Pregnancy complications (premature rupture of membranes, induction of labor)
Non-reassuring fetal heart rate
Epidural anesthesia
Macrosomia
Pelvic contraction
Occiputoposterior position
Nulliparity
Short stature (<150 cm)
High station at full dilatation
Chorioamnionitis
Postterm pregnancy
Obesity
High-risk patients (women with hypertensive disorders, gestational diabetes, polyhydramnios, fertility treatment)

Neuraxial anesthesia is generally associated with an increased duration of the first and second stages of labor, incidence of fetal malposition, use of oxytocin, and operative vaginal delivery. However, it has not been proven to increase CD rates.

Cephalopelvic Disproportion

A disproportion in the size of the fetus relative to the mother can lead to a diagnosis of dystocia. The diagnosis of cephalopelvic disproportion (CPD) is inexact and is often based on an observation of protracted or arrested labor. These are often due to fetal malposition (extended or asynclitic fetal head) or malpresentation (mentum posterior, brow), rather than a true disparity between fetal and maternal pelvic dimensions. Medicine's ability to predict maternal CPD leading to arrest of labor has been disappointing. Clinical or radiologic assessment of the maternal pelvis (pelvimetry) and fetal size is an inexact science with a poor predictive value.

Occiputoposterior Position

Persistent occiputoposterior (POP) position is associated with a longer duration of active labor and the second stage, as well as a higher risk of arrest of descent requiring operative delivery. The length of the second stage correlates with the degree of rotation away from occiputoanterior.

Management

When managing women with dystocia, there are four major issues to consider: (1) if the contractions are adequate; (2) if there is fetal malposition; (3) if there is CPD caused by suspected macrosomia or a contracted pelvis; and (4) if there are other coexisting clinical issues (e.g., chorioamnionitis, nonreassuring fetal monitoring) that will impact the treatment options.

Managing the First Stage of Labor

Latent phase: The latent phase could be managed by observation, sedation, or labor augmentation. Inducing labor may take a while. A cesarean delivery for dystocia should not be performed in women who remain in latent labor.

Active phase: Once in active labor, amniotomy before oxytocin use may be sufficient to augment a protracted labor. Amniotomy with early oxytocin augmentation shortens labor 2 hours compared with expectant management. Although amniotomy is a simple procedure, it

still carries a risk of causing increased variable decelerations because of cord compression.

An intrauterine pressure catheter, which calculates Montevideo units, can be used to evaluate the strength and frequency of uterine contractions in women with protracted or arrested labor. If contractions are inadequate, intravenous oxytocin can be administered to increase their frequency, duration, and strength. There are various protocols for dosage, dosing interval, and duration of oxytocin treatment. However, a high-dose regimen has been shown to increase hyperstimulation with no adverse fetal effects.

Traditionally, arrested labor has been defined as having adequate contractions for at least two hours without cervical change; therefore at least two hours of observation should go by before deciding on operative intervention. Extending the time to four hours before operative treatment has been shown to decrease the cesarean delivery rate for arrested labor from 26% to 8%.

Managing the Second Stage of Labor

Dystocia in the second stage of labor is characterized by prolonged duration or arrested descent. This may be caused by fetal malposition, inadequate contractions, poor maternal efforts, or true CPD. The most common fetal malposition is occipitoposterior. Usually, spontaneous rotation to the occipitoanterior position occurs before delivery. However, in 2–7% of nulliparous women, the fetus will remain in POP position. This position is associated with prolonged second stage of labor and increased oxytocin augmentation. Less than 30% of nulliparous women with a fetus in POP position will have a spontaneous vaginal delivery.

If a fetus remains in POP position in the second stage of labor, manual rotation can be attempted. A lower cesarean delivery rate has been reported with successful rotation compared with failed rotation.

A variety of maternal positions and movements have been proposed to resolve POP or asynclitic fetal positions. These include knee–chest, hands-and-knees, pelvic rocking, lunging, side-lying, or asymmetrical sitting or kneeling. None has been proven beneficial, however.

Intravenous oxytocin should be initiated or increased if contractions decrease in strength or frequency during the second stage of labor. Pushing in an upright or lateral position shortens the second stage of labor and decreases the risk of operative vaginal delivery, but this position increases the risk of second-degree perineal tears and blood loss of more than 500 mL in women without epidural analgesia. For women with epidural analgesia, delayed pushing increases the incidence of spontaneous deliveries.

A prolonged second stage of labor beyond a fixed time limit is no longer an indication for operative vaginal or cesarean delivery. Although the length of the second stage of labor is not associated with poor neonatal outcome, a prolonged second stage is associated with increased maternal morbidity and operative delivery rates.

Key Points

Labor can be divided into three stages: first (time from the onset of labor until complete cervical dilatation, latent and active phases), second (time from complete cervical dilatation to expulsion of the fetus), and third (time from expulsion of the fetus to expulsion of the placenta).

- Abnormal labor can result from one or more abnormalities of the cervix, uterus, maternal pelvis, or fetus (power, passenger, or pelvis).
- Progress should be monitored in active labor with cervical examinations at 1–2-hour intervals.
- Oxytocin administration is suggested for patients in active labor who fail to make adequate progress over 2 hours.
- As long as clinical assessment of fetal and maternal size is favorable and the fetal heart rate is reassuring, oxytocin administration should achieve at least three uterine contractions or more than 200 Montevideo units in 10 minutes.
- Labor progress should continue to be monitored for 2–4 hours.
- The decision to perform an operative vaginal delivery, cesarean delivery, or continue observation in the second stage of labor is based on clinical assessment of mother and fetus, and the skill and training of the obstetrician.

Evidence Box 15.1

High serum levels of CRH may be predictive of impending labor.
McLean et al. conducted a prospective cohort study that measured serum CRH concentrations between 17 and 30 weeks of gestation in 860 unselected pregnant women. They found that the median serum CRH in pregnancies that subsequently spontaneously delivered preterm (37 women) was two times higher than that of women of the same gestational age who went on to deliver at term. Further, they found exponential rise in maternal plasma CRH concentrations with advancing pregnancy is associated with a concomitant fall in concentrations of the specific CRH binding protein in late pregnancy. This leads to a rapid increase in circulating levels of bioavailable CRH at a time that coincides with the onset of parturition, suggesting that CRH may act directly as a trigger for parturition in humans.

McLean M, Bisits A, Davies J, Woods R, Lowry P, Smith RA. Placental clock controlling the length of human pregnancy. Nat Med 1995;1:460–463.

Further Reading

Barros FC, Victora CG, Matijasevich A, et al. Preterm births, low birth weight, and intrauterine growth restriction in three birth cohorts in Southern Brazil: 1982, 1993 and 2004. *Cad Saude Publica* 2008;24(Suppl 3):S390–S398

Chatterjee J, Gullam J, Vatish M, Thornton S. The management of preterm labour. *Arch Dis Child Fetal Neonatal Ed* 2007;92(2):F88–F93

Effect of corticosteroids for fetal maturation on perinatal outcomes. *NIH Consens Statement* 1994;12:1–24

Goldenberg RL, Hauth JC, Andrews WW. Intrauterine infection and preterm delivery. *N Engl J Med* 2000;342(20):1500–1507

Grimes-Dennis J, Berghella V. Cervical length and prediction of preterm delivery. *Curr Opin Obstet Gynecol* 2007;19(2):191–195

Iams JD, Romero R, Culhane JF, Goldenberg RL. Primary, secondary, and tertiary interventions to reduce the morbidity and mortality of preterm birth. *Lancet* 2008;371(9607):164–175

Lockwood CJ, Kuczynski E. Markers of risk for preterm delivery. *J Perinat Med* 1999;27(1):5–20

McIntire DD, Leveno KJ. Neonatal mortality and morbidity rates in late preterm births compared with births at term. *Obstet Gynecol* 2008;111(1):35–41

McLean M, Bisits A, Davies J, et al. Predicting risk of preterm delivery by second-trimester measurement of maternal plasma corticotropin-releasing hormone and alpha-fetoprotein concentrations. *Am J Obstet Gynecol* 1999;181(1):207–215

Menon R. Spontaneous preterm birth, a clinical dilemma: etiologic, pathophysiologic and genetic heterogeneities and racial disparity. *Acta Obstet Gynecol Scand* 2008;87(6):590–600

Romero R, Ghidini A, Mazor M, Behnke E. Microbial invasion of the amniotic cavity in premature rupture of membranes. *Clin Obstet Gynecol* 1991;34(4):769–778

Salafia CM, Vogel CA, Vintzileos AM, Bantham KF, Pezzullo J, Silberman L. Placental pathologic findings in preterm birth. *Am J Obstet Gynecol* 1991;165(4 Pt 1):934–938

Schrag S, Gorwitz R, Fultz-Butts K, Schuchat A. Prevention of perinatal group B streptococcal disease. Revised guidelines from CDC. *MMWR Recomm Rep* 2002;51(RR-11):1–22

Wen SW, Smith G, Yang Q, Walker M. Epidemiology of preterm birth and neonatal outcome. *Semin Fetal Neonatal Med* 2004;9(6):429–435

16 Pre-Eclampsia–Eclampsia Syndrome

E. Albert Reece

Pre-eclampsia and eclampsia are part of the same disorder, which occurs only during pregnancy and the postpartum period and affects both the mother and the unborn baby. Typically, it occurs after 20 weeks of gestation (in the late second or third trimester or middle to late pregnancy), though it can occur earlier.

Proper prenatal care is essential to diagnose and manage pre-eclampsia, otherwise it can rapidly progress to severe pre-eclampsia and ultimately eclampsia, a serious, life-threatening condition. It is important to note, however, that research shows that more women die from pre-eclampsia than eclampsia, and one is not necessarily more serious than the other. Fortunately, it is a condition that, if detected early, can be properly managed with minimal negative consequences for mother and baby.

Definition and Diagnosis

Pre-eclampsia—sometimes referred to as pregnancy-induced hypertension—is defined by high blood pressure measured on two occasions at least 6 hour apart and excess protein in the urine after 20 weeks of pregnancy. (Note that both hypertension and proteinuria must be present for the diagnosis of preeclampsia to be valid). Often, pre-eclampsia causes only a modest increase in blood pressure. However, if pre-eclampsia is left untreated it can lead to more severe complications, including cerebral and vascular disturbances, edema, pain, liver dysfunction, and a low platelet count (**Table 16.1**). At this stage, it is known as severe pre-eclampsia.

Eclampsia is the final and most severe phase of pre-eclampsia and occurs if severe pre-eclampsia is left untreated. It is characterized by convulsions and usually occurs after the onset of pre-eclampsia, although sometimes there are no recognizable symptoms. The convulsions characteristic of eclampsia may appear before, during, or after labor. However, eclamptic seizures are relatively rare and occur in less than 1% of women with pre-eclampsia.

Table 16.1 Criteria for Pre-eclampsia and eclampsia

Pre-eclampsia
Blood pressure: 140 mmHg or higher systolic or 90 mmHg or higher diastolic after 20 weeks of gestation in a woman with previously normal blood pressure
Proteinuria: 0.3 g or more of protein in a 24-hour urine collection (usually corresponds with 1+ or greater on a urine dipstick test)

Severe pre-eclampsia
Blood pressure: 160 mmHg or higher systolic or 110 mmHg or higher diastolic on two occasions at least 6 hours apart in a woman on bed rest
Proteinuria: 5 g or more of protein in a 24-hour urine collection or 3+ or greater on urine dipstick testing of two random urine samples collected at least 4 hours apart
Other features include: oliguria (less than 500 mL of urine in 24 hours), cerebral or visual disturbances, pulmonary edema or cyanosis, epigastric or right upper quadrant pain, impaired liver function, thrombocytopenia, intrauterine growth restriction

Eclampsia
Cerebral accidents: — Cerebrovenous thrombosis — Cerebroarterial embolism
Hypertensive disorders: — Hypertensive encephalopathy — Pheochromocytoma
Space-occupying central nervous system lesions: — Tumor — Abscess
Infectious diseases: — Meningitis — Encephalitis
Metabolic diseases: — Hypoglycemia — Hypocalcemia — Water intoxication — Epilepsy

Table 16.1 (continued)

HELLP Syndrome	
Hemolysis	
Abnormal peripheral blood smear (burr cells, schistocytes)	
Elevated bilirubin ≥ 1.2 mg/dL	
Increased LDH more than twice the normal upper limit	
Elevated liver enzymes	
Elevated ALT or AST ≥ twice the normal upper limit	
Platelet count < 100 000/µL	

The four recognized stages of eclampsia are as follows:

1. *Premonitory stage*, which is usually missed unless constantly monitored; the woman rolls her eyes while her facial and hand muscles twitch slightly.
2. *Tonic stage*, soon after the premonitory stage, in which the twitching turns into clenching. The patient may bite her tongue as she clenches her teeth, while her arms and legs become rigid. Her respiratory muscles also may spasm, causing her to stop breathing. This stage continues for around 30 seconds.
3. *Clonic stage*, in which the spasm stops but her muscles start to jerk violently. Frothy, slightly bloodied saliva appears on her lips and can sometimes be inhaled. After a few minutes the convulsions stop, leading into the final stage: a coma. In some cases, there is heart failure as well.
4. *Comatose stage*: the patient falls deeply unconscious and exhibits noisy, labored breathing, which can last only a few minutes or may persist for hours.

The HELLP (hemolysis, elevated liver enzymes, and low platelets) syndrome is a variant of pre-eclampsia, although considerable controversy exists regarding its definition, diagnosis, incidence, etiology, and management. Thrombocytopenia with a platelet count of ≤100 000/µL is considered to be a hallmark of HELLP.

Pre-eclampsia Versus Chronic Hypertension

It is important to distinguish between pre-eclampsia and chronic hypertension. Chronic hypertension is defined by an elevated blood pressure that predates the pregnancy, is documented before 20 weeks of gestation, or is present 12 weeks after delivery. In contrast, pre-eclampsia–eclampsia is defined by elevated blood pressure and proteinuria occurring after 20 weeks of gestation (**Fig. 16.1**).

However, chronic hypertension may be complicated by superimposed pre-eclampsia (or eclampsia), which is diagnosed when there is an exacerbation of hypertension and the development of proteinuria that was absent earlier in the pregnancy. Approximately 15–30% of chronically hypertensive women develop superimposed pre-eclampsia. Conditions necessary for the diagnosis of superimposed pre-eclampsia include:

- the sudden exacerbation of blood pressure in a woman with previously well-controlled hypertension on antihypertensive medication
- the new onset of proteinurea (≥0.5 g of protein in 24-hour urine collection) in a woman with chronic hypertension but no proteinurea prior to 20 weeks gestation
- a worsening of proteinurea in a woman with chronic hypertension and proteinurea prior to 20 weeks' gestation
- a new onset of aspartate aminotransferase (AST) or alanine aminotransferase (ALT) anomalies in the liver
- a new onset of thrombocytopenia with a platelet count of ≤100 000/µL

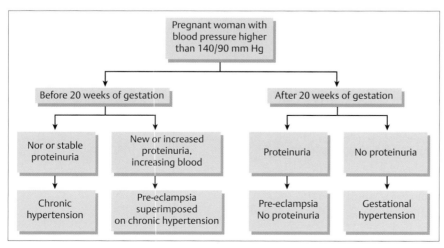

Fig. 16.1 An algorithm for differentiating among hypertensive disorders in pregnant women. Reproduced with permission from Wagner LK. Diagnosis and management of preeclampsia. American Family Physician 2004; 70(12):2318 (Fig. 1).

- a new onset of symptoms of severe pre-eclampsia (e.g., persistent headache, right upper quadrant pain, epigastric pain, scotomata, nausea, and vomiting)

Prevalence and Epidemiology

Pre-eclampsia is a complication of an estimated 7–10% of all pregnancies in the developed world. Eclampsia affects just under 1 in 50 women, with 1 in 14 fetuses of affected women dying despite best-available medical care.

Etiology and Pathophysiology

The exact causes of pre-eclampsia and eclampsia are still being investigated. Although some researchers suspect maternal constitutional factors, such as genetics, poor nutrition, or high body fat as potential contributors, other theories focus on problems of placental development and perfusion, oxidative stress, or immune factors (**Fig. 16.2**).

It is important to remember that although hypertension and proteinuria are the diagnostic criteria for pre-eclampsia, they are only symptoms of the underlying pathophysiologic changes that occur in the disorder.

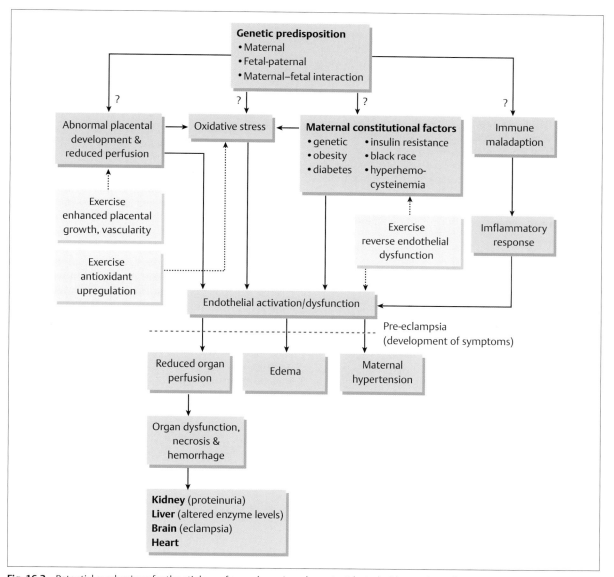

Fig. 16.2 Potential mechanisms for the etiology of pre-eclampsia–eclampsia. Adapted with permission from Weissgerber TL et al. The role of regular physical activity in preeclampsia prevention. Medical Science and Sports Exercise 2004; 36(12):2028 (Fig. 1).

One of the most striking physiologic changes that occur in pre-eclampsia–eclampsia is intense systemic vasospasm, which is responsible for decreased blood flow to virtually all of the organ systems of the mother's body. This reduced blood flow to major organs is further exacerbated by the activation of the blood's coagulation cascade, which results in the development of microthrombi.

History

As part of their initial prenatal assessment, pregnant women should be asked about potential risk factors for pre-eclampsia, including their obstetric history and specifically whether they have experienced hypertension or pre-eclampsia during a previous pregnancy. The medical history also should include questions to identify any pre-existing medical conditions that increase the risk for pre-eclampsia, including diabetes mellitus, hypertension, vascular and connective tissue disease, nephropathy, and antiphospholipid antibody syndrome.

After 20 weeks of gestation, pregnant women should be asked during each prenatal visit about specific pre-eclampsia symptoms, including whether they may be experiencing any visual disturbances, persistent headaches, epigastric or right upper quadrant pain, and increased edema. Questions about these symptoms are included in many standardized prenatal documentation forms.

Physical Examination

The chief complaints of women presenting with pre-eclampsia may include acute headache, visual disturbances, and vomiting with upper abdominal pain. On examination, their reflexes will be very brisk, even to the state of clonus. Their blood pressure will be high, and they will have elevated proteinuria. Some women, however, are asymptomatic at the time they are found to have pre-eclampsia, making it sometimes difficult to detect.

They also may have epigastric pain, which reflects liver involvement and is typical of the HELLP syndrome. Patients often describe it as the worst pain they have ever experienced. This symptom is often is confused with heartburn, a very common problem of pregnancy. However, it is fairly easy to distinguish from normal heartburn because it does not spread upward, toward the throat, is associated with hepatic tenderness, may radiate through the back, and is not relieved by antacid therapy. Because of the high risk of pre-eclampsia among pregnant wom-

en, blood pressure should be measured at each prenatal visit. Previously, increases above the patient's baseline (>30 mmHg systolic or >15 mmHg diastolic) were considered to be criteria for the diagnosis of pre-eclampsia. However, this is no longer the case. Nevertheless, such increases warrant close observation.

To ensure accurate readings, an appropriate-size blood pressure cuff should be used. Blood pressure should be measured only after a rest period of 10 minutes or more. The patient should be in an upright or left lateral recumbent position with the arm level with the heart when the blood pressure measurement is taken.

In addition, at each prenatal visit, fundal height should be measured because a small fundal in relation to the length of gestation may indicate intrauterine growth retardation or oligohydramnios, conditions that may become apparent long before diagnostic criteria for pre-eclampsia are met. It is necessary also to make note of any increasing maternal facial edema and rapid weight gain, because fluid retention is associated with pre-eclampsia. Although such symptoms are not unique to pre-eclampsia, they need to be closely monitored. Of less concern is swelling in the extremities, which is a frequent and normal complication of pregnancy.

Laboratory Testing

There is currently no single, reliable, cost-effective screening test for pre-eclampsia. Although an elevated serum uric acid level may be of some use in identifying pregnant women with chronic hypertension with an increased likelihood of having superimposed pre-eclampsia, it is not a definitive test for the condition.

In women who are at high risk for pre-eclampsia, a baseline laboratory evaluation should be taken that includes hepatic enzyme levels, a platelet count, a serum creatinine level, and a 12 to 24-hour urine collection for total protein measurement. Once the diagnosis of pre-eclampsia has been made, an expanded set of laboratory tests should be performed (**Table 16.2**). In women who have pre-eclampsia with no suspected progression, all laboratory tests should be conducted weekly. If progression to eclampsia is suspected, such tests should be repeated more frequently.

Table 16.2 Laboratory tests for pre-eclampsia–eclampsia

For women who develop hypertension after 20 weeks' gestation
Hemoglobin level
Hematocrit
Platelet count
Urine protein collection (12 or 24 hour)
Serum creatinine level
Serum uric acid level
Serum transaminase level
Serum albumin level
Lactic acid dehydrogenase level
Peripheral blood smear
Coagulation profile
For women at high risk of eclampsia
Same tests as preeclampsia but more frequently

Adapted from National High Blood Pressure Education Program. Working Group on High Blood Pressure in Pregnancy. Bethesda, Md.: U.S. Dept. of Health and Human Services, Public Health Service, National Institutes of Health, National Heart, Lung, and Blood Institute, 2000; NIH publication no. 00-3029.

Treatment of Pre-eclampsia

The single, most effective therapy for pre-eclampsia, severe pre-eclamsia, eclampsia, or HELLP syndrome is to deliver the fetus and placenta. If mild pre-eclampsia is diagnosed prior to term, it may be managed conservatively either at home or in the hospital.

The essential elements of conservative management are bed-rest, initial assessment and ongoing surveillance, fetal assessment including nonstress tests, and/or ultrasound surveillance. Steroids should be used to accelerate fetal lung maturation if the condition occurs before 34 weeks of gestation.

Daily assessment by the physician is an integral part of conservative management, with close attention to:
- weight gain
- blood pressure variation over the previous 24 hours
- proteinuria levels
- fetal movement
- general symptoms

Conservative management of mild or severe pre-eclampsia beyond term is not beneficial to the fetus because blood flow to the uterus and placenta may be severely restricted. Therefore, after 37 weeks of gestation, labor should be induced as soon as the cervix is ready. Conservative management of preterm patients with severe pre-eclampsia is an option. However, these patients need to be hospitalized for treatment with magnesium sulfate to prevent seizures and antihypertensive medication to control blood pressure (see Evidence Box 16.1).

Although the threshold for deciding when to manage a woman with pre-eclampsia as a hospital in-patient remains low, it is reasonable to offer outpatient surveillance to women whose systolic blood pressure (sBP) is <140 mmHg and diastolic blood pressure (dBP) is <90 mmHg, with 1+ or less proteinuria on dipstick on one occasion, a normal platelet count, and without adverse features.

In the presence of any of the above signs, closer surveillance should include: frequent office visits (every 3–4 days), close maternal and fetal assessment, and patient education regarding decreased activity and home/childcare assistance. In addition, several weekly laboratory tests are needed, including:
- complete blood cell count, including platelets
- uric acid (an elevated uric acid helps with the diagnosis of gestational hypertension)
- liver enzymes

Indications for hospitalization and/or delivery of a patient with mild pre-eclampsia include worsening maternal or fetal parameters, a favorable cervix at term, or spontaneous rupture of membranes.

Once hypertension and proteinuria have evolved, it is likely that a woman will be delivered for either maternal or fetal indications within two weeks. **Table 16.3** lists the major indicators for when hospitalization should be considered as well as the criteria for conservative versus aggressive management once the patient is hospitalized.

The presence of gestational hypertension with proteinuria at a late gestational age (i.e., ≥34 weeks) may signify the need for immediate delivery of the fetus, depending upon progression of the disease, assessment of the fetus, and status of the cervix.

If the gestational age is less than 34 weeks, management must balance maternal risks against fetal benefits. Delivery may be delayed if blood pressure is controlled (i.e., sBP <160 mmHg and dBP <110 mmHg), fetal assessment remains within tolerable limits (see above), platelet count remains >50 000–100 000 μL, and depending on the practitioner's expertise, training, and comfort in managing pre-eclampsia.

Studies suggest that attempts at conservative management of patients who develop pre-eclampsia at gestational ages 24 weeks or less are associated with serious maternal complications. Pregnancy termination should be considered in these cases.

On the other hand, there is good evidence that conservative management of patients with adverse features be-

Table 16.3 Indicators for hospitalization and conservative management of women with pre-eclampsia

Major indicators for hospitalization of pre-eclamptic women	Indicators for conservative management once patient is hospitalized
A sBP ≥140 mmHg and /or dBP ≥90 mmHg	A stable, well-controlled blood pressure (sBP <160 mmHg / dBP <110 mmHg), and on less than maximal oral antihypertensive therapy for at least two agents (i.e., 1200 mg labetalol/d + 2000 mg methyl-dopa/d + nifedipine [Adalat PA/XL formulations] 90 mg/d)
A repeated 1+ or greater proteinuria 1+ on dipstick or protein	Proteinuria ≤2+ on dipstick (<1g/d or <100 mg/mmol by PCR); this marker of disease severity may not exclude conservative management at gestational ages remote from term, a plasma albumin <20g/L places the patient at greatly increased risk of pulmonary edema and should be considered a contraindication for conservative management
A creatinine ratio >30 mg protein per mmol creatinine	A platelet count ≥100 × 10⁹/L; this marker of disease severity may not exclude conservative management at gestational ages remote from term, depending on the rate of platelet count fall, and the presence or absence of concomitant liver enzyme abnormalities or coagulopathy
Hyperuricemia	
A platelet count ≤100 000/µL	
Any adverse features and/or ultrasound evidence of oligohydramnios or inadequate fetal growth (see Chapter 19)	

dBP, diastolic blood pressure; sBP, systolic blood pressure; PCR, polymerase chain reaction.

tween gestational ages of 24 to 32 weeks produces better outcomes. This is particularly true if the patient is closely monitored in a tertiary care setting staffed with physicians who are very familiar with the disease process.

Treatment of Severe Pre-eclampsia

Women with severe pre-eclampsia should be assessed and managed in a quiet room in an intensive-care situation. Ideally, there should be one-on-one nursing care, at least initially, when the stability of the condition is being assessed. After initial assessment, transfer should be considered for maternal or perinatal reasons depending on the capacity of the local facility.

Proper management requires intense surveillance to lessen risks to the patient. Critical care flow charts should record all physiological results, and all treatments must be carefully recorded. When oral antihypertensive treatment is possible, it should be regarded as the route of choice.

Blood pressure and pulse should be measured every 15 minutes for a minimum of 4 hours until stabilized and then every 30 minutes. At least initially, an indwelling catheter should be inserted and urine output measured hourly whenever intravenous fluids are given. All urine should be tested for proteinuria. Urine outputs as low as 10 mL/h should be considered adequate in the absence of pre-existing renal disease.

An intravenous cannula should always be inserted to administer intravenous fluids by a controlled volumetric pump. Fluid administration should be judicious and fluid balance should be monitored very carefully. Detailed input and output recordings should be charted hourly.

Careful fluid balance is aimed at avoiding fluid overload. Total intravenous input should be limited to 80 mL/h (approximately 1 mL/kg per hour, using current weight). If oxytocin is used, it should be at high concentration (20 U per 500 mL normal saline or Ringer solution). As these women are at high risk of cesarean section, oral fluids should be limited.

Oxygen saturation should be measured continuously and charted with the blood pressure. If oxygen saturation drops below 95%, medical review is needed. Respiratory rate should be measured every hour and temperature should be measured every 4 hours. When present, central venous pressure should be measured continuously and charted with the blood pressure.

Fetal Assessment

A baseline nonstress test should be performed, prior to administration of $MgSO_4$, if possible. Unless the situation mandates immediate delivery, an initial ultrasound assessment is advised for growth, amniotic fluid assessment, and umbilical artery Doppler flow velocity waveform.

Thromboprophylaxis

Women with pre-eclampsia are at particularly increased risk for thromboembolic disease as their condition resolves. Thus, all pre-eclampsia patients should be given antiembolic stockings and/or heparin while they are immobile during the entire antenatal, intrapartum, and postpartum periods. Unfractionated heparin 5000 IU subcutaneously twice daily should be given until the woman is fully mobile. A prophylactic dose of low molecular weight heparin can be used postpartum.

The use of mini-heparinization is not a contraindication to the insertion of an epidural, providing there is no evidence of a coagulopathy. Ideally, the epidural should be inserted 1 hour prior to the next dose of unfractionated heparin, as a subset of patients may become therapeutically anticoagulated during subcutaneous heparin therapy. Since unfractionated heparin reaches its peak effectiveness between 2 and 6 hours following its administration, one should avoid inserting an epidural during that time period unless the activated partial thromboplastin time (APTT) is normal. Of course, such clinical decisions will be assessed by the anesthesiologist on a case-by-case basis.

Treatment of Eclampsia

The treatment of seizures in eclampsia consists of:
- preventing convulsions
- controlling blood pressure
- delivering the fetus

A bolus of magnesium sulfate 20% solution, 4 g intravenously over 5 minutes is the first-line method for preventing convulsions. This is followed by a maintenance dose of magnesium sulfate (10% solution) administered at a rate of 1000 mL/h.

To control elevated blood pressure, hydralazine is given intravenously (5 mg, slowly) every 5 minutes until blood pressure is lowered. This is repeated hourly as needed.

Another option is to administer hydralazine 12.5 mg intramuscularly every 2 hours as needed (see next section for more options).

As soon as the woman's condition stabilizes, delivery should be initiated immediately. Delaying delivery to increase the maturity of the fetus will only risk the lives of both the mother and the fetus. Delivery should occur regardless of the gestational age.

In severe pre-eclampsia, delivery should occur within 24 hours of the onset of symptoms. In eclampsia, delivery should occur within 12 hours of the onset of convulsions. Delivery should be by caesarean section, if vaginal delivery is not anticipated within 12 hours (for eclampsia) or 24 hours (for severe pre-eclampsia).

In the absence of convulsions, prolonging the pregnancy may be possible to improve the outcome of a premature fetus but only if the mother remains stable. This type of management is associated with markedly improved outcomes for the fetus, but does incur some, as yet unquantified, maternal risk. Continued close-monitoring of mother and fetus is needed. It seems ideal to achieve delivery, particularly of premature infants, during normal working hours (i.e., 8 a.m. to 5 p.m.).

Delaying delivery by just a few hours may be helpful if it allows the neonatal unit to be more organized or to transfer a mother to a place where an ICU bed is available, assuming the mother is stable before transfer.

Antihypertensive Therapy

Antihypertensive agents such as labetalol, hydralazine, nifedipine, and sodium nitoprusside are used for the acute reduction of blood pressure in women with severe pre-eclampsia to prevent maternal morbidity. The use of angiotensin-converting enzyme inhibitors is contraindicated in pregnant women.

The aim of antihypertensive is to decrease the dBP to <110 mmHg. This approach is based on the assumption that a significantly lower dBP will cause decreased placental perfusion and fetal compromise.

After severe hypertension has been addressed, the optimal blood pressure for promoting the best outcomes for both mother and fetus is less clear. "Less tight" control (i.e., dBP 90–109 mmHg) is associated with more transient hypertension, which adversely impacts the mother. There is evidence, however, that tighter control (i.e., dBP <90 mmHg) can adversely affect fetal growth. Thus, the aim of blood pressure management should be to reduce sBP to <160 mmHg and dBP to <110 mmHg, slowly and carefully.

Irrespective of pre-existing conditions, blood pressure should be lowered if either sBP is ≥160 mmHg and/

Table 16.4 Management of hypertension

Clinical Diagnosis	Management Plan
If one or more of the following:	Conservative management
Controlled hypertension	
Urinary protein > 5000 mg/24 hr	
Oliguria (< 0.5 mL/kg/h) that resolves with routine fluid and food intake	
AST or ALT more than twice the upper limit of normal with epigastic pain or right upper quadrant tenderness	
If one or more of the following:	Delivery of the fetus within 72 hours
Uncontrolled, severe hypertension	
Eclampsia	
Platelet Count <100 000 cells/μL	
AST or ALT more than twice the upper limit for normal with epigastric or upper right quadrant tenderness	
Pulmonary edema	
Comprised renal function	
Persistent severe headache or visual impairment	

Table 16.5 Drugs commonly used in the treatment of acute severe hypertension during pregnancy

Hydralazine (Apresoline)
Initial dose: 5 mg IV or 10 mg IM
When blood pressure is controlled, repeat initial dose as needed (usually about every 3 hours; maximum, 400 mg per day).
If blood pressure is not controlled in 20 minutes, repeat initial dose every 20 minutes until maximum dosage is reached, or go immediately to next step.
If blood pressure is not controlled with a total of 20 mg IV or 30 mg IM, consider using a different antihypertensive drug (labetalol,† nifedipine [Procardia], sodium nitroprusside [Nitropress]).
Labetalol (Normodyne, Trandate)
Initial dose: 5–10 mg in IV bolus
If blood pressure is not controlled, give 40–80 mg over 20 minutes (maximum cumulative dose: 300 mg).
If blood pressure is not controlled, use a different antihypertensive drug (hydralazine, nifedipine, sodium nitroprusside).
Note: Labetalol is contraindicated in women with asthma or congestive heart failure.
Nifedipine
10–20 mg p.o. every 30 minutes
Nitroprusside
0.2–0.5 ug/kg/min

Reproduced with permission from Wagner LK. Diagnosis and management of preeclampsia. American Family Physician 2004; 70(12):2322 (Table 5).

or dBP is ≥110 mmHg. At sBP 140–159 mmHg and/or dBP 85–109 mmHg the choice of antihypertensive medication will be based on practitioner preference, training, and experience.

In the presence of prepregnancy renal disease or pregestational diabetes, every effort should be made to maintain normal blood pressure to protect renal function; therefore the threshold for intervention should be either sBP ≥140 mmHg and/or dBP ≥90 mmHg. **Table 16.4** displays the management options for hypertension and **Table 16.5** displays the major types of antihypertensive medications used for treating severe hypertension.

Key Points

- Pre-eclampsia, or pregnancy-induced hypertension, is a common problem during pregnancy.
- Eclampsia is the final and most severe phase of pre-eclampsia and can cause convulsions and death, if untreated.
- It is important to distinguish between pre-eclampsia and chronic hypertension as they may be managed differently.
- The most effective therapy for severe pre-eclamsia, eclampsia, or HELLP (hemolysis, elevated liver enzymes, low platelets) syndrome is to deliver the fetus and placenta immediately. However, mild pre-eclampsia diagnosed prior to term may be managed conservatively through bed-rest and ongoing, vigorous surveillance and assessment of the fetus.

Evidence Box 16.1

Conservative management of severe pre-eclampsia before 25 weeks of gestation is associated with considerable perinatal mortality and morbidity for the fetus.

Sezik et al. evaluated the outcome of expectant management of pre-eclampsia among 55 women presenting with severe pre-eclampsia at or before 24 weeks and 6 days of gestation. Indications for delivery were the development of severe maternal morbidity secondary to pre-eclampsia. Complications were identified from individual patient and infant records. Conservative management was associated with a 94.5% (52 of 55) intrauterine fetal loss rate. Of the three live-born infants, one died secondary to respiratory distress syndrome followed by neonatal sepsis and the other two survived with cognitive and motor developmental delay. HELLP (hemolysis, elevated liver enzymes, low platelets) syndrome was diagnosed in 12 women (21.8%). Nine women (16.3%) required transfusions with blood or blood products. There was 1 case (1.8%) of eclampsia. Overall, 15 women (27.2%) had developed some maternal morbidity without any significant differences between <23 weeks' and ≥23 weeks' gestation. None of the women died or required any long-term treatment.

Sezik M, Ozkaya O, Sezik HT, Yapar EG. Expectant management of severe preeclampsia presenting before 25 weeks of gestation. Med Sci Monit 2007 Nov;13(11):CR523–527.

Further Reading

Eruo FU, Sibai BM. Hypertensive diseases in pregnancy. In: Reece EA, Hobbins JC, eds. Clinical Obstetrics: the Fetus and Mother. Malden, Mass: Blackwell Synergy Publishing; 2007:683–699

Hibbard JU. Hypertensive disease and pregnancy. *J Hypertens Suppl* 2002; 20(2, Suppl)S29–S33

Roberts JM, Pearson GD, Cutler JA, Lindheimer MD; National Heart Lung and Blood Institute. Summary of the NHLBI working group on research on hypertension during pregnancy. *Hypertens Pregnancy* 2003;22(2):109–127

von Dadelszen P, Menzies J, Gilgoff S, et al. Evidence-based management for preeclampsia. *Front Biosci* 2007;12:2876–2889

Sezik M, Ozkaya O, Sezik HT, Yapar EG. Expectant management of severe preeclampsia presenting before 25 weeks of gestation. *Med Sci Monit* 2007;13(11):CR523–CR527

Wagner LK. Diagnosis and management of preeclampsia. *Am Fam Physician* 2004;70(12):2317–2324

17 Rhesus Isoimmunization

E. Albert Reece

Definition

Rhesus (Rh) isoimmunization occurs when a pregnant woman develops antibodies in her blood in response to antigens on the surface of fetal red blood cells that have traversed the placenta. These antibodies cross the placenta and coat the fetus' red blood cells, which are then destroyed in the fetus' spleen. This erythrocyte-destroying, or hemolytic, process is called isoimmunization, which can result in the fetus eventually developing severe anemia and other blood disorders (**Fig. 17.1**). In severe cases, it can even cause death.

An antibody isolated from human plasma, called RhoGAM (RH$_0$[D] Immune Globulin), can neutralize this isoimmunization reaction between an Rh-negative woman and her Rh-positive offspring. Before the widespread use of the RhoGAM, the most common cause of isoimmunization was sensitization to the Rh or D antigen. However, because prophylactic RhoGAM has been so successful in preventing women from becoming Rh(D) sensitive, cases of isoimmunization to other red blood cell antigens have become more prevalent.

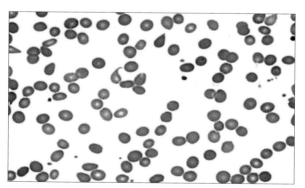

Fig. 17.1 A blood smear examination of patient with hemolytic anemia reveals red blood cell fragments, an unusually large number of reticulocytes (immature erythrocytes), or atypically small, round cells (darker cells).

Diagnosis

In the management of an Rh-sensitized pregnant patient, it is important to know the blood types of the father and of the fetus. Unless documented otherwise, fetal blood should be considered Rh-positive. If, after testing, the fetus is Rh-negative, the maternal antibody will not cause hemolytic disease.

If the father is homozygous Rh-positive, the fetus will be Rh-positive, and further fetal surveillance is mandatory. If he is heterozygous Rh-positive, there is a 50% chance that he has passed the D antigen to the fetus and further testing is warranted. If he is Rh-negative, further surveillance is unnecessary.

The most likely zygosity at the Rh(D) locus of a father can be estimated using race, serology, and the Rh-antigen status of his offspring from previous pregnancies. Recent evidence suggests that an Rh(D) deletion results in the majority of Rh(D)-negative phenotypes among Whites.

Increasingly, Doppler ultrasonography is being used to help diagnose severe hemolytic disease in the fetus, particularly of hydrops fetalis, a severe condition in which the fetus develops systemic edema and a build-up of fluid (perfusion) in body cavities such as the pericardium, thorax, and abdomen.

Doppler examination of the middle cerebral artery is performed to measure the intensity of blood flow (**Fig. 17.2**). This measurement has been shown to correlate with the severity of anemia in the fetus (Evidence Box 17.1).

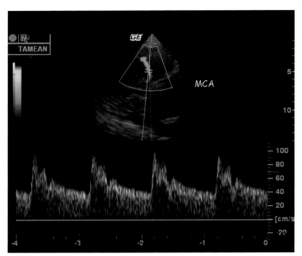

Fig. 17.2 Doppler ultrasonogram of the middle cerebral artery of a fetus.

Prevalence and Epidemiology

The incidence of Rh(D) hemolytic disease in newborns in the United States is approximately 10.6 per 10 000 total births, corresponding to approximately 4000 affected infants nationwide. However, approximately 15 % of the White female population are Rh-negative and, therefore, at risk for developing Rh isoimmunization when they become pregnant. Only 5–8 % of African-Americans are Rh-negative, and it is rare in other populations, except for the Basque region of Spain where it is extraordinarily high (**Table 17.1**).

Etiology

Historically, isoimmunization to the Rh(D) antigen has been the most common and clinically important form of immune sensitization occurring in pregnancy. As a result of the development of RhoGAM, there has been a dramatic decrease in the incidence of Rh isoimmunization among pregnant women in most developed countries.

Even with the substantial decrease in Rh(D) hemolytic disease over the past 40 years, Rh isoimmunization continues to be a problem among pregnant women. This is because some women become sensitive to other blood antigens for which there is no prophylactic treatment.

Maternal antibodies to all non-D antigens are collectively referred to as "irregular antibodies." Although they may occur naturally as a result of pregnancy, the majority develop as the result of blood transfusions. This type of sensitization occurs because most blood transfusions are compatible only with ABO and Rh(D) antigens.

Many of these irregular antibodies, similar to Rh(D), can produce severe disease in the neonate, including profound fetal anemia and hydrops fetalis. Because many others are likely, maternal antibody screening should at least search for those already demonstrated to cause problems.

Hemolytic diseases caused by sensitization to irregular antibodies now accounts for the largest percentage of isoimmunized pregnancies in the developed world. The presence of irregular antibodies is not related to the mother's ABO type or Rh status, and it is possible to become sensitized to more than one type of red blood cell antigen.

In addition to the clinically relevant Rh group, non-Rh groups such as Kell, MNS, Duffy, and Kidd (**Table 17.2**) have assumed increasing importance as the incidence of Rh (D) sensitization has decreased. Nonetheless, sensitization to Rh antigens (non-D) is still responsible for the largest proportion of hemolytic disease in the newborn.

In addition to blood antigen incompatibility, various other situations, such as an amniocentesis or an abortion, may increase the risk of an Rh-negative mother developing Rh isoimmunization (**Table 17.3**).

Table 17.1 Incidence of the Rh-negative blood group in various populations

Population	Incidence (%)
Chinese and Japanese	1
North American Indian and Inuit	1–2
Indo-Eurasian	2
African-American	4–8
Caucasian	15–16
Basque	30–35

Table 17.2 Antibodies commonly associated with hemolytic disease

Rh: D, E, c, C, Cw, e	Dia, Dib, PP1Pk, Far, Good,
Kell: K1, Kpa, k, Jsa, Jsb	Lan, LW, Mta, U, Wra, Zd
Duffy: Fya	
MNS: M, S, s, N	
Kidd: Jka	

Table 17.3 Incidence of significant antenatal fetomaternal hemorrhage for various potential causes of Rh(D) isoimmunization

Event	Incidence of significant fetomaternal hemorrhage (%)
Chorionic villus sampling (CVS) to identify chromosomal abnormalities and other inherited disorders	14–18
Amniocentesis	6–15
Cordocentesis	40
External cephalic version	1.8–6
Molar pregnancy	Sensitization has been reported
Spontaneous abortion	1.5–2.0
Elective termination	4–5
Threatened abortion	11
Third-trimester bleeding	4–8
Uneventful pregnancy	2.6–8

Pathophysiology

The initial maternal response to Rh isoimmunization is to develop large molecular weight antibodies that are unable to cross the placenta. This is followed by the synthesis of anti-Rh(D) immunoglobulin G (IgG) antibodies that do cross the placenta and stick to the fetal red cells, accelerating their destruction, or hemolysis, in the fetus' spleen.

The initial immune response of an Rh-negative mother to her fetus' D antigen-positive blood can sometimes take as long as 6 months to develop. The resulting immune response may be mild and only a relatively small number of the fetus' erythroblasts are hemolyzed. Thus, the consequences of the fetal red cell destruction may be minimal, with no demonstrable after-effects other than acute hyperbilirubinemia as a neonate.

When the immune response is stronger, however, and significantly more blood cells are hemolyzed, the fetus may begin to develop mild to moderate anemia in utero. As the severity of red cell destruction increases, it begins to exceed the ability of the bone marrow to produce new red cells. The more severe stage of the disease is known as erythroblastosis fetalis.

Mild to moderate hemolysis manifests as increased indirect bilirubin (red cell pigment). Severe hemolysis leads to red blood cell production by the spleen and liver. Subsequently, hepatic circulatory obstruction (portal hyper-

tension) with placental edema interferes with placental perfusion, and ascites may develop. This can lead to heart failure, massive edema, hepatosplenomegaly, hyperbilirubinemia, placental hypertrophy and, eventually, intrauterine death.

For babies that do make it to term, bilirubin is no longer cleared from their blood via the placenta and the symptoms of jaundice (yellowish skin and yellow discoloration of the whites of the eyes) typically increase within 24 hours after birth. In addition, there may be persistent anemia, which can cause high-output heart failure, with pallor, enlarged liver and/or spleen, generalized swelling, and respiratory distress.

The pathophysiology of hydrops fetalis is not fully understood, but extravascular hemolysis with fetal anemia plays a major role by stimulating erythropoiesis in the liver causing distortion of the hepatic vessels, which leads to portal hypertension and impaired albumin production. Profound hypoalbumin anemia leads to ascites, edema, and pleural pericardial effusions. Severe anemia leads to cardiac failure and tissue hypoxia, which damages the endothelial wall, leading to fluid extravasation to the extravascular space.

History

Chief Complaint

Diseases caused by anti-Rh(D) and antibodies to other blood antigens show a wide spectrum of severity. Not all D-positive infants born to mothers with anti-D antibodies in their serum, for example, are affected by hemolytic disease. Some infants are only mildly affected, with jaundice and anemia developing in the first week of life.

More severely affected infants develop profound hyperbilirubinaemia with signs of brain damage, leading to death within a week of birth in majority of cases. Those who survive have permanent brain damage characterized by choreoathetosis and spasticity and, in milder cases, by high-frequency deafness.

Profound anemia is the most severe manifestation of hemolytic disease. It can develop in utero as early as the 18th week of gestation. Unmanaged, it can quickly lead to hydrops fetalis with generalized edema, ascites, hepatosplenomegaly, erythroblastosis, and a high risk of mortality.

A thorough prenatal history must include questions about the many factors that can potentially put the patient at an increased risk of developing Rh isoimmunization (**Table 17.4**). The appearance of any of these factors in a medical history should trigger an extensive diagnos-

Table 17.4 Maternal and family history factors known to increase the risk of developing Rh isoimmunization and other hemolytic diseases

Maternal history factors	Family history factors
Rh-negative blood type	Jaundice in other family members or in previous child
Known presence of isoimmune blood group antibodies	Family history of twinning (specifically, monozygotic)
Prior administration of blood products	Family history of genetic disorders, chromosomal abnormalities, or metabolic diseases
Illicit drug use	Congenital malformation in previous child
Collagen-vascular disease	Previous fetal death
Thyroid disease or diabetes	Prior Rh isoimmunization
Organ transplant	Previous fetomaternal transfusion
Blunt abdominal trauma	Congenital heart disease in previous child
Coagulopathy	Hydramnios
Use of indomethacin, sodium diclofenac, or potentially teratogenic drugs during pregnancy	
Younger (<16 y) or older (>35 y) maternal age	
Sexually transmitted diseases	
Hemoglobinopathy	
Occupational exposure to infants or young children	
Owning a pet cat	
Current or recent community epidemic of viral illness	

tic follow-up, including physical assessments, laboratory tests, and imaging studies.

Physical Examination

A number of maternal or fetal physical factors that are related to Rh isoimmunization should prompt further diagnostic evaluation. These include any incidences of:

- twinning
- hydramnios
- exanthem or other evidence of intercurrent viral illness
- herpetic lesion or chancre
- decrease in fetal movements

Laboratory Testing

A maternal antibody titer, as detected by an indirect Coombs test, is used to select sensitized patients for further fetal assessment. The concept of a critical titer has evolved, meaning that the fetus is at significant risk of severe hemolytic disease when the titer is at this level or higher.

In most centers this titer is considered to be 1 : 16 or 1 : 32 in a first sensitized pregnancy, although some have set the level as low as 1 : 4. The choice of level depends on how the titer is obtained (albumin, indirect Coombs test, or other method), the laboratory where the test is run, and the antibody in question. In the past, it may have been possible for each laboratory to develop its own standards, but with the significant decline in the number sensitized pregnancies in recent years, this is no longer an option in most circumstances.

Currently, the American College of Obstetricians and Gynecologists (ACOG) recommends considering invasive testing (amniocentesis or cordocentesis) when the titer is 1 : 16 or greater in albumin or 1 : 32 or greater by indirect Coombs test. The ACOG recommends that using a titer of 1 : 8 may be more aggressive than the available data warrant.

In a woman who has already had a sensitized pregnancy, antibody titers become less reliable as a prognostic indicator, and fetal surveillance should be initiated at the earliest gestational age at which fetal transfusion is an option, usually 18 weeks.

At their first hospital visit, all pregnant women should have their ABO and D blood groups tested and their serum screened for alloantibodies. If no antibodies are present the D blood group, alloantibody testing is typically repeated at 28 weeks' gestation. However, if alloantibodies are detected, further testing should be carried out monthly, depending on the clinical significance and potency of the antibody. The evaluation of a positive antibody screen should include identification of the antibody and its titer.

There are several classes of antibodies. The two of interest are IgM and IgG. If the antibody can be identified as an IgM, then it does not cross the placenta and there is no risk of fetal hemolysis. If it is an IgG, then it does cross the placenta and can cause hemolytic disease. Antibodies directed against Rh antigens, as well as anti-K, anti-D, anti-E, anti-Fya, and anti-Jka antibodies comprise the majority of those responsible for hemolytic disease of the newborn (see **Table 17.4**)

A pregnant woman with titer of greater than 1 : 4 is considered sensitized. However, it is possible to encounter women with much higher titers, who have fetuses that are negative for the antigen to which the antibody is directed.

Cordiocentesis

Cordiocentesis should be performed for all patients with a history of severe disease and those with a hemolytic antibody level of more than 15 IU/mL or a titer of 1 : 128 or more (see Laboratory Testing).

First, obtain a fetal blood sample and then determine the hemoglobin concentration. If this is below the normal range, the tip of the needle is kept in the lumen of the umbilical cord vessel and fresh, packed, rhesus-negative blood compatible with that of the mother is infused manually into the fetal circulation (**Fig. 17.3**).

At the end of the transfusion, aspirate a further fetal blood sample to determine the final hemoglobin concentration. Give subsequent transfusions at intervals of 1 to 3 weeks until 34–36 weeks of gestation. Their timing should be based on the findings of noninvasive tests, such as Doppler ultrasonography. Following a fetal blood transfusion, the mean rate of decrease in fetal hemoglobin is approximately 0.3 g/dL per day.

A cord plasma bilirubin concentration of 4 mg/dL or more may also be an indication for exchange transfusion. If an immediate exchange transfusion is not indicated, monitor plasma bilirubin concentrations every few hours: levels above 306 mmol/L (18 mg/dL) in mature infants may lead to brain damage. In premature infants the criteria to assess severity are stricter.

Just as the partner of the Rh(D)-sensitized woman can be tested to determine if he is Rh(D)-positive, testing for the presence for any of these antigens can be performed in the partner of the woman who has developed irregular antibodies.

Serial Amniocentesis

Fetuses affected by hemolytic disease secrete abnormally high levels of bilirubin into the amniotic fluid. The amount of bilirubin can be quantitated spectrophotometrically by measuring absorbance at the 450-nm wavelength in a specimen of amniotic fluid that has been shielded from light. Alternatively, percutaneous umbilical blood sampling may be used to determine all blood parameters directly.

If amniocentesis is used to monitor the fetus, the results (delta 450) are plotted on a "Liley" curve. The Liley curve is divided into three zones (**Fig 17.4**). A result in zone I indicates mild or no disease. Fetuses in zone I are usually followed up with amniocentesis every 3 weeks, or sometimes less frequently. A result in zone II indicates intermediate disease. Fetuses in low zone II are usually followed up with amniocentesis every 1–2 weeks. A re-

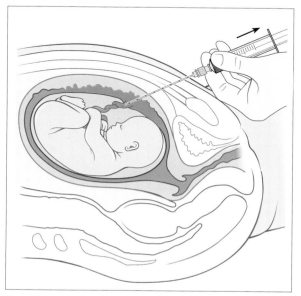

Fig. 17.3 Intrauterine transfusion can be accomplished with a 10-mL syringe or a transfusion set inserted in the umbilical cord.

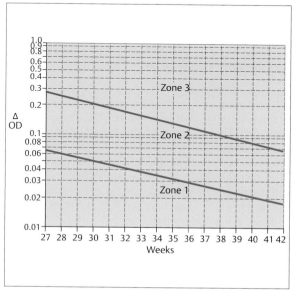

Fig. 17.4 A typical Liley Curve showing the three zones indicating mild to severe disease.

sult above the middle of zone II often requires immediate transfusion or delivery of the fetus.

Patients with results in zone I or low zone II can be allowed to proceed to term, at which point labor should be induced. In most cases, patients in the middle of zone II can progress to 36–38 weeks of gestation. Depending on gestational age, patients in zone III should either be delivered or receive intrauterine fetal transfusion.

Although serial determinations of delta optical density (DOD) at 450 nm and cordiocentesis are the most common methods for evaluating the status of the fetus, Doppler ultrasonography of the middle cerebral artery has also been used to identify fetuses at risk for moderate to severe hemolytic disease (see Evidence Box 17.1).

Treatment

In the first sensitized pregnancy, monthly indirect Coombs titer should be performed on the mother whose pregnancy is complicated by Rh(D) isoimmunization. If a critical titer is reached, paternal and fetal antigen status should be determined as appropriate.

If the fetus is known or likely to be Rh(D)-positive, either amniocentesis for DOD 450 or peak systolic velocity of the middle cerebral artery (as determined by Doppler) can be used to follow the sensitized mother. If DOD 450 is used as the prognostic indicator, an extended Liley curve is preferable.

In most instances, for the second or greater sensitized pregnancy, amniocentesis or Doppler scanning of the middle cerebral artery should be initiated at 18–20 weeks of gestation, because antibody titers are less reliable.

Intrauterine Transfusion

The most common site for intrauterine transfusion (IUT) at this time is the cord insertion into the placenta. These transfusions can also be intraperitoneal, at the intrahepatic portion of the umbilical vein, or even intracardiac. The ideal red cells used for IUT are type O, Rh(D)-negative, cytomegalovirus-negative, hemoglobin S-negative, irradiated, and leukocyte-poor. The red cells should be tightly packed to a hematocrit of 75% to 90% in an effort to avoid volume overload in the fetus.

Various formulas exist for calculating the amount of blood to transfuse. These usually consider the fetoplacental blood volume, the desired hematocrit (Hct), the starting fetal hematocrit, and the hematocrit of the transfused red cells. The most widely used formula is:

$$\text{Volume}_{\text{transfused}} = [\text{Fetal blood volume} \times (\text{Hct}_{\text{desired}} - \text{Hct}_{\text{initial}})] / [\text{Hct}_{\text{donor}} - \text{Hct}_{\text{desired}}].$$

The fetoplacental blood volume can be estimated based on gestational age and fetal weight. The desired hematocrit is based on the average hematocrit at a given gestational age.

Because red cell antibodies acquired across the placenta in utero persist in the infant's circulation at birth and for some time thereafter, neonates affected by red cell isoimmunization are at risk of needing blood transfusions in the immediate neonatal course. In addition, some neonates require late blood transfusions. It is, therefore, critically important that these babies be followed very closely in the first few months of life. The need for late neonatal transfusions is related to the extent and duration of bone marrow suppression resulting from IUT.

Key Points

- Isoimmunization to the Rh(D) antigen has been the most common and clinically important form of immune sensitization occurring in pregnancy, although there has been a dramatic decrease in the incidence of Rh isoimmunization among pregnant women in most developed countries.
- Adverse reactions to "irregular" antibodies also can produce severe disease in the neonate; hemolytic diseases caused by sensitization to irregular antibodies now accounts for the largest percentage of isoimmunized pregnancies in the developed world.
- A thorough prenatal history must include questions about the many factors that can potentially put the patient at an increased risk of developing isoimmunization diseases.
- The appearance of any of potential causative factors in a medical history should trigger an extensive diagnostic follow-up, including physical assessments, laboratory tests, and imaging studies.
- Treatment is based on the results of the follow-up diagnostic tests.

Evidence Box 17.1

Doppler measurement of the peak velocity of systolic blood flow in the middle cerebral artery can safely replace invasive testing in the management of Rh-allo-immunized pregnancies.

Oepkes et al. conducted a prospective, international, multicenter study including women with RhD-, Rhc-, RhE-, or Fy(a)-alloimmunized pregnancies with indirect antiglobulin titers of at least 1 : 64 and antigen-positive fetuses. The aim was to assess whether Doppler ultrasonographic measurement of the peak systolic velocity of blood flow in the middle cerebral artery was at least as sensitive and accurate as measurement of amniotic-fluid delta optical density (DOD) at 450 nm for diagnosing severe fetal anemia. Doppler ultrasonography of the middle cerebral artery had a sensitivity of 88% (95% CI, range 78% to 93%), a specificity of 82% (95% CI, range 73% to 89%), and an accuracy of 85% (95% CI, range 79% to 90%). In contrast, amniotic-fluid DOD 450 had a sensitivity of 76% (95% CI, range 65% to 84%), a specificity of 77% (95% CI, range 67% to 84%), and an accuracy of 76% (95% CI, range 69% to 82%). Doppler ultrasonography was more sensitive, by 12 percentage points (95% CI, 0.3 to 24.0), and more accurate by 9 percentage points (95% CI, 1.1 to 15.9), than measurement of amniotic-fluid DOD 450.

Oepkes D, Seaward PG, Vandenbussche FP, et al. Doppler ultrasonography versus amniocentesis to predict fetal anemia. N Engl J Med. 2006 Jul 13;355(2):156–164.

Further Reading

Alshimmiri MM, Hamoud MS, Al-Saleh EA, Mujaibel KY, Al-Harmi JA, Thalib L. Prediction of fetal anemia by middle cerebral artery peak systolic velocity in pregnancies complicated by rhesus isoimmunization. *J Perinatol* 2003;23(7):536–540

Contreras M, de Silva M. The prevention and management of haemolytic disease of the newborn. *J R Soc Med* 1994;87(5):256–258

Cunniff C; American Academy of Pediatrics Committee on Genetics. Prenatal screening and diagnosis for pediatricians. *Pediatrics* 2004;114(3):889–894

Harkness UF, Spinnato JA. Prevention and management of RhD isoimmunization. *Clin Perinatol* 2004;31(4):721–742

Kumar S, O'Brien A. Recent developments in fetal medicine. *BMJ* 2004;328(7446):1002–1006

Shaver SM. Isoimmunization in pregnancy. *Crit Care Nurs Clin North Am* 2004;16(2):205–209

18 Multifetal Pregnancy

E. Albert Reece

Because of their higher rates of perinatal morbidity and mortality compared with single-birth pregnancies, multifetal pregnancies present a significant challenge to OB/ GYN practitioners. Multifetal births are often complicated by low birth weight, fetal growth restriction, placental and cord abnormalities, pre-eclampsia, anemia, preterm labor, and an increased risk of infant mortality.

This increased risk of fetal morbidity and mortality associated with multifetal pregnancies is matched by a similarly increased maternal risk for a variety of complications, including hypertension, anemia, and abruption. For these reasons, pregnancies that involve more than one fetus require especially close monitoring, particularly during the antepartum period when intervention is most likely to be effective in minimizing such problems.

Definitions

Amnionicity: Refers to the number of amniotic sacs. The amniotic sac is the pouch, or sac, in which the fetus develops.

Aneuploidy: A genetic status characterized by cells having an abnormal number of chromosomes. Genetic syndromes caused by an extra or missing chromosome are among the most widely recognized genetic conditions. Down syndrome is a well known example.

Chorionicity: A chorionicity scan is used to distinguish between twins that share a placenta and those who have separate ones. For example, in a dichorionic twin pregnancy, each developing fetus has its own placenta.

Fraternal dizygotic siblings: This term refers to multiple-birth siblings resulting from the fertilization and implantation of more than one egg. Fraternal dizygotic siblings are not genetically identical. Instead they have what is known as "coequal" genetic similarity, which is the same as any other full siblings do.

Hydramnios: The condition of having excessive amniotic fluid, sometimes referred to polyhydramnios. Inadequate volume of amniotic fluid is referred to as oligohydramnios.

Identical montozygotic siblings: This refers to one egg being fertilized and the resulting zygote splitting into more than one embryo. Identical siblings therefore have the same genetic material.

Multiple birth: This expression is used only when more than one fetus is carried to term in a single pregnancy. Different names have been assigned to babies that are born to a woman giving birth to multiples, depending on the number of live offspring, such as twins, triplets, quadruplets, quintuplets, etc.

Multifetal pregnancy: This term is used for a pregnancy that involves more than one fetus.

Placentation: This term refers to the formation, structure, or arrangement of a placenta or placentas. The function of placentation is to transfers nutrients from the mother to the growing embryo.

Polyzygotic birth: In some multiple births, it is possible for a combination of identical and nonidentical births. For example, a set of triplets may have one fraternal baby from one egg, plus two identical twins from a second egg.

Diagnosis

The ability to diagnose a multifetal pregnancy early on is crucial to developing an effective antepartum management strategy. Once a multifetal pregnancy is suspected, ultrasonography, which is very sensitive for this purpose and has a detection rate approaching 99.3%, should be performed at the earliest possible gestational age. It will not only detect the number of fetuses but also other fetal health indicators, including placentation, amnionicity, and chorionicity.

It is easiest to determine amnionicity and chorionicity in the first trimester and becomes increasingly difficult and less accurate as the gestation matures due to progressive thinning of the membrane and fetal crowding. Ascertaining these parameters is important because monochorionic pairs, which account for 20–33% of twin gestations, have a 2.5 greater relative risk of perinatal mortality than single-fetus pregnancies. They also are at increased risk of neurologic problems associated with twin–twin transfusion syndrome (see Etiology and Pathogenesis below) and demise of a co-twin in utero.

Dichorionicity is established by ultrasound imaging of two separate placentas or fetuses of different gender. If these characteristics are not easily discernable, another tell-tale sign of dichorionicity is a piece of chorionic tissue projecting between the layers of the dividing membrane (i.e., the lambda or twin-peak sign) (**Fig. 18.1**). If this feature is absent, then it indicates monochorionicity.

The thickness of the intertwin membrane has been used to predict chorionicity. However, this method is much less reliable. If chorionicity cannot be reliably established, the physician should consider more invasive testing. Monoamnionicity can ruled out by visualizing the presence of a membrane between the fetuses. Ultrasound imaging also is valuable for detecting the presence of any fetal anomalies.

Prevalence and Epidemiology

In the past several decades, multiple births have become significantly more prevalent due to the greater reliance on assistive reproductive technology (ART), especially among women delaying childbirth until their 30s and 40s. The most common form of human multiple birth is twins (two babies). Twins are relatively common and occur on average 13 times per 1000 maternities, though the **twinning** frequency varies over time and geographic location.

Due to the dramatic increase in the use of ART between 1981 and 1997, the overall twinning birth rate in

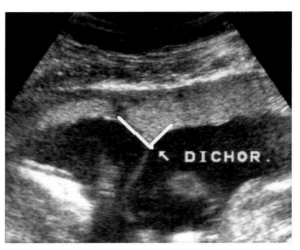

Fig. 18.1 Ultrasound image of a dichorionic pregnancy. The arrow points to the characteristic lambda peak.

the United Stated has increased almost 40%, while that rate of higher order births has increased almost 360%. This same trend for twins and higher order births has been seen in other developed countries, including Great Britain, France, and Canada (**Table 18.1**).

There have been a few cases of higher order births up to octuplets (eight babies), with all siblings being born alive. However, the largest multiple birth delivery in which the babies survived more than a few days were septuplets, the first of which occurred in 1997. The largest set to have even a single member survive is octuplets, which were born in 1998 to a couple in Texas (seven of the eight babies survived).

There have been a few sets of nonuplets (nine) in which a few babies were born alive, though none lived longer than a few days. There even have been cases of human pregnancies that started out with ten, eleven, twelve, and even fifteen fetuses. However, there are no known instances of a live birth in such pregnancies. Most of these higher-order pregnancies were the result of fertility medications and ART, although in 1992 a set of duodecaplets (twelve) was conceived spontaneously (without the aid of fertility treatments) in Argentina.

The birth rate of monozygotic twins is approximately 4 per 1000 births and is constant worldwide. In contrast, dizygotic twinning is associated with multiple ovulation, and its frequency varies among races within countries and is affected by maternal age. It increases from 3 per 1000 births in women younger than 20 years old to 14 per 1000 births in women aged 35–40 years and declines thereafter.

The highest birth rate of dizygotic twins occurs in African nations, and the lowest birth rate of dizygotic twins occurs in Asia. The Yorubas of western Nigeria have a birth rate of 45 twins per 1000 live births, and approximately 90% are dizygotic.

Table 18.1 Multiple births: rate and time trends between 1981 and 1997

	Twins				Triplets or more		
	Total No. live births	No.	Rate per 1000	% increase	No.	Rate per 1000	% increase
Canada							
1981	238 937	4304	18.0		84	0.3	
				+28			+197
1997	210 174	4849	23.1		218	1.0	
England/Wales							
1982	625 931	12 154	19.4		230	0.4	
				+41			+273
1997	643 095	17 551	27.3		890	1.4	
France							
1982	797 223	15 550	19.5		423	0.5	
				+45			+111
1997	726 768	20 585	28.3		814	1.1	
USA							
1981	3 629 238	70 049	19.3		1385	0.4	
				+39			+358
1997	3 884 329	104 208	26.8		6752	1.7	
				+28			+197
1997	210 174	4849	23.1		218	1.0	

Reproduced with permission from Blondel B et al. The impact of the increasing number of multiple births on the rates of preterm birth and low birthweight: an international study. Am J Public Health 2002; 92(8):1323–1330 (Table 1).

Etiology

Many factors contribute to the recent increase in the prevalence of multiple pregnancies. The principal causes, however, are advancing maternal age and infertility treatments. As women get older, their chance of having "multiples" doubles. Women between 20 and 24 years of age have twins at the rate of approximately 22.4 per 1000 live births, whereas women between 40 and 44 years have twins at the rate of 51.3 per 1000 births.

Women are also having children later in life. For example, in 2003 the birth rate for women between 40 and 44 years of age was approximately 8.7 births per 1000 compared to 3.9 births per 1000 among women in the same age group in 1980.

Both environmental and genetic factors contribute to the tendency to conceive spontaneous dizygotic twins. Variations in these two factors are mostly attributed to the differences in dizygotic **twinning** rate, since the mo-

nozygotic **twinning** rate is relatively constant. For example, mothers of dizygotic twins report significantly more female family members also with dizygotic twins than mothers of monozygotic twins.

In addition to genetics, advanced age and increased parity also are known risk factors for dizygotic twins. Recent research has demonstrated that taller mothers and mothers with a high body mass index (BMI >30) are at greater risk of dizygotic **twinning**. Seasonality, smoking, oral contraceptive use, and folic acid also have been associated with an increased risk of twinning. However, these associations have not been found to be highly statistically significant.

Genomic analysis has identified multiple genes that appear to contribute to the risk of **twinning**. Mutations in one of these genes—known as growth differentiation factor 9, or GDF9—occur significantly more frequently in mothers of dizygotic twins. However, the mutations are rare and only account for a small part of the genetic contribution for **twinning**.

According to studies, 30–40% of pregnancies in the United States with three or more births occur because physicians implant more than the recommended number of embryos during in vitro fertilization. This practice places both the mother and fetus at greater risk for adverse outcomes. Multiple births are linked to a greater risk of premature birth, low birth weight, and other complications, such as cerebral palsy in the infant and pregnancy-related high blood pressure and postpartum depression in the mother.

A number of European countries, including the United Kingdom, Germany, Sweden, and Switzerland, have banned the implantation of more than three embryos in the womb. In contrast, the United States only offers a voluntary guideline, which many doctors choose not to follow. Some doctors say they implant more than three embryos if a woman's embryos are inferior. However, competition with other clinics and pressure from patients for high success rates also appear to play a role in this decision.

Pathophysiology

Mother

A woman's body must make many more physiological adjustments to multiple gestations than to a singleton pregnancy. For example, the size of her uterus must increase much more, which results in the abdominal organs becoming more compressed or displaced. Also, the diaphragm can be elevated, compressing the lungs.

As a result of the abnormal size and weight of the larger uterus required for multiple pregnancies, the mother often experiences more pressure symptoms and more difficulty in ambulating and performing daily tasks. Furthermore, with a single fetus, a woman's blood volume will increase by 40–50% in late pregnancy. In contrast, if she is carrying twins, her blood volume will increase by 50–60% (an extra 500 mL). In addition, compared with a singleton pregnancy, the increase in red cell mass in multiple gestations is less, thus producing a more pronounced "physiological anemia."

A woman carrying more than one fetus must also increase her cardiac output compared with a singleton gestation. This increased cardiac output in a twin pregnancy occurs primarily during the second and third trimesters and is the result of increased heart rate and higher stroke volume. Multifetal pregnancies also are complicated by an increase in the incidence of hypertensive disorders, which tend to occur earlier and be more severe than in singleton pregnancies.

Fetus

In a multifetal pregnancy, all of the fetuses are at increased risk of premature delivery, abnormal presentation and position, and hydramnios. In addition, they all have an increased risk for a prolapsed cord, premature separation from the placenta, and hypoxia. Also, during delivery, they may be injured by manipulation or may suffer ill-effects from prolonged anesthesia.

Twinning and higher order pregnancies also are more prone to restriction, competition for nutrients, and cord compression and entanglement compared with singleton pregnancies. Monozygotic twins tend to be smaller and are significantly more prone to fetal demise in utero than dizygotic twins.

Although it is well known that twin pregnancies carry higher risks for adverse consequences than single pregnancies, some types of twins—particularly those connected to a single (monochorionic) placenta—may face even higher risks. For monochorionic twins, the risks of serious, life-threatening complications are up to 10 times higher than for those twins who have one placenta each (i.e., dichorionic twins). The dangers in monochorionic twins are caused by the fact that the circulations of the twin pair are usually connected with each other via the placenta.

The most serious complication with monochorionic placentas is a condition known as "twin-to-twin transfusion syndrome" in which blood is shunted from one fetus to the other through blood vessel connections in a shared placenta (**Fig. 18.2**). Over time, the recipient fetus receives too much blood, which can overload the cardiovascular system and cause too much amniotic fluid to develop. The smaller donor fetus meanwhile receives inadequate blood flow and has low amounts of amniotic

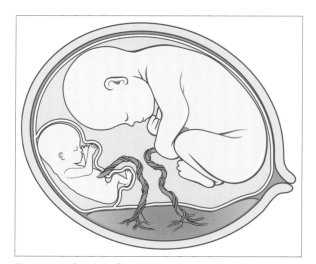

Fig. 18.2 When twin fetuses share a single placenta, it can lead to twin-to-twin transfusion syndrome, in which one twin receives too much blood while the other receives too little, leading to potentially severe complications for both.

fluid. This syndrom occurs in about 15% of twins with a shared placenta. Fortunately, it is possible to distinguish between monochorionic and dichorionic twins by ultrasound exam in the first and early second trimesters and to take steps to prevent such complications.

History

In places where ultrasound exams are not routinely administered during the first trimester of a pregnancy, the early diagnosis of a multifetal pregnancy is highly dependent on the physician's ability to recognize predisposing factors during history-taking. A uterine size clinically estimated to be greater than expected, a history of assisted reproduction, or an elevated maternal serum α-fetoprotein level (see below) are enough to warrant further investigation.

Chief Symptoms

There are a number of tell-tale signs that a woman is carrying more than one fetus. She often will exhibit earlier and more severe symptoms of a normal pregnancy, including pressure on the pelvis, nausea, backache, constipation, hemorrhoids, varicosities, abdominal distention, and breathing difficulties. Fetal activity often is greater and more persistent as well.

Physical Examination

The following physical symptoms are indications that a mother is carrying more than one fetus and is in need of immediate follow-up examinations and laboratory evaluations:

- She has a larger-than-expected uterus (>4 cm) for gestational date.
- She has excessive weight gain that is not explained by obesity or edema.
- She has polyhydramnios.
- Her uterus contains three or more large parts.
- Her uterus has a multiplicity of small parts.
- She displays a simultaneous recording of different fetal heart rates, each one asynchronous with her pulse rate.

To be safe, it is prudent to consider all pregnancies as potentially multiple until it can be proven otherwise. By doing so, 75% of multifetal pregnancies can be identified before the second trimester by physical examination alone.

Ultrasonography

The vast majority of multiple pregnancies are identified by ultrasound imaging, which can diagnose a twin pregnancy as early as the 10th week of gestation. Ultrasonography also has an important role in diagnosing abnormalities and providing fetal surveillance throughout the duration of gestation. This determination, as well as dating the pregnancy, is most accurate during the first 12–14 weeks of gestation, particularly if transvaginal sonography (TVS) is the method of detection.

The proper management of a multifetal pregnancy hinges on both an accurate determination of the date of conception, as well as chorionicity and amnionicity. Monochorionic multifetal pregnancies are associated with higher perinatal morbidity and mortality than are dichorionic twin pregnancies. Perinatal mortality in monoamniotic twins has been reported to be as high as 30–70%. However, mortality can be significantly reduced by early diagnosis and fetal surveillance. Although ultrasound imaging cannot predict zygosity with a high degree of accuracy, it is highly effective in predicting chorionicity and determining placentation.

Chorionicity

The ideal time to determine chorionicity of a twin or higher order multiple pregnancy and the number of embryos is during the first trimester when the chorionic sacs can be counted. TVS provides better resolution and detail than transabdominal sonography (Evidence Box 18.1). This is particularly true in obese patients.

The number of chorionic sacs can be determined as early as 4–5 postmenstrual weeks by TVS. The sacs, which measure between 2 mm and 4 mm at this stage of gestation, are round sonolucent structures with a brightly echogenic rim (chorion). By simply counting the number of chorionic sacs, one can determine whether the pregnancy will be dichorionic, trichorionic, and so on. It is, thus, possible to determine precisely the chorionicity of a multifetal pregnancy by the fifth postmenstrual week of the gestation.

By the sixth postmenstrual week, the chorionic sacs are large enough that the yolk sacs and embryos can be seen within them. The yolk sacs are almost attached to the fetal pole (**Fig. 18.3**).

The embryonic heartbeats start on day 21 after conception but only become detectable by ultrasound scan at the end of the fifth or in the sixth postmenstrual week. Initially, the frequency of the heartbeats is about 80 to 90 beats per minute. As the pregnancy progresses, the heart rate reaches around 150 to 160 beats per minute at around the ninth postmenstrual week. It is prudent to wait until the embryonic heartbeats are visible to determine the number of fetuses in the pregnancy. The

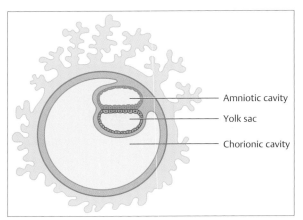

Fig. 18.3 Illustration of the chorionic sac showing the developing yolk sac and amniotic cavity.

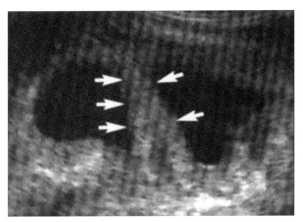

Fig. 18.4 Ultrasound image displaying two chorionic sacs. The thick intertwin membrane (arrows) indicates dichorionicity.

presence of cardiac activity is crucial for accurately determining the number of viable fetuses.

In monoamniotic twins, the number of yolk sacs detected may be variable. A single yolk sac, a partially divided yolk sac, or two yolk sacs may be present, depending on the timing of cell division.

By approximately 10 weeks' gestation, chorionicity can be determined by visualizing the junction between the two amniotic sacs and the chorion or uterus. In pregnancies with a single fused placenta, the junction between the two placentas will be thick and wedge-shaped ("lambda sign" or "twin-peak sign"), confirming dichorionicity .

If this junction appears thin and T-shaped and meets the uterine wall at a 90° angle, the pregnancy is monochorionic. This criteria can also be used in higher order multiples with mixed chorionicity.

Multiple studies have confirmed the accuracy of these sonographic techniques in predicting chorionicity. As confirmed by pathological findings, first-trimester sonography has 100 percent accuracy in determining chorionic and amniotic type.

Amnionicity

When multiple chorionic sacs are visualized each with a single yolk sac (**Fig. 18.4**), a diagnosis of dichorionic–diamniotic pregnancy can be made reliably by the seventh week of gestation. If a single chorionic sac is visualized, and two yolk sacs are seen within this chorionic sac, it is difficult to determine amnionicity until the eighth week of pregnancy. This is because prior to the eighth postmenstrual week, the amnion rests too close to the fetus to make a reliable diagnosis. However, at about the eighth week, with increasing amniotic fluid volume, the amnion separates from the fetal body and becomes easier to image.

Caveats

Determining both chorionicity and amnionicity in a woman diagnosed with a twin gestation during the second trimester is more difficult. Although first-trimester sonography has up to 100% accuracy in determining chorionicity, second-trimester sonography is only about 90% accurate. The following findings can assist in making an accurate diagnosis after the first trimester:

1. *The gender of the fetus.* Determining fetal gender is an important component of assessing chorionicity. In the vast majority of cases, twins of different genders indicates dichorionicity; however, in approximately 50% of dichorionic–diamniotic (Di-Di) twin pregnancies, like-sex twins will be present, which requires further evaluation. In such cases, it is necessary to scrutinize the placentas to make the diagnosis.

2. *The number of placental masses.* The ability to image separate placental sites suggests dichorionicity. However, only about one-third of all twin gestations will have placentas that are widely separated from each other. Thus, this approach has limitations. In cases of concordant sex and a single placental mass, further evaluation is necessary. At 11 weeks, monochorionic–diamniotic twin pregnancy demonstrates the T-shaped junction between the chorionic sac and the two amniotic sacs (**Fig. 18.5**).

3. *The intertwin membrane*
   - *Thickness:* When evaluating fetal gender and placental mass fail to detect chorionicity, the intertwin membrane thickness can be measured. In monochorionic–diamniotic twins, the dividing membrane consists of two layers of amnion and this membrane is very thin and hairlike, measuring less than 2 mm. In dichorionic–diamniotic twins, the dividing membrane consists of four layers—two layers of amnion and two layers of chorion. Thus, a dichorionic dividing membrane will be significantly thicker

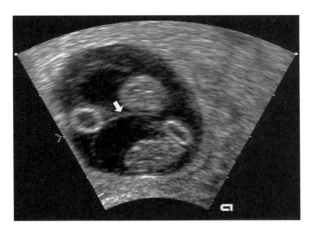

Fig. 18.5 In monochorionic twins, the intertwin membrane is relatively thin, approaches the placenta at approximately 90°, and takes on a characteristic T shape (arrow).

when measured by ultrasonography. Counting the latter two layers can be achieved by enlarging the picture for better imaging.

- *Membrane origin:* Often the view of the membrane origin, or take-off, is obscured by the fetus. However, if it can be detected, it is the most useful and reliable marker of chorionicity. When it is shaped like a triangle, it is a consistent marker of dichorionicity. The accuracy of this sign in determining chorionicity has been reported to be 100%. When the take-off has a T shape or the membrane approaches the placenta at or close to 90°, this becomes a dependable sign of monochorionicity (**Fig. 18.5**).

Given the current limitations of second and third trimester ultrasonography in predicting chorionicity and amnionicity, the optimal time for determining these characteristics is during the first trimester of pregnancy. Thus, all women suspected of carrying a multiple gestation should be imaged sonographically during the first trimester.

Laboratory Testing

In a multiple pregnancy, a mother's urinary chorionic gonadotropin, estriol, and pregnanediol titers will be elevated as will her mean serum values for cystine, leucine aminopeptidase, oxytocinase, and alkaline phosphatase. However, these values will not be high enough or elevated early enough to be useful in diagnosing a multifetal pregnancy. Thus, testing for these biomarkers is not recommended for diagnosing multiple fetuses in pregnancy.

On the other hand, maternal serum alpha fetal protein (MSAFP) can be used in multifetal pregnancies to screen for fetal neural tube defects. An elevated MSAFP value that is 4.5 times the median in an uncomplicated twin gestation is abnormal for most laboratories and requires further testing. This value gives a detection rate for NTDs of 50–85% based on a 5% false-positive rate.

It is possible to successfully perform an amniocentesis of all gestational sacs for genetic determination in most patients with an ultrasound-guided, double-needle approach. Injecting 1–2 mL of indigo carmine dye into the first amniotic sac, followed by removal of clear fluid with a different needle from the second sac, ensures an adequate sample of both sacs. If the twins are monozygotic, as determined ultrasonically, only one sac needs to be sampled. The rate of pregnancy loss after genetic amniocentesis in twins is considered similar to that in singletons.

An alternative to amniocentesis in multiple gestations is chorionic villous sampling (CVS) under ultrasound guidance performed between 10 and 13 weeks. In experienced centers, twin–twin contamination occurs in 4–6% of samples.

Management

Antepartum Management

The ultimate goals of antepartum management of a twin or other multifetal pregnancies is to prevent preterm delivery of the fetuses, to identify growth restriction in one or more fetuses, to deliver the fetuses without significant trauma, and to ensure that expert anesthesia and neonatal care are available.

Weight Gain and Nutritional Supplementation

Since multiple pregnancies significantly increase the mother's requirements for calories, protein, minerals, and vitamins, evidence suggests that it is beneficial to incorporate dietetic services into antenatal care. For a twin gestation, for example, a woman should gain between 16 and 18 kg (35–40 lb) of total weight whereas a woman with triplets should gain a minimum of 23 kg (50 lb) during her pregnancy.

To achieve such a gain in weight requires, on average, an additional 150 kcal per day above the level for singleton pregnancy. In addition, as a result of the increased need for red blood cells, a woman carrying multiple fetuses will need to increase her intake of iron and folic acid. Thus, current recommendations are that a woman with a multifetal pregnancy should take 30 mg of iron as well as 300 µg of folate after the 12th week of gestation.

Genetic Testing

With increasing maternal age, the incidence of both twin gestations and fetal aneuploidy increases. In monozygotic twin gestations, in which both fetuses have the same karyotype, the risk of fetal aneuploidy is the same as the age-related risk for a singleton. However, in dizygotic twin pregnancies the risk of fetal aneuploidy is twice the maternal age risk for a singleton pregnancy.

There is little available information on maternal serum screening for aneuploidy in twin gestations. However, the average serum α-fetoprotein level in twins is approximately 2 times higher than that of singleton pregnancies. In addition, the mean unconjugated estriol level is approximately 1.6 times higher, and the average human chorionic gonadotropin is almost two times higher. Currently, the reliability of the serum screening for Down syndrome in twins is unknown.

Midtrimester amniocentesis and first-trimester CVS are used for prenatal diagnosis in twin gestations. Second trimester amniocentesis under direct ultrasound guidance is not associated with an excess pregnancy loss. When administered by an experienced clinician, CVS is at least as safe and effective as amniocentesis for prenatal diagnosis of twin gestations.

In performing genetic amniocentesis in twin pregnancies, care must be taken to sample each sac separately and not to sample the same sac twice. Genetic amniocentesis should be done under direct ultrasound guidance to map and label the positions of the fetuses relative to the maternal orientation, fetal membranes, and placental localizations (see Chapter 5). Injecting indigo carmine or Evan blue into the first sac sampled can be used to differentiate between the two fetal sacs before the second sample is taken. Methylene blue dye should not be used because of the risks of fetal hemolytic anemia, small intestinal atresia, and fetal demise.

Hypertension

As noted earlier, multifetal pregnancies are complicated by an increase in the incidence of hypertensive disorders, which tend to occur earlier and be more severe than in singleton pregnancies (see Chapter 21 for a detailed discussion of hypertension management in pregnancy).

Antepartum Ultrasound Surveillance

After 30 weeks of gestation, the growth of the fetuses in twin and other multifetal pregnancies typically lags significantly behind the growth of the fetus in singleton pregnancies. Also, there can be unequal or intrapair discordant growth. Therefore, serial ultrasound imaging at 2–4-week intervals is done to monitor the interval growth of twin gestations in the third trimester. Normal interval growth is reassuring, but discordant growth warrants further evaluations to check the status of the fetus.

Amniotic fluid volume is another parameter that should be evaluated by ultrasonography. Oligohydramnios may indicate uteroplacental insufficiency, requiring additional testing to check for fetal wellbeing. In twin pregnancies, it often is difficult to quantify the volume of amniotic fluid of both fetuses. The amniotic fluid volume can be assessed by measuring the deepest vertical pocket in each sac, or by measuring the amniotic fluid index (AFI). If the AFI is abnormal, then the clinician needs to discover which sac is responsible and the possible cause.

Antepartum Tests of Fetal Wellbeing

Ultrasound surveillance is the mainstay of monitoring fetal growth of multifetal pregnancies and determining amniotic fluid volume. The estimated fetal weight provides the best indicator of discordant growth, but estimating the amniotic fluid volume, as stated earlier, is often difficult in multifetal pregnancies.

Tests for fetal wellbeing in twin gestations include: 1) assessing fetal growth and amniotic fluid volume by ultrasonography; 2) Doppler velocimetry of the umbilical artery; 3) nonstress testing; and 4) determining the biophysical profile. Of the four, the nonstress testing and Doppler velocimetry are better predictors of fetal wellbeing than determing the amniotic fluid volume and biophysical profile.

However, in higher order multiple gestations (triplets, quadruplets, etc.) the biophysical profile is a very reliable test for fetal wellbeing. Measuring umbilical venous blood flow and systolic/diastolic ratios with duplex Doppler ultrasound imaging is useful in predicting and confirming concordant and discordant growth in multifetal pregnancies.

Preventing Preterm Delivery

One of the major complications of multifetal pregnancies is preterm delivery. Several management plans and/or techniques and procedures have been proposed to delay preterm labor and delivery in multifetal.

Routine hospitalization with bed-rest does not appear to help prolong multifetal pregnancies but may increase birth weight at delivery. However, monitoring the cervical length does appear to be an effective means of determining whether a preterm birth is imminent. The cervical length is best measured by TVS when the mother's bladder is empty (see Chapter 19). Although cervical length measurement by TVS is helpful as a predictor of preterm delivery, its clinical usefulness as a routine evaluation is questionable because of the lack of proven treatments affecting outcome.

Tocolytic Therapy

Most randomized trials using beta-mimetics in multifetal gestations have not shown any benefit in reducing preterm deliveries. Furthermore, complications occur more often with the use of tocolytic therapy in multiple gestations than in singletons. This is the result of a greater increase in plasma volume and cardiac output that occurs in multiples compared with single gestations.

Preterm Corticosteroids

The Consensus Development Conference on the Effect of Corticosteroids for Fetal Maturation sponsored by the National Institutes of Health recommended the use of corticosteroids to enhance fetal lung maturation in multiple gestations in preterm labor and impending delivery (<34 weeks' gestation). Participants in this conference concluded that the data supported the use of corticosteroids between 28 and 34 weeks for triplet pregnancies to reduce the incidence of hyaline membrane disease of the newborn. However, the data in the literature concerning acceleration of fetal lung maturation in twin pregnancies are conflicting.

Preterm Premature Rupture of the Membranes

As in singleton pregnancies, twin gestations complicated with preterm premature rupture of the membranes (pPROM) are managed expectantly (see Chapter 20).

Fetal Reduction

In recent years, fetal reduction has become more clinically and ethically acceptable as a therapeutic option in pregnancies with four or more fetuses. It also is considered appropriate in multifetal pregnancies in which one or more of the fetuses has congenital abnormalities. In cases of triplet gestations, however, this procedure remains controversial.

Complicating the clinical and ethical discussion surrounding this procedure in triplet gestations are reports of the improving outcome of triplet pregnancies as well as the failure to demonstrate an improvement in the outcome of triplet pregnancies reduced to twins as compared with those managed expectantly. There have also been reports that this procedure increases the risk of losing the entire pregnancy.

When considering the clinical options and the ethical issues involved in the management of triplet or higher order gestations, it is necessary to include the probability of achieving a successful pregnancy outcome.

The most commonly technique for multifetal pregnancy reduction (MPR) is the intrathoracic injection of potassium chloride by the transabdominal approach at 10–12 weeks' gestation. It has been reported that MPR performed at later weeks of pregnancy may be accompanied by increased risk of pregnancy loss. If an MPR is performed at around 14 weeks' gestation, a detailed ultrasonographic fetal anomaly scan should be done prior to the reduction. This allows the reduction to be performed more selectively and decreases the risk of delivering a fetus with a chromosomal or structural anomaly.

Other methods of MPR have been proposed. Some clinicians have used transcervical aspiration of the gestational sac. This method, however, may be associated with an increased incidence of fetal loss due the introduction of bacteria from the cervix causing infection, or due to cervical incompetence brought about by cervical dilatation.

There have been reports of successful pregnancy outcomes with fetal reduction used very early in gestation (6–8 weeks) by the transvaginal puncture and embryo aspiration. However, this method also has limitations, such as: 1) the need to use general anesthesia; 2) the possibility of spontaneous fetal reduction at this stage of gestation; 3) the inability to perform early fetal screening, such as a nuchal translucency test, which is done later on in pregnancy; and 4) the possibility of introducing infections.

Labor and Delivery in Multifetal Births

Managing the labor and delivery of a woman with multiple gestation presents many potential complications including fetal malpresentation, a prolapsed umbilical cord, dysfunctional uterine contractions, preterm labor, abruptio placentae, premature rupture of the membranes, uterine atony, and immediate postpartum hemorrhage. Thus, it is critical to anticipate such complications and more appropiate precautions so they can be properly managed. Such precautions include:

1. Monitoring the patient in labor with a multiple gestation using an external twin monitor or simultaneous monitoring by internal and external electronic fetal monitoring, if the membranes of the presenting twin are ruptured.
2. Making sure that blood and blood component products are immediately available.
3. Installing a large-bore intravenous catheter, so it is available during the labor and delivery process.
4. Administering an appropriate intravenous antibiotic for group B Streptococcus prophylaxis, if indicated.
5. Delivering the multiple gestation babies in an operating room or in the cesarean section area of a delivery room.

6. Ensuring that ultrasound equipment is easily available in the delivery room to determine the lie, presentation, and position of the second twin after the delivery of the first fetus.

7. Ensuring that an experienced anesthesiologist/anesthetist is present in the delivery room to provide appropriate anesthesia, if an urgent cesarean section is necessary, or to administer a tocolytic agent, such as nitroglycerin, to relax the uterus for extraction and delivery of the second twin.

8. Ensuring that a trained pediatrician or neonatologist skilled in neonatal resuscitation is available for each fetus immediately after delivery.

9. Ensuring that delivery is attended by an obstetrician who is skilled in evaluating the presentation and position of the second twin and also skilled in intrauterine manipulation to expedite the delivery of the second twin.

Stimulating Labor and/or Induction

The first stage of labor is shorter in twin gestations than in singleton pregnancies. However, the labor in twin gestations can sometimes be dysfunctional and characterized by ineffective or inefficient uterine contractions. In this situation, labor can be safely and effectively stimulated using dilute intravenous oxytocin.

Multifetal gestation is not a contraindication for induction of labor provided the criteria for labor induction are met as outlined by the American College of Obstetricians and Gynecologists (ACOG Education Pamphlet AP154).

Fetal Monitoring

In a twin gestation, it is critical to monitor both fetuses during labor, which is possible with the newer fetal monitors. Both twins can be monitored at the same time, externally, using just a single monitor. However, there are several potential problems using a single monitor including: 1) inadvertently monitoring one twin twice, and 2) mistaking the maternal heart rate for fetal bradycardia.

To assure that either or both of these situations does not occur, it is important to take the mother's pulse and to use ultrasonography to adjust the cardiotransducers, so that each fetus is accurately monitored. Once the membranes of the first twin have ruptured, a spiral electrode can be placed internally to monitor its fetal heart rate. The second twin can continue to be monitored simultaneously using the external monitor.

If it is necessary to monitor the contractions more closely, an intrauterine pressure catheter can be used. After the delivery of the first twin, it is essential to continue monitoring the second twin. This can be done with an external monitor or, if there is no contraindication to rupturing the membrane, a spiral electrode can be applied to directly monitor fetal heart rate of the second twin.

Anesthesia

Adequate analgesia and anesthesia are necessary for the optimum intrapartum management of a multifetal gestation. Epidural anesthesia provides excellent analgesia and flexibility to cover the various anesthetic needs of a multifetal pregnancy during labor and delivery.

Epidural anesthesia provides a number of benefits during labor, including: 1) pain relief, 2) inhibition of early pushing, 3) a relaxed pelvic floor and perineum at delivery, and 4) the option to extend anesthesia for emergency cesarean section, if needed.

Since the patient with a multifetal gestation is at an increased risk for supine hypotension from aortocaval compression, she should first receive a bolus of intravenous fluids and then be placed in the full lateral position during and after the induction of epidural anesthesia.

Mode of Delivery: Twins

Deciding on the mode of delivery is a critically important aspect of the management of a twin pregnancy in labor. The factors that determine the route of delivery include: 1) the fetal presentation or lie; 2) estimated fetal weight (EFW) of the fetuses, particularly of twin B; 3) EFW of twin B relative to twin A; 4) the skill of the obstetrician in intrauterine manipulation and vaginal breech delivery; and 5) fetal status.

However, the fetal presentation or lie is the most significant factor that determines the mode of delivery. Twin pregnancies can present with various combinations of fetal presentation at term. The most common combination is cephalic–cephalic, followed by cephalic–breech and cephalic–transverse. The combination of breech–breech is the least common.

Vertex–Vertex

The safety of vaginal delivery for cephalic–cephalic twin gestations is well supported in the literature. Immediately after the delivery of twin A, the presentation and status of twin B should be determined by vaginal examination, fetal monitoring, and ultrasound imaging. If it is safe to do so, artificially rupture the membranes of twin B. Then, with continuous fetal monitoring and reassuring fetal status, allow labor to continue in anticipation of vaginal delivery of the second twin. Cesarean section should be performed, however, if there is nonreassuring fetal status of twin B or prolapse of the umbilical cord.

Vertex–Nonvertex

There is evidence in the literature to support vaginal delivery of the nonvertex second twin weighing >1500 g by primary breech extraction. On the other hand, there are insufficient data to advocate either routine abdominal or routine vaginal delivery of the second twin whose birth weight is <1500 g, although cesarean section is frequently performed in such cases.

After vaginal delivery of twin A, ultrasound and vaginal exam should be used immediately to assess the presentation, lie, and status of the second twin. If twin B is <1500 g and is in a breech presentation or transverse lie, it is reasonable to attempt an external cephalic version. If successful, the membranes can be ruptured, if it is safe to do so. With continuous fetal monitoring and reassuring fetal status, the fetus can be delivered vaginally. A cesarean section should be performed if the external cephalic version is unsuccessful or the fetal status is nonreassuring, or in the event that the umbilical cord prolapses.

If twin B is >1500 g, external cephalic version could be tried and delivered vaginally as a cephalic presentation. Another option, in the case of a frank breech presentation, is a spontaneous or assisted vaginal breech delivery with continuous fetal monitoring during labor. If the second twin is in a transverse lie or a footling breech presentation, the fetus can be delivered by breech extraction.

To accomplish this, the feet are grasped and then brought down and out of the vagina before the membranes are ruptured to reduce the risk of cord prolapse. Fundal or suprapubic pressure should be applied by an assistant to keep the fetal head flexed to facilitate the vaginal delivery. However, to perform these intrauterine manipulations safely, there has to be adequate anesthesia and uterine relaxation.

If the uterus is contracted, intravenous nitroglycerin, which is a short-acting smooth muscle relaxant, can be administered to induce a transient and prompt uterine relaxation without affecting maternal and fetal prognosis. Cesarean section should be performed for nonreassuring fetal status of twin B, or in the event of prolapse of the umbilical cord. Furthermore, if the second fetus is in a breech presentation or in a transverse lie and is much larger than the first, a cesarean section of twin B may be necessary.

Twin A Nonvertex

The potential for locked twins (**Fig. 18.6**) exists when the first twin is breech and the second twin is cephalic. In general, when this occurs, the recommended mode of delivery is cesarean section.

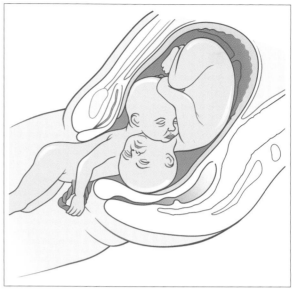

Fig. 18.6 If one twin is in the breech position and the other is cephalic, the potential exists for their heads to become "locked." In such cases, cesarean section is the only option for delivery.

Timing of Delivery

The ideal time of delivery for an uncomplicated twin pregnancy is still uncertain. However, the literature appears to support delivery by 38 weeks of gestation. After 38 weeks of gestation, the growth of twins begins to decline. In addition, the lowest incidence of perinatal death (10.5 per 1000 infants) is seen at 38 weeks in twin pregnancies, which corresponds to the incidence of perinatal death in singleton pregnancies at 43 weeks of gestation. Thus, the data would therefore suggest that twins are "postterm" after 38 weeks. If elective delivery is considered before 38 weeks of gestation, fetal lung maturity should be assessed.

Time Interval Between Deliveries

If there is continuous fetal and uterine monitoring, it is unnecessary to place a time restriction on the delivery interval between the first and second twin.

Triplets

The management of labor and delivery of triplets and higher order multifetal pregnancies is significantly more difficult than the management of twin gestations, because it is difficult to adequately monitor all fetuses simultaneously. Furthermore, after vaginal delivery of the first triplet, the delivery of the remaining fetuses requires a complicated set of intrauterine maneuvers and possibly a cesarean section.

There is also an increased risk for other complications, including abruptio placentae, fetal obstruction, and cord prolapse. As a result, most triplet or higher order multifetal pregnancies are delivered by cesarean section.

Key Points

- Multiple births have become significantly more prevalent due to the greater reliance on assistive reproductive technology.
- Once a multifetal pregnancy is suspected, ultrasound surveillance, which has a greater than 99% detection rate, should be performed at the earliest possible gestational age.
- The ultimate goals of the antepartum management of a multifetal pregnancy are to prevent preterm delivery of the fetuses, to identify growth restriction in one or more fetuses, and to deliver the fetuses without significant trauma.
- Weight restriction and nutritional supplementation, careful monitoring of fetal health, and prophylactic corticosteroid therapy to enhance fetal lung maturation may all be of benefit in preventing or delaying preterm birth and its complications.

Evidence Box 18.1

The transvaginal approach is the safest procedure for multifetal pregnancy reduction, whereas the transcervical procedure should be excluded from clinical practice owing to higher rate of fetal loss.

To evaluate efficacy and safety of first-trimester fetal reduction in the management of multifetal pregnancies, Dechaud et al. analyzed 33 studies from an international review of the literature that included 2756 multifetal pregnancy reduction procedures (2145 transabdominal, 363 transcervical, and 248 transvaginal procedures). The researchers found a difference between fetal loss rates between the different procedures: 16.7% for the transabdominal, 24.8% for the transcervical and 10.9% for the transvaginal ($P = 0.03$). The risk of fetal loss was 12% for the transabdominal, 20% for the transcervical, and 10% for the transvaginal approach at <24 weeks of gestation ($P = 0.04$).

Dechaud H, Picot MC, Hedon B, Boulot P. First-trimester multifetal pregnancy reduction: evaluation of technical aspects and risks from 2756 cases in the literature. Fetal Diagn Ther 1998 Sep–Oct;13(5):261–265.

Further Reading

American College of Obstetrics and Gynecology. Multifetal pregnancy reduction and selective fetal termination. ACOG Committee opinion: Committee on Ethics. Number 94–April 1991.

ACOG Education Pamphlet AP154—Labor Induction. American College of Obstetricians and Gynecologists, 1991

Ayres A, Johnson TR. Management of multiple pregnancy: prenatal care-part I. *Obstet Gynecol Surv* 2005;60(8):527–537

Ayres A, Johnson TR. Management of multiple pregnancy: prenatal care—part II. *Obstet Gynecol Surv* 2005;60(8):538–549

Bortolus R, Parazzini F, Chatenoud L, Benzi G, Bianchi MM, Marini A. The epidemiology of multiple births. *Hum Reprod Update* 1999;5(2):179–187

Effect of corticosteroids for fetal maturation on perinatal outcomes, NIH Consensus Statement 1994, Feb 28–Mar 2; 12(2):1–24

Keith L, Oleszczuk JJ. Iatrogenic multiple birth, multiple pregnancy and assisted reproductive technologies. *Int J Gynaecol Obstet* 1999;64(1):11–25

Modena AB, Berghella V. Antepartum management of multifetal pregnancies. *Clin Perinatol* 2005;32(2):443–454, vii

19 Preterm Birth and Fetal Growth Restrictions

E. Albert Reece

During pregnancy, a mother and her fetus act in harmony. The mother provides for the needs of the developing fetus, while at the same time the fetus lends support to the mother as she experiences a myriad of physiologic changes. The growth of a normal fetus is, thus, controlled by a delicate balance of genetic, placental, and maternal factors.

The prevailing view in embryology is that a fetus has an inherent growth potential. Under normal circumstances, it will develop into a healthy, appropriately sized newborn. However, if there is an imbalance in one or more of these critical growth and development factors, the baby may fail to reach its appropriate size and weight.

Inhibition of the fetus' growth potential, particularly its growth in weight, is analogous to "failure to thrive" in the infant. However, low birth weight is not necessarily associated with long-term adverse consequences for the infant (**Fig. 19.1**). In the absence of obvious risk factors, a small but otherwise normally developed fetus should not be considered pathologic, and every effort should be made to distinguish that from a truly abnormal condition.

Approximately 40% of growth-restricted fetuses develop serious complications (**Fig. 19.1**). Infants who are born weighing less than 2500 g (5 lb, 8 oz) at term have a perinatal mortality rate that is 5 to 30 times greater than that of infants whose birth weights are at the 50th percentile. The mortality rate is 70 to 100 times higher in infants who weigh less than 1500 g (3 lb, 5 oz) compared to normal-weight babies. Two major pathological conditions associated with poor fetal development are preterm birth and fetal growth restriction, which are the focus of the rest of this chapter.

Preterm Birth

Definition

Most pregnancies last around 40 weeks, and babies born between 37 and 42 completed weeks of pregnancy are considered full term. Babies born before completion of 37 weeks of pregnancy are called premature, or preterm.

Most preterm babies (71.2%) are born between 34 and 36 weeks of gestation. These are known as "late" preterm births. Almost 13% of preterm babies are born between 32 and 33 weeks of gestation, about 10% between 28 and 31 weeks, and about 6% at less than 28 weeks.

Diagnosis

A number of biochemical markers of preterm labor and delivery have been studied and most are associated with overall poor predictive values (**Table 19.1**), except the level of fetal fibronectin (fFN).

In symptomatic women, a positive fFN test (defined as >50 ng/mL) in cervicovaginal secretions after 20 weeks of gestation indicates potential decidual disruption. It does not guarantee, however, that a woman is about to give birth or that she will deliver early.

The fFN test has an even higher negative predictive value (as high as 99.7% or a one in 333 chance of deliv-

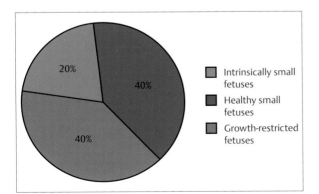

Fig. 19.1 Proportion of low birth weight babies with normal (purple and green) and abnormal (blue) medical profiles.

Table 19.1 Ability of biochemical markers to predict preterm labor*

Marker	Test	Sensitivity (%)	Specificity (%)	PPV (%)	NPV (%)
Fibronectin	Cervical or vaginal	69–93	72–86	13–83	81–99
Cytokine (Interleukin-6)	Serum	50	73–85	47–57	67–86
	Amniotic fluid	52	100	100	79
Estradiol-17ß	Serum	12	71–76	12–14	–
Estriol	Salivary	71	77	27	77
Progesterone	Serum	6–35	67–69	7–32	–

NPV, negative predictive value; PPV, positive predictive value.
*Values are a summary of ranges noted in the cited articles.
Reproduced with permission from Von Der Pool B. Preterm Labor: diagnosis and treatment. American Family Physician 1998; 57(10):2457–2464 (Table 2).

Table 19.2 Maternal, lifestyle, and medical factors that increase a woman's risk of preterm labor

Maternal factors	Lifestyle factors	Medical factors
Previous preterm birth	Smoking	Late or no prenatal care
Pregnant with twins, triplets or more	Drinking alcohol	Infections (including urinary tract, vaginal, sexually transmitted, and possibly other infections)
Having certain uterine or cervical abnormalities	Taking illicit drugs	High blood pressure
Short periods between pregnancies (<6–9 months between birth and beginning of next pregnancy)	Domestic violence (including physical, sexual, or emotional abuse)	Diabetes
Pregnant with a single fetus after in vitro fertilization	Exposure to the drug DES	Clotting disorders (thrombophilia)
Being underweight before becoming pregnant	Lack of social support	Certain birth defects in the baby
Being overweight or obese	Extremely high levels of stress	Bleeding from the vagina
	Standing for long periods	

ery within 1 week of a negative test result). A negative result on the fFN test means it is highly unlikely that the woman will give birth in the next week or two (See Evidence Box 19.1).

This negative predictive value is extremely useful, because in the early stages of preterm labor, it is very difficult to tell if a woman really is in labor based on her symptoms and a pelvic exam (see History Taking section below). The test's greatest value in the future may be to identify symptomatic women who may be able to continue their pregnancies without drug intervention.

Fetal Growth Restriction

Definition

The most widely used definition of fetal growth restriction (FGR) is a fetus whose estimated weight is below the 10th percentile for its gestational age, and whose abdominal circumference is below the 2.5th percentile. The birth-weight cutoff for being classified as fetal-growth restricted is 2500 g (5 lb, 8 oz) at term.

FGR is usually the result of placental insufficiency and is associated with a high rate of perinatal mortality. In the United States, for example, it is linked to a 6–10-fold increased rate of perinatal mortality. Often referred to in the scientific literature as intrauterine growth restriction, FGR is classified typically as either symmetric or asymmetric. Symmetric growth restriction refers to a fetus with a small, but proportionally developed, body. Asymmetric growth restriction refers to an undernourished fetus that is forced to use up all of its energy to just maintain the growth of its vital organs, such as the brain and heart, at the expense of its liver, muscle, and fat.

The greatest risk of adverse perinatal outcomes with FGR occurs among growth restricted fetuses/infants with weights below the third percentile for gestational age. In addition, FGR appears to be a precursor of some cases of hypertension, hyperlipidemia, coronary heart disease, and diabetes mellitus when the child reaches adulthood.

Diagnosis

Diagnosing FGR is heavily dependent on accurate dating in early pregnancy. It is based on a certain date for the last menstrual period in a woman with regular cycles or ultrasound assessment of gestational age performed no later than the 20th week, when the margin of error is only 7–10 days. The most accurate method for estimating gestational age is to perform a sonographic evaluation at 8–13 weeks of gestation. Although ultrasonography performed later in the pregnancy is valuable for estimating fetal weight, it is only accurate in predicting gestational age within about 3 weeks when performed at term.

A common—and potentially dangerous—medical error is changing a patient's due date based on a third-trimester ultrasound assessment. Doing so can, and often does, result in failure to recognize FGR.

Prenatal screening for FGR in general obstetrical populations also involves identifying risk factors for impaired fetal growth (**Table 19.2**) and physically assessing fetal size. Once FGR is suspected, based upon risk factors or physical examination, it should be followed by a detailed sonographic assessment of the fetus, placenta, and amniotic fluid.

Fortunately, advances in obstetrics and neonatology (the branch of pediatrics that deals with newborns) have improved the chances of survival for even the smallest babies. Late preterm babies generally have few or mild problems. Babies born before about 32–34 weeks' gestation, however, may have a number of complications, ranging from mild to severe. These babies usually are very small, and their organs are less developed than those of babies born later. Their symptoms may include:

- respiratory distress syndrome
- apnea
- intraventricular hemorrhage
- patent ductus arteriosis
- necrotizing enterocolitis

- retinopathy
- jaundice
- anemia
- chronic lung disease (also called bronchopulmonary dysplasia)
- infections

Although a fetus with asymmetric FGR has normal head dimensions, its abdomen will be proportionally small due to decreased liver size. It also will have spindly limbs due to decreased muscle mass, and thin skin due to decreased fat.

If growth-restricting conditions are sustained long enough, or are severe enough, the fetus may lose the ability to compensate and will become symmetrically growth-restricted. Of greatest concern to the developmental potential of the fetus is arrested head growth, which offers a poor prognosis for mental development.

Prevalence and Epidemiology

Preterm labor and FGR are the two leading causes of perinatal morbidity and mortality. In the United States, preterm birth affects 8–10% of births each year—totalling more than half a million babies, and causes at least 75% of neonatal deaths, excluding those related to congenital malformations.

Despite four decades of research, the rate of premature births has not changed, and some data indicate that the rate may be worsening. Because of technological advances in perinatal and neonatal medicine, survival rates have increased and morbidity has decreased. On the other hand, costs have soared. The health care expenditures for management of preterm labor and preterm birth account for more than $3 billion per year.

FGR is the second leading cause of perinatal morbidity and mortality, with an estimated incidence of approximately 5% of births. However, the incidence varies, depending on the population under examination (including its geographic location) and the standard growth curves used as reference.

Etiology and Pathophysiology

Preterm Birth

Preterm labor is characterized by cervical effacement and/or dilatation, and increased uterine irritability that occurs before 37 weeks of gestation. In most cases, the precise causes of preterm labor are not known. The strength of the association of each identified risk factor has been shown to vary, which has evoked a significant amount of debate in the literature. Women with a history of previous preterm delivery have the highest recurrence risk, estimated to be between 17% and 37%.

Most preterm births result from spontaneous preterm labor, either by itself or following spontaneous premature rupture of the membranes (PROM), when the amniotic sac inside the uterus that holds the baby breaks prematurely. The causes of preterm labor and PROM are not fully understood. The latest research suggests that many cases are triggered by the body's natural response to certain infections, including infections involving the amniotic fluid and fetal membranes (see Chapter 20). However, in about 40% of all cases of preterm birth, the cause cannot be determined.

About 25% of preterm births result from early induction of labor or cesarean delivery due to pregnancy complications or health problems in the mother or the fetus. In most of these cases, early delivery is probably the safest approach for mother and baby.

Nevertheless, preterm birth is a serious health problem for the baby. In the short term, many preterm babies are at increased risk for common newborn health complications. They often must be cared for in a neonatal intensive care unit, which has specialized medical staff and equipment that can deal with the multiple problems they face. In the longer term, preterm babies may face lasting disabilities, such as mental impairment, cerebral palsy, lung and gastrointestinal problems, vision and hearing loss, and even premature death.

Any woman can deliver a preterm baby, but some women are at greater risk than others. Certain groups of women, certain life style factors, or certain medical conditions may put a woman at greater risk for preterm labor (**Table 19.2**).

Fetal Growth Restriction

It is important to identify the etiology of FGR whenever possible because such information additionally benefits the patient. For instance, knowing that there may be a chromosomal or genetic etiology may enable the patient to prepare better for her delivery, as well as plan for future pregnancies. This is also true when fetal anomalies are present.

FGR may be caused by fetal, placental, or maternal factors. There is significant overlap among these entities. Fetuses with trisomies, particularly for chromosomes 13 and 18, often have FGR. Triploidy also is a risk factor for FGR (**Fig. 19.2**). Others, including sex chromosome abnormalities such as 45 XO fetuses, and those with mosaic cell lines, are often seen with growth restriction. Overall, chromosomal and genetic causes of FGR account for 5–15% of growth restricted fetuses and are more often seen with symmetric rather than asymmetric FGR.

Congenital abnormalities with or without chromosomal abnormalities are also seen with FGR. Most common are cardiac malformations such as tetralogy of Fallot and transposition of the great vessels. Other abnormalities, including gastroschisis and omphalocele, are also seen with altered fetal growth.

Among the agents that cause FGR, some of the strongest associations are infections caused by rubella, cytomegalovirus, and toxoplasmosis (see also Chapter 23). These infections involve multiple organs of the fetus that lead to growth restriction. Infections account for 5–10% of all FGR cases.

In multiple gestation pregnancies, FGR results from abnormal placental development and possibly abnormal cord insertions. In addition, nutritional factors and uteroplacental blood flow variations contribute to the growth restriction in such pregnancies (see Chapter 18).

Nutritional deficiencies, particularly protein intake, are among the most significant maternal factors associated with FGR, as are maternal medical pthologies, including cardiovascular, endocrine (e.g., diabetes, thyroid disorders), autoimmune, and renal diseases.

Environmental agents can pose significant risks to fetal growth as well, and include adverse effects from cigarette

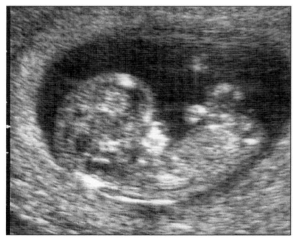

Fig. 19.2 Utrasonogram of severe asymmetrical growth restriction in a 13-week-old fetus with triploidy, showing normal head but small, underdeveloped torso and limbs.

smoking, alcohol, and cocaine abuse. Women exposed to organic solvents and other toxins in the workplace have similar, elevated risks for FGR. High altitude, another risk factor for FGR, leads to an increase in the fetal hematocrit and results in fetal hypoxia. **Table 19.3** lists some of the most common causes of FGR.

On a physiological level, FGR occurs when the exchange of gas and delivery of nutrients to the fetus are not sufficient to allow it to thrive in utero. This process can occur primarily because of maternal disease causing decreased oxygen-carrying capacity (e.g., cyanotic heart disease, smoking, hemoglobinopathy), a dysfunctional oxygen delivery system secondary to maternal vascular disease (e.g., due to diabetes with vascular disease, hypertension, autoimmune disease affecting the vessels leading to the placenta), or placental damage resulting from maternal disease (e.g., from smoking, thrombophilia, various autoimmune diseases).

Unfortunately, significant obstacles remain in terms of defining the population of growth-restricted fetuses at high risk of adverse outcome, accurately identifying these fetuses in utero, and determining interventions to improve outcome.

History Taking: Preterm Labor

Chief Complaints

Women in preterm labor often present with lower abdominal discomfort as their chief complaint. They may describe this discomfort as painful, menstrual-like cramps, periodic tightening of the abdomen, suprapubic pain, or pelvic pressure. Another common discomfort is low back pain. Changes in vaginal secretions, especially a bloody discharge, also may be an ominous indication of preterm labor.

Prior to the onset of preterm labor, the woman may note an increase in uterine activity and may complain or grimace with pain simultaneously with the contractions. Although slightly more than a quarter of all pregnant women report uterine contractions before 37 weeks' gestation, about a third of those women who present with preterm contractions resolve on their own without treatment.

Preterm labor may be the result of ruptured membranes. If suspected, a digital examination is contraindicated. A sterile speculum exam should be given to detect the presence of amniotic fluid. If found, immediate consultation or referral for medical management is required.

If the membranes are not ruptured, a pelvic exam can now be performed. If the cervix is soft with some dilation and/or shortening, that is a warning sign that preterm labor is about to begin.

Once preterm labor is suspected, a complete history should be taken, including ascertaining the patient's present symptoms, expected date of delivery, past medical history, medication use, and allergies. **Figure 19.3** presents a typical route for triaging a woman suspected of being in preterm labor.

Table 19.3 Common causes of fetal growth restriction

Placental insufficiency	Fetal malformations
Unexplained elevated maternal α-fetoprotein level	Immunological factors
Idiopathic	Antiphospholipid syndrome
Pre-eclampsia	Infections
Chronic maternal disease	Cytomegalovirus
Cardiovascular disease	Rubella
Diabetes	Herpes
Hypertension	Toxoplasmosis
Abnormal placentation	Metabolic disorders
Placental abruption	Phenylketonuria
Placenta previa	Poor maternal nutrition
Infarction	Substance abuse (smoking, alcohol, drugs)
Circumvallate placenta	Multiple gestation
Placenta accretia	Low socioeconomic status
Hemangioma	
Genetic disorders	
Family history	
Trisomy 13, 18, or 21	
Triploidy	
Turner syndrome (some cases)	

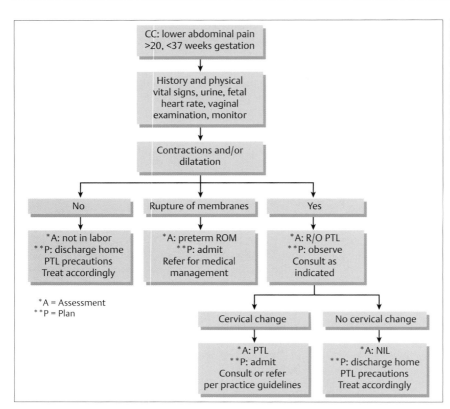

Fig. 19.3 A typical triage diagram for preterm labor screening. PTL, preterm labor; NIL, not in labor; CC, chief complaint; ROM, rupture of membranes; R/O, rule out Reproduced with permission of Elsevier, from Peck D, Griffis N. Preterm labor in the triage setting. Journal of Nurse-Midwifery 1999; 44(5):449–457.

History Taking: Fetal Growth Resriction

Chief Complaints

Most cases of FGR present during the third trimester, which makes them difficult to diagnose accurately. This is especially true if the patient presents for prenatal care at a late stage. FGR is frequently detected in a pregnant woman whose third trimester weight gain was less than expected (100–200 g [3.5–7 oz] per week), or if weight begins decreasing. Small maternal weight gains in pregnancy may correspond with a small baby. FGR also may be an incidental finding on ultrasound examination when fetal measurements are smaller than expected for gestational age.

Timely diagnosis and management of FGR is one of the major achievements in contemporary obstetrics. If the growth-restricted fetus is identified and appropriate managed, perinatal mortality can be significantly reduced.

Physical Examination: Preterm Labor

Before the physical examination, a clean-catch or catheterized urine specimen should be obtained from the mother for laboratory analysis and culture. A general physical examination, including a vaginal examination using a sterile speculum, can then be performed.

After the pelvic exam is complete, the patient should be placed in the lateral recumbent position and externally monitored for fetal heart tones and contractions. If uterine contractions occur at least every 15 minutes, an intravenous bolus of 500 mL of normal saline or Ringer lactate can be administered. This causes rapid intravascular expansion and can diminish the contractions of an irritable uterus in many women. It also helps the physician differentiate the latter condition from preterm labor.

If the initial bolus is effective, the rate of intravenous fluid replacement can then be adjusted to 100 mL per hour. If contractions persist, however, a single dose of terbutaline sulfate (Brethine, Bricanyl) 0.25 mg, can be given subcutaneously to allow time to discuss treatment options, to transfer the patient, or to differentiate preterm labor from an irritable uterus.

Diagnostic Ultrasonography

There is a great deal of controversy currently as to whether weekly cervical assessment is a useful predictor of preterm labor in women with uncomplicated pregnancies. The lack of overwhelming evidence that routine cervical examination is effective in reducing preterm deliveries suggests that such examinations do not identify women at risk for preterm delivery, or that the interventions prompted by the test are ineffective.

Cervical length, however, may be a useful predictor of the risk of premature delivery, with a shorter cervix predicting a higher risk. Cervical dilatation has been demonstrated with some accuracy up to 4 cm. Cervical effacement and lower uterine segment changes may predate cervical dilatation. The unaffected cervix in the third trimester usually measures between 3.5 cm and 4.8 cm in length. Fifty-percent effacement corresponds to a cervical length of 1.5 cm, and 75 % effacement corresponds to a length of 1.0 cm.

Given the substantial intra-observer and inter-observer variations that occur with digital examinations, transvaginal ultrasonography, which is highly reproducible, provides a more reliable method of measuring cervical length. Short cervical length on transvaginal ultrasonography in women with uterine anomalies has been associated with a 13-fold increased risk for preterm birth.

Physical Examination: Fetal Growth Restriction

Accurate knowledge of gestational age is critical to diagnosing FGR, given that normal and abnormal fetal size are defined, in part, by comparing the fetal weight of the index fetus to that of other fetuses of the same gestational age.

Clinical assessment is a reasonable screening tool for FGR in low risk pregnancies, as there is no high-quality evidence that alternative approaches, such as routine ultrasound examination, improve outcome over clinical assessment alone. However, if available, an ultrasound examination may be performed to determine the gestational age, presentation, placental location, and presence of fetal anomalies.

A detailed anatomical survey of the fetus is recommended in all cases, since major congenital anomalies are frequently associated with failure to maintain normal fetal growth. Among malformed infants, the frequency of FGR ranges from 20 % to 60 %, with the highest risk in infants with multiple anomalies. Approximately 10 % of FGR is accompanied by congenital anomalies.

Anomalies associated with FGR include omphalocele, diaphragmatic hernia, skeletal dysplasia, and congenital heart defects; thus, examination of the fetal heart (fetal echocardiogram) and skeleton are particularly important. Microcephaly, although rare, is associated with several syndromes manifesting growth restriction. Polyhydramnios is associated with trisomy 18 and several congenital anomalies.

The size of the uterus should be assessed at each prenatal visit. If the measurements are performed by the same person, techniques such as serial measurement of the uterine fundus are helpful in documenting continued growth. A tape-measure should be used to measure the distance from the top of the pubic symphysis to the dome of the uterine fundus. Between 20 and 38 weeks of gestation, this measurement, in centimeters, is normally accurate to within 3 weeks of the gestational age.

A fundal height that lags by more than 3 cm, or is increasing in disparity with the gestational age, may signal FGR. A lag of 4 cm or more is suggestive of FGR.

Increased surveillance is particularly important in patients with a previous history of FGR. A history of a previous small-for-gestational-age infant has been reported to be among the most predictive factors for subsequent FGR. Such women have up to a twofold to fourfold increased risk of giving birth to another similarly affected fetus.

Ultrasound Biometry

Currently, the "gold standard" for assessing fetal growth is ultrasound biometry of the fetus. The biparietal diameter, head circumference, abdominal circumference, and femur length are the measurements most commonly taken. Fetal weight is calculated based on percentiles that have been established for each of these parameters.

The most sensitive indicator of symmetric and asymmetric FGR is the abdominal circumference, which has a more than 95 % sensitivity if the measurement is below the 2.5th percentile.

In the absence of reliable dating, it is critical to perform serial scans at intervals of two or three weeks to accurately identify FGR. Each measured parameter has an error potential of about 1 week up to 20 gestational weeks, about 2 weeks from 20 to 36 weeks of gestation, and about 3 weeks thereafter.

Doppler Flow Velocimetry

Another way to diagnose FGR during pregnancy is with Doppler flow velocimetry. This technique uses sound waves to measure blood flow. The sound of moving blood produces waveforms that reflect the speed and amount of the blood as it moves through a blood vessel.

The waveforms may show that blood flow in the umbilical vessels of a fetus with suspected FGR is decreased, indicating that the fetus may not be receiving enough

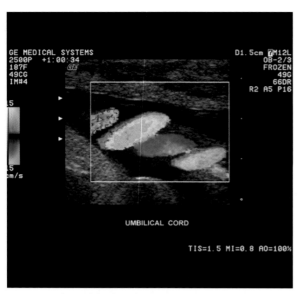

Fig. 19.4   The umbilical cord. Color Doppler flow image in a normal three-vessel cord with a left twist.

blood, nutrients, and oxygen from the placenta. Blood vessels in the fetal brain and the umbilical cord blood flow can be checked with Doppler flow studies (**Fig. 19.4**).

Laboratory Testing: Preterm Labor

Vaginal discharge or pooled fluid should be checked for ferning. If PROM is suspected, a nitrazine test can be performed for pH of the vaginal fluid. The normal pH for vaginal fluid is between 4.5 and 5.5, and normal pH of amniotic fluid usually lies between 7.0 and 7.5. If a sample of vaginal fluid is more alkaline (has a higher pH) than normal, then it is very likely that the membranes have ruptured and amniotic fluid has leaked into the vagina.

If preterm PROM is documented, digital examination should not be performed. Dilatation and effacement of the cervix can be estimated during the vaginal examination. If there is no evidence of preterm PROM, a careful, gentle digital examination may be performed.

If an amniocentesis is performed, amniotic fluid can be sent to obtain a Gram stain, glucose level, lecithin/sphingomyelin ratio, and culture and sensitivity testing.

Bacterial vaginosis also is strongly associated with preterm labor. Thus, a wet preparation and a potassium hydroxide preparation should be obtained for testing. In addition, cervical culture for Chlamydia trachomatis and Neisseria gonorrhoeae is recommended, because of their association with preterm labor. A rectovaginal culture for group B Streptococcus should also be obtained.

Treatment Options

Preterm Labor

Parenteral Tocolytic Therapy

Parenteral tocolytic agents are clearly effective in delaying delivery for 24–48 hours. Such a delay increases the time for adjunctive corticosteroid therapy (see below) to take effect, or for the patient to be transferred to a well-equipped, tertiary treatment center.

Drugs used for tocolysis include magnesium sulfate, ritodrine (Yutopar), terbutaline, nifedipine (Adalat, Procardia), and indomethacin (Indocin). Antocin (Atosiban), an oxytocin receptor inhibitor (not labeled by the US Food and Drug Administration [FDA] for this purpose), may also be effective.

The efficacy of these drugs has been difficult to measure oweing to the lack of a definitive diagnosis of preterm labor and a consensus regarding the optimal treatment approach. Furthermore, tocolytic therapy has not been definitively shown to improve fetal outcome, and most of these drugs are associated with significant complications (see **Table 19.4**).

Table 19.4   Potential complications of tocolytic agents

Beta-adrenergic agents
Hyperglycemia
Hypokalemia
Hypotension
Pulmonary edema
Cardiac insufficiency
Arrythmias
Myocardial ischemia
Maternal death

Magnesium sulfate
Pulmonary edema
Respiratory depression*
Cardiac arrest*
Maternal tetany*
Profound muscular paralysis*
Profound hypotension*

Indomethacin (Indocin)
Hepatitis†
Renal failure†
Gastrointestinal bleeding†

Nifedipine (Adalat, Procardia)
Transient hypotension

* Effect is rare and occurs with toxic levels.
† Effect is rare and is associated with chronic use.
Adapted from American College of Obstetricians and Gynecologists. Preterm labor. Technical Bulletin No. 206. Washington, DC: ACOG; 1995.

Before initiating parenteral tocolytic therapy, however, the practitioner must thoroughly evaluate the patient's history, physical examination, laboratory tests, and ultrasonography results to determine whether she meets the criteria for preterm labor. If she is an appropriate candidate for this therapy, it should be initiated only after the practitioner advises her and her family of its risks as well as its potential benefits and involves them in the decision.

Furthermore, several absolute and relative contraindications must be considered before initiating therapy with any of these compounds, which are listed in **Table 19.5**.

Magnesium Sulfate

Magnesium sulfate is often used as a first-line therapy for tocolysis because it is highly effective and is associated with fewer side effects compared to beta-mimetic agents (see below). Magnesium decreases seizures and blocks neuromuscular transmission. The mechanism by which it prevents uterine contraction is unknown but may be related to calcium antagonist activity. An initial loading dose of 4–6 g is usually given intravenously over 15 to 30 minutes, followed by continuous infusion of 1–4 g per hour to maintain a magnesium level between 4 and 6 mEq.

Table 19.5 Contraindications to tocolysis for treatment of preterm labor

General contraindications
• Acute fetal distress (except intrauterine resuscitation)
• Chorioamnionitis
• Eclampsia or severe pre-eclampsia
• Fetal demise (singleton)
• Fetal maturity
• Maternal hemodynamic instability

Contraindications for specific tocolytic agents
Beta-mimetic agents
• Maternal cardiac rhythm disturbance or other cardiac disease
• Poorly controlled diabetes, thyrotoxicosis or hypertension
Magnesium sulfate
• Hypocalcemia
• Myasthenia gravis
• Renal failure
Indomethacin (Indocin)
• Asthma
• Coronary artery disease
• Gastrointestinal bleeding (active or past history)
• Oligohydramnios
• Renal failure
• Suspected fetal cardiac or renal anomaly
Nifedipine (Adalat, Procardia)
• Maternal liver disease

Adapted from American College of Obstetricians and Gynecologists. Preterm labor. Technical Bulletin No. 206. Washington, DC: ACOG; 1995.

The infusion is continued until the uterus is quiescent for 12–24 hours. Thirty minutes before discontinuing the magnesium sulfate infusion, administer 2.5–5.0 mg of terbutaline orally and repeat every 2–4 hours thereafter to control contractions.

Maternal side effects of magnesium sulfate include nausea, vomiting, hypotension, and headaches; more severe side effects include respiratory depression and pulmonary edema. Because it crosses the placenta, it effects the fetus as well: magnesium sulfate has caused decreased muscle tone and lethargy in the fetus. Magnesium toxicity in the fetus is treated with an immediate infusion of calcium gluconate.

Beta-Mimetic Agents

Intravenous ritodrine and terbutaline are the most commonly used beta-mimetic drugs. These two drugs act similarly by stimulating the β2 receptors, resulting in relaxation of the uterine muscles and the smooth muscles of the lung. Most importantly, they appear to have few effects on the β1 cardiac receptors. Intravenous ritodrine, which is the only drug of the two specifically approved by the FDA for tocolysis, is typically given at an initial dose of 0.05–0.1 mg per minute then increased at 15-minute intervals to 0.35 mg per minute. The usual dosage of terbutaline is 0.25 mg administered subcutaneously every 1–6 hours.

Terbutaline also can be given orally every few hours in a dosage of 2.5–5.0 mg to prevent uterine contractions that result in cervical change. The dosage is adjusted to minimize fetal contractions and to maintain the maternal heart rate between 90 and 105 beats per minute. If used, oral tocolytic therapy should be continued until 35–37 weeks of gestation.

Because beta-mimetic therapy can cause severe tachycardia and hypotension, the patient's blood pressure should be monitored frequently. Intravenous administration of ritodrine can also lead to myocardial ischemia. Thus, if the patient has chest pain or develops an arrhythmia, an electrocardiogram should be obtained immediately.

In such cases, ritodrine therapy should be discontinued immediately. Monitoring of fluid input and output, daily weight, hourly respiratory rate, and signs of pulmonary fluid accumulation should begin immediately. Pulmonary edema, a common complication, can be prevented by limiting the sodium and total fluid load to a maximum of 2500–3000 mL per 24 hours.

Hyperglycemia and ketoacidosis have occurred in some patients receiving beta-mimetic therapy. Therefore, it is necessary to measure serum glucose at baseline and repeat it at 12-hour intervals in patients without diabetes. Patients with diabetes who receive intravenous fluids should have their serum glucose checked at 2-hour intervals. Other medical problems should be treated appropriately.

Second-Line Agents for Tocolysis

Indomethacin and calcium channel blockers are used as "second-line" therapies for treating preterm labor. Indomethacin is a prostaglandin inhibitor, which acts by inhibiting the production of cytokines that may trigger labor, and it can inhibit preterm labor for 48 hours in pregnancies of less than 32 weeks of gestation.

Indomethacin is typically administered rectally as a 100-mg dose, repeated after one to two hours if contractions persist. Because of potential fetal side effects, such as oligohydramnios and transient constriction of the ductus arteriosus, oral indomethacin (25 mg every 4–6 hours) should not be given for longer than 48 hours.

Calcium channel blockers, such as nifedipine, inhibit the contraction of smooth muscle, resulting in uterine relaxation. Typically, nifedipine is administered orally in a loading dose of 30 mg, followed by 20 mg given every 4–8 hours for 24 hours. This is followed by a maintenance dose of 10 mg every 8 hours until 35–37 weeks of gestation, or delivery.

Emerging Treatments

Oxytocin inhibitors offer a potential new therapeutic agent for the treatment of preterm labor. Although the exact mechanism of action is not known, uterine oxytocin receptors and/or oxytocin may have etiologic roles in the development of uterine hyperactivity in women with preterm labor. Studies of the two oxytocin antagonists, antocin and an orally active nonpeptidyl oxytocin antagonist, have demonstrated a high level of efficacy with few side effects (primarily nausea and vomiting).

Antibiotic Therapy

Certain maternal infections, which were previously discussed, play a potential etiologic role in preterm labor. Therefore, women with sexually transmitted diseases, urinary tract infections, severe respiratory infections, or vaginitis should be treated appropriately. Patients with intact amniotic membranes and a history of positive group B streptococcal culture are usually treated with intravenous penicillin. Pregnancy and delivery may be prolonged in women treated with erythromycin, ampicillin, and clindamycin.

Corticosteroid Therapy

In addition to considering treatment options for the mother experiencing preterm labor, the practitioner also must consider how to potentially treat the premature infant. Not only are preterm babies often small and sick, but also they may look and behave very differently compared to full-term babies. For example, their skin may be thin and wrinkled, and their heads may look too large for their bodies. But these babies look the way they should at their stage of development. They will begin to appear and act more like full-term babies as they continue to develop and grow.

Throughout their first year of life, these babies should be evaluated according to their adjusted age (which takes the extent of their prematurity into account). Corticosteroid therapy is presently the only treatment shown to improve fetal survival when given to a woman in preterm labor between 24 and 34 weeks of gestation. Studies have shown a decrease in intraventricular hemorrhage, respiratory distress syndrome, and mortality, even when treatment lasts for less than 24 hours. Optimal benefits begin 24 hours after therapy and last for 7 days.

Corticosteroid therapy also may be beneficial when given to pregnant women of less than 30–32 weeks of gestation with preterm PROM and no evidence of chorioamnionitis. Treatment regimens typically include 12 mg betamethasone given intramuscularly every 24 hours for 2 days, or 6 mg dexamethasone given intramuscularly every 12 hours for 2 days.

Fetal Growth Restriction

The treatment of FGR must be individualized for each patient. In addition to managing any maternal illness, a detailed sonogram should be performed to search for fetal anomalies. To rule out aneuploidy, karyotyping should be considered (see Chapters 5 and 7).

Symmetric restriction may be due to a fetal chromosomal disorder or infection. On the other hand, many infants with evidence of growth restriction are constitutionally small. Serial ultrasound examinations are important to determine the severity and progression of FGR.

The timing of delivery to prevent intrauterine demise because of chronic oxygen deprivation is still controversial. Preterm delivery is indicated if the growth-restricted fetus demonstrates abnormal fetal function tests, or in the absence of demonstrable fetal growth. The risks of prematurity must be weighed against the complications unique to FGR.

General management measures include treatment of maternal disease, getting her to quit abusing substances such as alcohol, good nutrition, and bed rest, the latter which may maximize uterine blood flow. Antenatal testing also should be instituted. Options include the nonstress test, the biophysical profile and an oxytocin (Pitocin) challenge test. The biophysical profile involves assessing fetal well-being with a combination of the nonstress test and four ultrasonographic parameters (amniotic fluid volume, respiratory movements, body movements and muscle tone).

Doppler flow velocimetry, usually of the umbilical artery, will identify the growth-restricted fetus at greatest risk for neonatal morbidity and mortality. In controlled

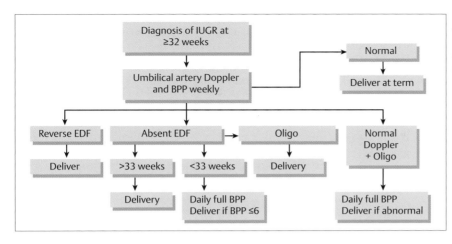

Fig. 19.5 Approach for managing fetal intrauterine growth restriction (IUGR). BPP, biophysical profile; EDF, end diastolic flow (through umbilical artery)

trials, Doppler analysis has been found to improve outcomes, although it is considered experimental by the American College of Obstetricians and Gynecologists. Each of these tests has a relatively high false-positive rate (i.e., 50%) in the low-risk patient.

Given the high false-positive rate of nonstress tests, the significance of a nonreactive nonstress test should be further evaluated before making any management decision. A nonreassuring nonstress test followed by assessment of the biophysical profile has been shown to lead to lower rates of intervention when compared with the oxytocin contraction test, with no impact on perinatal outcome.

Combination testing is thought to predict more accurately the status of the fetus. For this reason, close antenatal surveillance is encouraged, with a well-timed delivery. A proposed management approach for FGR is shown in **Fig. 19.5**. This approach is based on outstanding advances in neonatal care and improved outcome for the low birth weight infant.

Key Points

- Growth-restricted fetuses, particularly individuals born weighing less than 2500 g, have a significantly higher risk for developing serious medical complications and/or dying than normal weight infants.
- Prenatal screening for fetal growth restriction involves identifying risk factors for impaired fetal growth and continuously assessing fetal size by physical examination and sonographic assessment, if warranted.
- Accurate knowledge of gestational age also is critical to accurately diagnosing fetal growth restriction.
- Preterm birth is another major cause of fetal morbidity and mortality.
- Certain groups of women, certain life style factors, or certain medical conditions may put a woman at greater risk for preterm labor.
- The fetal fibronectin test is a powerful tool for determining whether a woman is in labor, or whether labor is imminent.

Evidence Box 19.1

A negative fetal fibronectin test is associated with fewer admissions to an antepartum ward and a shorter hospital stay for preterm labor.

Lowe et al investigated the effect of the rapid fetal fibronectin test on the length of hospital stay and the rate of admission for preterm labor in a group of women randomly assigned to receive fetal fibronectin ($N = 46$ women) testing or to preterm labor management without fetal fibronectin ($N = 51$ women) testing.

There was no difference between groups in demographic or obstetric characteristics, the hours spent in labor and delivery, the number of women who were admitted to the antepartum service, the length of stay, or medical interventions. However, when the results for women with a negative fetal fibronectin test were compared to women with a positive fetal fibronectin test, the investigators found a statistically significant difference in admissions to the antepartum service ($P = 0.032$) and the length of stay ($P = 0.008$).

Lowe MP, Zimmerman B, Hansen W. Prospective randomized controlled trial of fetal fibronectin on preterm labor management in a tertiary care center. Am J Obstet Gynecol 2004 Feb;190(2):358–362.

Further Reading

Airoldi J, Berghella V, Sehdev H, Ludmir J. Transvaginal ultrasonography of the cervix to predict preterm birth in women with uterine anomalies. *Obstet Gynecol* 2005;106(3):553–556

Alberry M, Soothill P. Management of fetal growth restriction. *Arch Dis Child Fetal Neonatal Ed* 2007;92(1):F62–F67

Fact sheet: Preterm Birth. Available from the March of Dimes website at: http://www.marchofdimes.com/professionals/14332_1157.asp, accessed October 9, 2008.

Lowe MP, Zimmerman B, Hansen W. Prospective randomized controlled trial of fetal fibronectin on preterm labor management in a tertiary care center. *Am J Obstet Gynecol* 2004;190(2):358–362

McCormick MC. The contribution of low birth weight to infant mortality and childhood morbidity. *N Engl J Med* 1985;312(2):82–90

Peck D, Griffis N. Preterm labor in the triage setting. *J Nurse Midwifery* 1999;44(5):449–457

Peleg D, Kennedy CM, Hunter SK. Intrauterine growth restriction: identification and management. *Am Fam Physician* 1998;58(2):453–460, 466–467

Papageorghiou AT, Leslie K. Uterine artery Doppler in the prediction of adverse pregnancy outcome. *Curr Opin Obstet Gynecol* 2007;19(2):103–109

Von Der Pool BA. Preterm labor: diagnosis and treatment. *Am Fam Physician* 1998;57(10):2457–2464

Weismiller DG. Preterm labor. *Am Fam Physician* 1999;59(3):593–602

Yanney M, Marlow N. Paediatric consequences of fetal growth restriction. *Semin Fetal Neonatal Med* 2004;9(5):411–418

20 Premature Rupture of Membranes and Third Trimester Bleeding

E. Albert Reece

Premature rupture of membranes (PROM) and third trimester bleeding represent two of the most serious complications of pregnancy. Preterm PROM is responsible for approximately one-third of preterm deliveries.

Similarly, few obstetric emergencies cause greater concern than bleeding in late pregnancy and the immediate postpartum period. Third trimester bleeding is a major cause of maternal and fetal mortality. Massive bleeding can occur without forewarning, and there are few reliable clinical indicators available to predict those at greatest risk. Patients may remain hemodynamically stable until a sudden deterioration in condition takes place. In many cases the extent of the bleeding can be unclear, as the bleeding may be concealed behind the placenta.

Definitions

Placental abruption (abruptio placentae): This term is used to describe a partial or complete separation of the placenta from the wall of the uterus.

Placenta previa: Placenta previa is a placental implantation that overlies or is within 2 cm (0.8 in) of the internal cervical os. A complete previa is placenta that covers the os. A marginal previa occurs when the edge lies within 2 cm of the os. When the edge is 2–3.5 cm (1.4 in) from the os, the placenta may be described as low lying.

Premature rupture of membranes (PROM): This is a membrane rupture that occurs before the onset of labor.

Uterine rupture: This term describes anything in a continuum of events that can occur to the uterus during pregnancy, from a weak spot in the uterine wall noticed by the surgeon at the time of cesarean to the catastrophe of the uterus tearing open and the fetus, placenta, and a lot of blood extruding into the mother's abdomen.

Vasa previa: A condition that occurs when the fetal blood vessels are situated across the entrance to the birth canal and rupture when the cervix begins to dilate at the start of birth or during labor.

Diagnosis

Premature Rupture of Membranes

The diagnosis of PROM is generally based on a suspicious history, combined with physical examination and, when indicated, additional laboratory tests. If there is a suspicious history (see below), the first confirmatory steps include performing a sterile speculum examination, visually evaluating cervical dilatation and effacement, and obtaining appropriate cervical cultures for infectious diseases, such as *Chlamydia trachomatis* and *Neisseria gonorrhoea*.

In most cases, PROM can be confirmed by documentation of fluid passing from the cervical os with visualization of a pool of fluid in the posterior vaginal fornix. Although helpful, nitrazine and ferning tests are not always accurate. A false-positive nitrazine test may occur if there is blood, semen, alkaline antiseptics, or bacterial vaginosis present in the vagina. Alternatively, if membrane rupture is chronic and little amniotic fluid is present, the nitrazine test can be falsely negative. Causes of false-positive and false-negative ferning tests include cervical mucus and prolonged leakage.

Alternate adjunctive tests include vaginal prolactin, α-fetoprotein, human chorionic gonadotropin (HCG), and fetal fibronectin. If negative, these tests may be helpful. However, a positive test is not specific to the diagnosis of membrane rupture. Digital examination should be avoided unless delivery is anticipated, because of the increased risk of infection and the scant additional information about the mother's condition obtained with this procedure.

As previously mentioned, cervical weakness is one primary causes of PROM. Although pregnant women are routinely monitored for weakness in the lower half of the cervix, most practitioners do not routinely screen for changes in the upper half of the cervix, which can also dilate and shorten, giving it a funnel-like appearance (**Fig. 20.1**). This cervical "funneling" is the result of the internal portion of the cervix closest to the baby beginning to open. A funneling cervix can allow the bag of waters to slip down into the cervix and rub against it, which could cause PROM.

Late Pregnancy Bleeding

Bleeding during pregnancy is a common occurrence. Cervical dilation during normal labor is commonly accompanied by a small amount of blood or blood-tinged mucus (bloody show), and many pregnant women experience spotting or minor bleeding after sexual intercourse or a digital vaginal examination. Minor versus serious causes of vaginal bleeding can usually be differentiated by the history, a physical examination, ultrasonography for placental location, and a brief period of observation.

The use of transvaginal ultrasonography for the diagnosis of placenta previa is accurate as well as safe. In the past, the placental location was ascertained by clinical examination and digital palpation of the placental edge from the internal cervical os. However, currently the diagnosis is based on the findings of the ultrasound examination. It is well established that the use of transvaginal ultrasonography is superior to transabdominal ultrasonography in defining the relationship of the placental edge and the internal cervical os.

Cervicitis, cervical ectropion, cervical polyps, and cervical cancer are possible underlying causes (see Pathophys-

iology below). Evaluation with a sterile speculum may be performed safely before ultrasonographic evaluation of placental location; however, digital examination should not be performed unless ultrasonography excludes a placenta previa.

Prevalence and Epidemiology

Premature Rupture of Membranes

PROM complicates approximately 3–5% of pregnancies. The higher rates of perinatal morbidity and mortality associated with PROM are related both independently and by increased rates of preterm birth. Prospective research has shown that there are higher rates of severe neonatal morbidity in pregnancies complicated by PROM than in those caused by idiopathic preterm labor (27% vs.15.1%, $P = 0.02$). It has also been demonstrated that PROM affects from 32% to 40% of preterm deliveries, with 60% to 80% of these patients entering spontaneous labor within 48 hours, with the ensuing neonatal sequelae of preterm delivery.

Third Trimester Bleeding

Third trimester bleeding occurs in approximately 4% of patients. Approximately 50% of these will have an inconsequential cause and 50% will have a life-threatening event. Placental abruption occurs in approximately 1 in 120 births and accounts for 15% of perinatal mortality. Placenta previa occurs in about 1 in 200 live births. However, it rarely causes maternal hemorrhage, unless instrumentation or digital exam is performed.

Spontaneous uterine rupture occurs in 0.03% to 0.08% of all delivering women, but is much more prevalent in patients with a history of uterine scarring (0.3–1.7%).

Etiology and Pathophysiology

Premature Rupture of Membranes

Recently, it has become clear that PROM is not merely the result of the stretch and shear forces of uterine contractions, although they are contributors to the process. Rather, a "programmed" weakening of the placenta appears to

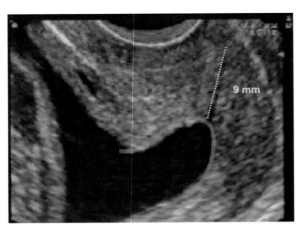

Fig. 20.1   Ultrasound image of a short cervix (9 mm) with funneling.

be a more significant contributor to the process. Research in rats has demonstrated that collagen remodeling, with activation of matrix metalloproteinases, and apoptosis (programmed cell death) increase markedly in the amnion of a woman with PROM, suggesting the involvement of these pathways in fetal membrane weakening.

The management of PROM is challenging, because once the membranes have broken, the risk of fetal or maternal infection, or both, increases. Preterm PROM adds to this management challenge, mainly because of the added problem of prematurity.

PROM can also result from: infections in the ascending genital tract, which initiate a cytokine cascade that enhances membrane apoptosis; protease production and dissolution of the extracellular matrix; placental abruption with decidual thrombin expression triggering thrombin–thrombin receptor interactions and increasing choriodecidual protease production; and membrane stretch that may increase amniochorionic cytokine and protease release.

Known clinical risk factors for preterm PROM include low socioeconomic status, low body mass index, prior preterm birth, cigarette smoking, urinary tract infection, sexually transmitted disease, cervical conization or cerclage, uterine overdistention, amniocentesis in the current pregnancy, and prior preterm labor or symptomatic contractions in the current pregnancy. In many cases, the ultimate cause of membrane rupture cannot be determined, however.

Various other mechanisms have been proposed as causes of PROM, including mechanical, infectious, and inflammatory processes. It is apparent that a no single pathophysiological mechanism is responsible for all cases of PROM, but rather a combination of processes is in operation.

Third Trimester Bleeding

Vaginal bleeding during any given time during pregnancy is not normal and is always of concern. Third trimester bleeding is often the result of the four potentially serious conditions: 1) placental abruption, 2) placenta previa, 3) vasa previa, or 4) uterine rupture. Though the exact etiology of the bleeding often cannot be determined, the onset of bleeding may provide clues to indicate the etiology. Due to the variable mechanisms for bleeding, the amount of blood loss will vary anywhere from spotting to extensive hemorrhaging requiring aggressive emergency measures.

Placental Abruption

Placental abruption can be caused by trauma, hypertension, and coagulopathies. Any of these conditions can lead to the avulsion of the anchoring villi of the placenta from the expanding lower uterine segment. This leads to bleeding into the decidua basalis and can push the placenta away from the uterus and cause further bleeding.

Placental abruptions are classified by grade (0 to 3) according to severity:
- **Grade 0:** Asymptomatic and only diagnosed through post partum examination of the placenta.
- **Grade 1:** The mother may have vaginal bleeding with mild uterine tenderness or tetany, but there is no distress of mother or fetus.
- **Grade 2:** The mother is symptomatic but not in shock. There is some evidence of fetal distress, which can be found with fetal heart-rate monitoring.
- **Grade 3:** Severe bleeding (which often is dark, or occult) leads to maternal shock and fetal death. There may be maternal disseminated intravascular coagulation, and blood sometimes forces its way through the uterine wall into the serosa, a condition known as Couvelaire uterus.

Placenta Previa

To date, research has identified no specific cause of placenta previa. However, it is believed that it may be related to abnormal vascularization of the endometrium caused by scarring or atrophy from previous trauma, surgery, or infection. Risk factors for placenta previa include prior placenta previa, prior cesarean delivery, increased maternal age, large placentas (e.g., multiple gestations or erythroblastosis), and a maternal history of smoking.

In the last trimester of pregnancy the isthmus of the uterus unfolds and forms the lower segment. In a normal pregnancy the placenta does not overlie it, so there is no bleeding. If the placenta does overlie the lower segment, it may shear off and a small section may bleed. Placenta previa is itself a risk factor of placenta accreta, another type of bleeding disorder.

Placenta previa is classified in four stages (**Fig. 20.2**) according to the placement of the placenta as follows.
- **Type I** or low lying: The placenta encroaches the lower segment of the uterus but does not infringe on the cervical os.
- **Type II** or marginal: The placenta touches, but does not cover, the top of the cervix.
- **Type III** or partial: The placenta partially covers the top of the cervix.
- **Type IV** or complete: The placenta completely covers the top of the cervix. This type of previa often will not bleed until labor starts.

Vasa Previa

Vasa previa is caused by the fetus' blood vessels traversing the fetal membranes over the internal cervical os (**Fig. 20.3**). These vessels may originate from either a vela-

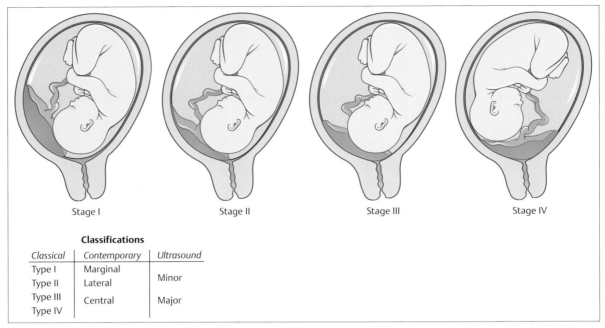

Stage I   Stage II   Stage III   Stage IV

Classifications

Classical	*Contemporary*	*Ultrasound*
Type I	Marginal	Minor
Type II	Lateral	
Type III	Central	Major
Type IV		

Fig. 20.2   Illustrations of the four stages of severity of placenta previa.

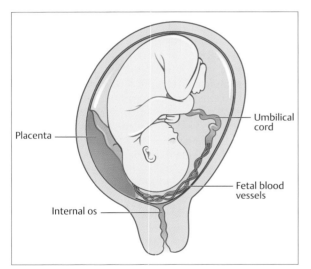

Placenta

Umbilical cord

Fetal blood vessels

Internal os

Fig. 20.3   In cases of vasa previa, some of the fetus' blood vessels block the opening to the internal cervical os, presenting an extremely dangerous obstacle to vaginal delivery.

mentous insertion of the umbilical cord or may be joining an accessory (succenturiate) placental lobe to the main disk of the placenta. If these fetal vessels rupture during delivery, fetal exsanguination can occur extremely rapidly, causing fetal death.

Uterine Rupture

Uterine rupture is a catastrophic tearing open of the uterus into the abdominal cavity. Its onset is often marked only by sudden fetal bradycardia, and treatment requires rapid surgical attention for good neonatal and maternal outcomes.

Excessive uterine stimulation can cause rupture. Cocaine abuse during pregnancy, thus, is associated with uterine rupture as is over-use of oxytocin (Pitocin). **Table**

Table 20.1   Conditions associated with uterine rupture

Uterine scars
• Prior cesarean section
• Prior rupture
• Trauma
• Injury from instrumentation during an abortion
• Significant myomectomy
• Any cause of uterine perforation

Uterine anomalies (i.e., undeveloped uterine horn)

Prior invasive molar pregnancy

History of placenta percreta or increta

Difficult forceps delivery

Malpresentation

Fetal anomaly

Obstructed labor

Induction of labor (suspected association)

Excessive uterine stimulation
• Prostaglandin E1 (misoprostol [Cytotec])
• Prostaglandin E2 (dinoprostone [Cervidil])
• Oxytocin (Pitocin), especially high infusion rates
• Alkaloidal/crack-cocaine abuse

20.1 lists all the conditions and drugs believed to be risk factors for this condition.

History

A medical history for either PROM or third trimester bleeding should include questions about:
- past OB history
- prior episodes of PROM or bleeding
- abdominal pain
- uterine contractions
- recent intercourse
- tobacco / substance abuse
- past medical history

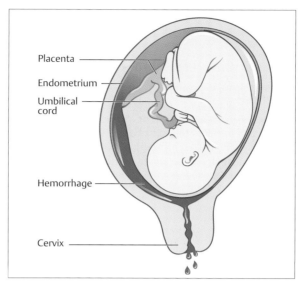

Fig. 20.4 The most common symptom of placental abruption is visible vaginal bleeding. However, in some cases, signs of bleeding may be obscured or may be dark or intermixed with amniotic fluid.

Chief Complaints

Premature Rupture of Membranes

The chief complaints of women with PROM include leaking or a gush of watery fluid from the vagina and/or constant wetness in underwear garments. However, the symptoms of PROM may resemble other medical conditions.

Third Trimester Bleeding

Placental abruption: Also referred to as abruptio placentae, this usually occurs during the third trimester or after 20 weeks of gestation, when something causes the placenta to separate either partially or completely from the wall of the uterus. Bleeding through the vagina, called overt or visible bleeding (**Fig. 20.4**), occurs 80% of the time. However, in some cases, the blood will pool behind the placenta. This is known as concealed, or internal, placental abruption.

This condition may present with blood loss, ranging from very little to severe. The patient will most likely complain of severe pain characterized as a severe "tearing" sensation. The more extensive the abruption (tear), the more likely will there be a greater severity of pain and blood loss. Preterm labor, growth restriction, and intrauterine fetal death are the major fetal risk factors associated with placental abruption.

Placenta previa: The chief symptoms of placenta previa include "painless" bright-red vaginal bleeding. As a general rule, all incidents of painless vaginal bleeding during pregnancy are considered to be placenta previa until proven otherwise. Another complication of a placenta previa is that the placenta may be the presenting part

during delivery and, thus, the patient requires an emergency cesarean section.

Vasa previa: This condition is rarely diagnosed before delivery. Rather, the diagnosis is usually confirmed, on examination of the placenta and fetal membranes after delivery. Most often the fetus is already dead when the diagnosis is made due to massive blood loss. Vasa previa can also present with fetal bradycardia when the velamentous vessels are compressed by the presenting part. Occasionally, fetal vessels are palpated at the time of digital examination, and compression of the vessel may cause deceleration of the fetal heart rate.

Uterine rupture: A significant uterine rupture is commonly accompanied by a severe, localized pain and abnormalities of the fetal heart rate. There may or may not be vaginal bleeding. When uterine rupture occurs outside a hospital setting, even if the mother is transported quickly to the emergency room for stabilization and emergency surgery, it is more likely to lead to severe outcomes. However, when a uterine rupture is diagnosed in a hospital setting during labor, and an emergency cesarean can be performed immediately, the baby's life usually can be saved.

Physical Examination

Premature Rupture of Membranes

A typical diagnostic approach will begin with an aseptic speculum examination. The observation of amniotic fluid passing through the cervical os and pooling in the posterior vaginal fornix is the most useful and definitive diagnostic test. If no fluid is passed spontaneously, the patient is asked to cough or bear down to induce passage of amniotic fluid through the os.

Placental Abruption

Patients with placental abruption typically present with abdominal pain and bleeding. The abdomen is usually tender and the uterus is contracted or hard (woody). Back pain may also be present. It is often difficult to palpate fetal parts, and a fetal heart beat may be absent. Preterm labor, growth restriction, and intrauterine fetal death also may occur. Bleeding may be completely or partially concealed or may be bright, dark, or intermixed with amniotic fluid.

Placenta Previa

Historically, placenta previa was diagnosed via digital palpation of the placental tissue through the cervical canal. The slightest amount of manipulation, however, may result in a substantial amount of hemorrhage. Physical examination, therefore, should be performed only with a fetus that has achieved pulmonary maturity and only in a fully staffed operating room. Maternal bleeding may be so severe that immediate delivery is necessary.

Vasa Previa

Vasa previa can only be diagnosed prenatally by ultrasound examination. The specificity of ultrasonographic diagnosis of vasa previa has been reported to be as high as 91%, and antenatal diagnosis has been shown to prevent the catastrophic outcomes commonly associated with this condition. Thus, good outcomes for women with vasa previa depend on prenatal diagnosis and cesarean delivery before the membranes rupture.

Uterine Rupture

In the past, caregivers were taught to look for classic signs of uterine rupture, such as sudden tearing, uterine pain, vaginal hemorrhage, cessation of uterine contractions, and regression of the fetus. However, such signs have been demonstrated to be unreliable or absent. Uterine contraction patterns often appear normal in women with uterine rupture, and even ruptures monitored with an intrauter- ine pressure catheter often fail to show a loss of uterine tone or contractile pattern after uterine rupture.

Rather, the most reliable presenting clinical symptom of uterine rupture is fetal distress. Prolonged, late, or variable decelerations and bradycardia seen on fetal heart rate monitoring are the most common symptoms of uterine rupture.

Laboratory Testing

Premature Rupture of Membranes

If attempts to observe amniotic fluid passing through the cervical os fail to confirm PROM, a fluid specimen from the posterior vaginal fornix can be obtained with a sterile swab and smeared onto a glass slide. This sample is then tested with nitrazine paper, which turns blue when saturated with fluid that has a pH greater than 6.4. Vaginal fluid with an alkaline pH (any pH greater than 7) may be indicative of PROM.

Bacterial vaginosis, trichomoniasis, or the presence of blood, semen, or alkalinized urine in the vaginal fluid also can lead to the alkalinization of the vaginal secretions. Thus, this pH test can give rise to false-positive test results. False-negative reactions can occur if there is insufficient passage of amniotic fluid to increase the vaginal pH.

The glass slide also can be examined under a microscope for the presence of a characteristic arborization, or ferning, pattern (**Fig. 20.5**). The fluid specimen must be obtained from the posterior vaginal fornix rather than from the cervical canal, as approximately 30% of women

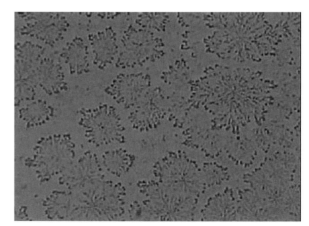

Fig. 20.5 Amniotic fluid, when dried, creates a fern-leaf–like pattern that can be seen microscopically. The presence of this pattern is a strong indicator that the bag of waters has broken.

will have persistent ferning of cervical mucus throughout pregnancy.

Less useful diagnostic tests for PROM include instillation of a dye solution into the amniotic cavity with transabdominal amniocentesis and subsequent assessment of the cervix and vagina for the presence of dye-stained fluid. Biochemical assessment of vaginal or cervical fluid is also possible, with detection of high levels of α-fetoprotein or fetal fibronectin providing evidence of the presence of amniotic fluid. These tests are somewhat expensive and are not readily available in all centers, nor are they usually necessary for the diagnosis of PROM at term. In the rare event that bedside testing is equivocal, it is acceptable to repeat the physical examination and bedside testing after several hours, rather than resort to laboratory evaluation or invasive procedures.

Although maternal white blood cell count may increase in amnionitis, such test results may be artificially elevated if antenatal corticosteroids have been administered within 5–7 days. Alternatively, an increasing white blood cell count in the presence of suspicious clinical findings may be useful in identifying patients who require closer observation—including continuous contraction and fetal monitoring—or who require delivery. If the clinical diagnosis is not sufficiently clear, additional information can be gained with amniocentesis, provided an adequate amniotic fluid pocket is accessible. When amniocentesis is performed, care should be taken to avoid inadvertently sampling the umbilical cord. Color flow ultrasonography may be helpful in differentiating a small amniotic fluid pocket from umbilical-cord arterial or venous flow.

Third Trimester Bleeding

Laboratory evaluation for third trimester bleeding should include blood type and cross match (in case a transfusion is needed), as well as a complete blood count and coagulation status (e.g., prothrombin and thromboplastin time). When a placental abruption is suspected, d-Dimer and fibronectin are the most sensitive tests for confirming a coagulopathy. Unfortunately, they are only useful for detecting abruptions, not their severity.

Treatment

Premature Rupture of Membranes

PROM carries an extremely high risk of preterm delivery (see Chapter 19). However, in the absence of infection, abruption, advanced labor, or fetal compromise, patients with preterm PROM between 23 and 31 weeks' gestation are generally managed conservatively to prolong their pregnancy and reduce the risk of morbidity to the preterm infant. Even women with preterm PROM who are amenable to conservative management only have a 50% chance of remaining pregnant for at least 1 week after membrane rupture (**Fig. 20.6**).

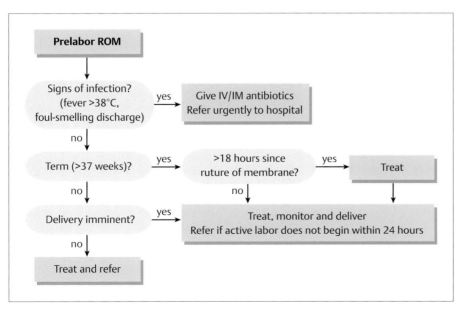

Fig. 20.6 Word Health Organization's medical management flowchart for premature (prelabor) rupture of membranes (ROM).

On the other hand, a small number of women (2.6–13%), especially those with preterm PROM subsequent to amniocentesis, will experience a spontaneous resealing of the membranes and restoration of a normal amniotic fluid volume. Women being managed conservatively for preterm PROM remote from term should generally be managed as hospital in-patients, so that problems such as amnionitis, vaginal bleeding, nonreassuring fetal heart-rate patterns, and labor can be detected early and managed appropriately. The facility should be capable of providing emergency care to both mother and infant.

Avoid digital examinations to reduce the risk of intrauterine infection and enhanced latency. Assess uterine contraction and fetal heart rate at least once daily to assess for occult contractions, fetal wellbeing, and umbilical cord compression. Additional tests may be needed based on these findings.

If a nonstress test is unreactive, it may be helpful to conduct a biophysical profile to assess fetal wellbeing. Because pregnancy and inactivity are significant risk factors for thromboembolic complications, a pregnant woman prescribed bed-rest should be administered preventive measures, such as leg exercises, antiembolic stockings, and prophylactic doses of subcutaneous heparin.

The combination of fever with uterine tenderness or maternal or fetal tachycardia in the absence of another evident source of infection is suggestive of intrauterine infection and should lead to consideration of delivery. Some patients will not demonstrate classical symptomatology of amnionitis, however. Increasing uterine discomfort or menstrual cramps may be an early finding.

Antenatal corticosteroids: It is recommended that women managed conservatively with preterm PROM remote from term be administered antenatal corticosteroids for fetal maturation, if they have not previously received corticosteroids in the current pregnancy to reduce the risk of intraventricular hemorrhage. Research suggests that antenatal corticosteroid administration given concurrently with antibiotic administration (see below) reduces the incidence of respiratory distress as well as perinatal death in preterm newborns.

Harding et al. analyzed data from 15 controlled trials of corticosteroid treatment among more than 1400 women with PROM. Their analysis found that antenatal corticosteroid administration, compared with controls, reduced the incidence of respiratory distress (20% vs. 35.4%), intraventricular hemorrhage (7.5% vs. 15.9%), and necrotizing enterocolitis (0.8% vs. 4.6%), without significant increased risks of maternal infection (9.2% vs. 5.1%) or neonatal infection (7.0% vs. 6.6%).

Prophylactic antibiotic treatment: It is well established that intrapartum antibiotic prophylaxis is effective against the vertical transmission of group B Streptococcus from mother to infant. Adjunctive antibiotic therapy is often administered during conservative management of preterm PROM to treat or prevent any ascending subclinical decidual infection, to prolong pregnancy, to reduce infectious morbidity, and to reduce neonatal infectious and gestational, age-dependent morbidity.

The efficacy of aggressive, limited-duration, broad-spectrum antibiotic therapy to reduce of infant morbidity after PROM has been supported by a number of clinical trials (Evidence Box 20.1). The protocol recommended by the National Institute of Child Health and Development—Maternal Fetal Medicine Unit, for the prophylactic antibiotic management of PROM, is a 7-day protocol. Initially, antibiotics are administered intravenously for 48 hours (2 g ampicillin and 250 mg erythromycin every 6 hours). This is followed by 250 mg of oral amoxicillin and 333 mg of oral enteric-coated erythromycin every 8 hours for 5 days.

Although there are reports that shorter-duration antibiotic treatment is appropriate during conservative management of women with preterm PROM, the studies conducted to date in this area lacked enough subjects, and thus statistical power, to properly evaluate equivalency regarding infant morbidity or latency.

When preterm PROM occurs at 34–36 weeks' gestation, the risk of severe acute neonatal morbidity and mortality with expeditious delivery is low. Conversely, conservative management at 34–36 weeks has been associated with an eightfold increase in amnionitis (16% vs. 2%, $P = 0.001$) and only brief prolongation of latency and maternal hospitalization (5.2 days vs. 2.6 days, $P = 0.006$), without significant reduction in perinatal morbidity related to prematurity.

Hence these women are best served by expeditious delivery with labor induction, in the absence of contraindication to labor or vaginal delivery. Intrapartum group B Streptococcus prophylaxis should be given in the absence of a recent, negative anal–vaginal culture. Broad-spectrum antibiotics should be given intravenously, if amnionitis is suspected.

Management of Premature Rupture of Membranes Near Term

When preterm PROM occurs at 32–36 weeks' gestation, fetal pulmonary maturity assessment can be helpful in determining the optimal approach to management.

In the presence of fetal pulmonary maturity documented by either vaginal pool sampling or amniocentesis after 32 weeks, there is little risk of severe neonatal morbidity with expeditious delivery. Indeed, women with documented fetal pulmonary maturity after preterm PROM at 32–36 weeks' gestation are best served by expeditious delivery with intrapartum antibiotic administration, as described earlier.

Expeditious delivery should be considered unless the fetus is considered to be at significant risk for gestational age-dependent morbidity, in which case measures should be taken to reduce the risk of infection and enhance fetal maturation. If antenatal corticosteroids and antibiotics cannot be administered in this setting, the woman may be better served by expeditious delivery with appropriate intrapartum antibiotic therapy.

When amniotic fluid testing reveals an immature result, or when amniotic fluid is unavailable after preterm PROM at 32–36 weeks' gestation, conservative management, rather than delivery, may be appropriate. The infant delivered with documented pulmonary immaturity is at an increased risk of respiratory distress and other complications. Antenatal corticosteroids have been demonstrated to benefit populations at high risk for fetal immaturity. Antibiotic treatment in the setting of preterm PROM has been shown to reduce the risk of infectious morbidity. Given these general principles, conservative management with antenatal corticosteroid administration and concurrent antibiotic therapy may be appropriate.

Third Trimester Bleeding

Placental Abruption

Expectant management of preterm placental abruption with marginal placental requires careful fetal monitoring with close follow-up of the maternal hematologic and coagulation profile. Early maternal management should focus on improving the airway, breathing (oxygenation), and circulation. Treatment must be aimed at the prevention of shock disseminated intravascular coagulopathy. A wide-bore intravenous line should be set up and blood sent for cross matching of at least six units of blood. Blood should also be taken to check hemoglobin, platelets, and clotting. The laboratory should be informed of the urgency and a hematologist involved, if necessary. Until this blood arrives, other plasma expanding fluids, such as Gelofusine, should be used. In severe cases, resuscitation can begin with O-negative blood.

If gestation is sufficiently advanced and the fetus is viable, a caesarean section is the best management approach. However, if the fetus is dead, conservative management can be pursued provided that the woman does not continue deteriorating, for example, by developing a coagulopathy. Most women with a severe placental abruption that kills the fetus will go into spontaneous labor soon and have an easy delivery. However, cesarean section is occasionally necessary for maternal indications alone.

Placenta Previa

Caesarean section is the traditional mode of delivery for major placenta previa, whereas minor previa is most often managed by vaginal delivery. The placenta is considered "too low" for cesarean section due to bleeding, or the risk of hemorrhagic complications.

However, the translation of this management strategy is far from clear when the diagnosis is based only on ultrasonography. Oppenheimer et al. attempted to establish criteria for the diagnosis of placenta previa, based on ultrasonographic results of 127 women with suspected placenta previa. They found that the mean distance of the placental edge from the internal cervical os in women requiring a cesarean section for placenta previa was 1.1 cm (range 0.0–2.0 cm). No patient with a placental edge greater than 2 cm from the internal cervical os required cesarean section for the indication of placenta previa, whereas seven of eight patients with a distance of less than or equal to 2 cm underwent a cesarean section because of bleeding.

Thus, a low-lying placenta can be delivered vaginally. However, appropriate precautions must be taken to prevent hemorrhagic complications (**Fig. 20.7**).

Vasa Previa

Vasa Previa is usually managed by immediate emergency cesarean delivery.

Uterine Rupture

As the presenting signs of uterine rupture are frequently nonspecific, the initial management is the same as for other causes of acute fetal distress—urgent surgical delivery. Research suggests the best outcomes are achieved when surgical delivery occurs within 17 minutes of the onset of fetal distress as detected by electronic monitoring.

Key Points

- Premature rupture of membranes (PROM) and third trimester bleeding represent some of the most serious complications of pregnancy.
- Preterm PROM is responsible for approximately one-third of preterm deliveries, and bleeding in the third trimester can present as a life-threatening event for both mother and baby.
- The cause of these two conditions varies, so treatment must be tailored to match a woman's symptoms.
- Women with third trimester bleeding require careful fetal monitoring with close follow-up of maternal hematologic and coagulation profiles.
- Most cases of third trimester bleeding that are determined to be not normal and where the fetus is still viable are treated by cesarean section.

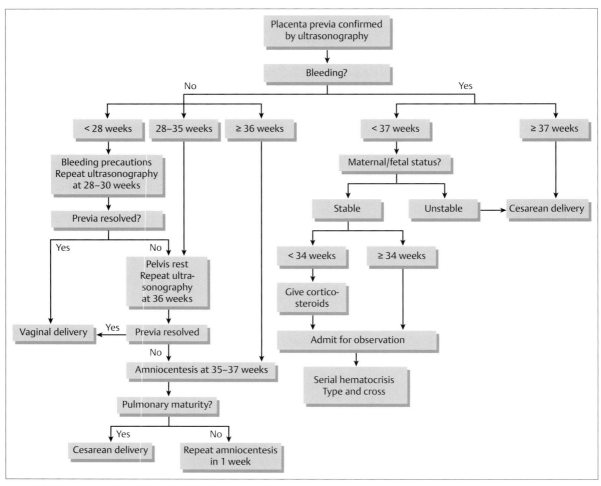

Fig. 20.7   Schematic of placenta previa clinical management.

Evidence Box 20.1

Expectant mothers with preterm premature rupture of membranes may benefit from antibiotics to prolong pregnancy and reduce infant morbidity.

Mercer et al. conducted a randomized, double-blind, placebo-controlled trial to determine whether antibiotic treatment during expectant management of preterm premature rupture of membranes (PROM) could reduce infant morbidity. A total of 614 women with preterm PROM between 24 and 32 weeks of gestation were randomized to receive either intravenous antibiotics for 48 hours followed by oral antibiotics for 5 days, or to receive a matching placebo regimen. In the total study population, overall morbidity (44.1% vs. 52.9%; $P = 0.04$), respiratory distress (40.5% vs. 48.7%; $P = 0.04$), and necrotizing enterocolitis (2.3% vs. 5.8%; $P = 0.03$) were significantly less frequent in those women taking antibiotics. Furthermore, among women who were negative for Group B streptococcus, the researchers found a significant prolongation of pregnancy among women treated with antibiotics versus placebo ($P < 0.001$).

Mercer BM, Miodovnk M, Thurnau GR, et al. Antibiotic therapy for reduction of infant morbidity after preterm premature rupture of the membranes. A randomized controlled trial. National Institute of Child Health and Human Development Maternal-Fetal Medicine Units Network. JAMA. 1997 Sep 24;278(12):989–995

Further Reading

Bhide A, Thilaganathan B. Recent advances in the management of placenta previa. *Curr Opin Obstet Gynecol* 2004;16(6):447–451

Harding JE, Pang J, Knight DB, Liggins GC. Do antenatal corticosteroids help in the setting of preterm rupture of membranes? *Am J Obstet Gynecol* 2001;184(2):131–139

Lee T, Silver H. Etiology and epidemiology of preterm premature rupture of the membranes. *Clin Perinatol* 2001;28(4):721–734

Lijoi AF, Brady J. Vasa previa diagnosis and management. *J Am Board Fam Pract* 2003;16(6):543–548

Main DM, Gabbe SG, Richardson D, Strong S. Can preterm deliveries be prevented? *Am J Obstet Gynecol* 1985;151(7):892–898

Mercer BM, Miodovnik M, Thurnau GR, et al; National Institute of Child Health and Human Development Maternal-Fetal Medicine Units Network. Antibiotic therapy for reduction of infant morbidity after preterm premature rupture of the membranes. A randomized controlled trial. *JAMA* 1997;278(12):989–995

Mercer BM, Goldenberg RL, Meis PJ, et al; The National Institute of Child Health and Human Development Maternal-Fetal Medicine Units Network. The Preterm Prediction Study: prediction of preterm premature rupture of membranes through clinical findings and ancillary testing. *Am J Obstet Gynecol* 2000;183(3):738–745

Mercer BM. Preterm premature rupture of the membranes. *Obstet Gynecol* 2003;101(1):178–193

Oppenheimer LW, Farine D, Ritchie JW, Lewinsky RM, Telford J, Fairbanks LA. What is a low-lying placenta? *Am J Obstet Gynecol* 1991;165(4 Pt 1):1036–1038

Sakornbut E, Leeman L, Fontaine P. Late pregnancy bleeding: a review. *Am Fam Phys* 2007;75:1199–1206

21 Hypertension in Pregnancy

E. Albert Reece

Hypertension is a complicating feature of 6–8% of pregnancies. It causes some of the most serious complications for both the fetus and the mother during pregnancy. Fetal complications include severe growth restriction and stillbirth. In addition, hypertensive disorders account for nearly 15% of maternal deaths in the United States, ranking second only to embolism as a leading cause of maternal mortality. Other complications for the mother can affect heart (**Fig. 21.1**), kidney, liver, and central nervous system functions.

For these reasons, it is critical to accurately diagnose the type of hypertension that the patient has and to prescribe an appropriate therapeutic intervention.

Definition

Hypertension in pregnancy is not a single entity. Rather, it is classified into four main categories, as recommended by the National High Blood Pressure Education Program Working Group on High Blood Pressure in Pregnancy:

1. Chronic hypertension
2. Pre-eclampsia–eclampsia
3. Pre-eclampsia superimposed on chronic hypertension
4. Gestational hypertension (transient hypertension of pregnancy or chronic hypertension identified in the latter half of pregnancy)

This terminology is preferred over the older but widely used term, pregnancy-induced hypertension (or PIH), because it is more accurate.

Chronic hypertension: This is defined as a blood pressure (BP) greater than 140/90 mmHg that either predates pregnancy or develops before 20 weeks' gestation. When hypertension is first identified during a woman's pregnancy and she is at less than 20 weeks' gestation, BP elevations usually represent chronic hypertension.

Pre-eclampsia: This condition—which occurs in approximately 5% of all pregnancies, 10% of first pregnancies, and 20–25% of women with a history of chronic hypertension—is pregnancy-induced hypertension in association with proteinuria or edema, or both. Virtually any organ system may be affected.

Pre-eclampsia superimposed on chronic hypertension: Pregnant women with pre-existing chronic hypertension may develop pre-eclampsia. Superimposed pre-eclampsia is suspected when proteinuria develops or increases suddenly; when previously controlled hypertension exhibits a sudden increase; or when the patient develops thrombocytopenia or elevated liver enzyme levels. Women with pre-eclampsia superimposed on chronic hypertension have a significantly poorer prognosis than women with either condition alone.

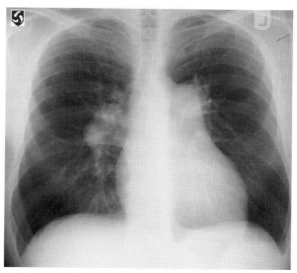

Fig. 21.1 A radiograph of a patient with an enlarged heart due to chronic hypertension.

Gestational hypertension: This condition is pregnancy-induced hypertension in isolation; it may reflect a familial predisposition to chronic hypertension, or it may be an early manifestation of pre-eclampsia. Pregnancy-induced hypertension, which develops after 20 weeks' gestation, complicates 5–10% of pregnancies (see Prevalence and Epidemiology).

Diagnosis

Sometimes, determining whether hypertension identified during pregnancy is due to chronic hypertension or to pre-eclampsia is a challenge. Clinical characteristics, such as history, physical examination, and certain laboratory examinations, are used to help clarify the diagnosis.

Chronic Hypertension

Chronic hypertension is diagnosed if there is a persistent elevation in BP to at least 140/90 mmHg on two occasions more than 24 hours apart prior to conception, prior to 20 weeks of gestation, or beyond 12 weeks postpartum. Other factors that may suggest the presence of chronic hypertension include:

- retinal changes on fundoscopic examination
- radiographic and electrocardiographic evidence of cardiac enlargement
- comprised renal function or associated renal disease, or
- multiparity with a previous history of hypertensive pregnancies

Chronic hypertension in pregnancy may be subclassified into mild hypertension (diastolic [d] BP ≥90 to <110 mmHg or systolic [s] BP ≥140 to <180 mmHg) or severe hypertension (dBP ≥110 mmHg to or sBP ≥180 mmHg). For the purpose of clinical management, chronic hypertension in pregnancy may be divided into a low-risk group (hypertension with no organ damage or association with other comorbidities) or a high-risk group (hypertension with organ damage and associated comorbidities). **Table 21.1** lists some of the major complications of chronic hypertension for both the mother and fetus.

Pre-eclampsia–Eclampsia

(See Chapter 16.)

Pre-eclampsia Superimposed on Chronic Hypertension

Chronic hypertension may be complicated by superimposed pre-eclampsia (or eclampsia), which is diagnosed when there is an exacerbation of hypertension and the development of proteinurea that was not present earlier in the pregnancy. Conditions for the diagnosis of superimposed pre-eclampsia on chronic hypertension are detailed in Chapter 16.

Gestational Hypertension

Gestational hypertension is defined as dBP ≥90 mmHg or sBP ≥140 mmHg (without proteinurea) measured on two occasions at least 6 hours apart and no more than 7 days apart after 20 weeks of gestation. It is usually a mild form of hypertension, late in onset, often occurs close to term, and occurs intrapartum or within 24 hours of delivery. It often resolves within 10 days of the postpartum period without treatment.

Severe gestational hypertension is defined as a sustained sBP ≥160 mmHg and/or a dBP ≥110 mmHg measured at least 6 hours apart with no proteinurea. Women with severe gestational hypertension have higher maternal and perinatal morbidities that those with mild gestational hypertension. However, women with mild gestational hypertension often progress to severe gestational hypertension and pre-eclampsia if not treated.

The rate of progression from severe hypertension to pre-eclampsia is dependent on the gestational age at the time of diagnosis; the rate reaches 50% when gestational hypertension develops before 30 weeks of gestation.

Table 21.1 Complications of chronic hypertension in pregnancy

Mother
Pregnancy aggravated hypertension
Superimposed preeclampsia
Placental abruption
Fetus
Prematurity
Placental insufficiency
Intrauterine growth restriction
Placental abruption

Prevalence and Epidemiology

Chronic hypertension occurs in up to 22% of women of childbearing age, with the prevalence varying according to age, race, and body mass index. Chronic hypertension complicates 1–5% of pregnancies. In the United States, for example, there are at least 120 000 pregnant women with chronic hypertension (3% of 4 million pregnancies) per year, a rate expected to increase with the obesity epidemic and as age at childbearing increases in the developed world (see below). Pre-eclampsia complicates about 5% of all pregnancies, 10% of first pregnancies, and at least 20% of pregnancies in women with a history of chronic hypertension.

Race

Black women have higher rates of pre-eclampsia complicating their pregnancies compared with other racial groups, mainly because they have a greater prevalence of underlying chronic hypertension. A study in the US found that among women aged 30–39 years, chronic hypertension is present in 22.3% of Blacks, 4.6% of Whites, and 6.2% of Hispanics, who generally have BP levels that are the same as or lower than those of non-Hispanic White women.

Age

Pre-eclampsia is more common at the extremes of maternal age (<18 years or >35 years). The increased prevalence of chronic hypertension in women older than 35 years can explain the increased frequency of pre-eclampsia among older gravidas.

Etiology and Pathophysiology

Chronic hypertension may be either essential (90%) of cases or secondary to some identifiable underlying disorder, such as renal disease, endocrine disorders, or vascular problems (**Table 21.2**).

About 20–25% of women with chronic hypertension develop pre-eclampsia during pregnancy. However, the exact cause of pre-eclampsia is unknown.

The widespread endothelial dysfunction that preeclampsia causes in the mother has the potential to cause

Table 21.2 Potential causes of chronic hypertension in pregnancy

Renal factors	Acute and chronic glomerulonephritis
	Acute and chronic pyelonephritis
	Polycystic renal disease
	Renovascular disease
Collagen disease with renal involvement	Lupus erythematosus
	Periarteritis nodosa
	Schleroderma
Endocrine factors	Diabetes with vascular involvement
	Thyrotoxicosis
	Aldosterone producing tumors
	Pheochromocytoma
Vascular system	Coarctation of the arota

catastrophic damage to the brain and the hepatic, pulmonary, renal, and hematological systems. Endothelial damage can lead to leakage of the capillaries, which, in the mother, manifests as rapid weight gain, edema of the face or hands, pulmonary edema, and/or hemoconcentration resulting in hemoglobin levels greater than 12 g/dL or creatinine levels greater than 0.8 mg/dL. A renal biopsy may uncover endotheliosis that is associated with proteinuria greater than 300 mg in 24 hours.

Although the exact pathophysiologic mechanism is not clearly understood, pre-eclampsia can be thought of as a disorder of endothelial function with vasospasm. In some cases, light microscopy demonstrates evidence of placental insufficiency associated with abnormalities, such as diffuse placental thrombosis, an inflammatory placental decidual vasculopathy, and/or abnormal trophoblastic invasion of the endometrium. This association suggests that abnormal placental development or placental damage from diffuse microthrombosis may be central to the development of this disorder (see Chapter 16).

When the placenta becomes involved, it can affect the fetus via decreased uteroplacental blood flow. This decrease in perfusion can manifest clinically as nonreassuring fetal heart rate testing, low scores on a biophysical profile, oligohydramnios, and, in severe cases, fetal growth restriction.

Hypertension occurring in pre-eclampsia is due to vasospasm, with arterial constriction and relatively reduced intravascular volume compared with normal pregnancy. Usually, the vasculature of pregnant women demonstrates decreased responsiveness to vasoactive peptides such as angiotensin II and epinephrine. Women who develop pre-eclampsia show a hyper responsiveness to these hormones, an alteration that may be seen even before the hypertension becomes apparent. In addition, their BPs are labile. Their normal circadian BP rhythms may be blunted or reversed.

Transient hypertension refers to hypertension occurring in late pregnancy without any other features of pre-eclampsia and with normalization of BP postpartum. The pathophysiology of transient hypertension is unknown, but it may be a harbinger of chronic hypertension later in life.

Medical History

Uncomplicated chronic hypertension in pregnancy is labeled low-risk, whereas the high-risk group includes patients with renal disease, diabetes mellitus, connective tissue disorders, etc. (**Table 21.3**).

Hypertension prior to 20 weeks' gestation almost always is due to chronic hypertension. New-onset or worsening hypertension after 20 weeks' gestation should lead to a careful evaluation for manifestations of pre-eclampsia (see Chapter 16). Pre-eclampsia is rare prior to the third trimester.

Physical Signs

Signs of a secondary medical cause of chronic hypertension include:
- centripetal obesity, "buffalo hump," and/or wide, purple abdominal striae indicative of glucocorticoid excess

- a systolic bruit heard over the abdomen or in the flanks indicative of renal artery stenosis
- radiofemoral delay or diminished pulses in lower versus upper extremities indicative of coarctation of the aorta
- hyperthyroidism, hypothyroidism, or growth hormone excess

Signs of end-organ damage from chronic hypertension include:
- S_4 on cardiac auscultation, which is not a normal finding in pregnancy. It is indicative of left ventricular hypertrophy or diastolic dysfunction due to pre-eclampsia-induced vasospasm. In the presence of pre-eclampsia, consider any cardiac gallop should be considered a pathological finding.
- diminished distal pulses due to peripheral vascular disease
- retinal changes of chronic hypertension
- carotid bruits

Laboratory Studies

Laboratory testing to evaluate chronic hypertension includes testing for target organ damage, potential secondary causes of hypertension, and other risk factors. **Table 21.4** lists both mandatory and optional laboratory tests for chronic hypertension during pregnancy.

Because serum lipids (i.e., total cholesterol, high-density lipoprotein, low-density lipoprotein, triglycerides) predictably increase during pregnancy, these tests should be deferred until the postpartum period. Furthermore, the increase in endogenous corticosteroid levels during normal pregnancy makes it difficult to diagnose secondary hypertension due to excess levels of adrenal hormones.

Table 21.3 Factors contributing to higher risks of chronic hypertension in pregnancy

Maternal age >40 years (may consider age ≥40 years)
Duration of hypertension >5 years
Blood pressure exceeding 160/110 mmHg early in pregnancy
Diabetes mellitus (classes B–F)
Cardiomyopathy
Renal disease
Connective tissue disorders
Morbid obesity (weight ≥36 kg [300 lb])

Table 21.4 Mandatory and optional laboratory tests for evaluating chronic hypertension in pregnancy

Mandatory lab tests	Optional lab tests
Urinalysis	Creatinine clearance
Complete blood cell count	Microalbuminuria
Serum sodium	24-hour urinary protein
Serum potassium	Serum calcium
Serum creatinine	Uric acid
Glucose levels	Glycosylated hemoglobin
	Thyroid-stimulating hormone

Treatment

In normal pregnancy, women's mean arterial pressure drops by 10–15 mmHg over the first half of pregnancy. Most women with mild, chronic hypertension (i.e., sBP 140–160 mmHg, dBP 90–100 mmHg) have a similar decrease in BPs and may not require any medication during this period. Conversely, dBP greater than 110 mmHg has been associated with an increased risk of placental abruption and intrauterine growth restriction.

Therefore, it is recommended to place pregnant patients on antihypertensive therapy if the sBP is greater than 160 mmHg or the dBP is greater than 100 mmHg. The goal of pharmacologic treatment should be a dBP of about 80–90 mmHg.

Three treatment options are available in cases of mild chronic hypertension in pregnancy:

- Antihypertensive medication may be withheld or discontinued, with subsequent close observation of BP. Because BP drops during normal pregnancy, begin treatment when BP exceeds 140/90 mmHg.
- If a woman is on pharmacologic treatment with an agent not recommended for use in pregnancy, she may be switched to an alternative antihypertensive agent recommended for use in pregnancy.
- If a woman is on pharmacologic treatment with an agent recommended for use in pregnancy, she may continue her current antihypertensive therapy.

Closely observe women with chronic hypertension in pregnancy for the development of worsening hypertension and/or the development of superimposed pre-eclampsia (the risk is approximately 20%). Repeat laboratory investigations for pre-eclampsia if the patient's BP increases or if she develops signs or symptoms of pre-eclampsia.

Promptly hospitalize women with suspected or diagnosed pre-eclampsia for close observation. When diagnosed with pre-eclampsia, delivering the baby always is in the mother's best interest. Any delay in delivery should be due to uncertainty about the diagnosis or immaturity of the fetus. When pre-eclampsia develops remote from term (i.e., <34–36 weeks' gestation), attempts are often made to prolong the pregnancy to allow for further fetal growth and maturation.

If the pregnancy is prolonged, it is necessary to monitor both maternal and fetal status closely. Perform fetal testing at least twice weekly, using a combination of biophysical profiles and nonstress testing supervised by an obstetrician. Facilitated delivery should occur if either maternal or fetal deterioration is noted, with the mode of delivery decided by obstetric indications.

Consultations

- An obstetrician should follow all cases of women with chronic hypertension throughout pregnancy; refer women with moderate or severe hypertension to a specialist in maternal–fetal medicine (perinatologist) or, if one is unavailable, to any physician experienced in obstetric medicine.
- A maternal–fetal medicine consultant is highly valuable in the care of women with chronic hypertension due to a secondary cause, women with target organ damage, and women in whom pre-eclampsia causes significant organ failure.
- Diagnosis of secondary hypertension during pregnancy can be difficult.
- Renal captopril scans involve radioactive isotopes and usually are deferred to the postpartum period.
- Hyperaldosteronism and hypercortisolism are difficult to diagnose during pregnancy, owing to the high levels of progesterone and the normal increase in endogenous cortisol output.

Diet

Multiple dietary interventions have been investigated for a role for diet in preventing pre-eclampsia, but none has shown any effect in trials.

Physical Activity

- Women with worsening hypertension during pregnancy are often placed on bed-rest or restricted activity, although no scientific evidence demonstrates that this is beneficial in prolonging gestation or reducing maternal or fetal morbidity/mortality.
- Women with hypertension and suspected pre-eclampsia typically are admitted to a hospital for close observation and investigation. Those with established pre-eclampsia must be observed very closely, either in hospital or in a comprehensive home monitoring program under the care of a high-risk obstetrician (e.g., a perinatologist or maternal–fetal medicine specialist).

Pharmacologic Therapy

Women with mild chronic hypertension often do not require antihypertensive therapy during most of their pregnancy. Pharmacologic treatment of mild hypertension does not reduce the likelihood of developing pre-eclampsia later in gestation and increases the likelihood of an adverse effect in the mother or the fetus. However, if maternal BP exceeds 140/90 mmHg, pharmacologic treatment is recommended.

If a pregnant woman's BP is sustained at greater than 170 mmHg systolic and/or 110 mmHg diastolic at any time, lowering her BP quickly with rapid-acting agents is indicated for maternal safety. Chapter 16 describes the various pharmacologic options for managing severe hypertension during pregnancy (**Table 16.5**).

Medications to avoid during pregnancy include angiotensin-converting enzyme (ACE) inhibitors, which are associated with fetal renal dysgenesis or death when used in the second and third trimesters. ACE inhibitors reduce angiotensin II levels, decreasing aldosterone secretion. Angiotensin II receptor antagonists/blockers are not used during pregnancy because they have similar mechanism of action as ACE inhibitors.

Breast-feeding

The available data suggest that all antihypertensive agents are excreted into human breast milk, but most are excreted to a negligible degree. In addition, all of these medications are believed to be compatible with breast-feeding. However, using medications with a well-established track record is preferred (Evidence Box 21.2). For example, atenolol, as well as the other beta-blocking agents nadolol and metoprolol, appear to be concentrated in breast milk. Labetalol and propranolol on the other hand do not share this behavior and are preferred agents if a beta-blocker is indicated.

Prognosis

Transient hypertension in pregnancy—that is, the development of isolated hypertension in a woman in late pregnancy without other manifestations of pre-eclampsia—is strongly linked with later development of chronic hypertension.

Special Concerns

When severe complications occur during pregnancy, the patient often feels bewildered and angry. Therefore, you should take all possible steps to adequately inform her and her family about the potential complications and remedies and involve them in the decision-making process.

Reassure the patient that, in most cases, the complications are not due to her actions or failure to act. Follow up by discussing plans for evaluation and treatment, providing her an opportunity to ask questions. It is important for you to make the patient feel comfortable in asking any question she may have, and you should feel comfortable providing her with honest, straightforward answers. You should also be comfortable consulting with other clinicians (e.g., specialists) who can help you to care for the patient, and let her know that you are willing to do so. This will reassure her that all avenues of treatment are being explored and will help to cement the bond of trust between you and the patient.

Key Points

- Hypertension is a complicating feature of 6–8 % of pregnancies and causes some of the most serious complications for both the fetus and the mother during pregnancy.
- Thus, it is critical to accurately diagnose the type of hypertension the patient has and to prescribe an appropriate therapeutic intervention.
- It is sometimes difficult to determine whether hypertension identified during pregnancy is due to chronic hypertension or to pre-eclampsia. Clinical characteristics, such as history, physical examination, and certain laboratory examinations, are used to help clarify the diagnosis.
- Pregnant patients should be prescribed antihypertensive therapy if their systolic blood pressure is greater than 160 mmHg or their diastolic blood pressure is greater than 100 mmHg. The goal of pharmacologic treatment should be a diastolic blood pressure of about 80–90 mmHg.

Evidence Box 21.1

Either intravenous hydralazine or intravenous labetalol is effective and safe in the management of severe hypertension in the postpartum period.

Vigil-De Gracia et al. compared the safety and efficacy of intravenous labetalol and hydralazine for acutely lowering blood pressure in pregnancy. Patients were randomized to receive hydralazine (5 mg as a slow bolus dose given intravenously, and repeated every 20 min to a maximum of five doses) or labetalol (20 mg in an intravenous bolus dose followed by 40 mg if not effective within 20 min, followed by 80 mg every 20 min to a maximum dose of 300 mg). The primary endpoint was the successful lowering of blood pressure. Secondary endpoints were maternal complications and side effects. Forty-two women were enrolled in the hydralazine group and 40 in the labetalol group. Women were similar with respect to characteristics at randomization. There were no significant differences for persistent severe hypertension or maternal side effects. There was only one case of persistent, severe hypertension in the labetalol group. There were no maternal deaths in any of the women studied.

Vigil-De Gracia P, Ruiz E, López JC, et al. Management of severe hypertension in the postpartum period with intravenous hydralazine or labetalol: a randomized clinical trial. Hypertens Pregnancy 2007;26(2):163–171.

Further Reading

Frederick UE, Sibai BM. Hypertensive diseases in pregnancy. In: Reece EA, Hobbins JC, ed. Clinical Obstetrics: the Fetus and Mother. Malden, Mass: Blackwell Synergy Publishing; 2007:251–260

Magee LA, Ornstein MP, von Dadelszen P. Fortnightly review: management of hypertension in pregnancy. *BMJ* 1999;318(7194):1332–1336

Seely EW, Maxwell C. Chronic hypertension in pregnancy. *Circulation* 2007;115:188–190

Sibai BM. Caring for women with hypertension in pregnancy. *JAMA* 2007;298(13):1566–1568

22 Postpartum Hemorrhage and Infection

Gustavo Leguizamòn and Alberto Fernández

Postpartum hemorrhage is excessive bleeding following the birth of a baby. It is one of the most life-threatening complications following birth. There are many types and causes of abnormal bleeding in a pregnant woman. This chapter discusses the many types of bleeding events that can occur in pregnancy, their frequency, their common symptoms, and the most effective approaches to management. Also briefly discussed in this chapter are measures needed to prevent the introduction of naturally occuring bacteria into the hemorrhage site and further complicating management of these serious conditions. Chapter 28 contains a more extensive discussion of the prevention and management of a wide vaiety of infections that can occur in pregnancy.

Definitions

Placental abruption (abruptio placentae): This term is used to describe the premature separation, either partial or total, of the placenta from the uterus during pregnancy or in labor. Placental abruption can be classified as:

- **Grade 1:** Mild clinical symptoms with no laboratory abnormalities and normal hemodynamic parameters.

- **Grade 2:** Partial abruption with mild to moderate vaginal bleeding. Contractions and uterine symptoms are significant. Maternal and fetal tachycardia are usually present. Resting blood pressure is normal but orthostatic hypotension is frequent. Fibrinogen levels may be decreased.
- **Grade 3:** Complete abruption accompanied by moderate to severe bleeding, or a concealed hemorrhage associated with a tetanic uterus. It is frequently associated with maternal hypotension, coagulopathy, and fetal death.

Placenta acreta: This refers to an abnormal attachment of the placenta to the uterine wall, secondary to the absence of the decidua basalis. When this abnormal attachment extends to or through the myometrium it is called placenta increta or placenta percreta, respectively.

Placenta previa: This condition occurs when the placenta locates either over, or in close proximity to, the internal os. Three types have been traditionally recognized (**Fig. 22.1**).
- *complete*: when the cervical os is completed occluded by placental tissue
- *partial*: when the cervical os is partially covered by placental tissue

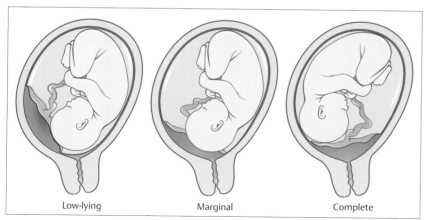

Fig. 22.1 Classification scheme for placenta previa.

Low-lying   Marginal   Complete

- *marginal*: when the margin of a low-lying placenta is 2–3 cm from the internal os

Puerperal endometritis: This term describes a polymicrobial infection caused by bacteria from the genital tract.

Uterine atony: The lack of an effective contraction after the delivery of the placenta. It is the most common etiology of postpartum hemorrhage.

Vasa previa: This term refers to the velamentous insertion of fetal vessels over the cervical os. The condition is a grave one, since vessel rupture is a frequent event with subsequent fetal exanguination.

Diagnosis

Placenta Acreta

Identifying risk factors is of the outmost importance to enable prompt diagnosis of this condition. Few situations are as dangerous for the patient and stressful for the health care team as diagnosing an unsuspected placenta acreta during a cesarean section.

The best approach to early detection of placenta acreta is to identify risk factors (see Etiology and Risk Factors below) and, if present, conduct an ultrasonographic evaluation of placental insertion. The loss of the normal hypoechoic limit between placenta and myometrium is indicative of a possible acreta.

Placenta Previa

This condition is usually asymptomatic until membranes are ruptured and vessels start bleeding. Occasionally, it is diagnosed antenatally with Doppler ultrasonography. Intensive fetal monitoring and early admission as well as delivery should be considered.

Puerperal Endometritis

Symptoms usually manifest during the first 48 hours after delivery. The most frequent findings are:
- fever, tachycardia, malaise
- fundal tenderness
- malodorous lochia
- nonspecific abdominal pain

If diagnosis is not clear, conduct a vaginal exam to confirming pain on uterine palpation and an increase in temperature of the vaginal mucosa.

Uterine Atony

Uterine atony is typically diagnosed after delivery when there is excessive bleeding and a large, relaxed uterus. The doctor may perform an examination to be certain that there are no tears of the cervix or the vagina, and that all fragments of placenta have been removed from the uterus.

Vasa Previa

The diagnosis often is not made antepartum. Patients usually present with bleeding at the time of spontaneous or artificial rupture of membranes. However, bleeding can occur before the rupture of membranes. Vasa previa can also present with fetal bradycardia when the velamentous vessels are compressed by the presenting part.

Most often, the fetus is already dead when the diagnosis is made due to massive blood loss.

Prevalence and Epidemiology

Placental Abruption

The prevalence of placental abruption depends on the population studied. It has been reported as ranging from 1 in 75 to 1 in 226 deliveries. Risk of recurrence is between 5% and 17% after one placental abruption. After two consecutive episodes, the recurrence risk is approximately 25%.

Although a significant decrease in perinatal mortality has been observed in many populations, placental abruption is still of significant concern. There is a ninefold increase in intrauterine demise and fourfold increase in preterm delivery associated with this condition.

Placenta Acreta

This condition occurs with a frequency of approximately 1 in 500 deliveries.

Placenta Previa

The overall incidence has been reported to be 0.4%. It is more frequent in the second trimester, with an incidence of 4–6%.

Puerperal Endometritis

The lowest risk corresponds to normal vaginal delivery (3%), followed by planned cesarean section (10–15%), and intrapartum cesarean section (between 20% and 35%, depending on the use of prophylactic antibiotics).

Uterine Atony

Overall, this condition occurs in 5% of deliveries.

Vasa Previa

The prevalence of vasa previa ranges from 1 in 2761 pregnancies to 1 in 5000 pregnancies.

Etiology and Risk Factors

Placental Abruption

Although the etiology of this condition is unknown there are identifiable risk factors:
- multiparity and advanced maternal age
- history of previous abruption
- cocaine use
- cigarette smoking
- abdominal trauma
- preterm premature rupture of membranes
- inherited thrombophilia
- maternal hypertension

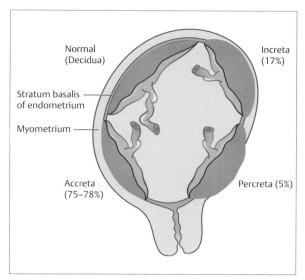

Fig. 22.2 Placenta acreta is thought to be caused by damage to, or the absence of, the decidua basalis. Placenta increta and percreta also may occur. However, acreta is the predominant location.

Placenta Acreta

The exact etiology for placenta acreta is unknown. There is some evidence that it is caused by damage to the decidua basalis, which is a fertile implantation site for the enlarging placenta and also acts as a barrier between the placental tissue and uterine muscle. If this decidual tissue is somehow damaged or absent, placenta acreta or placenta increta may result (**Fig. 22.2**).

Certain risks factors can significantly increase its incidence:
- placenta previa
- previous cesarean delivery or uterine surgery
- multiparity
- advanced maternal age

Placenta Previa

Although the etiology of placenta previa has not been elucidated, previous endometrial damage could be involved. Numerous risk factors have been identified, including:
- increasing parity and maternal age
- cigarette smoking
- residence at high altitude
- multiple gestation
- history of placenta previa
- prior curettage
- prior cesarean section

Puerperal Endometritis

Puerperal endometritis is a uterine infection, typically caused by bacteria ascending from the lower genital or gastrointestinal tract. The infections tend to be polymicrobial and may develop after chorioamnionitis during labor, or postpartum. The most common pathogens include Gram-positive cocci (predominantly group B streptococci, *Staphylococcus epidermidis*, and *Enterococcus* sp.), anaerobes (predominantly peptostreptococci, *Bacteroides* sp., and *Prevotella* sp.), and Gram-negative organisms (predominantly *Gardnerella vaginalis*, *Escherichia coli*, *Klebsiella pneumoniae*, and *Proteus mirabilis*).

Many risk factors have been identified, including:

- premature rupture of membranes
- cesarean section (especially intrapartum)
- low socioeconomic background
- multiple vaginal examinations
- genital infection

Uterine Atony

Uterine atony is the most common cause of postpartum hemorrhage and the most common indication for postpartum hysterectomy or blood transfusion. After a woman delivers, bleeding typically stops on its own by the action of strong uterine contractions and compression of the vessels. If the uterine contractions are insufficiently strong, the bleeding will continue. In most cases, this deficiency is due to the uterine muscle simply failing to contract adequately.

However, some cases are caused by pieces of the placenta remaining in the uterus after delivery, or benign growths such as fibroids preventing the uterus from contracting effectively. In these cases, the term "atony" is usually not applied.

Risk factors include:

- multiple pregnancies
- macrosomia
- polyhydramnios
- multiparity
- prolonged second stage with prolonged use of oxytocin
- placenta previa

Vasa Previa

Vasa previa is present when fetal vessels traverse the fetal membranes over the internal cervical os. These vessels may either arise from a velamentous insertion of the umbilical cord, or be joined by an accessory placental lobe to the main disk of the placenta. If they rupture, the bleeding is from the fetoplacental circulation. Fetal exsanguination will occur rapidly, leading to fetal death.

History

Chief Complaint

The typical symptom of postpartum bleeding is painless vaginal bleeding during the second or third trimester. The lack of pain and the absence of abnormal uterine tone assist in the differential diagnosis of placental abruption. The signs and symptoms are very important in the diagnosis of placental abruption, since they can arouse suspicion and instigate the procurement of supportive sonographic and laboratory tests.

The most frequent presentation, vaginal bleeding, is concealed in up to 20% of cases. Furthermore, among those women with bleeding, the profuseness of bleeding is not necessarily related to the severity of the abruption. Abdominal pain, labor, and increased uterine tone are also frequent findings that assist in the differential diagnosis of other etiologies for vaginal bleeding.

When labor is present in a bleeding placenta previa, a differential diagnosis is not possible. Diagnosis, thus, must rely exclusively on the ultrasonographic examination. The so-called sentinel bleeding is the first episode of hemorrhage, and it occurs generally at the beginning of the third trimester. One-third of the patients are symptomatic before 30 weeks of gestation and one-third after 33 weeks. Usually, the bleeding is spontaneous with no identifiable cause for its onset. Absence of bleeding does not rule out placenta previa, however, since 10% of such patients become symptomatic only after onset of labor. Finally, vaginal digital examination must be avoided, since cervical manipulation has been associated with massive bleeding in pregnant women with placenta previa.

Physical Evaluation

Every pregnant patient with vaginal bleeding must undergo ultrasonographic evaluation. If placenta previa is the cause of the bleeding, ultrasound imaging gives the definitive diagnosis. Some pitfalls in the diagnosis are related to fetal position. Occasionally, the fetal head makes visualization of placental margins difficult. In fact, false negatives have been reported to be as high as 7% of cases (see also Evidence Box 22.1).

Although initial evaluation can be performed with transabdominal scanning (a fundal placenta rules out placenta previa), definitive diagnosis frequently requires transvaginal ultrasonography. This approach is very safe in the hands of experienced operators and decreases significantly both false-positive and false-negative results.

Sonographic finding can give supportive information for the diagnosis of abruption, and the magnitude and location of the hematoma can be identified. Early hemorrhage is viewed as hyperechogenic; resolving hematomas are hypoechoic, and after a week they become sonolucent. Ultrasonographic evaluation can identify different types of abruption according to hematoma location:

- *retroplacental abruption* is located between the placenta and the myometrium
- *subchorionic abruption* is located between the placenta and the fetal membranes
- *preplacental abruption* is located anterior to the placenta, within the chorioamniotic layer

Management

The most widely used measures to manage patients with postpartum bleeding and associated complications include:

- serial ultrasonographic scanning to determine appropriate fetal growth
- pelvic rest (avoiding cervical examination and intercourse)
- restriction of physical activity
- iron supplementation to decrease incidence and severity of maternal anemia

Outpatient versus in-patient management

Asymptomatic patients can be managed as outpatients. Patients with a history of a small bleed that ceased spontaneously, and who have been stable, can be managed as outpatients, if the following conditions are met:

- they reside in close proximity to the hospital
- they have transportation availability 24 hours per day
- they are compliant patients who understand the potential complications of bleeding

Patients with active bleeding, or who have had clinically significant bleeding, as well as those not able to fulfill the outpatient profile, must be managed in the hospital.

Once vaginal bleeding is established, the following measures should be instituted:

- admit to labor and delivery
- begin continuous fetal monitoring
- insert IV line with a large bore
- begin basic laboratory work-up: complete blood cell count (CBC), platelets, coagulation studies, fibrinogen, and fibrinogen degradation products, which rise in level after a bleeding event
- if the mother is of less than 34 weeks gestation, administer steroids to promote fetal lung maturity
- if the mother is Rhesus negative, administer the antibody RhoGAM (see Chapter 17) and a Kleihauer–Betke analysis to determine the appropriate dose.

Delivery

Delivery should be performed by cesarean section in every case of complete previa. If the placental previa is marginal, vaginal delivery can be considered. However, since there is high incidence of intrapartum complications secondary to bleeding, precautions must be taken.

The timing of delivery varies with the wide spectrum of clinical presentation; however, since the vast majority of the bleeding events are self-limited, attempts should be made to deliver a mature infant. Consider on amniocentecis at 37 weeks of gestation to ascertain fetal lung maturity.

Placental Abruption

- Admit to labor and delivery.
- Obtain basic lab tests: CBC, platelet count, fibrinogen, fibrin degradation products, and coagulation studies.
- Insert IV line with large bore.
- Continue fetal electronic monitoring.
- Do blood typing and cross.
- Evaluate the patient close to the operating room.
- Communicate with the neonatal team.
- Abruption in term or near-term pregnancies is an indication for delivery irrespective of the severity.
- In mild preterm abruption with reassuring maternal and fetal wellbeing, expectant management can be attempted. Steroid administration must be considered.

Placenta Acreta

Once a diagnosis of placenta acreta is suspected the patient must be counseled and informed that it is needed to avoid massive bleeding. Informed consent must be obtained for this intervention, followed by:

- transfer to an adequate facility
- type and cross with at least 4 units of blood
- insert two IV lines with a large bore

Access to the uterus should avoid placental incision. Sometimes, if the placenta is anterior and low lying, a fundal incision is necessary. After the delivery of the baby and cord clamping, a hysterectomy may be indicated.

Puerperal Endometritis

The cornerstone of treatment is antimicrobial therapy. Most frequently used regimes for broad-spectrum antibiotics include: 1) clindamycin/gentamicin, 2) clindamycin/aztreonan, 3) metronidazole/penicillin, 4) ampicillin/gentamicin. Treatment is associated with clinical improvement after the initial 48–72 hours. Once the patient is asymptomatic for 24 hours, therapy must be stopped and the patient discharged.

If fever persists other etiologies must be considered such as: wound infection, pelvic abscess, pelvic septic thrombophlebitis, or mastitis.

Uterine Atony

Two prophylactic measures are known to reduce the risk of postpartum bleeding secondary to uterine atony:
1. Oxytocin administration during the third stage of labor
2. Spontaneous removal of the placenta at cesarean section

If such preventive measures are unsuccessful, therapeutic intervention should start promptly, including:

- *bimanual uterine massage*
- *pharmacologic therapy*: oxytocin, methylergonovine, prostaglandins $F_{2\alpha}$ and E_2, and misoprostol (**Table 22.1**)
- *uterine packing*
  A long gauze is introduced into the uterine cavity to fill the uterus. A urinary Foley catheter is also applied to avoid urinary retention. If the bleeding stops, the tamponade should be retrieved within 24 hours.
- *selective arterial embolization*
  If the patient is hemodynamically stable, and previous measures were unsuccessful, she is a candidate for embolization. The bleeding vessels are identified by pelvic angiography and occluded with an embolization of Gelfoam.
- *surgical interventions*
  Surgical measures have to be considered if the less invasive techniques were unsuccessful. Surgical repair or tamponade is the treatment of choice (**Fig. 22.3**). Laparotomy is required to reach the uterus. The B-Lynch technique involves the placement of a compression suture over the uterus. Another surgical approach consists of ligating different pelvic vessels such as uterine, utero-ovarian, the infundibulopelvic ligament, and the hypogastric arteries.

Vasa Previa

This condition calls for *immediate* treatment with an emergency cesarean delivery.

Table 22.1 Pharmacologic therapy of uterine atony

Agent	Dose	Route	Dosing frequency	Side effects	Contra-indications
Oxytocin (Pitocin)	10–80 units in 1000 mL of crystalloid solution	First line: IV Second line: IM or IU	Continuous	Nausea, emesis, water intoxication	None
Methylergonovine (Methergine)	0.2 mg	First line: IM Second line: IU or PO	Every 2–4 h	Hypertension, hypotension, nausea, emesis	Hypertension, preeclampsia
15-Methyl prostaglandin $F_{2\alpha v}$ (Hemabate)	0.25 mg	First line: IM Second line: IU	Every 15–90 min (8-dose max)	Nausea, emesis, diarrhea, flushing, chills	Active cardiac, pulmonary, renal or hepatic disease
Prostaglandin E_2 (Dinoprostone)	20 mg	PR	Every 2 h	Nausea, emesis, diarrhea, fever, chills, headache	Hypotension
Misoprostol (Cytotec)	600–1000 mcg	First line: PR Second line: PO	Single dose	Tachycardia, fever	None

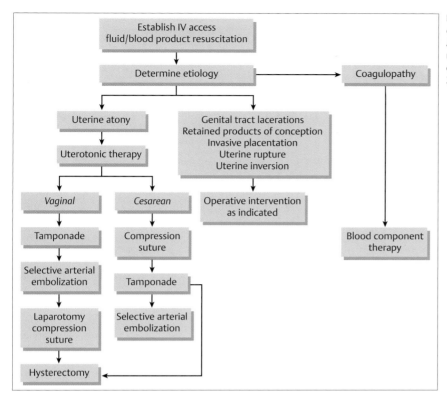

Fig. 22.3 Schematic for the surgical management of uterine atony. Adapted from Gabbe SG et al. Obstetrics. Normal and Problem Pregnancies. New York: Churchill Livingstone; 2007.

Key Points

- Placenta previa occurs when the placenta locates either over, or in close proximity to, the internal os. If severe, it can be associated with maternal and fetal morbidity.
- Risk factors for developing placenta previa are: increasing parity and maternal age, cigarette smoking, residence at high altitude, multiple gestation, history of placenta previa, prior curettage, and prior cesarean section.
- Placenta previa can be managed expectantly remote from term. When bleeding occurs near term, cesarean section is indicated.
- The severity of placental abruption (abruptio placentae) is assessed by ultrasonographic evaluation, laboratory work-up, and hemodynamic adaptation.
- Uterine atony is the most common cause of puerperal bleeding.
- Prophylactic antibiotics are effective in decreasing puerperal endometritis.

Evidence Box 22.1

Color flow Doppler imaging is more sensitive than magnetic resonance imaging in diagnosing placenta previa.

Moodley et al. assessed the sensitivity and specificity of Gray scale ultrasonography, magnetic resonance imaging (MRI), and color flow Doppler imaging in the diagnosis of placenta previa by prospectively examining 30 cases of placenta previa. Delivery by elective caesarean section was carried out at the 38th week, before the onset of labor, unless obstetric complications supervened. Three patients had a morbid adherence of the placenta at delivery, two of whom required cesarean hysterectomy and the other an internal iliac artery ligation. One patient was delivered at 33 weeks' gestation due to uncontrollable bleeding, and the remainder were delivered at 38 weeks. All mothers and infants were well at the time of discharge. Color flow Doppler was more specific in diagnosing morbidly adherent placenta previa than MRI. Doppler had a negative predictive value of 95%.

Moodley J, Ngambu NF, Corr P. Imaging techniques to identify morbidly adherent placenta praevia: a prospective study. J Obstet Gynecol 2004 Oct;24(7):742–744.

Further Reading

Ananth CV, Oyelese Y, Prasad V, Getahun D, Smulian JC. Evidence of placental abruption as a chronic process: associations with vaginal bleeding early in pregnancy and placental lesions. *Eur J Obstet Gynecol Reprod Biol* 2006;128 (1-2):15–21

Reece EA, Hobbins JC, eds. Clinical Obstetrics: the Fetus and Mother. 3rd ed. Malden, Mass: Blackwell Synergy Publishing, 2007

Kaminsky LM, Ananth CV, Prasad V. The influence of maternal cigarette smoking on placental pathology in pregnancies complicated by abruption. Am J Obstet Gynecol 2007;197(3):275.e1–275.e5

Kramer MS, Usher RH, Pollack R, Boyd M, Usher S. Etiologic determinants of abruptio placentae. *Obstet Gynecol* 1997;89(2):221–226

Moodley J, Ngambu NF, Corr P. Imaging techniques to identify morbidly adherent placenta praevia: a prospective study. *J Obstet Gynaecol* 2004;24(7):742–744

Naeye RL. Abruptio placentae and placenta previa: frequency, perinatal mortality, and cigarette smoking. *Obstet Gynecol* 1980;55(6):701–704

Gabbe SG, Niebyl JR, Simpson JL. Obstetrics—Normal and Problem Pregnancies. New York: Elsevier/Churchill Livingstone; 2007

23 Infectious Diseases in Pregnancy

Felicitas von Petery and Gustavo Leguizamón

When a woman is pregnant, an infection can be more than just a problem for her. Some infections can imperil her baby as well. For example, when a pregnant woman becomes infected with cytomegalovirus, which is normally a benign infection in adults and even children, she can pass the virus on to her fetus. In a small, yet significant, number of cases, cytomegalovirus-infected newborns develop serious illnesses or lasting disabilities, and even die.

Due to the ever-present risk of infectious pathogens, pregnant women often need to take medicines or get vaccinated to prevent their babies from also becoming infected. However, only a selected number of medicines and vaccines are safe to take during pregnancy. Thus, OB/GYN physicians need to understand not only the potential consequences for the mother of various types of infections during pregnancy, but also the potential negative consequences for the baby of available medicines and treatment approaches.

This chapter covers the major types of infections that occur during pregnancy and are likely to cause complications for the fetus—excluding human papilloma virus, which is covered in Chapter 6, and puerperal endometritus (Chapter 22). Also covered are the most recent, evidence-based approaches for diagnosing and managing major infectious diseases in pregnancy.

Definitions

Avidity index: This indicates the degree of antibody avidity toward a specific antigen, helping to differentiate between a recent versus an old infection.

Hematogenous: This means spread by the blood.

Latency: This word describes the dormant asymptomatic state observed after the clearance of an acute infection.

Lymphadenopathy: This is a disease state that is characterized by abnormally enlarged lymph nodes.

Malaise: This condition presents a general feeling of fatigue or vague discomfort.

Myalgia: This is a term for pain in one or more muscles.

Paresthesia: This is a term given to an abnormal neurological sensation, usually perceived as numbness, tingling, burning, or prickling.

Thrombocytopenia: This term is used to describe an abnormal decrease in the number of platelets in the blood.

Vertical transmission: Transmission of an infection from mother to child during the prenatal period, during delivery, or via breast feeding.

Viral titer: This expression is used for the measurement of the amount of virus present in blood.

Viremia: This describes the presence of a virus in the blood.

Viral Infections

Viruses are very tiny capsules with genetic material inside. Some cause familiar infectious diseases such as the common cold, influenza, and warts. They also cause more severe illnesses such as AIDS, hepatitis, and cancer. Viruses invade living, normal cells and use those cells to multiply and produce other virus particles like themselves. This process eventually kills the cells, which can make the infected person sick. If that person is pregnant, her baby can become sick as well.

Viral infections are hard to treat because viruses live inside the body's cells, and they are often "protected" from treatments by their host cells. Antibiotics do not gnerally work against viral infections. Although a few antiviral medicines are available. However, vaccines are the best way to prevent a woman from getting many viral diseases. In addition to human papilloma virus (see Chapter 6), other major viral infections for which pregnant women need to be monitored include cytomegalovirus, herpes simplex virus, and human immunodeficiency virus (HIV).

Cytomegalovirus

Cytomegalovirus (CMV) is a double-stranded DNA virus and a member of the herpes virus family. It is endemic throughout the world, affecting individuals in all social and demographic areas. It represents the most common cause of congenital viral infection.

Clinical Manifestations

Among healthy individuals, viral transmission typically requires repeated and prolonged contact. Infection is mainly asymptomatic, with incubation periods varying from 20 days to 2 months. The infection may result in complications throughout the body (**Fig. 23.1**). Symptoms usually involve fever, malaise, headache, and my-

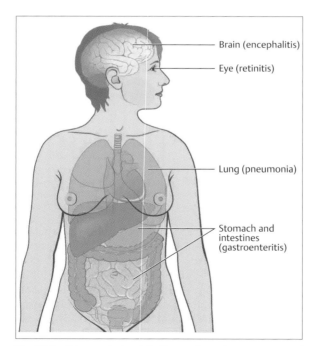

Fig. 23.1 Cytomegalovirus infection can impact many organs and systems in the body, including the brain, eyes, lungs, stomach, intestines, and liver.

algia. Lymphadenopathy may be present. Laboratory findings may include elevated liver enzymes, atypical lymphocytes, and thrombocytopenia. Individuals with chronic CMV infection may develop pneumonia, gastroenteritis, retinitis, or encephalitis.

During the initial infection, viremia occurs. Peak titers of immunoglobulin M (IgM) antibodies can usually be detected 1–3 months after the onset of infection. Viral titers decline to undetectable levels by 12 months, but they can persist up to 18 months.

After the resolution of the primary infection, the virus establishes latency within host tissues and can be isolated in blood and secretions. Most infections resolve spontaneously within 2–6 weeks. Secondary complications of primary CMV infection include hepatitis and pneumonia.

Diagnosis of Maternal and Fetal Infection

Approximately 50% of pregnant patients are seropositive for CMV antibodies. The incidence of primary infection during pregnancy ranges from 1% to 4%, with 5% to 68% of patients presenting clinical symptoms.

Initially, diagnosis of maternal infection is established by determining the IgG, IgM, and IgG avidity indexes in the blood (**Fig. 23.2**). When these results indicate high probability of a recent infection, the mother should be counseled and offered more invasive diagnostic testing for fetal infection.

A first-time (primary) CMV infection during pregnancy results in a 30–40% risk of vertical transmission to the fetus. In contrast, the risk of transmission with recurrent maternal infection is between 0.2% and 1.8%.

The most likely pathway for congenital CMV is via blood transmission to the fetus. Placental infection occurs first, followed by replication of the virus and transfer to the fetus. Once the fetal infection occurs, the virus replicates in the renal tubular endothelium and is excreted into the amniotic fluid. The cycle then can repeat itself. Finally, neonates can acquire the infection through breastfeeding.

Only 10–15% of infected neonates are symptomatic at birth. Among infected infants, asymptomatic at birth, 5–15% will develop sequelae later in life (**Table 23.1**; Evidence Box 23.1).

The symptoms of congenital, fetal CMV infection appear to be related to the timing of maternal infection. Infection during the first half of pregnancy, for example, is associated with symptomatic disease, whereas infection in the latter half is more commonly associated with initially asymptomatic disease.

Prevention

Because there are no effective therapies for congenital CMV infection, prevention in the mother is ideal. Several vaccines have been developed that prevent maternal CMV

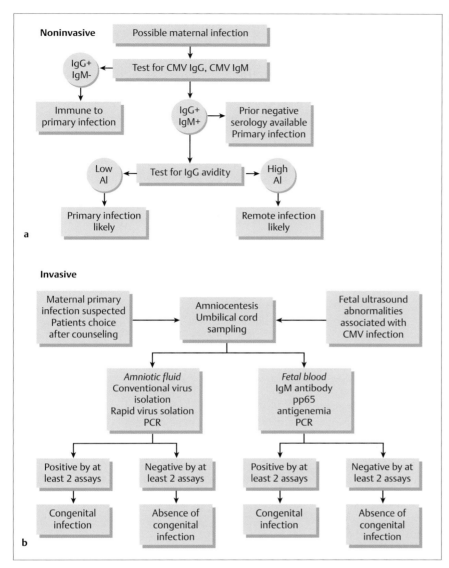

Fig. 23.2a, b Diagnostic options flowchart, if maternal cytomegalovirus (CMV) infection is suspected.

Table 23.1 Abnormalities associated with congenital cytomegalovirus infection

Antenatal ultrasonographic findings	Early postnatal findings	Late findings
Microcephaly	Microcephaly	Developmental delay
Periventricular calcifications	Periventricular calcifications	Mental retardation
Intracranial hemorrhage	Ventriculomegaly	Seizures
Ventriculomegaly	Chorioretinitis	Visual impairment
Echogenic bowel	Hyperbilirubinemia	Sensorineural hearing loss
Hepatosplenomegaly	Hepatosplenomegaly	
Fetal Growth Restriction	Hepatitis	
	Growth delay	

infection. However, many physicians are reluctant to use these vaccines to immunize women of childbearing age, because their safety has not been properly established. Also, reports of new infections in previously immune patients have raised questions about the efficacy of CMV vaccination in general.

Thus, women of childbearing age need to be educated about CMV and how it is transmitted, so they are not at risk. They should also be taught how to be careful in handling potentially infected articles, such as diapers, and about the need to thoroughly wash their hands if they are exposed to young children or immunocompromised individuals. Although universal screening is not currently recommended, high-risk women need to be counseled about serologic screening before pregnancy.

Herpes Simplex Virus

Herpes simplex virus (HSV) is a double-stranded DNA virus (**Fig 23.3**) transmitted by direct and intimate contact. Following primary infection, the virus remains latent in neuronal ganglia to reactivate at later times. There are two identified strains of HSV: type 1, which causes oropharyngeal lesions; and type 2, which is responsible for genital tract infections. Twenty-two percent of pregnant women are seropositive for HSV-2 and more than 2% of women acquire the infection during pregnancy.

Clinical Manifestations

Only 30% of pregnant women are symptomatic to primary infection, with manifestations ranging from mild

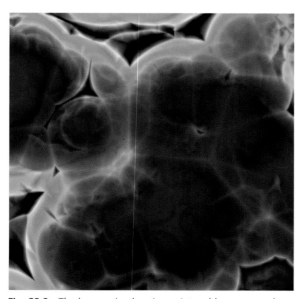

Fig. 23.3 The herpes simplex virus, pictured here, causes long-term persistent infection in most affected individuals.

discomfort to widespread genital lesions associated with pain, dysuria, tender regional lymph node enlargement, fever, and malaise.

HSV infections are classified as primary, nonprimary first episode, and recurrent (**Table 23.2**). Lesions are usually preceded by paresthesias, followed by the eruption of vesicles, which rupture forming a shallow-based ulcer that develops into a crust. Eventually all lesions heal without scarring.

Diagnosis

Isolation of HSV in cell culture is performed in patients who present with genital lesions. The sensitivity of viral culture is low, and decreases with reactivations and as lesions begin to heal.

Commercially-available polymerase chain reaction (PCR) assays for HSV are more sensitive and can be used instead of cell cultures. The lack of HSV detection both by PCR and in culture does not exclude HSV infection, because viral shedding is intermittent.

In women who lack lesions, use type-specific serology for HSV, or diagnostic culture and/or PCR assay. If infection is suspected and all tests are negative, repeat serology in 6 weeks.

Perinatal Transmission

Transmission to the fetus can occur during the antepartum or intrapartum period by different mechanisms. Antepartum infections are associated with a potential risk for hematogenous spread to the fetus. On the other hand, when intrapartum transmission occurs, it is usually secondary to direct exposure to maternal viral shedding in vaginal secretions. Finally, neonatal transmission may occur secondary to close contact with infected individuals.

Perinatal transmission rates vary according to the type of infection:

- primary: 50%
- nonprimary first episode: 33%
- recurrent: 0–4%

Table 23.2 Criteria for classifying herpes simplex virus infections

Primary	First clinical infection
	No pre-existing antibody
Nonprimary/ first episode	No history of genital infection
	Positive antibody to the other type of virus (HSV-1/HSV-2)
Recurrent	Prior history of clinical infection
	Positive antibody to same type of virus

Table 23.3 Recommended doses of antiviral medication for herpes simples virus (HSV) in pregnancy

Indication	Acyclovir	Valacyclovir
Primary of first episode HSV	400 mg p.o., t.i.d. for 7–14 days	1 g b.i.d. for 7–14 days
Symptomatic recurrent HSV	400 mg p.o., t.i.d. for 5 days	500 mg bid for 5 days
Daily suppressive therapy	400 mg p.o., b.i.d.	500 mg p.o. daily

Treatment and Preventive Strategies

All pregnant women must be asked during prenatal care about any history of genital herpes and counseled to avoid intercourse with infected individuals. If they do become infected, either one of the antiviral drugs acyclovir or valacyclovir may be administered, depending on the scenario (**Table 23.3**).

At the onset of labor, women should be questioned about symptoms of genital herpes and carefully evaluated for presence of vaginal or cervical lesions. Women without evidence of genital herpes can deliver vaginally, while those with either primary or recurrent lesions should undergo cesarean section to decrease the risk of perinatal transmission (**Fig. 23.4**).

Pregnancy in the HIV Era

Women account for a disportionately increasing number of new cases of HIV infection throughout the world. The prevalence of infected women of childbearing age has also increased as a result of the decreasing mortality associated with the advent of combined antiretroviral therapy and higher rates of heterosexual transmission.

In 2005, UNAIDS (the Joint United Nations Program on HIV/AIDS) estimated that 38.6 million people had HIV, of whom 17.3 million were women (with most being in their reproductive years). At least 3.28 million pregnant women infected with HIV are estimated to give birth each year, with more than 75% of these in sub-Saharan Africa. Most of the annual 700 000 new infections of HIV in children in sub-Saharan Africa occur via vertical transmission.

The management of HIV infection during pregnancy involves two major goals: the prevention of disease progression in the mother, and vertical transmission to the new born.

Human Immunodeficiency Virus

The HIV virus particle is 100–120 nm in diameter, with a spherical morphology. Its cone-shaped core is surrounded by a lipid matrix containing key surface antigens and glycoproteins. The viral core contains two copies of genomic RNA, reverse transcriptase, integrase, and proteases (**Fig. 23.5**). Gp120, a glycoprotein present in the viral surface, binds to cells bearing CD4 receptors, causing a change in their shape. This allows the virus to bind to other receptors on the cell and to fuse its membrane with the cell's membrane. Once this occurs, HIV empties it contents into the cytoplasm of the cell.

Shortly after HIV's entry into the host cell, it takes over the cellular machinery in order to make copies of itself. Later on, the virus will integrate into the host cell's DNA and remain there indefinitely. It is this ability of HIV to integrate into the host cell's genomic DNA that makes it so difficult to treat. There is no cure for HIV. However, there are many medicines, such as reverse transcriptase inhibitors and protease inhibitors, presently available which can interrupt the life cycle of the virus and, thus, prolong the lives of people who are infected with HIV. When several such drugs, typically three or four, are taken in combination, the approach is known as highly active antiretroviral therapy (HAART). Today, HAART therapy is greatly extending the lives of tens of millions of people worldwide, who otherwise would have died from this disease just a few years ago.

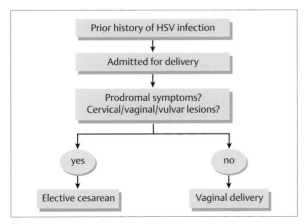

Fig. 23.4 Intrapartum approach for women with herpes simplex virus.

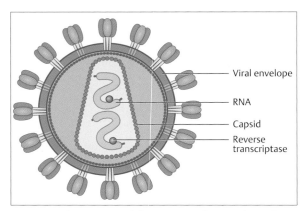

Fig. 23.5 The structure of the HIV virus, showing the viral core containing two backward S-shaped strands of RNA, as well as reverse transcriptase and other enzymes which are key to the virus' ability to invade and take over host cells.

Antenatal Testing

There is ample evidence that appropriate treatment of HIV infection during pregnancy modifies disease progression and greatly reduces vertical transmission. Therefore, universal screening should be offered to all pregnant women, while giving them the chance to opt-out. In areas of high prevalence, negative HIV testing can be repeated later in pregnancy.

The initial serologic screening consists of detecting specific antibodies. It is typically performed by an enzyme-linked immunosorbant assay (ELISA). In the event of a positive ELISA result, a repeat test is performed. If positive, a "Western blot" analysis is conducted to confirm the diagnosis.

For women going into labor with unknown HIV status, rapid testing is now available and, if positive, treatment can be initiated without waiting for confirmatory results.

Transmission

HIV infection is transmitted by sexual contact with an infected person or by sharing needles and/or syringes—usually for drug injection—with someone who is infected or a less common route (and rarely in countries where blood is systematically screened for HIV antibodies) is through transfusion of infected blood or clotting factors.

Babies born of HIV-infected mothers may become infected before or during birth or through breast-feeding after birth. This is known as vertical transmission. Certain factors increase the risk of vertical transmission:
- previous child with HIV
- mother with AIDS
- preterm delivery
- low maternal CD4 count
- high maternal viral load
- first-born twin

- chorioamnionitis
- excessive intrapartum bleeding (e.g., episiotomy)

Current data consistently demonstrate that HAART therapy combined with low or undetectable viral load (<1000 copies of the virus per mL of blood) limit perinatal transmission of HIV to approximately 1%. Another effective intervention to reduce perinatal transmission is to perform an elective cesarean section in certain clinical scenarios. Women with viral loads greater than 1000 copies/mL who deliver by cesarean section at 38 weeks before rupture of membranes or going into labor have lower perinatal transmission. Vaginal delivery is a reasonable alternative for women with undetectable viral load, however,

In candidates for vaginal delivery, the risk of perinatal transmission can be decreased if the physician avoids:
- artificially rupturing the membranes
- sampling the fetal scalp
- using fetal electrodes
- performing an episiotomy
- instrument delivery

Finally, infected women should receive intravenous zidovudine with a loading dose of 2 mg/kg in 1 hour followed by a maintenance dose of 1 mg/kg per hour.

Postpartum Measures

During the postpartum period, breast-feeding should be avoided since it significantly increases vertcal transmission risks. Newborns of HIV-infected mothers should receive oral azidothymidine (syrup 2 mg/kg every 6 hours, for the first 6 weeks of life).

Antenatal Measures

Currently, the standard of care is to treat pregnant HIV-infected women with HAART. This strategy includes three agents from at least two different classes of antiretrovirals. **Table 23.4** depicts relevant features of some of the most frequently used drugs in the United States.

Besides specific antiretroviral therapy, delivery, and neonatal strategies, management during the antenatal period is also of utmost importance to achieve successful maternal and fetal outcomes. The chart shown in **Fig. 23.6** depicts a general strategy for antepartum care in HIV-infected women.

Table 23.4 Most commonly used antiretroviral therapies for treating pregnant women, their regulatory designations, and important clinical features

Drug	Class	FDA category	Features
Zidovudine	RTI	C	300 mg b.i.d.
			Well tolerated
			No evidence of teratogenicity
Lamivudine	NRTI	C	150 mg b.i.d.
			Well tolerated
			No evidence of teratogenicity
Nelfinavir	Protease inhibitor	B	1250 mg b.i.d.
			Well tolerated
			No evidence of teratogenicity

FDA, US Food and Drug Administration; NRTI, non-nucleoside reverse transcriptase inhibitor; RTI, reverse transcriptase inhibitor.

Bacterial Infections

Group B Streptococcal Infection

Group B streptococci (GBS) are facultative, Gram-positive diplococci that colonize the lower gastrointestinal tract and vagina and can be isolated from swabs of vagina and rectum. An estimated 20–30% of pregnant women are GBS carriers. Prenatal screening between 35 and 37 weeks of gestation is currently recommended.

Neonatal Infection

In newborns, GBS can cause sepsis, pneumonia, meningitis, and localized infections, such as osteomyelitis, septic arthritis, or cellulitis. Early onset disease occurs within the first week of life. GBS is the leading cause of neonatal sepsis, which is an extremely preventable cause of death if the maternal risk factors (**Table 23.5**) are recognized and ameliorated before infection can occur.

Maternal Infection

In women, GBS can cause urinary tract infection, endometritis, chorioamnionitis, bacteriemia, and stillbirth. When amniotic fluid is cultured from cases of clinically evident amnionitis, GBS is isolated in 15% of cases. GBS also can be isolated in 2–15% of infected abdominal wounds after cesarean delivery. It is responsible for 15% of maternal bacteremia cases.

Diagnosis

Definitive microbiologic identification is done by the detection of the group B antigen. Presumptive identification of GBS is based on colonial morphology, its hemolysis pattern, and its Gram stain within 24 hours of plating on blood agar. A final report is usually available after 48 hours.

Therapy

Penicillin remains the agent of choice for GBS prophylaxis, followed by ampicillin as an alternative regimen. Re-

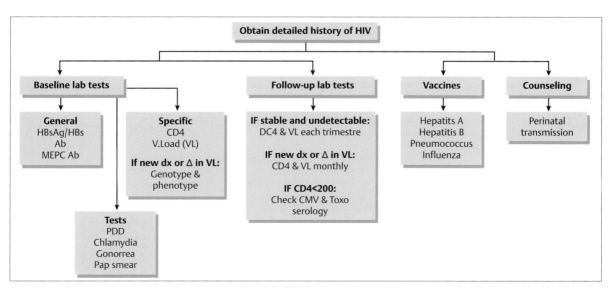

Fig. 23.6 Antepartum management strategy for women with HIV.

Table 23.5 Risk factors for early onset neonatal group B streptococcal (GBS) disease

Maternal GBS colonization
Preterm delivery
GBS bacteriuria during pregnancy
Prolonged rupture of membranes
Birth of a previous infant with invasive GBS disease
Maternal chorioamnionitis (intrapartum fever)
Young maternal age
African-American race
Hispanic ethnicity
Low levels of antibody to type-specific capsular polysaccharide antigens

Table 23.6 Recommended regimens for intrapartum antimicrobial prophylaxis for perinatal group B streptococcal (GBS) disease prevention

Recommended	Penicillin G 5 million units IV initial dose, then 2.5 million units IV every 4 hours until delivery
Alternative	Ampicillin 2 g IV initial dose, then 1 g IV every 4 hours until delivery
If penicillin allergic:	
Patients not at high risk for anaphylaxis	Cefazolin 2 g IV initial dose, then 1 g IV every 8 hours until delivery
GBS susceptible to clindamycin and erythromycin	Clindamycin 900 mg IV every 8 hours until delivery *Or* Erythromycin 500 mg IV every 6 hours until delivery
GBS resistant to clindamycin or erythromycin or susceptibility unknown	Vancomycin 1 g IV every 12 hours until delivery.

sistance to erythromycin has been increasing among isolates of GBS. For example, in 2003, 37 % of invasive GBS isolates were resistant to erythromycin and 17 % to clindamycin. **Table 23.6** gives the recommended, alternative treatment approaches to GBS infection based on its sensitivity to first-line therapy.

Prevention of Perinatal Infection

In 2002, the US Centers for Disease Control and Prevention (CDC) revised the strategy to prevent perinatal infection with GBS. The finding that universal screening culture and treatment of all colonized women prevented 78 % of the neonatal cases of GBS infection versus only 41 % with selective screening was a strong foundation from which to recommend universal screening for GBS. **Figure 23.7** depicts current recommendations for screening and prophylactic antibiotic administration to prevent neonatal GBS infection.

Syphilis

Syphilis is caused by the spirochete *Treponema pallidum* and transmitted, typically, by intimate contact with an infected partner. Minute abrasions in the vaginal mucosa provide a portal of entry for the spirochete, and the cervical changes associated with pregnancy increase the risk of spirochete entry. Local replication occurs and lymphatic dissemination leads to the systemic nature of syphilis.

The syphilitic infection is staged according to the disease duration and its clinical features. The early stages—primary, secondary, and early latent syphilis—are associated with the highest spirochete loads and transmission rates (30–50 %). Transmission rates in the "late syphilis," namely, late latent and tertiary stages, are much lower.

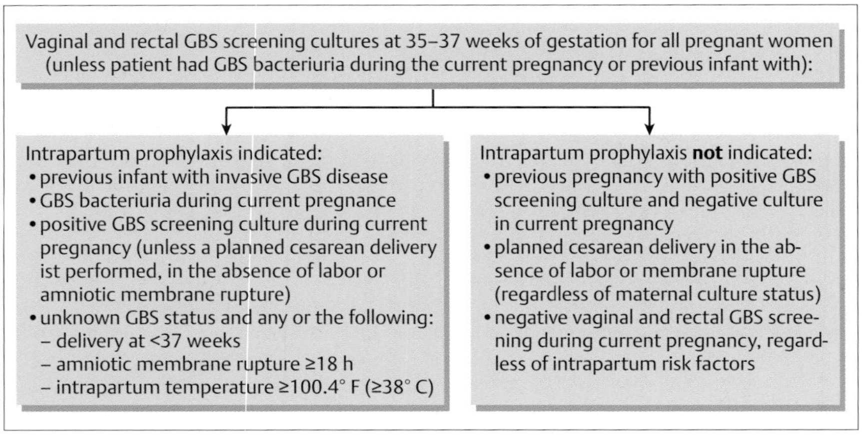

Vaginal and rectal GBS screening cultures at 35–37 weeks of gestation for all pregnant women (unless patient had GBS bacteriuria during the current pregnancy or previous infant with):

Intrapartum prophylaxis indicated:	Intrapartum prophylaxis **not** indicated:
• previous infant with invasive GBS disease	• previous pregnancy with positive GBS screening culture and negative culture in current pregnancy
• GBS bacteriuria during current pregnance	• planned cesarean delivery in the absence of labor or membrane rupture (regardless of maternal culture status)
• positive GBS screening culture during current pregnancy (unless a planned cesarean delivery ist performed, in the absence of labor or amniotic membrane rupture)	• negative vaginal and rectal GBS screening during current pregnancy, regardless of intrapartum risk factors
• unknown GBS status and any or the following: – delivery at <37 weeks – amniotic membrane rupture ≥18 h – intrapartum temperature ≥100.4° F (≥38° C)	

Fig. 23.7 Current recommendations for screening and prophylactic antibiotic administration to prevent neonatal group B streptococcal disease.

A fetus may become infected with syphilis via several routes, including transplacental passage, infection of fetal membranes, or through direct contact with lesions at delivery. The risk of fetal infection increases as pregnancy advances, but infection may occur at any gestational age.

Clinical Features

Pregnancy has little effect on the clinical course of syphilis; however, syphilis does have a major impact on pregnancy. Syphilis increases the risk of preterm delivery, spontaneous abortion, stillbirth, neonatal demise, and congenital infection in pregnancies. The fetal risk appears to be directly correlated with the degree of maternal infection and the duration of the disease.

Primary syphilis: Primary syphilis represents the initial infectious stage. Its hallmark lesion, the *syphilitic chancre*, develops at the site of inoculation. It is often a solitary, painless, smooth-based, red lesion with raised borders (**Fig. 23.8**). In 80% of women, the chancre is associated to a painless, nonsupurative lymphadenopathy. If untreated, the chancre will disappear in 3–8 weeks. Despite this, the woman will progress to the systemic or secondary stage of syphilis.

Secondary syphilis: The clinical manifestations of this stage of syphilis are the reason why it was named *"The Great Simulator;"* developing, on average, 6 weeks after the appearance of the chancre. The most common findings are dermatologic and genital lesions (**Table 23.7**), but almost any organ can be involved.

Table 23.7 Secondary syphilis: clinical features

Dermatologic (90%)	Constitutional symptoms (70%)	Gastrointestinal
Macular/ maculo-papular rash	Low-grade fever	Hepatitis
Palmar/plantar target lesions	Pharyngitis	Pancreatitis
Pruritus	Malaise	Uveitis
Mucous patches	Arthralgias/my-algias	
Patchy alopecia	Anorexia	
	Headache	
	Generalized lymphadenopathy	
Genital tract (20%)	Central nervous system	Renal
Condyloma lata	Aseptic meningitis	Glomerulone-phritis
Mucous patches	Vertigo	Nephrotic syn-drome
	Cranial nerve in-volvement	
	Diplopia	
		Bone/joint
		Osteitis
		Periostitis
		Synovitis

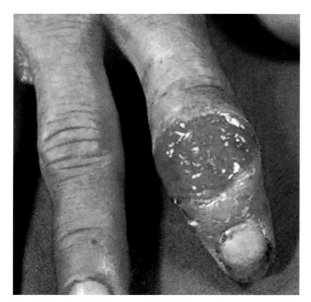

Fig. 23.8 Syphilis is a complicated disease. It can cause widespread lesions like the one pictured here throughout the body, or it can cause no symptoms at all.

Dermatologic lesions and genital *condyloma lata* in secondary syphilis are highly infectious. An epitrochlear lymphadenopathy should alert the physician of the possibility of syphilis.

Late syphilis: The lesions of secondary syphilis will resolve without treatment in 3–12 weeks. After this, the woman enters an asymptomatic phase which may last for many years. Arbitrarily latent syphilis is divided into *early* and *late* according to its duration (more or less than 12 months, respectively). During this time, relapses may occur frequently, resembling secondary syphilis. Relapses are uncommon in the late stages of latent syphilis.

Late/tertiary syphilis: Twenty to thirty percent of untreated women will develop tertiary syphilis, years after the initial infection. Its hallmark feature is the *gumma*, a locally destructive granulomatous lesion that may involve any organ, varying in size and distribution. Medial necrosis of the aorta will lead to the development of a saccular aneurysm in 10% of infected women. Neurosyphilis will occur in 7% of untreated women, mostly asymptomatic. Symptoms of CNS involvement include paresis, tabes dorsalis, hemiplegia, seizures and/or aphasia.

Congenital syphilis: Congenital syphilis is a severe, disabling, and often life-threatening infection seen in infants. A pregnant mother who has syphilis can spread the disease through the placenta to the unborn infant. The disease is divided into early and late stages, each with its own set of distinct symptoms (**Table 23.8**).

Despite the fact that this disease is curable with antibiotics if caught early, rising rates of syphilis among pregnant women throughout the world have recently increased the number of infants born with congenital syphilis. All pregnant women, therefore, should be screened for syphilis in their first prenatal visit. High-risk patients should be retested at 28 weeks of gestation and at delivery.

Diagnosis

Syphilis can be diagnosed using dark-field microscopy of skin lesions. However, because the strain of *Treponema pallidum* that causes syphilis cannot be readily cultivated in vitro, the accurate diagnosis of syphilis most often requires screening with a nontreponemal test and confirmed with a treponemal-specific test (**Table 23.8**).

Nontreponemal tests detect nonspecific treponemal antibodies. These include the Venereal Diseases Research Laboratory (VDRL) and rapid plasma reagin (RPR) tests. *Treponemal* tests detect specific treponemal antibodies. These include the *Treponema pallidum* hemagglutination assay (TPHA), the fluorescent treponemal antibody-absorbed test (FTA-abs), and most enzyme immunoassay (EIA) tests.

An important aspect of syphilis serology is the detection of treponemal antibody by a screening test, followed by confirmation of a reactive screening test result by further testing. The confirmatory test, or tests, should ideally have equivalent sensitivity and greater specificity than the screening test and be independent methodologically, so as to reduce the chance of coincident false-positive reactions. Indeed, false-positive nontreponemal tests occur in up to 1% of patients. They are associated with viral and

Table 23.8 The differential symptoms of syphilis, early vs. late stages

Early congenital syphilis (>2 years)	Late congenital syphilis (>2 years)
Hepatosplenomegaly	Hutchinson's teeth
Rash	Instertitial keratitis
Anemia	Viii nerve deafness
Thrombocytopenia	Mental retardation
Osteochondritis	Seizures
Periostitis	Cranial nerve palsies
Rhinitis	Saddle nose deformity
	Frontal bossing
	Saber shins

bacterial infection, intravenous drug use, malignancy, chronic disorders, and autoimmune and connective tissue disorders. **Table 23.9** lists the currently available tests for syphilis infection. **Table 23.10** compares the sensitivity and specificity of various nontreponemal and treponemal-specific tests.

Prenatal diagnosis of congenital syphilis is sometimes possible using untrasonography, as a syphilis infection in a fetus can lead to hydrops fetalis, placental thickening, hepatomegaly, and hydramnios. However, an infected fetus frequently will have a normal ultrasonogram.

Sampling the fetus' blood also may be used to confirm an infection, as there are characteristic physiologic markers, including anemia, thrombocytopenia, and elevated liver enzymes. Serologic testing of cord blood is diagnostic of syphilis if nontreponemal test titers are at least fourfold higher than maternal titers.

PCR assays also can be perfomed on amniotic fluid to detect a syphilis infection. Studies have shown that PCR results correlate well with serology results for detecting syphilis. In addition, PCR provides an earlier diagnosis than serology in some cases. It also offers a confirmatory diagnosis or a differential diagnosis between *Treponema pallidum* and HSV in other cases.

Table 23.9 The various methods used for diagnosing syphilis

Direct detection methods	Nontreponemal tests	Treponemal tests
Rabbit infectivity test (RIT)	Venereal Disease Research Laboratory (VDRL)	Fluorescent Treponemal Antibody Absorption (FTA-abs)
Darkfield microscopy	Rapid Plasma Reagin (RPR)	Microhemagglutination Assay (MHA-TP)
Silver impregnation		
Direct Fluorescent Antibody stains (DFA-Tp)		
PCR		

Table 23.10 The sensitivity and specificity of various nontreponemal and treponemal tests for syphilis

Stage of infection	Sensitivity (%)	Specificity (%)
Nontreponemal tests		97–99
Primary	78–86	
Secondary	100	
Latent	95–98	
Tertiary	71–73	
Treponemal tests		97–99
Primary	76–84	
Secondary	100	
Latent	97–100	
Tertiary	94–96	

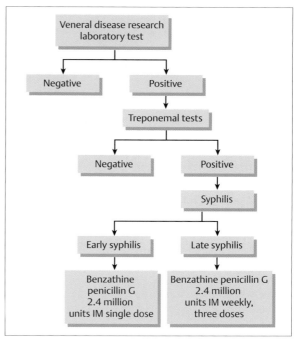

Fig. 23.9 Syphilis management scheme in pregnancy.

Management

Figure 23.9 provides a scheme for managing pregnant women with syphilis infections based on the results of specific laboratory tests and whether or not early or late stage syphilis is diagnosed.

Treatment

Penicillin remains the drug of choice for the treatment of syphilis in pregnancy, as penicillin resistance has not been reported for *Treponema pallidum*. It is effective in almost 100 % of cases. No other agent is currently recommended, owing to the high rate of treatment failure associated with other therapeutic agents.

Follow-up evaluation of the pregnant patient should be performed monthly to assess antibody titers via nontreponemal tests. Repeat treatment is required if symptoms persist, recur, or if nontreponemal test titers increase or decrease inappropriately.

Toxoplasmosis

Toxoplasmosis is caused by the protozoan *Toxoplasma gondii*, which is an obligate intracellular parasite. Although infection in immune-competent adults is usually asymptomatic or associated with self-limited symptoms posing as a mononucleosis-like syndrome, primary infection during pregnancy may cause serious health complications, if the parasite is transmitted transplacentally to the fetus.

Indeed, congenital toxoplamosis can lead to a wide array of manifestations and sequelae, ranging from mild chorioretinitis to miscarriage, mental retardation, mycrocephaly, hydrocephalus, and seizures.

Life Cycle

The life cycle of *Toxoplasma gondii* has three stages: 1) tachizoite, 2) bradizoite, and 3) sporozoite. Infective sporozoites are contained in oocytes. Oocytes are the product of sexual reproduction, which occurs in the small intestine of a cat that has recently ingested tissue cysts—usually via uncooked meat. Cats excrete unsporulated oocytes (i.e., noninfective) in their feces, which become infective 1–5 days later, depending on environmental conditions.

Tachizoites are rapidly dividing products of asexual reproduction occurring in macrophages following the invasion of the host's intestinal wall by either sporozoites (from oocysts) or bradizoites (from tissue cysts). Macrophages then serve as the vehicle for hematogenous dissemination of tachizoites in an intermediate host until an adequate immune response occurs in 7–10 days.

Hence, the protozoan becomes contained within tissue cysts as bradyzoites, and these cysts can remain dormant for the lifetime of the intermediate host in various tissues such as lymph nodes, retina, muscle, brain, liver, etc. If a person's immunity wanes, bradyzoites can resume rapid division and disseminate as tachizoites again via the blood.

Transmission

There are three main routes by which humans can acquire *Toxoplasma gondii* infection. First, humans can ingest tissue cysts present in infected, undercooked meat. Cooking meat to an internal temperature of 67 °C or freezing meat to below −12 °C kills bradyzoites, eliminating the risk of this mode of infection.

Second, infective oocytes can be ingested inadvertently through oral contact with feline feces from a litter box or from soil (e.g., soil from gardening, unwashed fruits and vegetables, or unfiltered water), releasing sporozoites that cause infection after they have invaded the human intestinal wall.

Third, a pregnant woman with toxoplasmosis can transmit tachizoites to her fetus via the placenta. Assuming a normal immune system, this form of infection only occurs when a pregnant woman develops a primary infection.

The risk of congenital toxoplasmosis infection from a mother with primary toxoplasmosis infection increases during pregnancy from 0–9% in the first trimester to 35–59% in the third trimester. Fortunately, the later in pregnancy the congenital infection occurs, the less severe the consequences are to the fetus.

Primary Prevention

Since more than 90% of acute toxoplamosis infections are asymptomatic, primary prevention is the best way to lower the risk of congenital infection. **Table 23.10** contains the most recent recommendations for women to follow.

Diagnosis

In asymptomatic women, the only sign of primary infection during pregnancy is seroconversion via detection of IgG or IgM antibodies. IgG antibodies become detectable 1–2 weeks after infection and remain elevated indefinitely, while IgM antibody levels increase within days and remain elevated for 2–3 months following acute infection. IgM levels, however, can remain detectable for more than two years in up to 27% of women when using the immunosorbent agglutination assay (ISAGA).

The detection of IgG in a woman at the beginning of pregnancy indicates previous infection, thus eliminating the risk of congenital toxoplasmosis.

Screening

Whether or not a woman should be screened for primary *Toxoplama gondii* infection remains a matter of controversy in many countries, because the false-positive rate of IgM antibody detection has been estimated to be as high as 1.3%. Such a high false-positive rate could result in early requests for pregnancy termination of many uninfected fetuses (**Table 23.11**).

Moreover, the incidence of maternal primary infection in many developed countries is relatively low, making screening ineffective. However, certain groups of women should be screened for acute infection if thought to be at high risk of exposure to risk factors such as raw meat, soil, or cat feces.

Congenital Toxoplasmosis

The classic triad of signs suggestive of congenital toxoplasmosis comprises chorioretinitis, hydrocephalus, and intracranial calcifications. However, other clinical manifestations are associated with this disease (**Table 23.12**).

Congenital toxoplasmosis can mimic diseases caused by other organisms, such as herpes simplex virus, cytomegalovirus, and rubella virus. Most neonates born with congenital toxoplasmosis are asymptomatic as determined by routine examination of the newborn.

Management

If acute toxoplasmosis is confirmed during pregnancy, treatment with spiramycin (with or without pirimethamine–sulfadiazine) is indicated to reduce the risk of congenital infection and decrease the incidence of late sequelae. An alternate treatment, pirimethamine, however, is teratogenic and contraindicated for women in the first trimester.

Table 23.11 Current recommendations for lowering the risk of primary toxoplasmosis infection among pregnant women

1. Avoid consumption of undercooked meat
2. Wash hands and all utensils thoroughly after handling raw meat
3. Wash all uncooked vegetables thoroughly
4. Wear gloves when gardening or working in soil. Wash hands immediately after contact with soil
5. If possible, keep cats indoors throughout pregnancy. Do not feed cats undercooked meat
6. Use gloves while, and wash hands immediately after, changing cat litter

Table 23.12 Clinical manifestations of congenital toxoplasmosis

Abnormal spinal fluid
Anemia
Chorioretinitis
Convulsions
Deafness
Fever
Growth retardation
Hepatomegaly
Hydrocephalus
Intracranial calcifications
Jaundice
Lymphadenopathy
Maculopapular rash
Mental retardation Microcephaly
Spasticity & palsies
Splenomegaly
Thrombocytopenia
Visual impairment

Key Points

- Cytomegalovirus (CMV) primary infection results in a 30–40 % risk of vertical transmission to the fetus. In contrast, the risk of transmission with recurrent maternal infection with CMV is between 0.2 % and 1.8 %. Only 10–15 % of infected neonates are symptomatic at birth, which manifests as growth restriction, ventriculomegaly, microcephaly, and cerebral calcifications.
- An estimated 20–30 % of pregnant women are carriers of group B streptococci (GBS). Prophylaxis of GBS with penicillin is highly effective in preventing neonatal morbidity and mortality. Universal screening should performed between 35 and 37 weeks of gestation.
- Women with vulvar–vaginal lesions due to herpes simplex virus infection at the time of delivery should undergo cesarean section to decrease perinatal transmission.
- Every pregnant woman should be offered HIV testing with an opt-out policy.
- Treatment with highly active antiretroviral therapy (HAART) during pregnancy, with the objective to achieve undetectable maternal viral load, reduces significantly the risk of HIV transmission to the fetus.
- Breast-feeding should be avoided in mothers with HIV infection.
- Cesarean delivery should be the mode of delivery if maternal viral load is greater than 1000 copies/mL.

- All pregnant women should be screened for syphilis in their first prenatal visit. High-risk patients should be retested at 28 weeks of gestation and at delivery.
- If syphilis is diagnosed, penicillin is the only accepted treatment during pregnancy.
- The risk of congenital toxoplasmosis infection from a mother with primary toxoplasmosis infection increases during pregnancy from 0 % to 9 % in the first trimester, and from 35 % to 59 % in the third trimester. The later in pregnancy the congenital infection occurs, the less severe the consequences are to the fetus.
- Since acute toxoplamosis infections are asymptomatic, primary prevention is the best way to lower the risk of congenital infection.
- The classic triad of signs suggestive of congenital toxoplasmosis include chorioretinitis, hydrocephalus, and intracranial calcifications.

Evidence Box 23.1

Congenital cytomegalovirus has an impact on child health but its effects can easily be overlooked owing to lack of signs in the neonatal period.

Engman et al. investigated the prevalence of congenital cytomegalovirus (CMV) infection among 6060 newborns in southern Stockholm during a 12-month period. Only 12 infants out of 6060, or 0.2 % (95 % CI, 0.1 % to 0.3 %), had congenital CMV infection. One boy among the 12 infected infants had unilateral hearing loss, indicating that the risk of hearing loss is greatly increased (about 20 times) in CMV-infected infants. No child developed ocular complications such as chorioretinopathy during 3 years of follow-up.

Engman ML, Malm G, Engstrom L, et al. Congenital CMV infection: prevalence in newborns and the impact on hearing deficit. Scand J Infect Dis 2008;40(11-12):935–942.

Further Reading

ACOG Committee on Obstetric Practice. ACOG committee opinion number 304, November 2004. Prenatal and perinatal human immunodeficiency virus testing: expanded recommendations. *Obstet Gynecol* 2004;104(5 Pt 1):1119–1124

Engman ML, Malm G, Engstrom L, et al. Congenital CMV infection: prevalence in newborns and the impact on hearing deficit. *Scand J Infect Dis* 2008;40(11-12):935–942

Malm G, Engman ML. Congenital cytomegalovirus infections. *Semin Fetal Neonatal Med* 2007;12(3):154–159

Minkoff H. Human immunodeficiency virus infection in pregnancy. *Obstet Gynecol* 2003;101(4):797–810

Reece EA, Hobbins JC, eds. Clinical Obstetrics: the Fetus and Mother. 3rd ed. Malden, Mass: Blackwell Synergy Publishing; 2007

Schrag S, Gorwitz K, Fultz-Butts K, et al. Prevention of perinatal group B streptococcal disease. Revised guidelines from CDC. *MMWR Recomm* Rep. 2002;51:1–22

Wendel GD. Gestational and congenital syphilis. *Clin Perinatol* 1988;15(2):287–303

24 Perinatal and Maternal Mortality

Eyal Sheiner and Arnon Wiznitzer

Among the more than 130 million babies born worldwide every year, more than 10 million die before their fifth birthday; almost 8 million die before their first. In addition, an estimated half a million women die each year worldwide owing to pregnancy-related complications, most of them in the developing world. Millions of other women sustain serious health problems due to pregnancy and childbirth. Many of these deaths and illnesses are preventable.

Clearly, the management and prevention of factors that increase women's risk for perinatal mortality as well as their own mortality is an important public health concern globally. Other chapters in this book deal with approaches and protocols for preventing and managing specific conditions that increase the risks for perinatal and maternal mortality. The purpose of this chapter, therefore, is to define these phenomena and broadly outline their scope and strategies for dealing with them.

Definitions

Perinatal mortality: Perinatal mortality refers to deaths that occur in the period following birth of infants weighing at least 500 g or born after 20 completed weeks of gestation until they reach 28 completed days after birth. The *perinatal mortality rate* refers to the number of stillbirths and neonatal deaths per 1000 total births. If an infant dies during the first 7 days following birth, this is considered an *early neonatal death*. Death of a live-born infant after 7 days but before 29 days following birth is considered a *late neonatal death*. The term *Infant death* refers to deaths of live-born infants from birth until 1 year of age.

Maternal mortality: Maternal mortality is maternal deaths that result from the reproductive process. The maternal mortality rate is the number of deaths per 100 000 live births (also known as the maternal mortality ratio).

Maternal deaths: Deaths that result from an obstetric complication, treatment, or intervention during pregnancy, delivery, or the puerperium are considered *direct maternal deaths*. Maternal deaths that are not the direct result of the reproductive process, but rather are due to a previously existing conditions or a disease that developed during pregnancy and was aggravated by physiological adaptation to pregnancy, are considered *indirect maternal deaths*.

Epidemiology and Etiology

Perinatal Mortality

Perinatal mortality is an important indicator of the level of health care provision in a society. Different definitions hamper direct comparisons between countries with regard to perinatal mortality rates. There has, however, been a dramatic decline in perinatal mortality rates in the Western world over the past several decades. In the United Kingdom, for example, there was a decline from 62 deaths per 1000 births to only 13 deaths per 1000 births during the 1990s.

Mortality rates have declined in much of the developing world. However, perinatal mortality rates and those of children under 5 years of age are significantly higher in Africa and the Middle East compared with the Americas and Western Europe (**Fig. 24.1**).

Premature birth (see Chapter 15) accounts for up to 70% of perinatal mortality cases in Western countries. There are many causes of premature birth, including infections, bleeding, and the stretching or overdistension of the uterus as a result of multiple births (**Fig. 24.2**). Whatever the cause, about 25% of all preterm births to mothers with one baby are ended early for maternal or fetal wellbeing. This is achieved either through the induction of labor or by planned cesarean section, depending on

Part II Obstetrics

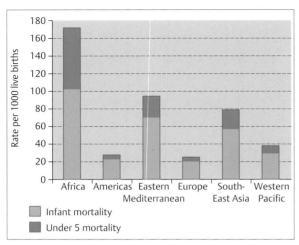

Fig. 24.1 Under-5 (years old) and infant mortality rates by region, 2003. Source: World Health Organization.

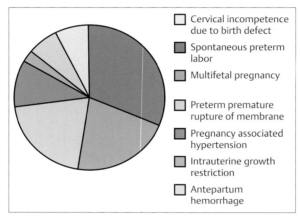

Fig. 24.2 Various conditions leading to overall premature birth rates.

the reason for the early arrival and the conditions of the mother and baby.

According to American College of Obstetricians and Gynecologists (ACOG) guidelines, labor should not be induced should prior to 39 weeks without a valid medical reason because of the increased risks. That leaves 75% of preterm labors as spontaneous. About a quarter of spontaneous preterm labors are due to premature rupture of membranes (see Chapter 20).

Besides premature birth, other causes of perinatal mortality include congenital malformations, growth problems such as intrauterine growth restriction, multiple pregnancies, maternal low socioeconomic status (including social deprivation), lack of prenatal care, teenage pregnancies, and pregnancies of older women (above 40 years of age).

Maternal Mortality

Maternal mortality is difficult and complex to monitor, particularly in settings where the levels of maternal deaths are highest. Information is required about deaths among women of reproductive age, their pregnancy status at or near the time of death, and the medical cause of death—all of which can be difficult to measure accurately, particularly where vital registration systems are incomplete.

The best estimate, according to the United Nations Children's Fund (UNICEF), is that more than 500000 women worldwide die each year from maternal causes. And for every woman who dies, approximately 20 more suffer injuries, infections, and disabilities in pregnancy or childbirth.

The vast majority (99%) of the 536000 estimated maternal deaths in 2005 occurred in developing countries. Slightly more than half of the maternal deaths (270000) occurred in the sub-Saharan Africa region alone, followed by South Asia (188000). Thus, sub-Saharan Africa and South Asia accounted for 86% of global maternal deaths.

The four most important causes of maternal death past mid-pregnancy are hemorrhage (severe bleeding), infection, eclampsia-induced hypertension, and unsafe abortions (**Fig. 24.3**). Ectopic pregnancies also are a significant cause of maternal death, predominantly from hemorrhage and infection (see Chapter 13).

There are also genetic and personal factors, such as race and age, that make pregnancy more risky for certain women. The maternal mortality rate for Black women (22.0 per 100000 live births), for example, is almost three times the rate for White women (7.5 per 100000 live births). Hispanics and other non-White women face significantly higher risks as well (**Fig. 24.4**).

Being pregnant too young or too old also increases a woman's mortality risks. Adolescents girls under age

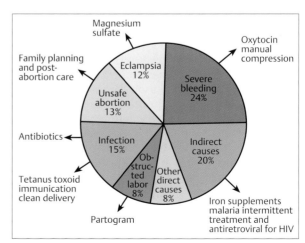

Fig. 24.3 Most common causes of maternal death past mid-pregnancy and potential interventions to prevent them from occurring.

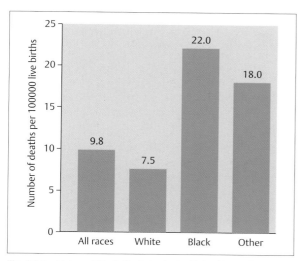

Fig. 24.4 Maternal Mortality Rates in the United States by Race of Mother: 2000. National Center for Health Statistics.

15 years are five times more likely to die during pregnancy or childbirth than women over the age of 20. If they get pregnant between 15 and 19 years old, they are twice as likely to die than pregnant women 20–30 years old.

After women reach age 30 years, their mortality risk begins to increase regardless of race. Women aged 35–39 years have approximately twice the risk of maternal death comapred with women aged 20–24 years.

Management and Prevention

Perinatal Mortality

Since more than two-thirds of perinatal deaths occur in preterm infants, the appropriate management and/or prevention of preterm labor is likely to have a significant impact on perinatal mortality. Unfortunately, progress in the management of preterm labor has been hampered by our lack of understanding of the process of parturition in humans. Progress also has been hampered by the unavailability of drugs capable of inhibiting uterine contractility efficiently, without causing potentially serious side effects for the mother or the baby.

Pharmacological Management

Numerous studies have shown that beta-mimetics are effective at delaying delivery in women in preterm labor for 48 hours. However, there is no evidence that this relatively short delay provides any benefit in terms of perinatal mortality or morbidity. Studies also have found increased

risk for various side effects in mothers, including chest pain, breathing difficulties, heart irregularities, headaches, and shaking. The potential for these multiple side effects must be shared with the patient before initiating any therapy.

Short-term tocolysis with intravenous ritodrine may improve the outcome for the baby if it prevents delivery until the patient can be transferred to a hospital with better neonatal facilities or if it allows time for the mother to complete a course of antenatal glucocorticoids. Both human and animal studies have confirmed that glucocorticoids promote pulmonary maturation and reduce mortality in fetuses. Several studies indicate that prenatal glucocorticoids also stimulate renal maturation.

Although single courses of antenatal glucocorticoids clearly decrease respiratory distress syndrome and mortality, there is growing concern that repetitive courses of antenatal glucocorticoids are being given to women at risk of preterm delivery without evidence of benefit or appreciation of potential risks. Although human studies are just beginning, evidence from animal studies suggests that repeated exposure to glucocorticoids has long-lasting deleterious effects on cardiovascular, metabolic, and neuroendocrine function. Thus, prevention remains an important strategy for addressing preterm labor and other contributors to perinatal mortality.

Preventive Methods

Preventive methods, such as drug and alcohol cessation, infection control, promoting healthy nutrition, and the quality of prenatal care of pregnant mothers, all significantly impact perinatal mortality.

Cessation of smoking: Smoking is one of the single most important preventable factors associated with low birth weight, preterm birth, and perinatal death. A recent review of 64 smoking cessation trials, representing close to 60 000 women, found that promoting smoking cessation in pregnancy reduced the proportion of women who continued to smoke and reduced low birth weight and preterm birth.

Cessation of alcohol and other drugs: Maternal alcohol consumption during pregnancy can lead to placental abruption as well as fetal alchohol syndrome in the developing infant. Furthermore, pregnant women who drink, often smoke. Therefore, women must be advised to abstain from drinking during pregnancy. Studies suggest the use of cannabis during pregnancy is not associated with increased risk of perinatal mortality or morbidity. However, frequent and regular use of cannabis throughout pregnancy may be associated with small but statistically detectable decrements in birth weight. Thus, cannabis should be avoided as well.

Infection control: Infection control also is important in reducing perinatal mortality. Women with abnormal genital tract flora diagnosed by bacterial vaginosis on Gram stain of vaginal secretions in pregnancy are at increased risk of late miscarriage and preterm birth (see also Chapter 19).

The earlier in pregnancy that spontaneous preterm labor occurs, the more likely it is to be due to a pathological signal or trigger, such as an infection. Recent randomized controlled trials have shown that the antibiotic clindamycin used in early pregnancy can reduce the risk of preterm birth by 40–60%.

The most severe common adverse effect of clindamycin is diarrhea associated with overgrowth of the bacterium *Clostridium difficile* (the most frequent cause of pseudomembranous colitis, a severe infection of the colon). This side effect is often linked primarily to clindamycin use, although it occurs with almost all antibiotics.

Diabetes control: Women with insulin-dependent diabetes are at increased risk for a variety of adverse pregnancy outcomes such as stillbirths, obstetric complications, and congenital malformations. Perinatal mortality and prevalence of congenital anomalies also are common in the babies of women with type 2 diabetes and gestational diabetes.

General improvements in prenatal care and in obstetric management of women with diabetes have led to a substantial decline in perinatal mortality rates among their infants. With these improvements, however, congenital malformations have emerged as the most common cause of perinatal mortality, particularly for infants of women with insulin-dependent diabetes, who account for approximately 50% of all perinatal deaths. Thus, diabetes control in pregnant women is critical to preventing adverse outcomes in their offspring.

Providing adequate prenatal care: The chief objective of prenatal care is to ensure good pregnancy outcomes. As advances in medical knowledge and practice in the 20th century contributed to dramatic reduction in maternal and perinatal mortality and morbidity, this concept has grown and evolved.

Analyses of mortality data in the United States have found that improvements in prenatal health care in general have contributed at least in part to declines in perinatal mortality due to avoidable conditions. Studies also have shown that the lack of prenatal care is an independent risk factor for perinatal mortality, and supplying adequate prenatal care to women in low income areas significantly decreases the rate of low birth weight babies and perinatal mortality. The qualities of adequate prenatal care are discussed extensively in many other chapters in this book.

Unfortunately, however, minorities continue to experience disproportionately high rates of miscarriage and newborn mortality, despite early access to prenatal care.

Thus, minority women may require a more comprehensive assessment and intervention strategy to help lower their perinatal mortality risk.

Maternal Mortality

Maternal mortality affects not only women, but also their families and communities. The risk of an infant dying increases significantly with the mother's death. The death of a woman of reproductive age also brings significant economic losses and setbacks to community development.

Accordingly, strategies to reduce a woman's mortality risk when she becomes pregnant must include:
- adequate prenatal care, including nutritional support
- early detection of anemia and other complications
- the assistance of a trained personnel at births
- appropriate referral of high-risk pregnancy to a fully equipped medical facility

Adequate preconception and prenatal care are covered extensively in Chapter 9. Protocols for detecting anemia and other life-threatening complications are discussed in Section II, Abnormal Obstetrics. The remainder of this chapter discusses the general interventions/approaches that the practitioner can take to prevent or to address the known risk factors for maternal mortality.

Magnesium Sulfate Administration for Pre-eclampsia

Studies have shown that calcium supplementation during pregnancy appears to almost halve the risk of pre-eclampsia, one of the leading causes of maternal morbidity (see Chapter 16). The administration of magnesium sulfate to women experiencing severe pre-eclampsia is highly effective in stopping convulsions and in lowering the risk of mortality.

Uterogenic Agents for Severe Bleeding

Postpartum hemorrhage is another leading cause of maternal morbidity and mortality. Thus, active management of the third stage of labor, including the use of methods to reduce blood loss, can have a significant impact on reducing maternal mortality.

For example, the use of routine uterotonic agents to prevent postpartum hemorrhage can reduce maternal mortality by 40%. For years, the uterotonic agent of choice has been oxytocin, which is given intramuscularly by injection.

Misoprostol, an oral preparation of prostaglandin E_1 analogue, is an alternative uterotonic with some advantages over oxytocin, including ease of use as an oral, vaginal, or rectal preparation, relative low cost in some areas, and stability at high temperature. Several randomized controlled trials have been conducted to examine whether misoprostol is a suitable alternative to oxytocin in low-resource settings for prevention of postpartum hemorrhage (Evidence Box 24.1). Although controversial, those studies suggest that misoprostol is equally as effective as oxytocin in preventing postpartum hemorrhage.

Iron Supplementation

Iron is an essential mineral and an important component of proteins involved in oxygen transport and metabolism. Iron is also an essential cofactor in the synthesis of neurotransmitters such as dopamine, norepinephrine, and serotonin. About 15% of the body's iron is stored for future needs and mobilized when dietary intake is inadequate. The body usually maintains normal iron status by controlling the amount of iron absorbed from food.

Iron supplements have been shown to help prevent iron deficiency anemia in pregnant women. Anemia in pregnant women is associated with adverse outcomes such as low birth weight, premature birth, and maternal mortality. Screening by a qualified health care provider is needed. Low doses of iron are generally well tolerated and associated with better compliance.

Obstructed Labor

Obstructed labor is an important cause of **maternal** deaths in communities where undernutrition in childhood is common, resulting in small pelves in women, **and** where there is no easy access to functioning health facilities with the capability of carrying out operative deliveries

(, cesarean section). **Obstructed** labor also causes significant **maternal** morbidity in the short term (notably, infection) **and** long term (notably, obstetric fistulas).

The development of the partograph (or partogram) has provided health professionals with a pictorial overview of the labor to allow early identification **and** diagnosis of pathological labor. Studies have shown that using the partograph (**Fig. 24.5**) can be highly effective in reducing complications from prolonged labor for the mother (postpartum hemorrhage, sepsis, uterine rupture and its sequelae) and for the newborn (death, anoxia, infections, etc.).

When there is clear evidence of obstruction in the first stage of labor, delivery by cesarean section is usually required. The maternal mortality rate after cesarean section is currently very low. However, cesarean section is more hazardous than vaginal delivery by a factor of 2 to 11. Infection is the most common cause of morbidity after a cesarean, blood transfusion being the second. A large number of factors modify the risk of infection, the most important being prophylactic antibiotics.

Symphysiotomy is a surgical procedure in which the cartilage of the symphysis pubis is divided to widen the pelvis to allow childbirth where there is a mechanical problem. It results in a temporary increase in pelvic diameter (up to 2 cm) by surgically dividing the ligaments of the symphysis under local anesthesia. This procedure should be carried out only in combination with vacuum extraction. Symphysiotomy in combination with vacuum extraction can be a life-saving procedure in areas of the world where cesarean section is not feasible or immediately available.

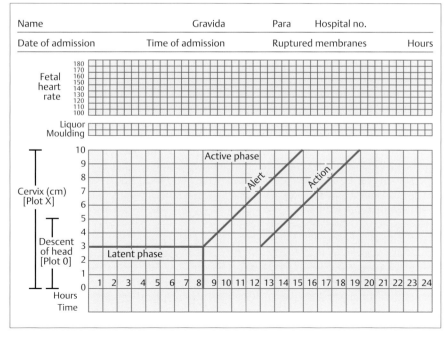

Fig. 24.5 The partograph is used to plot the multiple parameters for the progress of labor, including cervical dilatation, descent of fetal head, and uterine contractions. It also is used for monitoring fetal and maternal conditions.

An important advantage of this procedure is that women who are suitable will not enter future pregnancies with a scar on their uterus. However, the procedure does have risks, including urethral and bladder injury, infection, pain and long-term walking difficulty. Symphysiotomy should, therefore, be carried out only when there is no safe alternative. This procedure also should not be repeated in the same woman, owing to the risk of gait problems and continual pain.

Infection Control

Bacterial vaginosis: Approximately 10–30% of pregnant women will experience bacterial vaginosis (BV) during their pregnancy. BV is caused by an imbalance in the normal bacteria that exist in a woman's vagina. It is not transmitted sexually but is associated with having vaginal intercourse.

One of the symptoms of BV is a gray or whitish discharge that has a foul fishy odor. However some women do not experience any symptoms. Diagnosis is made through a pelvic exam. Vaginal discharge is tested through a wet mount (microscopic slide test), pH test (BV often causes a pH level of 4.5 or higher), KOH slide (microscopic slide test) or a whiff test (a mixture that causes a strong fishy odor). There is significant evidence linking BV with preterm labor and, thus, an increased risk for maternal and fetal morbidity and mortality.

Treatment is therefore highly recommended to avoid any chance of preterm labor. There are various treatment options, including oral medications (clindamycin 300 mg or metronidazole 500 mg twice daily for 7 days) and topical medications (clindamycin 5 g or metronidazole at bedtime for 5 days). However, topical medications for BV may give only symptomatic relief and may be inefficient at preventing pregnancy complications.

Listeria: *Listeria monocytogenes* is a type of bacterium that is found in water and soil. Vegetables can become contaminated from the soil, and animals can also be carriers. Listeria has been found in uncooked meats, uncooked vegetables, unpasteurized milk, foods made from unpasteurized milk, and processed foods. Listeria is killed by pasteurization and cooking.

According to the U.S. Centers for Disease Control and Prevention (CDC), an estimated 2500 persons become seriously ill with listeriosis each year in the United States, of whom 500 will die. According to research, pregnant women account for 27% of these cases. The CDC claims that pregnant women are 20 times more likely to become infected than nonpregnant, healthy adults. Symptoms in pregnant women include mild flulike symptoms, headaches, muscle aches, fever, nausea and vomiting. If the infection spreads to the nervous system it can cause stiff neck, disorientation, or convulsions. Infection can occur

at any time during pregnancy, but it is most common during the third trimester when a woman's immune system is somewhat suppressed. Listeriosis is treated with antibiotics during pregnancy. These antibiotics, in most cases, will prevent the infection from spreading to the fetus. These same antibiotics are also given to newborns with listeriosis.

Sexually transmitted diseases: Sexually transmitted diseases (STDs) can have many of the same consequences for pregnant women as for women who are not pregnant. STDs can cause cervical and other cancers, chronic hepatitis, pelvic inflammatory disease, infertility, and other complications. Many STDs in women are silent; that is, without signs or symptoms. Besides the risk of transmission to her baby, a pregnant woman with an STD may also have early onset of labor, premature rupture of the membranes surrounding the baby in the uterus, and uterine infection after delivery.

Most of these problems can be prevented if the mother receives routine prenatal care, which includes screening tests for STDs starting early in pregnancy and repeated close to delivery, if necessary (see Chapter 9). Other problems can be treated if the infection is found at birth.

Chorioamnionitis: Chorioamnionitis is a condition that can affect pregnant women in whom the chorion and amnion (the membranes that surround the fetus) and the amniotic fluid (in which the fetus floats) are infected by bacteria. This can lead to infection of both the mother and fetus, and means in most cases that the fetus has to be delivered as soon as possible.

If the mother has a serious case of chorioamnionitis, or if it goes untreated, she might develop complications, including:

- infections in the pelvic region and abdomen
- endometritis (an infection of the endometrium, the lining of the uterus)
- blood clots in the pelvis and lungs

The newborn might also have complications from a bacterial infection, including sepsis (infection of the blood), meningitis (infection of the lining of the brain and the spinal cord), and respiratory problems.

A woman with chorioamnionitis must be treated with antibiotics to address the infection. However, the ultimate cure is to deliver the fetus. In addition, if the newborn has an infection, he or she must given antibiotics as well.

Key Points

- Worldwide, an estimated half a million women die each year owing to pregnancy-related complications, and millions more sustain serious health problems during pregnancy and childbirth.
- Although rates have declined in much of the developing world as well, perinatal mortality rates and those of children under 5 years of age are significantly higher in Africa and the Middle East, in comparison with the Americas and Western Europe.
- The major causes of perinatal mortality are premature birth, congenital malformations, growth problems such as intrauterine growth restriction (IUGR), multiple pregnancies, maternal low socioeconomic status, lack of prenatal care, teenage pregnancies, and pregnancies of older women (above 40 years of age).
- The major causes of maternal mortality include hemorrhage (severe bleeding), infection, eclampsia-induced hypertension, unsafe abortions, and ectopic pregnancies.
- Many of these maternal and perinatal deaths and illnesses can be prevented with swift, appropriate intervention.
- Preventive methods, such as cessation of drug and alcohol use, infection control, promoting healthy nutrition, and the quality of prenatal care of pregnant mothers can significantly reduce perinatal mortality.
- Maternal mortality rates can be significantly reduced with adequate prenatal care, early detection of anemia and other complications, the assistance of trained personnel at births, and appropriate referral of a high-risk pregnancy to a fully-equipped medical facility.

Evidence Box 24.1

Rectal misoprostol is as effective as intramuscular injection of oxytocin in preventing hemorrhage during late labor.

Parsons et al. compared the effect of rectal misoprostol with intramuscular oxytocin in the routine management of the third stage of pregnancy in a rural developing country. They randomized 450 women living in Ghana, West Africa, who were in advance labor to receive rectal misoprostol 800 μg or intramuscular oxytocin 10 IU with delivery of the anterior shoulder. The main outcome measure was change in hemoglobin concentration from before to after delivery. Secondary outcomes included the need for additional uterotonics, estimated blood loss, transfusion, and

medication side effects. This study found no significant difference between treatment groups in change in hemoglobin (misoprostol 1.19 g/dL and oxytocin 1.16 g/dL; relative difference 2.6%; 95% confidence intervals [CIs]: 16.8% to 19.4%; $P = 0.80$). The only significant secondary outcome was shivering, which was more common in the misoprostol group (misoprostol 7.5% vs. oxytocin 0.9%; relative risk 8.0; 95% CI: 1.86 to 34.36; $P = 0.001$). Based on these findings, Parsons et al. concluded that rectal misoprostol 800 μg is as effective as 10 IU intramuscular oxytocin in minimizing blood loss in the third stage of labor and that rectal misoprostol has a lower incidence of side effects than the equivalent oral dose. They also concluded it is a safe and effective uterotonic for use in the rural and remote areas of developing nations where other pharmacologic agents may be less feasible.

Parsons SM, Walley RL, Crane JM, Matthews K, Hutchens D. Rectal misoprostol versus oxytocin in the management of the third stage of labour. J Obstet Gynaecol Can 2007 Sep;29(9):711–718.

Further Reading

López Bernal A. Overview. Preterm labour: mechanisms and management. *BMC Pregnancy Childbirth* 2007;7(Suppl 1):S2

Crowther CA, Doyle LW, Haslam RR, Hiller JE, Harding JE, Robinson JS; ACTORDS Study Group. Outcomes at 2 years of age after repeat doses of antenatal corticosteroids. *N Engl J Med* 2007;357(12):1179–1189

Parsons SM, Walley RL, Crane JM, Matthews K, Hutchens D. Rectal misoprostol versus oxytocin in the management of the third stage of labour. *J Obstet Gynaecol Can* 2007;29(9):711–718

Salinas AM, Coria I, Reyes H, Zambrana M. Effect of quality of care on preventable perinatal mortality. *Int J Qual Health Care* 1997;9(2):93–99

Su LL, Chong YS, Samuel M. Oxytocin agonists for preventing postpartum haemorrhage. *Cochrane Database Syst Rev* 2007; (3):CD005457

World Health Organisation. Maternal Mortality in 2000. Estimates developed by WHO, UNICEF and UNFPA. Available at: http://www.reliefweb.int/library/documents/2003/who-saf-22oct.pdf

Zupan J. Perinatal mortality in developing countries. *N Engl J Med* 2005;352(20):2047–2048

25 Psychiatric Issues during and after Pregnancy

Jill A. RachBeisel

A mother's mental health before, during, and following pregnancy is a key factor in her wellbeing and her baby's. It has been well established that the occurrence of an episode of mental illness during pregnancy has a significant influence on the health of the pregnancy, development of the fetus, and success of the mother and child following delivery. Caring for a woman with mental illness during pregnancy is complex and includes consideration of issues such as nutrition, the use of psychotropic medications, psychosocial supports, mother–infant bonding, and the care of both mother and child in the postpartum period.

Women with complicating conditions including anxiety, mood, and psychotic disorders face difficult decisions about whether or not to have a child or about treatment choices during pregnancy and while breast-feeding. Careful consideration must be given to the health and wellbeing of both mother and baby. The risk to the fetus of treating the mother's illness must be weighed against risk of no treatment at all to the mother and the baby. In such complicated situations it is critical that the obstetrician work closely with the psychiatrist in considering the best options to present to the expectant mother in managing her illness while maintaining the highest safety to her unborn child.

This chapter covers the essential critical issues in helping women with a history of mental health issues decide if they want to become pregnant as well as the assessment, diagnosis, and treatment of psychiatric disorders during and immediately following pregnancy. Because this subject matter is so vast, peripheral issues related to infertility, miscarriage, elective termination, loss of a child shortly following delivery, and menopause are not addressed in this chapter but are covered in other chapters of this book.

Family Planning

The too-often-voiced opinion that a woman with a mental illness should not get pregnant or attempt another pregnancy (if her first mental health episode was associated with a prior pregnancy) is simply not true. Although for some women with a history of psychiatric symptoms—either apart from or related to a prior pregnancy—becoming pregnant again may present too great a risk, for many, having a baby remains a viable option. However, careful attention must be paid to early signs and symptoms of illness, and appropriate monitoring is critical for a successful pregnancy and delivery of a healthy baby and happy mother. Equally important is the early detection of symptoms of emotional distress during or following delivery to ensure appropriate, timely treatment and to avoid long-term serious and, at times, potentially devastating complications for both mother and baby.

Discussing the possibility of having a baby is perhaps one of the most important issues to address when caring for a woman in her childbearing years with a history of mental illness. Ideally, such a discussion should occur when a couple is planning marriage and making future plans rather than after marriage or at the first prenatal visit, when the woman presents with an unexpected pregnancy. The discussion should cover several important topics including the heritability of the mental illness and risk factors to the mother and baby during and after delivery. The purpose of these discussions is to have a well-informed patient who can make the decision that is best for herself and her baby.

Genetics of Psychiatric Disorders

Since the 1970s, there has been growing interest in the inheritability of psychiatric illness. The likelihood that a particular psychiatric illness will be transmitted to the unborn child is determined by many factors, including the presence of biologic (susceptibility genes) and environmental (psychosocial stressors) factors.

To date, no single gene has been linked to the transmission of a mental illness from one generation to the next. On the other hand, studies have clearly demonstrated that many psychiatric disorders have a genetic component. Indeed, babies born to parents with schizophrenia, bipolar disorder, eating disorders, and anxiety disorders have a significantly greater risk of developing those illnesses in their lifetime compared to babies born to parents with little or no psychiatric illness.

Risk Factors for the Expectant Mother during Pregnancy

There has been a longstanding controversy regarding the impact of pregnancy on the course of mental illness. The theory that pregnancy protects the mother from an episode of illness directly conflicts with the idea that pregnancy is a time of increased vulnerability. Thus, the current clinical approach is one of individualization.

Factors that impact the effect of pregnancy on a woman's psychiatric illness include emotional stability, attitudes toward femininity and pregnancy, cultural attitudes, relationships with her significant other and her own mother, and degree of preparation for parenthood.

It has been shown that the less prepared for parenthood a mother is, the more stressful the pregnancy will be for her. Increased stress during pregnancy leads to an increased likelihood of emotional instability and an exacerbation any underlying mental illness. Careful assessment of these factors will help to identify patients at risk for more complications during the pregnancy, and whether they ultimately may require medications, enhanced psychosocial support, or acute psychiatric care.

Even among expectant mothers without a history of mental illness, 20% will experience an episode of depression sometime in their life. However, it is more likely that such an event will occur during a pregnancy, particularly in the face of psychosocial stressors such as poverty and poor interpersonal support.

Risk Factors for the Fetus during Pregnancy

For an expectant mother with mental illness, risks to the developing child come from two sources: exposure to the medications and the untreated psychiatric illness. Medication exposure can cause considerable risk, especially with the use of agents for bipolar illness. At the same time, it has been well documented that mothers who suffer from significant stress during pregnancy, including an exacerbation of their illness, are prone to have low birth weight babies, increased rates of schizophrenia, and preterm births. Further, a child's emotional, cognitive, and physical health and development are affected by their mother's mental health while pregnant. A more detailed discussion of impact of medicine versus lack of treatment of the mother's illness on the fetus is presented later in this chapter.

Postpartum Complications

The greatest postpartum complication for the mother is a sudden onset of existing or new psychiatric illness, typically referred to as postpartum depression. Approximately 20% of mothers experience some symptoms of depression within the first year after birth, most of whom are not identified or treated. The most severe forms of postpartum psychiatric illness typically occur within the first month following delivery and can greatly interfere with mother–infant bonding, self-care, and care of the baby.

The greatest risk for the newborn stems from two factors: 1) heightened medication exposure during breastfeeding due to an immature liver that no longer has the mother's liver to help with metabolism of the psychotropic medications, thus leading to toxicity and/or withdrawal phenomenon; and 2) onset or worsening psychiatric symptoms in the mother interfering with attachment, feeding, and basic care. In the worst cases, infants are unintentionally at risk for neglect or abuse due to the depressed mother's inability to care for her newborn child.

A rare but very real event is infanticide, a situation where the mother is most often depressed, has failed to attach or bond with her baby, and feels the baby would be better off dead and, thus, spared unhappiness and pain. The mother may attempt to kill herself as well. The majority of infanticides are not associated with psychosis but rather a severe depression.

Many of the risks factors are avoidable with close management, frequent assessment, and preventative strategies to minimize stress and promote a healthy, supportive pregnancy and postpartum periods.

Addressing Psychiatric Issues during Pregnancy

Pregnancy should be one of the most special and happiest times of a woman's life. However, for many women, it is a period of fearfulness, confusion, anxiety, stress, and, ultimately, depression. Complicating factors such as unexpected pregnancy, teenage pregnancy, poverty, lack of social support, and isolation create a psychological environment that is sometimes challenging for the expectant mother. At a time when she is most in need of expressing her feelings and being understood, many women find it difficult to reveal the conflicts they are experiencing.

Many times, fears of being seen as self-centered and thankless prevent them from speaking out about their emotional turmoil. As a result, depression in pregnancy remains under-recognized and under-treated, leaving the mother and developing fetus at greater risk for other adverse outcomes.

Depression

Etiology and Frequency

Depression occurs almost twice as often in women than men: a 21% lifetime prevalence of major depression in women versus 13% in men. This greater susceptibility to depression has been attributed to differences in monoamine transmitter function and processing between men and women.

Another possible underlying risk factor that may contribute to higher rates of depression in women is the fundamental requirement that the woman's brain must constantly adapt to fluctuating hormone levels. At no other time is this truer than during pregnancy and delivery. Although this is a topic of great research interest, it is still poorly understood, and effective preventative therapies have not been discovered. Thus, there is a need to carefully monitor, identify, and provide treatment of depression as it occurs.

Overall, the prevalence of all minor and major depressions ranges from 6.5% to 12.9% through pregnancy, while the prevalence of major depression only ranges from 1.0% to 5.6%. The major risk factors for depression during pregnancy are listed in **Table 25.1**.

Diagnosis

The diagnosis of depression during pregnancy can be difficult because many of its signs, such as decreased libido, poor appetite, and difficulty sleeping, often can be attributed to the pregnancy itself. Thus, the clinician must have a high level of suspicion and routinely ask the appropriate

Table 25.1 Risk factors for depression during pregnancy

Adolescence
Poverty or financial disadvantage
Unmarried status
African-American or Hispanic
Poor social support
Previous episode of depression
Recent negative life events

Table 25.2 Criteria for major depression

Five or more of the following lasting at least 2 weeks with at least one of the symptoms is either (1) depressed mood or (2) loss of interest or pleasure
Depressed mood most of the day, nearly every day
Markedly diminished pleasure or interest in most things, most of the day, nearly every day
Decrease or increase in appetite nearly every day
Difficulty concentrating
Psychomotor retardation or agitation
Insomnia or hypersomnia nearly every day
Fatigue or loss of energy nearly every day
Feelings of guilt or worthlessness
Reoccurring thoughts of death or suicide

screening questions concerning mood, appetite, level of energy, outlook regarding pregnancy, and outlook about the future in general.

Diagnosing depression during pregnancy is done via the clinical interview and by obtaining collateral information from the expectant mother's support system, if available. The *Diagnostic and Statistical Manual of Mental Disorders* (DSM-IVR) defines a major depressive episode as having sustained low mood or significant irritability for at least 2 weeks in addition to at least four other symptoms of depression (**Table 25.2**).

Treatment

Treatment of depression during pregnancy is a complicated issue with multiple factors to consider for both the mother and the developing child. Treatment consists of both medication and/or nonpharmacologic interventions. Although it is widely accepted that optimal treatment for a major depressive episode involves a combination of medicine and psychotherapy, in pregnancy this may not be the case. The first question that must be addressed is whether to treat with psychopharmacologic interventions at all. Either option can have serious consequences for both mother and fetus.

Decision not to use medications: It is important to understand the impact of untreated depression on the mother and fetus in order for the expectant mother and her doctor to decide the best course of action. Consequences of untreated depression can result in maternal behaviors that are particularly harmful to both herself and her child. These include a general disregard for a healthy life style or continued smoking, alcohol or substance use, poor prenatal care, and poor nutrition despite medical advice to the contrary.

The depression also can lead to an increased risk of suicide. Overall, untreated depression during pregnancy is a significant risk for postpartum depression, which also poses serious risks to mother and new baby.

The impact of untreated depression on the fetus is more complicated and may involve immediate and long-term developmental issues (**Table 25.3**).

Additionally, a number of behavioral problems in the child are correlated to untreated depression in the mother, including language and cognitive development, impulsivity, attention deficit disorder, behavioral dyscontrol, and sleep problems (Evidence Box 25.1). The reasons that maternal stress and depression lead to obstetric and post-term difficulties are still unclear. However, it is believed that there are strong connections to the role of the levels of placental corticotropin-releasing hormone on immune function, increased catecholamines, and uterine vascular changes.

Discontinuation of antidepressants: One question frequently arises with a pregnant woman who is on medication for depression and doing well: Should the medicine be discontinued? The answer, again, is complicated and highly case-specific. However, it is important for both the clinician and mother to understand that the risk of reoccurrence of depression following discontinuation of treatment is high, particularly in the first trimester.

Studies have shown that 68–75 % of patients experience return of depression following discontinuation of treatment. Nevertheless, discontinuation of antidepressant

Table 25.3 Impact of untreated depression on developing fetus

Preterm delivery
Miscarriage
Low Apgar scores
↓ birth weight
Small for gestational age
↑ neonatal cortisol levels

medication may be attempted with careful monitoring if a woman has been stable for years and has simply been hesitant to come off medication for fear of relapse prior to pregnancy. This may be particularly so in a depression that has been at the milder end of the spectrum.

Factors to consider in discontinuing medication include:
1. The severity of depression and any accompanying psychotic or suicidal symptoms
2. The impact on function, including work and home activities
3. Other children who are also dependent on the expecting mother for care

It is important to weigh the risks and the benefits of treating versus not treating, remembering that whatever decision is made at a given time can be reversed if the situation changes. However, a woman who opts to discontinue antidepressant medication must be closely monitored for return of symptoms, so that therapeutic interventions can be initiated quickly to prevent more serious complications later on.

Medications for depression: Understanding the impact of psychotropic medications on the developing fetus is confusing and complicated. The majority of studies are small and not well controlled. Often what appears in the literature are single case reports without clear correlation between the findings in the baby and other exposures or maternal factors. Further, replicating findings of drug effects have been inconsistent and contradictory, making the decision as to whether or not to use medications particularly challenging.

A comprehensive discussion of each medication with supporting data is beyond the scope of this chapter. Rather, it provides some generally accepted guidelines to follow when considering the use of medications in a pregnant woman, as well as the safety profile of common antidepressant medications.

The selective serotonin reuptake inhibitors (SSRIs) have become the mainstay of treatment for major depression. Research has clearly demonstrated that all antidepressants pass the placental barrier and are detectable in the umbilical cord blood and amniotic fluid, thus resulting in fetal exposure. Two recent meta-analyses done on SSRIs found that they were not associated with an increased risk of major or minor malformations above the general population baseline. Another study done in Denmark looking at the teratogenicity data from 151 800 births of mothers who took SSRIs early in pregnancy showed a 1.34 increased relative risk for congenital malformations. Thus, when considering all of the information available in the literature, the absolute risk is low.

The use of fluoxetine, sertraline, fluvoxamine, and citalopram is considered safe. In 2005, paroxetine was changed from class C to D due to some reports of increased risk of cardiac malformations with first-trimester exposure, although other studies have not shown this. The tricyclic antidepressants, venlafaxine, mirtazapine, bupropion, trazadone, and nefaxodone are thought to be equally low in risk for congenital malformations.

Another consideration when prescribing medications is their impact in the neonatal period. Due to low but detectable drug levels in the fetus at birth, coupled with a sudden discontinuation of exposure due to delivery and loss of maternal supply, both newborn toxicity and withdrawal reactions have been reported. Both of these complications result from third- trimester antidepressant use by the mother and are typically mild, short term, and manageable, if recognized and monitored carefully. Fluoxetine and paroxetine are more likely to be associated with these symptoms (**Table 25.4**).

Pulmonary hypertension: The newest concern with fetal exposure to SSRIs is persistent pulmonary hypertension of the newborn (PPHN). It has been established that maternal use of aspirin, anti-inflammatory drugs, smoking during pregnancy, and maternal diabetes are all risk factors for this SSRI-induced complication. First reported in the mid-1990s, more recent studies have demonstrated increased confidence in the association between SSRI exposure and PPHN.

A recent prospective study involving 506 infants in Sweden found that maternal use of SSRIs during pregnancy increased the risk for PPHN, and exposure after week 20 carries a higher risk than early pregnancy exposure. This effect was seen among infants born after 34 completed weeks of gestation. Although the general population risk for PPHN is 1–2 births per 1000, exposure during late pregnancy can raise this to 3 births per 1000, a small but statistically significant increase.

Strategies in the Use of Medications

When contemplating the use of antidepressant medication in pregnancy, several strategies are useful to consider in order to minimize the risk to the fetus while supporting the health and wellbeing of the mother.

Table 25.4 Symptoms of neonatal toxicity/withdrawal syndrome

Poor muscle tone
Weak cry
Respiratory distress
Hypoglycemia
Low Apgar score
Jitteriness
Irritability

1. When feasible and safe for the mother, avoid the use of antidepressants during the first trimester, as organ development is most critical during this time. If the expectant mother has been stable for a long period prior to pregnancy, has historically had a mild or moderate degree of depression, and is willing to taper offantidepressants for the first trimester, this may be reasonable to try. Further, if a pregnant woman begins to develop depressive symptoms during the first trimester but these remain manageable with non-pharmacologic treatments, it may be a good idea to hold off initiating antidepressants until she is past the first trimester.
2. Use the lowest, effective dose when prescribing antidepressants during pregnancy.
3. If it is safe for the mother, try to reduce neonatal complications by reducing exposure during the third trimester, particularly if fluoxetine or paroxetine is being used. Although anticipating delivery is almost impossible, tapering over several weeks starting approximately 3 weeks before the estimated date of delivery, usually provides enough time to eliminate the drug from circulation and reduce toxicity or withdrawal symptoms in the newborn.
4. Remember that all decisions can be reconsidered. If an attempt to minimize fetal exposure is made and the mother becomes increasingly depressed, the medication can always be resumed. It is critical, however, to look at the history of response to medication initiation and treatment of an individual before attempting a change in any treatment status. If a given patient has a history of severe relapse of symptoms following discontinuation of medication, then it should not be considered.

Bipolar Disorder

Bipolar Disorder is one of the most challenging psychiatric illnesses to manage during pregnancy. This is because the majority of medications used to treat bipolar illness are contraindicated during the first trimester of pregnancy. A woman who presents to the obstetrician and is actively being treated for, or has a history of, bipolar illness should be closely monitored by a psychiatrist. Most mood stabilizers, including lithium, valproic acid, and carbamazepine, have a significant risk for causing congenital malformations. It is strongly recommended to avoid the use of all of these in the first trimester. They should be used cautiously in subsequent trimesters, and only if no alternatives exist and the mother is at great risk.

Anxiety

Anxiety is a common disorder with a lifetime prevalence of 33% in women. However, peak onset of these symptoms is during the childbearing years. It is not uncommon for a woman to presenting to her obstetrician while being actively treated for generalized anxiety disorder (GAD), obsessive compulsive disorder (OCD), or more specific phobias.

The impact of untreated anxiety on the developing child is not insignificant and includes sleep disorders, altered electroencephalogram activation and increased heart rate. Furthermore, exposure to high maternal anxiety has been associated with developmental delays in newborns and increased risk for behavioral and emotional problems in young children.

Symptoms of anxiety include restlessness, insomnia, poor appetite, fatigue, and difficulty with concentration in the context of normal mood. First-line therapies for anxiety in pregnancy are nonpharmacologic and include interpersonal psychotherapy or cognitive behavioral therapy. Marital therapy is also helpful in the face of poor marital relationships that might be precipitating or aggravating a pre-existing state.

Pharmacologic treatments of anxiety can be used when other interventions are ineffective, and the anxiety is having a major impact on maternal function. SSRIs are the first-line pharmacologic treatment due to their lower teratogenic risk. The use of benzodiazepines is contraindicated in the first trimester due to increased risk of cleft palate malformation and during the third trimester due to neonatal toxicity and neonatal withdrawal. **Table 25.5** summarizes the signs and symptoms of each of these complications.

Table 25.5 Effects of benzodiazepine exposure on the neonate

Neonatal toxicity	Neonatal withdrawal symptoms
Hypothermia	Restlessness
Lethargy	Irritability
Poor respiratory effort	Abnormal sleep
Feeding difficulties	Suckling difficulties
	Growth retardation
	Hypertonia/ hyperreflexia
	Tremulousness
	Apnea
	Diarrhea/vomiting

Nonpharmacologic Treatments of Depression and Anxiety

The use of nonpharmacologic interventions during pregnancy, if effective, can reduce the risk of medication exposure to the unborn child and give the mother more of a sense of control over experience. Alternatives to medications include psychoeducation on stress management and relaxation, cognitive behavioral therapy for depression and anxiety, supportive psychotherapy focused on the dynamic issues of the impact of pregnancy on the mother, enhancement of social supports, and engaging the father as a supportive ally.

Schizophrenia and Other Psychotic Disorders

When presented with a pregnant woman who has a severe psychotic disorder, the obstetrician must carefully coordinate care of the patient with the treating psychiatrist to assist with maintaining stable mental health. Pregnancies in this population are often unplanned and are complicated by poor prenatal care, poor nutrition, and increased use of drugs or alcohol. They, thus, should be considered high risk.

Careful management of the mental illness is critical to the health of the pregnancy and wellbeing of the mother and child. A poorly managed psychotic illness during pregnancy places the mother and child at great risk after delivery, as worsening of a serious mental illness is often seen within the first 3 months.

When considering the selection of medications, the use of traditional antipsychotics to manage active symptoms is advised owing to their long track record of use in pregnant women with low risk. Haloperidol, although not completely risk free, is the medication of choice given its high potency with fewer sedation, anticholinergic, and cardiovascular effects than other antipsychotic medicines. The use of the more popular atypical antipsychotic medications have not been extensively studied, and there are no double-blind, controlled studies on their use in pregnancy.

To date there have been no reported congenital anomalies with the use of risperidone or quetiapine in pregnancy. However, the metabolic syndrome is associated with these medications, and its impact on pregnancy and the developing fetus has yet to be determined. Thus, these medications should be used with great caution, and the expecting mother should be referred to a psychiatrist who is able to provide specialized treatment during pregnancy.

Postpartum Mood Disorders

Screening

As previously stated, 20% of women will experience an episode of depression at some time in their life, and 13% of all women who carry a child to term will experience postpartum depression. Untreated mood disorders in the antenatal period have significant impact on the mother–infant relationship, which lays the groundwork for the psychological and physiological development of the child.

In addition to the impact of exposure to higher cortisol levels discussed earlier, the newborn of a depressed mother is at risk for neglect, which may result in insecure attachment, social interaction difficulties, and behavior problems. Signs of developing problems are evident as early as 2 months of age as the infant may demonstrate trouble engaging in social and object interactions, interact less with the mother, show less happy affect and more negative affect, and show lower activity levels.

Given the severe impact on the newborn and the prominence of mood disorders as well as the high rate of lack of identification and treatment, it is imperative that the obstetrician incorporate standard screening for depression.

There are many brief, easy to use, self-administered screening assessments. The Edinburgh Postnatal Depression Scale, for example, is a 10-question, easy to score, self-administered scale that has been validated in the US population. A cutoff score of 9 or 10 is recommended as a first-stage screen, and is a reliable indicator of the presence of postpartum depression in women. It should be administered within the first 4 weeks postpartum.

Postpartum Blues or the "Baby Blues"

Considered to be a self-limiting condition that occurs in 30–75% of new mothers, the postpartum blues is a transient mood disturbance. Symptoms typically occur within the first week of delivery, last a few hours to a few days and are characterized by mood lability and crying. A significant association between maternity blues and postpartum depression and anxiety disorders also has been reported, thus highlighting the importance of routine screening, early recognition, and treatment of postpartum mood disorders.

Postpartum Depression

Postpartum depression is an episode of major depression that begins within the first 3 months after delivery. Symptoms are similar to those of a Major Depression as described by the DSM-IV manual. Diagnosis follows the identical criteria shown in **Table 25.2**. Causes are thought to bear some relationship to decline in levels of reproductive hormones that occurs after delivery in susceptible women. Other risk factors include history of previous depression, poverty, unplanned pregnancy, poor social support, and adolescent pregnancy.

The greatest concern for a new mother suffering from a postpartum depression is the impact on the mother–child relationship and the mother's ability to care for herself and the child. In the worst-case scenarios, preoccupation with plans to harm oneself and possibly the newborn put the mother and child at great risk. Other consequences include general neglect of the infant leading to inadequate stimulation, nurturing, feeding, dressing, or attention to infant safety. Thus, it is critical for the physician to recognize the symptoms of postpartum depression early, and initiate appropriate treatment to sustain the function and wellbeing of mother and child.

Treatment

Treatment for a newly detected or a recurrent depression should be aggressive and comprehensive. Both medications and non-pharmacologic interventions should be discussed in the first visit. In recurrent cases of major depression, it is always wise to resume a course of treatment that has been effective in the past.

As stated earlier, the standard first-line treatment is an SSRI. Venlafaxine and bupropion, which are also safe and effective antidepressants, should be considered. Other adjunctive medications, including mood stabilizers and antipsychotics, must be carefully considered, particularly when the mother is breast-feeding.

Breast-Feeding and Psychotropic Medications

In addition to the well-known benefits of breast-feeding to the newborn—including decreased risk of otitis media, respiratory tract infections, atopic dermatitis, gastroenteritis, type 2 diabetes, sudden infant death, and obesity—the intimate nature of the breast-feeding process facilitates the bonding between mother and baby. Mothers who express a desire to breast-feed their babies should be encouraged to do so. It is the responsibility of the clinician to be knowledgeable and educate the new mother in how to best safely nurse her baby.

It has been well established that all psychotropic medications are excreted in the breast milk. However, resulting infant plasma concentrations vary widely, ranging from higher concentrations resulting in adverse events in the infant to nondetectable levels and no adverse events.

Most drugs are detected in the infant plasma but there have been no reports of adverse events. Thus, for a mother who desires to breast-feed, there are enough safe medications available to allow her to do so without placing her baby in harm's way. **Table 25.6** lists the most commonly used antidepressant medications, whether or not they enter the infant's blood through the breast milk, and whether or not there are any reported adverse events.

Table 25.6 Safety profile of commonly used antidepressants

Medicine	Infant plasma conc. detectable	Adverse events reported
Fluoxetine	Yes	Yes
Fluvoxamine	No	No
Paroxetine	No	No
Sertraline	Yes	No
Citalopram	Yes	Yes*
Venlafaxine	Yes	No
Bupropion	No	No
Mirtazapine	No	No

* One case report of a possible infant seizure following exposure to bupropion through maternal breast milk.

Of note, there have been only two case reports of infants experiencing colicky symptoms and toxicity following exposure to fluoxetine through breast milk. In both cases complications resolved with discontinuation of the maternal drug.

Postpartum Psychosis

The occurrence of a psychotic event in the postpartum period presents an even greater risk to the mother and child given the higher risk of hospital admission. Unlike nonpsychotic postpartum depression, genetic and psychosocial risk factors for postpartum psychosis have not yet been identified. A previous psychotic event related or unrelated to pregnancy is the most likely risk factor. A bipolar manic episode is the most likely cause. Symptoms are classified similar to any other psychotic event and include auditory hallucinations, delusions, and/or ideas of reference. Infanticide is often associated with a postpartum psychotic episode that is characterized by command hallucinations to kill the infant or delusions that the infant is demonic.

Postpartum psychosis is a very dangerous illness and is considered a psychiatric emergency that typically requires acute hospitalization. Rapid initiation of antipsychotic and mood stabilizing medications is needed to restore the mother's rational thinking and behavior.

The standard of care includes the use of atypical antipsychotic drugs along with lithium or valproic acid. The use of lithium during the postpartum period as a preventative measure reduces the risk of recurrent postpartum illness in women with histories of bipolar disorder or puerperal psychosis.

Breast-feeding issues

As with the antidepressants, all antipsychotic and mood stabilizing medications are excreted in the breast milk. Although this is naturally a major concern in women with major psychiatric symptoms who want to breast-feed, the risk to the infant is quite low. To date no relationship has been found between the infant's serum levels and neurobehavioral development. Even the use of lithium in the nursing mother, once contraindicated, is now considered an option. A recent study of 10 infants of mothers on lithium was followed up measuring maternal serum and breast milk concentrations, infant serum levels, and infant renal and thyroid functions. Serum levels in nursing infants were low and well tolerated. One cautionary note is that the clinician should avoid the use of clozapine, owing to the liability of inducing potential life-threatening events in the infant, and olanzapine, which is associated with an increased risk of inducing extrapyramidal reactions in infants.

Nonpharmacologic Approaches in the Postpartum Period

In addition to medication, there are several other interventions that are critical components of an approach to maximizing treatment outcomes. The first of these includes psycho-education for the mother and father as they come to understand what is happening to the woman psychologically, which treatments are available, estimated time lines to understand the course of the symptoms, and what this means for future pregnancies.

Letting a mother with psychiatric issues know that she isn't alone in this experience can be especially therapeutic for her. Thus, enhancing psychosocial support with extra help when the mother is feeling overwhelmed is critical to reducing stress, as are enhancing sleep and shortening the course of the illness. Individual and group therapy are also very useful interventions, as they may allow the woman to face psychological conflicts regarding motherhood and adapt to new role.

In the event that a woman's depression worsens, the new mother should never be left alone. Rather, she should be surrounded with support and plenty of understanding. Protection of the mother and the infant is of utmost priority while the illness is resolving. And finally, at the appropriate time, a discussion of what all of this means for future pregnancies is very important. Because a woman has had an episode of psychiatric illness during pregnancy, it does not mean that she can never have another child. Rather, she will have to be more closely monitored in the event of a subsequent pregnancy. Every effort to prevent a second episode is important to ensuring a happy experience and a positive outcome.

Key Points

- Caring for a woman with mental illness during pregnancy is complex and includes the care of both the mother and child in the postpartum period.
- Discussing the possibility of having a baby is perhaps one of the most important issues to address when caring for a woman in childbearing years with a history of mental illness.
- Increased stress during pregnancy leads to an increased likelihood of emotional instability and an exacerbation any underlying mental illness.
- Serotonin reuptake inhibitors have been shown safe in the treatment of depression in pregnancy, although there is a small risk of side effects in the infant.
- The majority of medications used to treat bipolar illness are contraindicated during the first trimester of pregnancy.
- The use of nonpharmacologic interventions during pregnancy, if effective, can reduce the risk of medication exposure to the unborn child and give the mother more sense of control over experience.

Evidence Box 25.1

Depression during pregnancy increases infants risk of sleep disturbances in the immediate postpartum period.

Armitage et al. evaluated whether sleep over the first 6 months of life was more disturbed in infants born to mothers who were depressed compared with infants from nondepressed women. The investigators recorded the sleep patterns of 18 babies (9 male and 9 female) for seven consecutive days starting at 2 weeks postpartum and monthly thereafter until 6 months of age. The babies mothers were asked to complete daily sleep/wake diaries. Seven infants were born to women with no personal or family history of depression; 11 infants were born to women diagnosed with depression or with elevated levels of depression symptoms. The researchers then computed total sleep time, sleep latency, sleep efficiency, and number and duration of sleep episodes for nocturnal and daytime sleep in each 24-hour block. This study found that infants born to the depressive mothers took longer to fall asleep, had lower sleep efficiencies, and had more sleep bouts in the nocturnal sleep period than did low-risk infants, and these effects persisted at 6 months postpartum. Based on this small study, the authors concluded that maternal depression is associated with significant sleep disturbance in infancy at 2 weeks postpartum and that this phenomenon persists at 24 weeks postpartum. They cautioned, however, that it remains to be determined whether sleep disturbance in infancy confers a greater risk of developing early-onset depression in childhood.

Armitage R, Flynn H, Hoffmann R, Vazquez D, Lopez J, Marcus S. Early developmental changes in sleep in infants: the impact of maternal depression. Sleep 2009 May 1;32(5):693–696

Further Reading

Armitage R, Flynn H, Hoffmann R, Vazquez D, Lopez J, Marcus S. Early developmental changes in sleep in infants: the impact of maternal depression. *Sleep* 2009;32(5):693–696

Einarson TR, Einarson A. Newer antidepressants in pregnancy and rates of major malformations: a meta-analysis of prospective comparative studies. *Pharmacoepidemiol Drug Saf* 2005;14(12):823–827

Gentile S. The safety of newer antidepressants in pregnancy and breastfeeding. *Drug Saf* 2005;28(2):137–152

Hale TW, Shum S, Grossberg M. Fluoxetine toxicity in a breast-fed infant. *Clin Pediatr (Phila)* 2001;40(12):681–684

Hollins K. Consequences of antenatal mental health problems for child health and development. *Curr Opin Obstet Gynecol* 2007;19(6):568–572

Källén B, Olausson PO. Maternal use of selective serotonin reuptake inhibitors and persistent pulmonary hypertension of the newborn. *Pharmacoepidemiol Drug Saf* 2008;17(8):801–806

Lester BM, Cucca J, Andreozzi L, Flanagan P, Oh W. Possible association between fluoxetine hydrochloride and colic in an infant. *J Am Acad Child Adolesc Psychiatry* 1993;32(6):1253–1255

Levey L, Ragan K, Hower-Hartley A, Newport DJ, Stowe ZN. Psychiatric disorders in pregnancy. *Neurol Clin* 2004;22(4):863–893

Moses-Kolko EL, Bogen D, Perel J, et al. Neonatal signs after late in utero exposure to serotonin reuptake inhibitors: literature review and implications for clinical applications. *JAMA* 2005;293(19):2372–2383

Nordeng H, Spigset O. Treatment with selective serotonin reuptake inhibitors in the third trimester of pregnancy: effects on the infant. *Drug Saf* 2005;28(7):565–581

Pearlstein T. Perinatal depression: treatment options and dilemmas. *J Psychiatry Neurosci* 2008;33(4):302–318

Petterson SM, Albers AB. Effects of poverty and maternal depression on early child development. *Child Dev* 2001;72(6):1794–1813

Rahimi R, Nikfar S, Abdollahi M. Pregnancy outcomes following exposure to serotonin reuptake inhibitors: a meta-analysis of clinical trials. *Reprod Toxicol* 2006;22(4):571–575

Viguera AC, Newport DJ, Ritchie J, et al. Lithium in breast milk and nursing infants: clinical implications. *Am J Psychiatry* 2007;164(2):342–345

Wogelius P, Nørgaard M, Gislum M, et al. Maternal use of selective serotonin reuptake inhibitors and risk of congenital malformations. *Epidemiology* 2006;17(6):701–704

Yaeger D, Smith HG, Altshuler LL. Atypical antipsychotics in the treatment of schizophrenia during pregnancy and the postpartum. *Am J Psychiatry* 2006;163(12):2064–2070

26 Other Medical Complications in Pregnancy

E. Albert Reece

This chapter discusses medical complications that commonly arise in pregnancy but are not covered elsewhere in this book. It includes a discussion of asthma, back pain, cholestasis and cholesytitis (two common, pregnancy-related liver disorders), diabetes, gastric motility disorders, and thyroid problems.

Definitions

Asthma: This is a chronic respiratory disease, in which the airways unexpectedly and suddenly narrow, often in response to an allergen, cold air, exercise, or emotional stress. Symptoms include wheezing, shortness of breath, chest tightness, and coughing.

Back pain: This term refers to a pain felt in the back that usually originates from the muscles, nerves, bones, joints or other structures in the spine.

Cholestasis: This is a condition in which the normal flow of bile in the gallbladder is affected by the high amounts of pregnancy hormones. It is more common in the last trimester of pregnancy when hormones are at their peak, but it usually goes away within a few days after delivery. Cholestasis is sometimes referred to as *extrahepatic cholestasis*, which occurs outside the liver, *intrahepatic cholestasis*, which occurs inside the liver, or *obstetric cholestasis*.

Cholecystitis: This is an acute or chronic inflammation of the gallbladder and the second most common nonobstetric surgical condition in pregnancy (after appendicitis). Acute cholecystitis is usually the result of a gallstone impacted in the cystic duct.

Diabetes: This is a disease in which the body doesn't produce or properly use insulin. There are three major kinds of diabetes: type 1, type 2, and gestational diabetes. *Type 1 diabetes* is attributed to about 5 to 10 percent of all diabetic patients in the United States and results from the body's failure to produce insulin. *Type 2 diabetes* accounts for about 90 to 95 percent of the all diabetic patients in the United States and results from the body's inability to produce sufficient amounts of insulin as well as the body's resistance to insulin, which means that the body doesn't use insulin effectively. *Gestational diabetes* is diabetes that arises or is diagnosed in pregnancy. It accounts for about 135 000 diabetic patients annually in the United States and occurs in approximately four percent of pregnant women. While most women recover from gestational diabetes after they give birth, they have an increased risk of developing type 2 diabetes in the future.

Gastrointestinal motility disorders: This phrase is used to describe a variety of disorders in which the gut loses its ability to coordinate muscular activity, owing to aberrant endogenous or exogenous causes. Intestinal motility disorders may be primitive or secondary and may manifest in a variety of ways including: abdominal distension and recurrent obstruction; severe abdominal colicky pain; severe constipation; and gastroesophageal reflux disease or intractable, recurrent vomiting.

Thyroid disorder: This disorder occurs when the thyroid gland is unable to supply the appropriate amounts of hormone to the body. As a result, the body's metabolism and growth functions may not operate properly. The most common types of thyroid disease include: 1) *hypothyroidism*, in which the thyroid gland does not release enough hormones, and 2) *hyperthyroidism*, in which the thyroid gland produces too much hormones.

Diagnosis

Asthma

Although the woman's symptoms, medical history, and physical examination may suggest that she has asthma, it may be necessary to perform lung function tests to confirm an asthma diagnosis. Lung function tests may include:

Spirometry. This is a noninvasive technique that measures how well a person breathes. During spirometry, the patient takes deep breaths and forcefully exhales into a hose connected to a machine called a spirometer (**Fig. 26.1**). Spirometry testing reveals two measurements that are important in diagnosing asthma: 1) forced vital capacity (FVC), which is the maximum amount of air someone can inhale and exhale, and 2) forced expiratory volume (FEV_1), which is the maximum amount of air a person can exhale in 1 second. If certain key measurements are below normal for a person's age, it may be a sign that that their airway is obstructed.

Challenge test. This test involves deliberately trying to trigger airway obstruction and asthma symptoms by having the patient inhale an airway-constricting substance or take several breaths of cold air. If the patient appears to have exercise-induced asthma, you may want to ask her to do vigorous physical activity to trigger symptoms. After triggering the symptoms, readminister the spirometry test. If the patient's spirometry measurements are still normal, it is likely that she does not have asthma. On the other hand, if her measurements have fallen significantly, it may mean she has asthma.

Back Pain

The most common, noninvasive diagnostic test performed in pregnant women with sacroiliac pain is the posterior pelvic provocation test (**Fig. 26.2**). The test is considered positive if it reproduces the woman's back pain; it has been shown to be 81% sensitive and 80% specific for sacroiliac pain. Other physical exams and findings used to localize pain to the sacroiliac joint include the following:

- The ventral gapping test reproduces pain in the region of the symptomatic sacroiliac joint when the pelvis is manually pressed apart.
- The dorsal gapping test reproduces pain when the pelvis is compressed together while the woman is lying supine.
- The sacroiliac joint fixation test evaluates the mobility of the sacroiliac joint as a standing woman flexes forward. It is positive if the posterior superior iliac spine on the side with pain is level or lower than the pain-free side while the woman is standing, and then is higher than the pain-free side as the woman flexes forward.
- The Patrick test, or FABERE maneuver, is another test to evaluate sacroiliac pain. The test is positive if back pain is reproduced when the examiner depresses the knee of the flexed leg. The term "fabere" is derived from the first letter(s) of the words involved in the maneuver: flexion, abduction, external rotation, and extension.
- The Derbolowski test is done first with the woman in a sitting position, then lying supine. The test is positive if the positions of the medial malleoli change in relation to one another when the woman is sitting or lying down.

In some cases, however, a computed tomography scan or magnetic resonance imaging scan is needed to get a better look at the underlying cause of back pain.

Cholestasis

Cholestasis is diagnosed by a complete medical history, physical examination, and blood tests that evaluate liver function, bile acids, and bilirubin.

Cholecystitis

Accurately diagnosing cholecystitis requires verification that the woman's abdominal pain is caused by gallstones and not by some other condition that can mimic a gallbladder attack, such as acute appendicitis, inflammatory bowel disease (Crohn disease or ulcerative colitis), pneumonia, stomach ulcers, gastroesophageal reflux and hiatal hernia, viral hepatitis, kidney stones, urinary tract infections, diverticulosis or diverticulitis, pregnancy complications, and even heart attack.

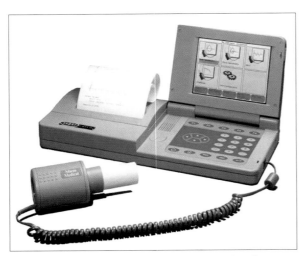

Fig. 26.1   A digital spirometer used for measuring lung function.

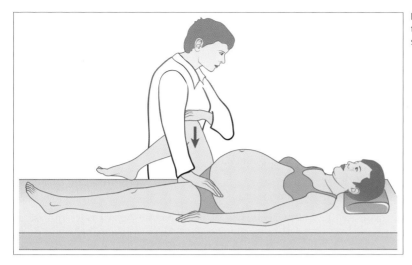

Fig. 26.2 The posterior pelvic provocation test is commonly used to help diagnose sacroiliac back pain in pregnancy.

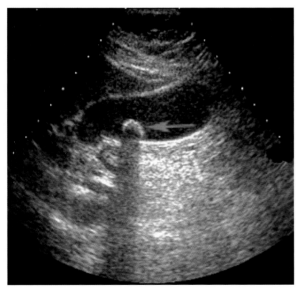

Fig. 26.3 A gallstone (red arrow) within the gallbladder produces a bright surface echo and causes a dark acoustic shadow (S).

Ultrasound or other imaging techniques can usually detect gallstones (**Fig. 26.3**). Nevertheless, because gallstones are common and most cause no symptoms, simply finding stones does not necessarily explain a patient's pain. In patients with known gallstones, the doctor can often diagnose acute cholecystitis (gallbladder inflammation) based on classic symptoms (constant and severe pain in the upper right quadrant of the abdomen). Imaging techniques are necessary to confirm the diagnosis. There is usually no tenderness in chronic cholecystitis.

Diabetes

The following tests are used to diagnose diabetes:

- A fasting plasma glucose (FPG) test measures blood glucose in a person who has not eaten anything for at least 8 hours. This test is used to detect diabetes and prediabetes.
- An oral glucose tolerance test (OGTT) measures blood glucose after a person fasts at least 8 hours and 2 hours after the person drinks a glucose-containing beverage. This test can be used to diagnose diabetes and prediabetes.
- A random plasma glucose test, also called a casual plasma glucose test, measures blood glucose without regard to when the person being tested last ate. This test, along with an assessment of symptoms, is used to diagnose diabetes but not prediabetes.

Test results indicating that a person has diabetes should be confirmed with a second test on a different day.

Gestational diabetes is also diagnosed based on plasma glucose values measured during the OGTT, preferably by using 100 g of glucose in the liquid for the test. Blood glucose levels are checked four times during the test. If blood glucose levels are above normal at least twice during the test, the woman has gestational diabetes. **Table 26.1** shows the above-normal results for the OGTT for gestational diabetes.

Gastrointestinal Motility Disorders

The modes of diagnosing motility disorders are as diverse as the disorders themselves and are beyond the scope of this chapter. However, the methods used to diagnose functional gastrointestinal disorders (including motility disorders) are chosen based on a patient's symptoms. To make the diagnosis as consistent as possible, a group of

Table 26.1 Gestational diabetes: above-normal results for the oral glucose tolerance test

When	Plasma glucose result (mg/dL)
Fasting	95 or higher
At 1 hour	180 or higher
At 2 hours	155 or higher
At 3 hours	140 or higher

more than 100 international experts created the Rome criteria. Rome III, published in 2006, provides the most current diagnostic criteria for all of the functional gastrointestinal disorders (see Further Reading).

Thyroid Disorder

If hypothyroidism is suspected in a pregnant patient, the physician can perform a thyroid stimulating hormone (TSH) blood test. Just as in nonpregnant women, the TSH level will be increased if hypothyroidism is present.

The diagnosis of hyperthyroidism in pregnancy can be complicated, however, since some of the blood tests used for the diagnosis are altered because of the pregnancy. The diagnosis is based on high levels of thyroid hormones, T3 and T4, and a low level of TSH.

Prevalence and Epidemiology

Asthma

Asthma is the most common lung disorder during pregnancy. At any given time, up to 8% of pregnant women have asthma. The factors that increase or decrease the risk of developing asthma during pregnancy are not entirely clear. The likelihood of these attacks is not constant throughout pregnancy. It is at its highest during weeks 17 through 24 of pregnancy.

Although the vast majority of pregnant women with asthma and their babies have no complications, pregnant women with asthma do have a small increase in the risk for certain complications of pregnancy. Compared to women who do not have asthma, women with asthma are slightly more likely to have high blood pressure or pre-eclampsia, a premature delivery, a cesarean delivery, or a baby that is small for its age.

Back Pain

Reports suggest that between 50% and 80% of all pregnant women have back pain sometime during their pregnan-

cy. It occurs more frequently later in the pregnancy as the weight of the baby increases. Although long-term pain is very rare, short-term pain tends to be dominant. Usually during the third trimester, 50% of pregnant patients will experience back pain. In contrast, by the postpartum period only about 9% of women experience back pain.

Cholestasis

Cholestasis occurs in about 1 of 1000 pregnancies but is more common in Swedish and Chilean ethnic groups.

Cholecystitis

The incidence of symptomatic biliary tract disease is 0.16% in pregnancy. However, approximately 80% of women with symptoms of gallbladder disease experience their first attack within one year of pregnancy, which seems to predispose women to developing biliary tract disease (see Etiology and Pathophysiology below).

Diabetes

Abnormal maternal glucose regulation occurs in 3–10% of pregnancies. Gestational diabetes mellitus accounts for 90% of cases of diabetes mellitus in pregnancy. Type 2 diabetes mellitus accounts for 8% of cases of diabetes mellitus in pregnancy. Given its increasing incidence, pre-existing diabetes mellitus now affects 1% of pregnancies. Studies suggest that the prevalence of diabetes among women of childbearing age is increasing in the United States. This increase is believed to be attributable to more sedentary life styles, changes in diet, continued immigration from high-risk populations, and the virtual epidemic of childhood and adolescent obesity that is presently evolving in United States (see Etiology and Pathophysiology below).

Gastrointestinal Motility Disorders

The average incidence is 3.5 per 1000 deliveries.

Thyroid Disorder

Thyroid disease is present in 2–5% of all women and 1–2% of women in the reproductive age group. Thus, thyroid problems are common in women who are pregnant.

Etiology and Pathophysiology

Asthma

Being pregnant has a significant impact on a woman's respiratory physiology. Although the respiratory rate and vital capacity do not change in pregnancy, there is an increase in tidal volume, minute ventilation, and minute oxygen uptake, which lead to a decrease in functional residual capacity and residual volume of air as a consequence of the elevated diaphragm. There is also an increase in airway conductance, while total pulmonary resistance is reduced, possibly as a result of progesterone.

Due to all of these physiological changes, pregnant women often have episodes of hyperventilation in the latter half of pregnancy. This may lead to a chronic respiratory alkalosis during pregnancy with a decreased Pco_2, decreased bicarbonate, and increased pH. The increases in minute ventilation and improved pulmonary function in pregnancy promote more efficient gas exchange from the maternal lungs to the blood. Therefore, changes in respiratory status occur more rapidly in pregnancy than in the nonpregnant patient.

Back Pain

The etiology of low back pain during pregnancy remains speculative. However, the scientific literature mentions as least three potential, pregnancy-related mechanisms: 1) biomechanical/musculoskeletal, 2) hormonal, and 3) vascular. In light of the variable clinical presentation of low back pain during pregnancy, a multifaceted etiology is an appropriate assumption.

Cholestasis

The etiology of choleostasis is not completely understood. Genetic, hormonal, and environmental factors may contribute to its pathogenesis. Clinical evidence suggests that estrogens play a role in the initiation of cholestasis. Indeed, cholestasis most commonly occurs in the last trimester, when estrogen levels reach their maximum. Also, the use of estrogen-containing oral contraceptives among women with a personal or family history of cholestasis could result in clinical features of cholestasis.

Progesterone and associated metabolites also may be involved in the pathogenesis of cholestasis, as significantly increased plasma levels of mono- or disulfated progesterone metabolites and an increased ratio of 3α-hydroxylated steroids to 3β-hydroxylated steroids have been found is some patients with cholestasis. High levels of the estrogens, glucuronides, and progesterone lead to the impairment of the function of major hepatocellular ABC transporters, such as the bile salt export pump, ABCB11, or the phospholipid transporter, and ABCB4 (MDR3), respectively. In addition, estrogens impair basolateral as well as canalicular bile acid transporter expression of liver cells *in vitro* by transcriptional mechanisms.

Thus, mutations in genes encoding hepatobiliary transport proteins as well as abnormal metabolites impairing hepatobiliary carriers may be involved in the pathogenesis of cholestasis.

Cholecystitis

Gallbladder function is sensitive to pregnancy hormones, which may cause a marked slowing down or stopping of the flow of bile. The gallbladder holds bile that is produced in the liver, which is necessary in the breakdown of fats in digestion. When the bile flow is slowed down or stopped, this causes a build-up of bile acids in the liver, which can spill into the bloodstream.

Since the developing baby relies on the mother's liver to remove bile acids from the blood, the elevated levels of maternal bile cause stress on the fetus's liver and can increase the risks for fetal distress, preterm birth, or stillbirth. Women with cholestasis need to monitored closely, and labor should be induced once the developing baby's lungs have reached maturity (see Management below).

Diabetes

Type 1 diabetes appears to stem from an inherited defect in the immune system, triggered by environmental stimuli. The exact cause of the disease is still unknown; however, scientists have identified a few factors that may be related to development of the disease, including genetic factors, diet, other environmental triggers, and viral infections.

Type 2 diabetes (formerly called noninsulin-dependent diabetes mellitus or adult-onset diabetes) is a metabolic disorder that is characterized by elevated blood glucose in the context of insulin resistance and relative insulin deficiency. Insulin resistance occurs when the cells of the body do not respond adequately to the presence of the insulin that is present. Unlike type 1 diabetes, the insulin resistance of type 2 diabetes is generally "post-receptor," meaning that the problem is with the cells that respond to insulin, rather than there being a problem with the production of insulin. The exact etiology of type 2 diabetes is presently unknown.

Gastrointestinal Motility Disorders

The digestion and propulsion of intestinal contents along the digestive tube requires coordinated movements of the stomach and intestines in a complex pattern of contractions and relaxations, a process known as peristalsis (**Fig. 26.4**). These contractions and relaxations of the gastrointestinal tract are generated by the nerves and muscles within the gastrointestinal walls.

Many factors can influence gastrointestinal motility (e.g., physical exercise, emotional distress). The pathogenesis of primitive intestinal motility disorders probably is multifactorial, but no biochemical or structural abnormality has been found, except in some forms of intestinal pseudo-obstruction.

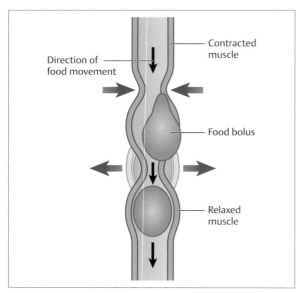

Fig. 26.4   The process of peristalsis.

Nausea: Alterations in gastric motility associated with elevated levels of progesterone are implicated in the nausea of pregnancy. Animal studies show inhibitory effects of progesterone on gastrointestinal smooth muscle, and research in rats found a significant reduction in contractile activity of excised esophageal, antrum, and colonic tissue pretreated with progesterone compared with nontreated tissue. Progesterone also has been shown to inhibit spontaneous contractile activity of human gastric muscles and the colon in vitro, whereas estradiol and corticosteroids do not affect these contractile responses.

Hyperemesis gravidarum: Hyperemesis gravidarum is characterized by intractable vomiting occurring early in pregnancy. Unlike the uncomplicated nausea and vomiting of pregnancy, hyperemesis gravidarum is associated with fluid and electrolyte imbalances. It is usually self-limited and disappears by the third month of pregnancy. Although it rarely persists throughout pregnancy, frequent relapses may occur.

The cause of hyperemesis gravidarum is poorly understood, but endocrine and psychological factors are suspected. Like the nausea and vomiting of pregnancy, abnormal levels of human chorionic gonadotropin, progesterone, estradiol, and even thyroid hormones may be important. Social and psychological factors have also been associated with hyperemesis gravidarum.

Gastroesophageal reflux disease: The pathogenesis of this disease during pregnancy involves both mechanical and intrinsic factors that adversely affect the lower esophageal sphincter tone. Early in pregnancy, lower esophageal sphincter pressure falls, returning to normal in the postpartum period. If the pressure falls too much, acid from the stomach enters the lower part of the esophagus (**Fig. 26.5**), causing intense heartburn.

Animal experiments have helped elucidate the important effects of female hormones on the lower esophageal sphincter. These experiments have demonstrated that the combination of progesterone and estradiol is more potent

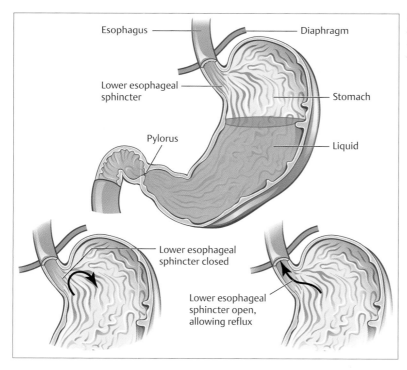

Fig. 26.5   The symptoms of gastroesophageal reflux disease are caused by the lower esophageal sphincter opening and allowing stomach acids to enter the lower esophagus.

than either hormone alone in reducing lower esophageal sphincter pressure.

Abdominal bloating and constipation: It is believed that abdominal bloating and constipation during pregnancy are caused by hormonally related changes in both small-bowel and colonic motility. Animal and human studies evaluating gastrointestinal transit during pregnancy and the menstrual cycle support this concept.

Thyroid Disorder

During the last few decades, growing evidence has emerged that adequate fetal thyroid hormone levels are critically important to ensure normal central and peripheral nervous system maturation. However, pregnancy has a significant effect on the thyroid and causes changes in iodine metabolism and serum thyroid binding proteins. This puts the fetus at risk for either hypo- or hyperglycemia, which carries a number of potentially adverse consequences for the fetus.

Low maternal levels of circulating thyroxine have been associated with a significant decrement in child IQ and development. Postpartum thyroid dysfunction occurs in 50% of women who were found to have thyroid peroxidase antibodies in early pregnancy. Thyroid peroxidase antibodies are present in 10% of women at 14 weeks' gestation, and are associated with: 1) an increased pregnancy failure (i.e., abortion) rate, 2) an increased incidence of gestational thyroid dysfunction, and 3) a predisposition to postpartum thyroiditis.

A high incidence (25–30%) of permanent hypothyroidism has been noted in these women. Women having transient postpartum thyroid disease with hypothyroidism should be monitored frequently, as there is a 50% chance of these patients developing hypothyroidism during the next seven years.

History

Chief Complaints and Physical Examination

Asthma

Predicting the course that asthma will follow in a woman's first pregnancy is extremely difficult. Asthma worsens in about one-third of women, improves in one-third, and remains stable in one-third. Other patterns that have been observed include:
- Among women whose asthma worsens, an increase in symptoms is often seen between weeks 29 and 36 of pregnancy.

- Asthma is generally less severe during the last month of pregnancy.
- Labor and delivery do not usually worsen asthma.
- Among women whose asthma improves, the improvement typically progresses gradually throughout pregnancy.
- The severity of asthma symptoms during the first pregnancy is often similar in subsequent pregnancies.

In general, pregnant women with asthma experience symptoms when the airways tighten, inflame, or fill with mucus. Common symptoms of asthma include:
- shortness of breath
- chest tightness or pain
- trouble sleeping caused by shortness of breath, coughing, or wheezing
- audible whistling or wheezing sound when exhaling
- bouts of coughing or wheezing that are worsened by a respiratory virus such as a cold or the flu

Back Pain

In approximately 80% of pregnancies, back pain is usually localized. However, the site often varies among patients. Although long-term pain is very rare, short-term pain tends to be dominant. Usually during the third trimester, 50% of pregnant patients will experience back pain.

Anatomically, pain during pregnancy presents itself most commonly in the following areas:
- sacroiliac joints at the posterior superior iliac spine
- groin area
- coccyx
- pubic symphysis anteriorly
- other areas of the pelvis and upper legs

The severity of back pain during pregnancy tends to be influenced by posture and is associated with a waddling gait. Rarely does pain occur below the knee. In addition to pain, other symptoms often include stiffness and limited range of motion of the back and legs. Research has demonstrated that women with fibromyalgia, a chronic type of muscle pain, experience a worsening of their symptoms during pregnancy.

Cholestasis

The chief complaints of a woman with cholestasis in pregnancy include:
- itching, particularly on the hands and feet (often this is the only symptom noticed)
- dark urine color
- light coloring of bowel movements
- fatigue or exhaustion
- loss of appetite
- depression
  Less common symptoms include:

- jaundice (yellow coloring of skin, eyes, and mucous membranes)
- upper-right quadrant pain
- nausea

Cholecystitis

A hallmark of cholecystitis is a colicky or stabbing pain in the right upper abdominal quadrant or epigastric area, radiating to the interscapular area, right shoulder, or scapula.

Diabetes

Symptoms of diabetes, whether type 1, type 2, or gestational, include:

- excessive thirst
- excessive urination
- thrush
- extreme hunger
- unusual weight loss
- extreme fatigue
- irritability
- nausea
- vomiting
- sweet-smelling breath
- blurred vision

However, the majority of women with gestational diabetes have no overt symptoms. For this reason, it is vitally important that all women be screened for gestational diabetes toward the end of the second trimester at around 24–28 weeks of pregnancy.

Gastrointestinal Motility Disorders

Abdominal bloating and constipation: Many women who are affected by constipation when they are not pregnant experience a worsening of this symptom during pregnancy.

Gastroesophageal reflux disease: The clinical features of gastroesophageal reflux in pregnancy do not differ from those found in the general population. Heartburn and regurgitation are the predominant symptoms, worsening as pregnancy advances.

Hyperemesis gravidarum: Hyperemesis gravidarum is characterized by intractable vomiting occurring early in pregnancy. Unlike the uncomplicated nausea and vomiting of pregnancy, hyperemesis gravidarum is associated with fluid and electrolyte imbalances.

Thyroid Disorder

Hypothyroidism: The symptoms of hypothyroidism are often difficult to detect during pregnancy, and may be mistaken for simple pregnancy-related inconveniences, including:

- fatigue and weakness
- weight gain
- frequent muscle aches
- cold intolerance

Once diagnosed, hypothyroidism typically requires daily treatment. Prompt treatment is especially important during pregnancy, because hypothyroidism can increase maternal risk of certain pregnancy complications including:

- miscarriage
- preterm labor
- hypertension

If left untreated, hypothyroidism can also put the fetus at risk for developmental problems. In fact, studies have shown that women with untreated hypothyroidism are four times more likely to give birth to a child with a low IQ.

Hyperthyroidism: Similar to hypothyroidism, the symptoms of hyperthyroidism are often difficult to diagnose during pregnancy, because the pregnancy itself frequently masks the symptoms, which may include:

- weight loss
- fatigue and weakness
- nausea and vomiting
- sweating
- heat intolerance

If properly managed throughout pregnancy, hyperthyroidism presents no increased risk for any health-related problems for a mother and her baby. Most women who are treated for the disease go on to experience normal pregnancies. In contrast, pregnant women with uncontrolled or untreated hyperthyroidism are at increased risk for:

- miscarriage or stillbirth
- pre-eclampsia
- iron deficiency-related anemia
- infection

Although hyperthyroidism usually does not affect labor and delivery, there is a slight risk of woman developing a "thyroid storm," which is associated with exacerbated hyperthyroidism symptoms, including:

- extremely high fever
- severe vomiting and diarrhea
- very high heart rate

Laboratory Testing

Asthma

Blood tests are sometimes taken to check on the overall health of a pregnant woman with asthma as well as to determine the status of her immune system. If she has low immune system function, it may mean that she is susceptible to catching lung infections, which might be the cause of her asthma symptoms. In contrast, a blood test that shows an active immune system with a high count of eosinophils can indicate allergic asthma. Eosinophils are classic signs of allergic reactions and inflammation in the airways.

Back Pain

Lab tests are used to find causes of back pain that are unrelated to mechanical or nerve dysfunction. For example, if an infection or cancer is responsible for a patient's back pain, lab tests may be done to analyze physiology. Generally, lab tests are performed by drawing blood.

Cholestasis

Blood tests for liver function, bile acids, and bilirubin often show changes which may also aid in the diagnosis of cholestasis.

Cholecystitis

Blood tests are usually normal in people with simple biliary colic or chronic cholecystitis. However, the following abnormalities may indicate gallstones or complications:
- Alkaline phosphatase and bilirubin levels are usually elevated in acute cholecystitis, and especially choledocholithiasis (common bile duct stones). Bilirubin is the orange-yellow pigment found in bile. High levels cause jaundice, which gives the skin a yellowish tone.
- The liver enzymes aspartate aminotransferase (AST) and alanine aminotransferase (ALT) are elevated when common bile duct stones are present. A threefold or more increase in ALT strongly suggests pancreatitis.
- A high white blood cell count is a common finding in many (but not all) patients with cholecystitis.

Diabetes

(See Definitions and Diagnosis sections above)

Gastrointestinal Motility Disorders

Gastroesophageal reflux disease: Physicians sometimes perform ambulatory pH monitoring to determine how much acid refluxes into the esophagus, how often, at what time of day or night, and whether the patient's symptoms occur at the same time as the reflux. Physicians also sometimes perform pH monitoring, to see whether the prescribed medicines are working, both in the stomach and the esophagus.

The test involves inserting a small tube, about 2 mm in diameter through the patient's nose into the esophagus. The tube is connected to a microcomputer which the patient wears around her waist or shoulder (**Fig. 26.6**). A small amount of tape holds the tube in place. The patient can then go home for 24 hours, after which she returns the monitor. Eating is possible, as is sleeping. A special diet is unnecessary—in fact, the patient should eat the things that provoke her symptoms. The tube may be uncomfortable, but is generally tolerated well enough, such that 98% of patients studied completed the procedure successfully.

Hyperemesis gravidarum: Patients with this disease are at significant risk of dehydration. Therefore, to check for signs of dehydration, a hematocrit and urine ketone test are often performed.

Thyroid Disorder

The TSH test is the "gold standard" for evaluating thyroid function and/or symptoms of hyper- or hypothyroidism. It is frequently ordered along with or preceding a T4 test, but other thyroid tests, such as a T3 test and thyroid anti-

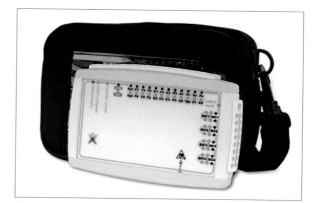

Fig. 26.6 Patients suspected of having gastroesophogeal reflux disease are sometimes given a lightweight, multi-modality ambulatory pH recorder attached to a small tube leading through the nose and into the esophagus.

bodies test (if autoimmune-related thyroid disease is suspected) may be ordered as well.

TSH testing is used to:

- diagnose a thyroid disorder in a person with symptoms
- screen newborns for an underactive thyroid
- monitor thyroid replacement therapy in people with hypothyroidism

Treatment

Asthma

The medications used to treat asthma during pregnancy are the same as those used to treat asthma at other times during a person's life. However, the types and doses of these medications will depend upon many factors. In general, inhaled drugs are recommended because of their limited body-wide effects in the mother and the baby. It may be necessary to adjust the type or dose of drugs during pregnancy to compensate for changes in the woman's metabolism and changes in the severity of asthma.

It is important to consider the unknown (but probably small) risks of asthma-controlling drugs compared to the potentially serious harm of undertreated asthma. Asthma attacks can reduce the oxygen supply to the fetus. Therefore, it is important to take asthma medications on a regular basis to prevent asthma symptoms.

With appropriate asthma therapy, most women can breathe easily, have a normal pregnancy, and deliver a healthy baby. Overall, the risk of poorly controlled asthma is much greater than the risk of taking medications to control asthma. In most cases, undertreated asthma poses a far greater risk to both the mother and the baby than the use of asthma-controlling drugs.

Back Pain

Back pain is no longer considered an "inevitable" part of pregnancy. With the use of proper prevention methods and appropriate diagnosis and management techniques, it can often be avoided altogether.

Education is a crucial component to managing back pain in pregnant women. A careful history should be obtained as to any prior low-back problems. If the patient has a positive history for back pain, then the physician should ask whether these problems have been completely worked up and treated in the past. She should also be educated as to the increased risk of developing recurrent symptoms during her pregnancy.

Ideally back-pain prevention strategies should be implemented before a woman becomes pregnant. Research has shown that women who engaged in 45 minutes or more physical activity per week and were physically fit prior to pregnancy are less likely to develop low-back pain during pregnancy (see Evidence Box 26.1). Pre-pregnancy fitness, however, does not seem to reduce the risk of sacroiliac pain.

There are a number of approaches to managing back pain in pregnant women. These include teaching them proper posture, how and when to exercise, and giving them an awareness of low-back biomechanics. Pregnant women also should be informed that weight gain and hormonal changes cause a redistribution of weight, which can exert more stress on the lower back and pelvis. They should also taught of the importance of proper posture in preventing unnecessary mechanical stress on the lower back. Further, pregnant women should be taught how to maintain a neutral spine posture—that is, how to avoid excessive lumbar lordosis and excessive reversal of lumbar lordosis—during all activities.

The local application of heat or ice has been shown to be beneficial and safe for lumbar and sacroiliac pain. Heat may also provide comfort, and cold may numb the pain. Transcutaneous electrical nerve stimulation (**Fig. 26.7**) may be safely prescribed by a knowledgable clinician, but whirlpool treatments and joint manipulation procedures are contraindicated.

Pregnant women with sacroiliac pain and objective evidence of biomechanical dysfunction may improve symptomatically with the use of a nonelastic trochanteric belt. This method of treatment has been shown to decrease pain when walking for prolonged periods of time. Although acetaminophen can be taken to relieve pain during pregnancy, nonsteroidal anti-inflammatory agents are generally contraindicated during pregnancy.

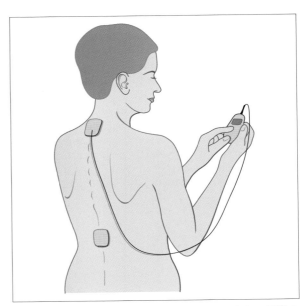

Fig. 26.7 Transcutaneous electrical nerve stimulation (TSE) is sometimes used to control low back pain in pregnant women.

Cholestasis

The treatment goals for cholestasis of pregnancy are to relieve the itching. Some treatment options include:

- topical anti-itch medications or medication with corticosteroids
- medication to decrease the concentration of bile acids such as ursodeoxycholic acid
- cold baths and ice-water slow down the flow of blood in the body by decreasing its temperature
- dexamethasone to increase the maturity of the baby's lungs
- vitamin K supplements administered to the mother before delivery, and again once the baby is born to prevent intracranial hemorrhaging
- dandelion root and milk thistle are natural substances that are beneficial to the liver
- bi-weekly nonstress tests which involve fetal heart monitoring and contraction recordings
- regular blood tests monitoring both bile serum levels and liver function

Treatments that should *not* be used for cholestasis include:
- antihistamines
- Aveeno
- Oatmeal Bath

Cholecystitis

Sometimes cholecystitis will resolve without treatment. However, most times treatment is needed. Treatments may include surgery to remove the gallbladder or draining the gallbladder, which is sometimes used in very ill patients.

Diabetes

To reduce the risk of adverse consequences of diabetes for both mother and baby, it is important to effectively manage hyperglycemia before, during, and after pregnancy. Self-glucose monitoring allows the pregnant woman with diabetes to know her blood glucose level at any time and to achieve tighter blood glucose control, which will prevent the immediate and potentially serious consequences of very high or very low blood glucose and decrease the long-term risks of diabetic complications for her and her baby.

Blood glucose meters are accurate, although there can be some variability from one manufactured unit to the next. They are less accurate during episodes of hypoglycemia (low blood glucose) compared with episodes of hyperglycemia. Researchers are evaluating the effectiveness of continuous glucose monitoring systems (CGMSs), which use a glucose sensor (contained in a small needle) to determine the level of glucose in the interstitial fluid, found between cells under the skin. Currently, CGMSs are recommended only for people with type 1 diabetes who use intensive insulin therapy, often with an insulin pump. However, because of the growing evidence that even short periods of hyperglycemia or hypoglycemia may be detrimental to the developing fetus, there is increasing interest in the effectiveness of CGMSs in managing type 2 and gestational diabetes as well.

Nutritional support during pregnancy can have a significant impact on the incidence and severity of diabetes. Specifically, a low-carbohydrate diet has been shown to significantly lower postprandial (after meal) glucose levels. Diabetic pregnant women also have been shown to benefit from taking multivitamins as well as folic acid supplements.

Human insulin has long been the preferred medication for treating diabetes in pregnancy. Short-acting insulin is given before breakfast, lunch, and dinner. In patients where the fasting value is over 100 mg/dL, intermediate-acting insulin is added before the evening meal. Some patients can even be managed on two doses of short-acting insulin (i.e., without a lunchtime dose). Insulin analogues, such as 28B-L-lysine-29B-L-proline insulin (Lispro) and 28B-aspartic acid *insulin* (Aspart), have an acceptable safety profile and studies have shown that several are clinically effective, with minimal transfer across the placenta and no evidence of teratogenesis. Although Lispro and Aspart have primarily been tested with type 1 diabetes, both have been shown to improve postprandial glucose excursions compared with human regular insulin and may be associated with lower risk of delayed postprandial hypoglycemia.

Oral diabetes drugs traditionally have not been used in pregnant women because of reports of fetal anomalies and other adverse outcomes in animal studies and in some human cases. However, more recent evidence suggests that some oral diabetes drugs, metformin in particular, may be useful in pregnancy.

Gastrointestinal Motility Disorders

The management and treatment of gastrointestinal ailments in pregnant women requires special attention and expertise to ensure the safety of the mother, fetus, and neonate. For example, castor oil can initiate premature uterine contractions, and there have been case reports of excessive use of mineral oil leading to a decrease maternal absorption of fat-soluble vitamins, resulting in neonatal hypoprothrombinemia and hemorrhage.

The use of laxatives during pregnancy has been shown to produce serious side effects to both mother and fetus. Laxitive use has been associated with an increased risk for congenital malformations, sodium retention in the mother, and diarrhea in the neonate.

Thus, the treatment of serious, persistent motility disorder symptoms must be done in consultation with a gastroenterologist who understands the unique clinical issues posed by pregnancy. The following offers a general overview of the treatment options for specific pregnancy-related motility disorders.

Gastroesophageal reflux disease: Because of potential teratogenicity of systemic drugs taken during gestation, life style modifications are particularly important in treating pregnant patients with this disease. Mild heartburn may be treated with life style and dietary modifications. Good posture while eating and avoiding lying down after meals may reduce the occurrence of heartburn. Smoking should also be avoided because it increases stomach acidity.

Nonsystemic drug therapy with antacids is the first step in treating the pregnant patient who does not respond to life style modifications. Animal studies show no teratogenic effects from constant ingestion of antacids during pregnancy.

Histamine-2 receptor blockers (H2RA) treat the discomfort of heartburn and acid indigestion by blocking histamine, which decreases acid secretion. They are also commonly used during pregnancy, and are available both over the counter and by prescription at higher doses.

Proton pump inhibitors decrease the stomach's production of acid more completely than the H2RAs by stopping the stomach's acid pump, which is the final step of acid secretion. Proton pump inhibitors are a relatively new class of treatment for gastroesophageal reflux disease, and less information is available about their safely profile in pregnancy.

Prokinetic agents hasten emptying of the stomach contents, resulting in less acid secretion available for reflux. Some agents also increase the "tone" of the lower esophageal sphincter, making it more difficult to open.

Hyperemesis gravidarum: Metabolic consequences of hyperemesis gravidarum occur as a result of fluid and electrolyte depletion. Treatment is directed at replacement of fluids and electrolytes and at correction of nutritional deficiencies, if present. Small, frequent meals high in carbohydrates are recommended. Although no anti-emetic is approved for use during pregnancy, promethazine or metoclopramide may be necessary to increase the patient's threshold for emesis. Total parenteral nutrition may be required in patients with persistent weight loss, acidosis, and malnutrition. In addition to medical therapy, adjunctive psychotherapy may be helpful in many cases.

Thyroid Disorder

If a woman was already being treated with thyroxine when she became pregnant, she should continue to take this medication during pregnancy. Thyroxine is safe to take and is well absorbed during pregnancy. Although there is usually no need for a dose change, some women require somewhat higher doses when they are pregnant. Physicians generally monitor the TSH level to detect even mild hypothyroidism and increase the thyroxine dose, if necessary.

The treatment of hyperthyroidism in pregnancy is limited because of safety concerns for the baby. Usually, drugs such as propylthiouracil (PTU) and methimazole (MMI) are used. Although both of these drugs do cross the placenta and can enter the fetal system, treatment is still preferred because of the poor outcomes associated with not treating these women. PTU is preferred because MMI has been associated with a rare scalp condition in the fetus known as "aplasia cutis."

Hyperthyroidic women who want to nurse their babies should be able to do so safely on PTU and MMI medications. Although the older literature discouraged breastfeeding for such women, newer studies indicated that it is safe since the concentration of drug that enters the breast milk is quite low. PTU is preferred since it has lower concentrations in breast milk.

Medications to slow the mother's heart rate down may also be necessary. The class of drugs recommended is called beta-blockers (metoprolol, propranolol). Although these drugs are not thought to be dangerous to the fetus (teratogenic), there have been associations with growth retardation. Low levels of blood sugars at birth and some respiratory problems have also been reported.

Key Points

- The most common "other" medical complications (not dealt with elsewhere in this book) in pregnancy include asthma, back pain, cholestasis and cholesytitis (two common pregnancy related liver disorders), diabetes, gastric motility disorders, and thyroid problems.
- The etiology for many of these other medical complications is unknown. However, the diagnostic and treatment methods for most have been well established.
- The medications used to treat asthma during pregnancy are the same medications used to treat asthma at other times during a person's life.
- Back pain is very common during pregnancy and is often the result of bad posture. Treatment typically involves correcting a woman's posture and prescribing a short course of daily exercise to relieve pain and stiffness.
- Pregnancy-related liver disorders are diagnosed by a complete medical history, physical examination, ultrasound imaging, and blood tests that evaluate liver function, bile acids, and bilirubin. Sometimes these conditions will resolve on their own without treatment. However, often drugs and/or surgical intervention are warranted.
- Test results indicating that a pregnant woman has diabetes should be confirmed with a second test on a different day to ensure accuracy.
- It is critical to tightly control blood levels of glucose during pregnancy, as hyperglycemia during pregnancy has adverse consequences for both mother and baby.
- The methods chosen to diagnose and treat functional gastrointestinal disorders (including motility disorders) are based on the patient's symptoms.
- The diagnosis of hypo- and hyperthyroidism in pregnancy can be complicated, since some of the blood tests used for the diagnosis are altered because of the pregnancy.

Evidence Box 26.1

Regular physical activity during leisure time significantly reduces the risk of low back pain and pelvic pain during pregnancy, whereas the risk is increased in those women who described their occupations as active or physically demanding.

Mogren investigated whether physical activity prior to pregnancy would impact low back pain and pelvic pain (LBPP) during pregnancy. He surveyed all women who gave birth at two hospitals in northern Sweden from January 1, 2002 to April 30, 2002. The response rate was 83% ($N = 891$).

Approximately 46% of the women reported visiting a physician as a result of LBPP. The mean number of visits was 2.0. One-third of the women with LBPP had received treatment, as had half of the women with "high pain score" for LBPP. A higher number of years of regular, leisure-time physical activity prior to pregnancy significantly decreased the risk of LBPP during pregnancy. On the other hand, the risk of LBPP was increased for women who characterized their occupation as "mainly active" (OR = 2.0, 95% CI: 1.1 to 3.5) and "physically demanding" (OR = 1.9, 95% CI: 1.1 to 3.2).

Mogren IM. Previous physical activity decreases the risk of low back pain and pelvic pain during pregnancy. Scand J Public Health 2005;33(4):300–306.

Further Reading

Borg-Stein J, Dugan SA. Musculoskeletal disorders of pregnancy, delivery and postpartum. *Phys Med Rehabil Clin N Am* 2007;18(3):459–476, ix

Carson MP, Ehrenthal D. Medical issues from preconception through delivery: a roadmap for the internist. *Med Clin North Am* 2008;92(5):1193–1225, xi

Keller J, Frederking D, Layer P; Medscape. The spectrum and treatment of gastrointestinal disorders during pregnancy. *Nat Clin Pract Gastroenterol Hepatol* 2008;5(8):430–443

Noble PW, Lavee AE, Jacobs MM. Respiratory diseases in pregnancy. *Obstet Gynecol Clin North Am* 1988;15(2):391–428

Okosieme OE, Marx H, Lazarus JH. Medical management of thyroid dysfunction in pregnancy and the postpartum. *Expert Opin Pharmacother* 2008;9(13):2281–2293

Rome III. *Gastroenterology* April 2006;130(5):

27 Post-Term Pregnancy

E. Albert Reece

A typical pregnancy lasts approximately nine months but can vary between 37 and 42 weeks and still produce a normal, healthy baby. On average, however, women give birth at approximately 40 weeks, or 280 days, from the first day of their last menstrual period.

Just as babies who are born preterm can have significant and long-lasting health problems, so can babies who stay too long in the womb. Indeed, a pregnancy that continues beyond 42 weeks is associated with adverse consequences for both the fetus and the mother. Thus, any physician caring for a pregnant woman who has passed her due date must have a management plan in place to prevent such complications from occurring.

Definition

The World Health Organization defines post-term, or prolonged, pregnancy as one that exceeds 42 completed weeks (294 days or more) from the onset of the last menstrual period (LMP).

Ideally, an accurate gestational age is determined early in the pregnancy. However, variations in when a woman ovulates can lead to errors in calculating the true duration of pregnancy and to overestimation or underestimation of when the baby is due.

Diagnosis

Traditionally, a woman's LMP was used to calculate the estimated due date (EDD). This typically involved using a pregnancy wheel (**Fig. 27.1**), in which the date of the patient's LMP was lined up with that date on the wheel, and an indicator on the wheel was used find the corresponding EDD. However, this method of dating a pregnancy is subject to many inaccuracies, particularly among women who have irregular cycles, have been on recent hormonal birth control, or who have first trimester bleeding.

Numerous studies have shown that dating a pregnancy early on via ultrasonography significantly improves the reliability of the EDD. However, the margin of error increases during each trimester of gestation. If an ultrasound scan is performed before 20 weeks' gestation, the margin of error is about 1 week. Between 20 and 30 weeks' gestation, the margin of error may increase to as much as 2 weeks. After 30 weeks' gestation, the margin of error may exceed 2 weeks.

In general, the margin of error is usually assumed to be 2 weeks. Thus, a pregnancy that is dated at 35 weeks' gestation by ultrasonography could actually be anywhere from 33 weeks to 37 weeks. A gestational age calculated by composite biometry from a sonogram (see below) must be considered only an estimate.

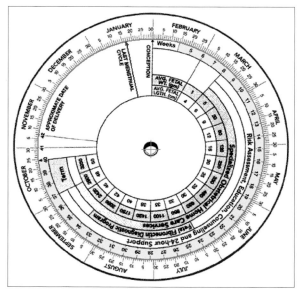

Fig. 27.1 A standard pregnancy wheel used to determine an estimated due date.

Prevalence

A great deal of controversy surrounds the prevalence of post-term pregnancies, with estimates ranging from 3% to 14% of all pregnancies. Because of inaccuracies in dating pregnancies, many "pseudo" post-term pregnancies, in fact, are not post-term.

Thus, it is important to accurately determine when a pregnancy begins, because errors in dating often lead physicians to deliver so-called term pregnancies prematurely, or to unnecessarily allow pregnancies to continue that are actually post-term.

Etiology

Inaccurate dating of conception is the most frequent cause of post-term pregnancy. However, there are other factors that can predispose a woman to carry a fetus past 42 weeks of gestation. These include primiparity, prior post-term pregnancy, the gender of the fetus (males are more likely to be post-term than females), and genetic factors. Studies of monozygotic and dizygotic twins and their subsequent development of prolonged pregnancies have found that maternal, but not paternal, genetic factors influence the rate of post-term pregnancies and account for in as many as 30% of these pregnancies.

Pathophysiology

A pregnancy that continues beyond 42 weeks is associated with significant adverse consequences to the fetus and the mother. The following provides an overview of the most common consequences.

Fetal Consequences

Pregnancies that continue beyond an actual 42 weeks of gestation have an increased risk of stillbirth or infant death. However, the increased risk is relatively small, with only 4 to 7 deaths per 1000 deliveries compared with 2 to 3 deaths per 1000 deliveries among women who deliver between 37 and 42 weeks.

On the other hand, true post-term fetuses do have a greater chance of developing complications related

to larger body size, or macrosomia, which is defined as weighing more than 4500 g, or about 10 pounds. Complications for the fetus can include prolonged labor, difficulty passing through the vagina, and birth trauma (e.g., fractured bones or nerve injury) related to shoulder dystocia (**Fig. 27.2**).

Post-term fetuses sometimes develop fetal dysmaturity syndrome—also called "post-maturity syndrome"—in which the fetus' growth in utero is restricted due to a problem with delivery of blood via the placenta. This puts the fetus at increased risk for umbilical cord compression in utero as well as problems after delivery, including long-term breathing and neurologic abnormalities.

One of the more severe consequences of a post-term pregnancy involves the fetus having a bowel movement of meconium into the amniotic fluid. If the fetus becomes stressed, it can inhale some of this meconium-contaminated amniotic fluid, which can cause breathing problems or infection when it is born.

Maternal Consequences

Adverse consequences to the mother of a post-term fetus are related to the larger size of the infant, and include difficulties during labor, an increase in injury to the perineum (including the vagina, labia, and rectum), and an increased rate of cesarean birth with its associated risks of bleeding, infection, and injury to surrounding organs.

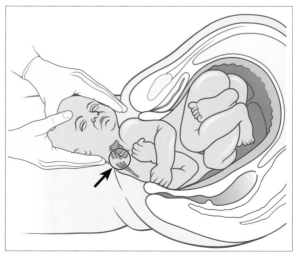

Fig. 27.2 Shoulder dystocia occurs when the infant's anterior shoulder has difficulty passing below the pubic symphysis, or significant manipulation is required to get it to pass.

History

Chief Complaints

A number of symptoms warrant an immediate evaluation in a woman who is nearing the term of her pregnancy or is suspected of being post-term. These include any perceived decrease in fetal movements or loss of fluid or any pain or other discomfort that appears abnormal.

Physical Examination

Antenatal Fetal Monitoring

The American College of Obstetricians and Gynecologists (ACOG) recommends initiating antenatal fetal monitoring only after 42 weeks, or 294 days, of gestation, followed by twice weekly monitoring, including a measurement of amniotic fluid volume. To be safe, however, many OB/GYN physicians prefer to begin fetal monitoring at 41 weeks. In most cases, testing is recommended if a pregnancy extends beyond the due date.

These tests, which may also include observing the fetus' heart rate using a fetal monitor (called a nonstress test) or its activity rate with ultrasound imaging (called a biophysical profile), give information about the health of the fetus and about the risks or benefits of allowing the pregnancy to continue.

Nonstress Testing

A nonstress test is typically performed two to three times weekly in a woman who is past her due date. It typically involves using sound waves (ultrasound) to measure the fetus' heart rate over a 20–30-minute period. A normal fetal baseline heart rate ranges between 110 and 160 beats per minute (bpm), and increases above its baseline by at least 15 bpm for 15 seconds when the baby moves. The ultrasound scan is considered normal, or "reactive," if two or more fetal heart rate increases are detected within a 20–30-minute period. If, after 40 minutes of testing, no increases are observed, further testing is urgently needed.

Biophysical Profile

A biophysical profile (BPP) score includes several tests which—when combined—give an assessment of the fetus' overall health. It consists of heart rate monitoring by nonstress testing plus ultrasound measurement of four additional fetal parameters: 1) fetal body movements; 2) breathing movements; 3) fetal tone (flexion and extension of an arm, leg, or the spine); and 4) amniotic fluid volume.

Each component of the BPP is scored individually. If the measured component is normal, it receives a score of 2 points, and 0 points if it is abnormal. The maximum possible score is 10.

Amniotic fluid volume, which can drop precipitously even within a few days, is an important variable in the BPP because a low volume (i. e., oligohydramnios) can significantly increase the risk of umbilical cord compression and may be indicative of potential problems in fetal circulation.

Contraction Stress Test

A contraction stress test (CST) checks fetal response to reduced oxygen levels, such as those that might normally occur during the contractions that accompany labor. A CST typically involves giving the mother oxytocin intravenously to induce uterine contractions combined with external fetal heart monitoring (**Fig. 27.3**). If the fetus' heart rate slows down during a CST, an immediate cesarean delivery may be indicated.

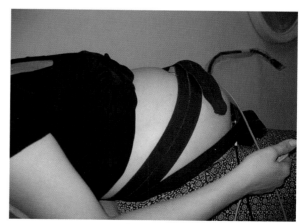

Fig. 27.3 If the fetus' heart rate slows down (decelerates) in a certain pattern instead of speeding up (accelerating) after a contraction, he or she may have problems with the stress of normal labor and an immediate cesarean delivery may be needed.

Management and Treatment

When managing an impending post-term pregnancy, a critical decision must be made whether to deliver the baby and, if so, by what route. In certain high risk cases, the decision is straightforward and is reached when the risks of remaining pregnant begin to outweigh the risks of delivery.

Perinatal morbidity and mortality do not increase appreciably between 40 and 41 weeks of gestation. However, at gestational ages greater than 42 weeks, the perinatal mortality rate is double that at term and increases sixfold at 43 weeks.

Babies born to mothers who carried them up to or beyond 42 weeks (post-term pregnancies) are at an increased risk for macrosomia, shoulder dystocia, cephalopelvic disproportion, and dysmaturity syndrome, which affects 20% of post-term fetuses. There are also maternal risks associated with post-term pregnancies. These include an increase in labor dystocia, perineal injuries, and cesarean deliveries. Such complications for baby and mother suggest that there are few benefits to be had from allowing well-dated pregnancies to progress beyond 42 weeks of gestation.

On the other hand, the approach to managing pregnancies between 41 and 42 weeks of gestation remains an open question (see Evidence Box 27.1). The main argument in the research literature against a policy of routine induction of labor at 41–42 weeks is that it increases the rate of cesarean delivery without decreasing maternal and/or neonatal morbidity.

The National Institute of Child Health and Human Development—part of the US National Institutes of Health—and the Canadian Multicenter Postterm Pregnancy Trial recently completed three prospective randomized studies on this question. These studies found no increase in the rate of cesarean delivery in patients who were randomized to routine induction of labor. In fact, more cesarean deliveries were performed in the noninduction groups. The most frequent indication for a cesarean section intervention was fetal distress.

The neonatal outcomes were similar in both the routine induction and noninduction groups. All three trials concluded that the incidence of adverse perinatal outcomes in low-risk pregnancies at or after 41 weeks' gestation is very low with either induction or expectant management.

Some data suggest that induction may be more beneficial than expectant management in patients at 41 weeks' gestation. One meta-analysis concluded that a policy of routine induction had a lower rate of perinatal morbidity and cesarean delivery, demonstrating both fetal and maternal benefit compared to expectant management. Another recent review concluded that routine induction in low-risk pregnancies at or after 41 weeks' gestation is associated with a reduction in perinatal mortality, with no increase in the rate of instrument deliveries or cesarean delivery.

Thus, the majority of data to date suggest that routine induction at 41 weeks' gestation does not increase the cesarean delivery rate, and may decrease it, without negatively affecting perinatal morbidity or mortality. There may be, in fact, both maternal and neonatal benefits to a policy of routine induction of labor in well-dated low-risk pregnancies at 41 weeks' gestation.

Once the decision to deliver the baby has been made, the route of delivery and the specifics of intrapartum management depend on individual obstetric circumstances. As many as 80% of patients who reach 42 weeks' gestation have an unfavorable cervical examination (i.e., a Bishop score <7). Many options are available for cervical ripening. However, the different preparations, indications, contraindications, and multiple dosing regimens of each require practitioners to familiarize themselves with several types of preparations.

Prostaglandin E_2 gel and suppositories for vaginal application were used extensively until the late 1990s. However, many pharmacies stopped manufacturing them because of the advent of commercially available and less labor-intensive preparations. Currently-available chemical preparations include prostaglandin E_1 tablets for oral or vaginal use (misoprostol), prostaglandin E_2 gel for intracervical application (Prepidil), and a prostaglandin E_2 vaginal insert (Cervidil).

Mechanical dilation is another method for ripening the cervix. These devices may act by a combination of mechanical forces and by causing the release of endogenous prostaglandins. Membrane sweeping or stripping, a Foley balloon catheter (**Fig. 27.4**) placed in the cervix, extra-amniotic saline infusions, and laminaria have all been shown to be effective as well.

Regardless of the method used for ripening the cervix, there are potential hazards surrounding the use of these agents in patients with a scarred uterus. In addition, care

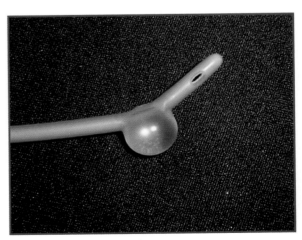

Fig. 27.4   A foley balloon catheter.

must be taken to avoid using too high or too short a dosing interval. Both can result in uterine tachysystole and subsequent fetal distress. Care also should be taken when using combinations of mechanical and pharmacologic methods of cervical ripening.

Once labor is induced, it is necessary to institute surveillance for the major potential complications associated with inductions beyond 41 weeks' gestation and to have a plan in place for dealing with each. Complications may include the presence of meconium, macrosomia, and fetal intolerance to labor.

The farther a pregnancy progresses beyond 40 weeks, the more likely it is that significant amounts of meconium will be present. This is due to increased uteroplacental insufficiency, which leads to hypoxia in labor and activation of the vagal system. In addition, the presence of less amniotic fluid increases the relative amount of meconium in utero.

Traditionally, saline amnioinfusion and aggressive nasopharyngeal and oropharyngeal suctioning at the perineum were used to decrease the risk of meconium aspiration syndrome. Recent studies, however, have concluded that amnioinfusion of thick, meconium-stained amniotic fluid does not decrease the risk of moderate-to-severe meconium aspiration syndrome, perinatal death, or other serious neonatal disorders compared with expectant management. Other recent studies also suggest that deep suctioning of the airway at the perineum does not effectively prevent meconium aspiration syndrome.

Recognizing the limitations of ultrasonography at term, it is still advisable to obtain an estimated fetal weight prior to induction of a post-term pregnancy. Abdominal palpation by an experienced practitioner is an acceptable alternative to ultrasonography for estimating fetal weight. However, any estimated fetal weight should be documented prior to beginning a post-date induction. In addition, mid-pelvic instrument deliveries should not be attempted.

Perhaps the most important part of a delivery plan is being prepared for shoulder dystocia in the event that this unpredictable, anxiety-provoking, and potentially dangerous condition arises.

Finally, it is critical to instigate intrapartum fetal surveillance in an attempt to document fetal intolerance to labor before it leads to acidosis. Whether continuous fetal monitoring or intermittent auscultation is used, it is critically important for a well-trained clinician to interpret the results. If the fetal heart rate tracing is equivocal, fetal scalp stimulation and/or fetal scalp blood sampling may provide the reassurance necessary to justify continuing the induction of labor. Without reassurance that the fetus is tolerating labor well, however, a cesarean delivery is highly recommended.

Key Points

- A pregnancy that continues beyond 42 weeks is associated with adverse consequences for both the fetus and the mother.
- Pregnancies that continue beyond an actual 42 weeks of gestation have an increased risk of a number of severe or fatal complications.
- Adverse consequences to the mother of a post-term fetus are related to the larger size of the infant.
- Ultrasound evaluation used early in a pregnancy can significantly improve the reliability of the estimating a woman's due date. However, the margin of error increases during each subsequent trimester of gestation.
- In most cases, further testing is recommended if a pregnancy extends beyond the due date.

Evidence Box 27.1

The optimal period for expectant management of pregnancies at 41 weeks and beyond is unknown.

Wennerholm et al. compared the perinatal and maternal outcomes between elective induction of labor versus expectant management of pregnancies by searching international literature for systematic reviews and randomized controlled trials comparing elective induction of labor versus expectant management of pregnancies at 41 weeks and beyond.

Elective induction of labor was not associated with lower risk of perinatal mortality compared with expectant management (relative risk (RR): 0.33; 95% confidence interval (CI): 0.10 to 1.09). Elective induction was, however, associated with a significantly lower rate of meconium aspiration syndrome (RR: 0.43; 95% CI: 0.23 to 0.79). Furthermore, women randomized to expectant management were delivered by cesarean section (RR: 0.87; 95% CI: 0.80 to 0.96).

Wennerholm UB, Hagberg H, Brorsson B, Bergh C. Induction of labor versus expectant management for post-date pregnancy: is there sufficient evidence for a change in clinical practice? Acta Obstet Gynecol Scand 2009;88(1):6–17.

Further Reading

ACOG. Practice Bulletin: Clinical management guidelines for obstetricians-gynecologists. No 55, September 2004 (replaces practice pattern No 6, October 1997). Management of Postterm Pregnancy. *Obstet Gynecol* 2004;104:639–646

Alfirevic Z, Walkinshaw SA. Management of post-term pregnancy: to induce or not? *Br J Hosp Med* 1994;52(5):218–221

Ananth CV. Menstrual versus clinical estimate of gestational age dating in the United States: temporal trends and variability in indices of perinatal outcomes. *Paediatr Perinat Epidemiol* 2007;21(Suppl 2):22–30

Gottlieb AG, Galan HL. Shoulder dystocia: an update. *Obstet Gynecol Clin North Am* 2007;34(3):501–531, xii

Norwitz ER, Snegovskikh VV, Caughey AB. Prolonged pregnancy: when should we intervene? *Clin Obstet Gynecol* 2007;50(2):547–557

Rand L, Robinson JN, Economy KE, Norwitz ER. Post-term induction of labor revisited. *Obstet Gynecol* 2000;96(5 Pt 1):779–783

Rosen MG, Dickinson JC. Management of post-term pregnancy. *N Engl J Med* 1992;326(24):1628–1629

Wennerholm UB, Hagberg H, Brorsson B, Bergh C. Induction of labor versus expectant management for post-date pregnancy: is there sufficient evidence for a change in clinical practice? *Acta Obstet Gynecol Scand* 2009;88(1):6–17

World Health Organization. WHO: recommended definitions, terminology and format for statistical tables related to the perinatal period and use of a new certificate for cause of perinatal deaths. Modifications recommended by FIGO as amended October 14, 1976. *Acta Obstet Gynecol Scand* 1977;56(3):247–253

Part III   Gynecology

Section I   General Gynecology

28 Contraception and Sterilization

Daniela Carusi

In the year 2001, over 3 million pregnancies in the United States were unintended, and half of these occurred among women using no contraception. Pregnancy prevention must be addressed in women's health care, as unplanned pregnancy may negatively affect a patient's psychological wellbeing and her health. Any woman of reproductive age should be considered at-risk for pregnancy, and the subject should be a routine part of her medical care.

Addressing Contraception with Patients

Women must consider a number of factors when choosing a contraceptive:
- mechanism of action (barrier, hormonal, behavioral)
- over-the-counter availability and cost
- reversibility
- level of effectiveness
- compliance requirements

Each patient's needs will vary in each of these categories, and medical providers have an important role in helping women to individualize their choices. At times these considerations may come into conflict. For example, a highly effective and reversible intrauterine device may have costs that seem prohibitive. It is important to maximize contraceptive effectiveness for each patient, which may require overcoming obstacles in cost and compliance.

When assessing an individual patient and helping her to find a method, the provider should investigate the following factors.

Compliance

There are many barriers to consistent contraceptive use. These might include financial cost, forgetting to obtain or take the contraceptive, failure to understand its correct use, concern about risks or side effects, or a partner's unwillingness to comply with a contraceptive plan.

Social Factors

Certain women may feel that family or cultural concerns limit their contraceptive choices. She should be reminded that this is a private, autonomous choice. Adolescents have the right to speak confidentially to health-care providers about contraception and sexuality; providers are not allowed to divulge these interactions to a teenager's parents or guardians. Similarly, a woman's partner may not have access to her medical or contraceptive records without her permission, and a partner's permission is not required for contraceptive or sterilization consent.

Medical Factors

Contraindications for various forms of contraception are listed in **Table 28.1.** Hormonal choices may be restricted by cardiovascular or stroke risk factors, and need to be avoided with certain cancers and liver disease. Additionally, physical abnormalities or infection of the pelvic organs may restrict use of an intrauterine device or sterilization. While barrier methods are very safe, their use may also be limited by allergy or sensitivity to the product. As a useful guide for health-care providers, the World Health Organization has classified contraceptive risks in the setting of different medical conditions.

Thus it is essential to take a careful medical history before prescribing contraception. Blood pressure must be measured before prescribing a hormonal method, and a

Table 28.1 Contraceptive contraindications

Contraceptive	Contraindications
Any method	Known allergy to the product Current or possible pregnancy (condoms are permissible)
Estrogen + progestin (combined) hormonal method	Current breast cancer Active liver disease or tumor Multiple cardiovascular risk factors* Poorly controlled hypertension Current vascular disease History of ischemia Advanced diabetes Known thrombophilia History of deep venous thrombosis or pulmonary embolism Major surgery or prolonged immobilization Migraine with aura
Progestin-only hormonal method	Current breast cancer
Intrauterine device	Active pelvic or genital tract infection Uterine anomaly (developmental) Distorted or obstructed uterine cavity Genital tract malignancy Unevaluated abnormal bleeding
Sterilization	Desire for future pregnancy Active pelvic infection
Emergency contraception: levonorgestrel	None (other than allergy)

* Cardiovascular risk factors include smoking, abnormal lipid profile, diabetes, hypertension, strong family history, age over 35 years, obesity.
Source: World Health Organization, *Medical Eligibility Criteria for Contraceptive Use*. 3rd ed. Reproductive Health and Research 2004. Geneva: World Health Organization.

pelvic exam is required prior to use of a diaphragm, intrauterine device, or sterilization technique.

As a good starting point, the provider should find out what method(s) the patient has previously used, and how well these worked for her. Staying with a tested method, and avoiding those methods she feels negatively about, can be extremely helpful.

Contraceptive Methods

Behavioral Methods

Behavioral contraception includes natural family planning, or the "rhythm method," withdrawal, and abstinence. All require a high degree of motivation and compliance on the part of the couple, and patients who choose these methods should be carefully educated on their correct use and risk of failure.

Abstinence

Many religions and cultures actively promote sexual abstinence until marriage. The US government has increasingly funded abstinence-only programs, though there is a paucity of evidence that it effectively prevents pregnancy.

While perfect abstinence is obviously very effective, it may be difficult to maintain. Even highly motivated patients should be encouraged to consider what method they will use when it eventually comes time to have intercourse, and may want to prepare in advance by having barrier methods available.

Withdrawal

With this method, the man removes his penis from his partner's vagina prior to ejaculation. While perfect use of this method may attain more than 80% effectiveness, the typical failure rate is closer to 30%. The man must not have any semen on his penis prior to ejaculation, and must be able to predict his ejaculation and pull out of the vagina prior to its occurrence.

Natural Family Planning

This method, also known as the "rhythm" method, requires that couples abstain from intercourse during fertile days of the cycle. These include the 5 days prior to, and 24 hours after, ovulation. Women with 26–32-day menstrual cycles may safely avoid intercourse on days 8–19 of the cycle. Alternatively, women may avoid intercourse on days in which they identify cervical mucus. The cervix will actively secrete mucus in the late follicular and ovulatory phases, when she is fertile.

Natural family planning may be 85–90% effective for women who have regular menstrual cycles and are highly compliant. It is generally inappropriate for women with very irregular cycles, those who are breast-feeding or perimenopausal, and those just coming off of hormonal birth control methods. For these women ovulation timing will not be predictable.

Barrier Methods

Barrier methods prevent contact between viable sperm and an egg without the use of hormones. All except the diaphragm are available without a prescription.

Chemical Methods: Spermicides

Spermicides act by killing viable sperm before they reach the upper genital tract. They are prepared as gels, foams, and films, which are inserted in the vagina. They must be applied prior to every act of intercourse, and may cause vaginal or urethral irritation. They have failure rates of 14–29% in clinical trials, with high rates of discontinuation. Furthermore, they do not protect against human immunodeficiency virus (HIV) acquisition when used alone. They are generally not recommended as the sole method of contraception, but rather are used in combination with a diaphragm, sponge, or condom.

The Contraceptive Sponge

The sponge, recently reintroduced to the American market, consists of a soft disk impregnated with a spermicide. It must be placed within the vagina prior to intercourse, and removed within 24 hours afterward. It is 70–85% effective with typical use.

Male Condom

The male condom consists of a flexible sheath, which the man applies to his erect penis prior to penetrating the vagina. It is most often made from natural rubber latex, though it can also be made from lambskin or polyurethane. Condoms are sold over the counter and are readily accessible. Most are lubricated with a spermicide, though unlubricated (spermicide-free) condoms are also available. They may be safely combined with a water-based lubricant for the couple's comfort. Oil-based products should be avoided as they may break the latex. With typical use the male condom is 85% effective, which may be increased by combining the condom with a spermicide or any other contraceptive method (such as a sponge, behavioral, or hormonal method).

Among contraceptive methods, the male latex condom has the strongest evidence for preventing HIV transmission, and appears to prevent transmission of herpes simplex virus, gonorrhea, and Chlamydia as well.

Female Condom

The female condom consists of a polyurethane sleeve with rigid rings at both ends. The closed end is inserted into the vagina, and placed in front of the cervix. The open end is left outside of the vagina. They are generally more difficult to use then male condoms, though they give women more control over both contraception and sexually transmitted disease (STD) prevention.

Diaphragm

The diaphragm consists of a rigid ring with an intervening, soft piece of impermeable latex rubber. The ring is placed into the vagina, and in proper position will extend from the posterior vagina to just behind the pubic symphysis. Spermicide must be generously placed within the diaphragm, and must be reapplied with each act of intercourse. The device must be left in place for six hours following the final act of intercourse, at which time it may be removed, cleaned and later reused. Unlike other barriers, the diaphragm is available by prescription only. It must be properly fitted to the patient by a health-care professional, and should be re-fitted after major change of body weight, vaginal surgery, or pregnancy. With typical use, the 1-year effectiveness is approximately 85%.

Hormonal Methods

Contraceptive hormones always contain a type of progestin, and often contain an estrogen as well. They come in many different forms, including the hormonal intrauterine device (IUD), which will be discussed separately. This is a very popular method of contraception, given its relatively high effectiveness (90–99%, depending on the method used), as well as a number of secondary, noncontraceptive benefits.

Mechanism of Action

Progestins can prevent pregnancy in three ways. They thicken the cervical mucus, limiting the ascent of sperm into the uterine cavity. Regular use will also cause the endometrial lining to atrophy, preventing successful implantation if an embryo enters the uterine cavity. In higher systemic doses the hormone also suppresses the hypothalamus. This prevents the monthly surge in luteinizing hormone, which ultimately suppresses ovulation.

Combination hormonal contraceptives contain an estrogen as well as a progestin. The estrogen component contributes to hypothalamic and ovulation suppression, and thus may add to the method's effectiveness. It also helps to prevent breakthrough bleeding and spotting, which can occur when progestins are used alone.

Formulations

The various dosing options for hormonal contraceptives are summarized in **Table 28.2**. As the dosing intervals, and consequently the compliance requirements, decrease, the effectiveness of the methods increases.

Table 28.2 Administration and effectiveness of hormonal contraceptives

Hormonal method	Dosing route	Dosing interval	1-year pregnancy rate (typical use)[*]
Combination hormonal contraceptives			
Pills	Oral	Daily	8% for all
Evra Patch	Transdermal	Weekly	
Nuvaring	Intravaginal	Monthly	
Progestin-only contraceptives			
Pills	Oral	Daily	8%
Depot medroxyprogesterone acetate	Intramuscular or subcutaneous	Every 3 months	3%
Implanon implant	Subdermal	Every 3 years	0.05%
Mirena IUD	Intrauterine	Every 5 years	0.2%

* From Hatcher RAJ et al., Contraceptive Technology. 19th ed. New York: Ardent Media; 2007

Combination Hormonal Contraceptives: These popular contraceptives contain both an estrogen (usually 20–35 mcg of ethinyl estradiol) and some type of progestin. All off them are considered similarly in terms of side effects, risks, and benefits.

Oral contraceptive pills (OCPs) are the most commonly used contraceptive in the United States. They are packaged in 28-day pill packs, with the days of the week labeled as an aid to compliance. They usually contain 21–24 days of hormonal, "active" pills, with the end of the pack filled with a placebo (or no pill in the last week). These hormone-free days allow a withdrawal bleed, which simulates a period.

Some combination pills are packaged in a "continuous" fashion, with no scheduled withdrawal bleed (that is, active pills are taken daily). This may help women avoid symptoms that occur with hormone withdrawal, such as cramping, headaches, and mood disruption.

Progestin-only Contraceptives: Progestin-only pills, or "minipills," contain a small dose of a progestin with no estrogen. They do not effectively suppress ovulation, and therefore women may have a natural menstrual cycle. Each pill pack contains 28 days of active medication with no scheduled "withdrawal" phase. It is important to instruct women to take all of the pills, as skipping the final pills in the pack or taking days "off" will diminish the pills' effectiveness.

Alternatively, the progestin injection (depot medroxyprogesterone acetate) and implant (Implanon) provide a relatively high dose of systemic hormone that suppresses ovulation. The lack of a "withdrawal" phase usually leads to the cessation of menstruation. Both may produce irregular breakthrough bleeding, though the injection is more likely to produce amenorrhea over time. The implant consists of a single plastic rod, which delivers a progestin over 3 years. The rod is placed under the skin of the upper inner arm with a minor office procedure. The rod may be removed at any time, or may be replaced after 3 years.

The 5-year progestin IUD (Mirena) acts locally within the uterine cavity, delivering lower systemic levels of progestin. Consequently, it does not suppress ovulation. This will be discussed in more detail in the IUD section.

Side Effects

Hormonal contraceptives may produce a wide range of minor side effects, which are usually transient. Often they produce no adverse effects at all. Rarely, the side effects will lead to discontinuation of the product.

Minor side effects: Some women notice nausea, headaches, breakthrough bleeding or spotting, or breast tenderness, which usually improves within the first or second cycle of use. While these side effects are not medically harmful, they are associated with skipping pills during a cycle and with discontinuation of the method. Women should be counseled about these side effects before starting their contraceptive, and encouraged to continue regular use.

Weight gain: Gain in body weight is uncommon with oral contraceptives, the patch, or the ring. Placebo-controlled trials have shown no effect of the combined pill or patch on weight gain. This side effect is more common with depot medroxyprogesterone acetate, with a median weight gain of 2 kg (4.5 lb) at 1 year, and 4.5 kg (10 lb) at 3 years of use.

Menstrual alterations: Because progestins cause the endometrium to atrophy, even in the presence of an estrogen, women on any hormonal method may become amenorrheic or have decreased menstrual bleeding. This is very common with depot-medroxyprogesterone acetate and the progestin IUD. The progestin implant leads to unpredictable bleeding patterns, ranging from frequent light bleeding to amenorrhea. Rarely do hormonal methods cause heavy bleeding.

Infection and cancer: There is some suggestion that OCP users have a higher risk for Chlamydial cervicitis when compared to users of other contraceptive methods (including both barriers and an IUD) or no method. However, among women with Chlamydia, those on OCPs are less likely than others to have an ascending, upper genital tract infection (pelvic inflammatory disease, PID). Women at risk for STDs should be encouraged to use condoms in addition to hormonal methods, and should undergo regular Pap screening.

Cervical cancer is the only malignancy linked to oral contraceptive use. Epidemiologic evidence has shown a lack of association between hormonal contraceptive use and lifetime breast cancer risk.

Serious side effects: Women who experience an increase in migraines (particularly with an aura), cholestasis or gallbladder dysfunction, major lipid alterations, liver adenomas, or hemangiomas should discontinue using the hormones.

Medical Complications and Contraindications

Estrogens are known to promote platelet adherence and blood clotting. Thus estrogen-containing contraceptives are contraindicated in women prone to arterial or venous clotting. This includes women with risk factors for stroke and cardiovascular disease, and those with thrombophilias. Women with well-controlled hypertension or diabetes may qualify for combination hormone use, but nonestrogen-containing methods should be considered.

Progestin-only methods have not been rigorously studied with regard to clotting and cardiovascular risk. However, epidemiologic research has suggested no increased risk of such events when progestin-only methods are used. In the absence of rigorous data, low-dose methods may be preferred for patients with cardiovascular risk (such as POPs or the progestin IUD).

The absolute risks of major cardiovascular events among healthy women are very low, and substantially lower than the risk of pregnancy. This should be explained to patients who are concerned about major risks. Women should be encouraged to avoid smoking while taking hormones, and combination hormones should be avoided in smokers over 35 years old.

Some breast and liver tumors are hormone sensitive, and women with a history of these tumors should be prescribed hormones only in consultation with an oncologist or gastroenterologist.

Noncontraceptive Benefits

Hormonal contraceptives may offer a number of benefits beyond contraception, and are frequently used by women who do not need contraception. These include regulation of the menstrual cycle (with controlled timing of a withdrawal bleed), management of dysmenorrhea, prevention of ovarian and endometrial cancer, and control of acne and hyperandrogenic symptoms.

Intrauterine Devices

There are two types of IUD approved for use in the United States: the TCu380A (Paragard), which uses copper, and the LNG-20 (Mirena), which uses the progestin levonorgestrel. Both IUDs are highly effective, long-lasting, reversible contraceptives, but remain underutilized in the United States. This may be due to misconceptions about IUD risks. Patient education and improved access may increase use of this valuable contraceptive method.

Both devices consist of a T-shaped piece of plastic with a long string attached to the base of the T. One is wrapped with copper, while the other is impregnated with the progestin. Either device may be inserted in a medical office without the use of anesthetics. The small, T-shaped device is placed within the endometrial cavity, with the string projecting through the cervix. The device is easily removed in the office by pulling on the string. Both methods are more than 99% effective, requiring no ongoing compliance on the part of the patient (other than having the device replaced after its expiration). Fertility rates after discontinuation of an IUD are similar to those following cessation of a hormonal method, and rates of infertility do not appear to be increased in this group.

Method of Action

Intrauterine devices may act in a number of ways. Both types alter the cervical mucus in ways that impede sperm from reaching the upper genital tract, and all types of IUD have effects on the endometrium that further inhibit the sperm. Copper IUDs accomplish this through a strong inflammatory response, while the hormonal IUD may inhibit sperm through endometrial and glandular changes. If fertilization should occur, both types of IUD can inhibit implantation through their endometrial effects. Neither type of IUD will inhibit ovulation.

Side Effects

The progestin IUD causes significant endometrial atrophy resulting in decreased bleeding when compared with a copper IUD or no IUD. This is often considered a benefit of the method, though it may be undesirable to women who prefer to have a monthly period. Serum progestin levels with the hormonal IUD are a fraction of that with oral progestins, and systemic hormonal side effects are uncommon.

Alternatively, users of the copper IUD are more likely to complain of heavy periods or dysmenorrhea. Both of these symptoms may be ameliorated with use of non-steroidal anti-inflammatory drugs (NSAIDs).

Risks and Contraindications

Many women are concerned that IUDs will cause infection. In fact, the risk of pelvic infection is less than 1 per 100 woman-years, and is negligible beyond the first 20 days postinsertion. Women who are at risk of STDs should be screened prior to device insertion, and some practices routinely screen for gonorrhea and Chlamydia prior to inserting the IUD. As with other methods, women using IUDs should be encouraged to actively avoid STDs by practicing monogamy or with condom use. Women with HIV may use the IUD with a low risk of infection, and the contraceptive effectiveness and avoidance of systemic hormones may be desirable in this group.

Though the IUD was long believed to cause tubal infertility, such an association has been essentially disproved. Correspondingly, nulliparity is no longer a relative contraindication to IUD use (Evidence Box 28.1)

There is a small (<1%) risk of uterine perforation with IUD insertion. In this situation, the IUD penetrates the myometrium, embedding in an incorrect location or migrating into the abdomen or pelvis. In this circumstance, the IUD may require removal with hysteroscopy or laparoscopy (see Chapter 38). An IUD cannot be properly placed in a unicornuate, bicornuate, or septate uterus. Additionally, large fibroids within the uterine cavity may interfere with proper placement and effectiveness.

Sterilization

Both women and men may undergo sterilization with minimally invasive methods. Its effectiveness is similar to the IUD at more than 99%, but its permanence obviates the need for replacement.

Female Sterilization

Female sterilization involves occlusion of the fallopian tubes through a variety of different methods. Though in selected cases it may be possible to later reconnect the tubes surgically, patients must understand that this is considered a permanent sterilization procedure. Effectiveness is over 99% in the first year after the procedures, but increases to an overall failure rate of about 1% after 4 years and close to 2% after 10 years. The long-term failure risk is higher for women sterilized at a younger age, as they have a longer fertile window in which to become pregnant.

Risks of sterilization include risks of the surgical procedure, which are very rare (less than 1% of procedures). Though the probability of any pregnancy is very low, a poststerilization pregnancy must always be considered ectopic (tubal or ovarian) until proven otherwise. The procedure's permanence can lead to feelings of regret, which occur in 6% of women 30 years and older, and 20% of sterilized women who are under 30. Thus it is especially important to counsel younger women about effective, reversible options, such as the IUD.

Postpartum tubal ligation: Immediately after birth the fallopian tubes are easily accessible for sterilization. Most postpartum methods involve removal of a fallopian tube segment with ligation of the cut tubal ends. These techniques may be performed immediately following uterine closure with a cesarean section, or through a mini-laparotomy incision after vaginal delivery. At this point, the uterine fundus is approximately at the level of the umbilicus, and the tubes may be accessed through a small, subumbilical incision. The most popular methods are the modified Pomeroy and the Irving procedures (**Fig. 28.1**). With the

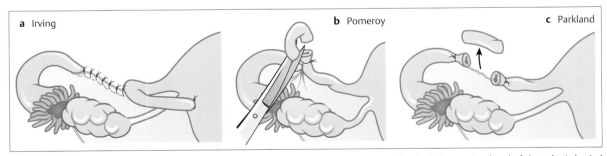

Fig. 28.1 Commonly used methods of postpartum tubal ligation. **a** Irving technique, with which the proximal end of the tube is buried within the uterine myometrium. **b** Pomeroy technique, whereby a knuckle of tube is formed and tied in place with an absorbable suture. The intervening loop of tube is then excised. **c** Parkland (or Modified Pomeroy) technique, with which absorbable sutures are placed proximally and distally, and the intervening segment of tube is excised.

latter, the proximal, cut end of the fallopian tube is buried within the myometrium at the time of cesarean section.

Laparoscopic tubal ligation: Fallopian tubes can usually be accessed easily during laparoscopy (see Chapter 38). The tubes may be occluded with cautery, permanent clips, or small bands (**Fig. 28.2**). Bands and cautery appear to have lower failure rates than clips. The procedure has the advantage of using very small incisions, and the surgery is almost always performed on an outpatient basis.

On the downside, laparoscopic tubal ligation almost always requires general anesthesia, and an operating room supplied with appropriate surgical equipment. When this arrangement is not available, or general anesthesia is deemed unsafe, the procedure may be performed through a mini-laparotomy incision with regional anesthesia.

Hysteroscopic tubal occlusion: More recently, an even less invasive technique has been developed for female sterilization. A hysteroscope is inserted into the uterine cavity, and small metal coils are threaded into each fallopian tube under direct visualization (see Chapter 38). Over the ensuing 3 months, fibrous scar tissue develops within these coils, completely occluding the tubes. A hysterosalpingogram—an X-ray with which a radiopaque dye is injected into the uterine cavity and fallopian tubes—will confirm final occlusion of the tubes (**Fig. 28.3**).

This procedure has the advantage of requiring minimal anesthesia, as it can be performed with intravenous sedation, or with intramuscular or oral analgesics alone. As an incision-free procedure, it avoids surgical risks that necessarily come with laparotomy and laparoscopy. It may also avoid technical limitations arising in women with pelvic adhesions or obesity. As a drawback, the procedure may be technically challenging or impossible to complete in 8–10% of patients. Pregnancy is extremely unlikely once the coils are placed and the tubes appear occluded by hysterosalpingogram.

Male Sterilization

Men may be sterilized with a vasectomy. With this minimally invasive procedure, a small puncture is made in the scrotum, through which the vas deferens is identified, cut, and occluded. Prior to having unprotected intercourse, the man must have a semen analysis to confirm azospermia, which will be present after three months and 20 ejaculations for the majority of men.

This is a very safe, outpatient procedure that may be performed with local anesthesia. It is also highly effective: 99.8% at 1 year. As with female sterilization, the couple should consider this a permanent procedure.

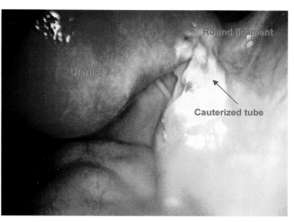
Fig. 28.2 Laparoscopic tubal ligation with cauterized right fallopian tube.

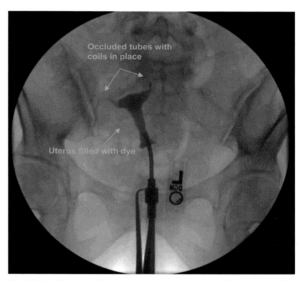
Fig. 28.3 Hysterosalpingogram showing bilaterally occluded fallopian tubes with metal coils in place.

Emergency Contraception

If couples engage in unprotected intercourse or misuse a contraceptive, they still have time to protect themselves from pregnancy. As suggested by the common name "morning-after pill," the most common method of emergency contraception (EC) involves taking high doses of progestins or, less commonly, combination OCPs. With the progestin-only method, the woman is traditionally instructed to take 0.75 mg of levonorgestrel within 72 hours of intercourse, and repeat the dose one time, 12 hours later. However, a randomized trial has shown that women may take the two tablets simultaneously, which may improve compliance, and that the method may still have an effect for up to 5 days postintercourse.

With the combination pill method, women must take a relatively high dose of estradiol and repeat it in 12 hours. This has the unpleasant side effect of nausea, which can limit its effective use. The levonorgestrel method largely removes this side effect, and has essentially replaced the combination method.

Hormonal EC is believed to work by delaying ovulation, though it may theoretically prevent implantation of a fertilized embryo as well. The method is most effective the sooner it is used, and women should be encouraged to use EC as soon as possible after unprotected sex. The method is approximately 80% effective at preventing pregnancy from a single act of intercourse (reducing the risk from 8% to 2%, though these numbers vary depending on the time of the cycle). It is extremely safe, with no contraindications except for a documented allergy to the medication. It is important to distinguish EC from medical abortion when counseling patients, as the two treatments may be confused by the uninformed.

Placement of a copper IUD within 5 days of unprotected intercourse reduces the pregnancy rate by over 90%. Unlike levonorgestrel, which is now available to adults over the counter, IUD access is limited by cost and the availability of a trained provider for insertion.

Key Points

- Many pregnancies are unintended. Adequate contraception will reduce the rate of unintended pregnancy. Adequate contraception is an important part of ensuring the health of women.
- Choosing an appropriate contraceptive requires balancing many factors including patient preferences, cost, efficacy, side effects, and potential medical contraindications.
- For couples requesting permanent sterilization, vasectomy is recommended for men or hysteroscopic tubal occlusion for women.
- For women desiring long-term reversible contraception, an intrauterine device is recommended with long-acting medroxyprogesterone injections or subdermal progestin implants as alternatives.
- For contraceptives that require daily use, we recommend estrogen–progestin contraceptives, either as a pill or vaginal ring for women, and the progestin-only pill as an alternative method.
- If used correctly and diligently, barrier contraceptives such as condoms for men or women and the diaphragm for women are very effective.
- The condom is the only method of contraception that is recommended for reducing the risk of sexually transmitted infections.

Evidence Box 28.1

Prior use of a copper intrauterine device is not associated with tubal infertility in nulligravid women.

Until recently, the intrauterine device (IUD) was indicated for parous women only. This stemmed from the belief that the IUD was an independent risk factor for infertility in nulliparous women. Unfortunately, this restricted the use of this highly effective contraceptive for thousands of otherwise eligible women.

In 2001 a large case–control study was published, which challenged the association between the IUD and infertility. In this study 1311 infertile, nulligravid women were identified prior to undergoing testing for tubal infertility. A control group of 584 primigravid women was selected from the same hospital system. All study subjects were interviewed about their contraceptive history, as well as other risk factors for tubal infertility. They also underwent serologic testing for *Chlamydia trachomatis*. Following the interview, the infertile women underwent hysterosalpingography to diagnose tubal occlusion.

Results of this study showed no association between infertility, with or without tubal occlusion, and prior use of a copper IUD. The fertile controls reported a higher number of lifetime sexual partners, and were more likely to suspect infidelity on the part of their partner. Alternatively, the infertile cases were more likely to report a history of pelvic inflammatory disease, and were more likely to carry antibodies to Chlamydia.

The authors concluded that Chlamydia exposure and a history of upper genital tract infection are risk factors for infertility, whereas IUD use is not. Correspondingly, the US Food and Drug Administration has changed its labeling of the copper IUD, making the device available to nulliparous women.

Hubacher D, Lara-Ricalde R, Taylor DJ, et al. Use of copper intrauterine devices and the risk of tubal infertility among nulligravid women. N Engl J Med 2001;345:561–567.

Further Reading

Arévalo M, Jennings V, Sinai I. Efficacy of a new method of family planning: the Standard Days Method. *Contraception* 2002;65(5):333–338

Bontis J, Vavilis D, Panidis D, Theodoridis T, Konstantinidis T, Sidiropoulou A. Detection of Chlamydia trachomatis in asymptomatic women: relationship to history, contraception, and cervicitis. *Adv Contracept* 1994;10(4):309–315

CDC. Primary Contraceptive Methods Among Women Aged 15–44 Years—United States, 2002. *MMWR* 2005;54(6):152

Cooper JM, Carignan CS, Cher D, Kerin JF; Selective Tubal Occlusion Procedure 2000 Investigators Group. Microinsert nonincisional hysteroscopic sterilization. *Obstet Gynecol* 2003;102(1):59–67

Farley TM, Rosenberg MJ, Rowe PJ, Chen JH, Meirik O. Intrauterine devices and pelvic inflammatory disease: an international perspective. *Lancet* 1992;339(8796):785–788

Finer LB, Henshaw SK. Disparities in rates of unintended pregnancy in the United States, 1994 and 2001. *Perspect Sex Reprod Health* 2006;38(2):90–96

Gallo MF, Lopez LM, Grimes DA, Schulz KF, Helmerhorst FM. Combination contraceptives: effects on weight. *Cochrane Database Syst Rev* 2006; (1):CD003987

Hannaford PCS, Selvaraj S, Elliott AM, Angus V, Iversen L, Lee AJ. Cancer risk among users of oral contraceptives: cohort data from the Royal College of General Practitioner's oral contraception study. *BMJ* 2007;335(7621):651

Hatcher RA, Trussell J, Nelson AL, et al. Contraceptive Technology. 19th ed. New York: Ardent Media; 2007

Hillis SDP, Marchbanks PA, Tylor LR, Peterson HB. Poststerilization regret: findings from the United States Collaborative Review of Sterilization. *Obstet Gynecol* 1999;93(6):889–895

Hubacher D, Lara-Ricalde R, Taylor DJ, Guerra-Infante F, Guzmán-Rodríguez R. Use of copper intrauterine devices and the risk of tubal infertility among nulligravid women. *N Engl J Med* 2001;345(8):561–567

Marchbanks PA, McDonald JA, Wilson HG, et al. Oral contraceptives and the risk of breast cancer. *N Engl J Med* 2002;346(26):2025–2032

National Institute of Allergy and Infectious Diseases, National Institutes of Health, et al. (2001). Scientific Evidence on Condom Effectiveness for Sexually Transmitted Disease (STD) Prevention. http://www3.niaid.nih.gov/about/organization/dmid/PDF/CondomReport.pdf (Accessed: August 19, 2009)

Sivin I, Stern J; International Committee for Contraception Research (ICCR). Health during prolonged use of levonorgestrel 20 micrograms/d and the copper TCu 380Ag intrauterine

contraceptive devices: a multicenter study. *Fertil Steril* 1994;61(1):70–77

Smith JS, Green J, Berrington de Gonzalez A, et al. Cervical cancer and use of hormonal contraceptives: a systematic review. *Lancet* 2003;361(9364):1159–1167

Wald A, Langenberg AG, Link K, et al. Effect of condoms on reducing the transmission of herpes simplex virus type 2 from men to women. *JAMA* 2001;285(24):3100–3106

Westhoff CJ, Jain JK, Milsom I, Ray A. Changes in weight with depot medroxyprogesterone acetate subcutaneous injection 104 mg/0.65 mL. *Contraception* 2007;75(4):261–267

Wølner-Hanssen PDA, Eschenbach DA, Paavonen J, et al. Decreased risk of symptomatic chlamydial pelvic inflammatory disease associated with oral contraceptive use. *JAMA* 1990;263(1):54–59

WHO. Medical Eligibility Criteria for Contraceptive Use. 3rd ed. Geneva: World Health Organization; 2004

World Health Organization Collaborative Study of Cardiovascular Disease and Steroid Hormone Contraception. Cardiovascular disease and use of oral and injectable progestogen-only contraceptives and combined injectable contraceptives. Results of an international, multicenter, case-control study. *Contraception* 1998;57(5):315–324

Zhou L, Xiao B. Emergency contraception with Multiload Cu-375 SL IUD: a multicenter clinical trial. *Contraception* 2001;64(2):107–112

29 Therapeutic Abortion

Melody Y. Hou

Definition

Therapeutic abortion is defined as the intended interruption of an established pregnancy. Under the landmark 1973 *Roe vs. Wade* decision, the United States Supreme Court ruled that abortion is a legal procedure up until the point when the fetus becomes viable, or "has the capability of meaningful life outside the mother's womb." Although individual States may regulate or prohibit abortion after viability, these actions are not permitted if abortion is deemed medically necessary to preserve the life or health of the woman seeking abortion. Prior to viability, States may enact restrictions if they do not create "undue burden" on the woman.

Abortion is an important issue in reproductive health, historically and worldwide, and few other topics in medicine have attracted as much debate. Some people feel that therapeutic abortion should be illegal because it destroys a developing human life. However, history has shown that a woman who has an undesired pregnancy will seek abortion despite the legal or social restrictions in her society, and that maternal mortality rate decreases significantly whenever and wherever abortion is safe and legal.

History and Legality

Abortion has been described as early as 2737 BC, and found in civilizations as diverse as the Chinese, Greek and Roman Empires. With the rise of Christianity, abortion and contraception became more controversial, culminating in the criminalization of abortion throughout the United States by the 1870s. Over the next century, thousands of women died or suffered serious injuries due to "back alley" abortions, and caring for women sick or dying from sepsis caused by these illegal and unregulated procedures became a common experience for medical

trainees. By 1970, the American Medication Association (AMA), which had originally supported the criminalization of abortion in order to establish physician dominance over nonphysician clinicians, reversed its stance on abortion and called for its legalization. Three years later, the US Supreme Court recognized the need for safe and legal abortion with its landmark decision in *Roe vs. Wade*. Since then, there has been an opposing movement in the United States to repeal or limit the abortion rights granted by this decision.

Epidemiology

Unintended pregnancy and abortion are important public health issues worldwide. The majority of the world's population lives in countries where abortion is restricted or generally prohibited. In 2008, 26% of all people resided in countries where abortion was permitted only to save a woman's life or is prohibited altogether, whereas 35% lived in countries where abortion was permitted only to preserve either physical or mental health or for socioeconomic grounds. The remaining 39% resided in countries where there were no restrictions as to reason for the procedure.

Wherever she lives, a woman's likelihood of having an abortion is the same, whether abortion be considered legal or illegal. In countries where abortion is legal and accessible, abortions are safe and complications are rare. In countries where abortion is restricted, abortions are unsafe, performed by persons lacking in necessary skills or in an environment that does not meet minimal medical standards, or both. Methods of unsafe abortion that are practiced include drinking bleach or turpentine, inserting foreign objects such as coat hangers or sticks into the uterus, or jumping off stairs or roofs. One in four women undergoing unsafe abortion will face serious complications. Complications from unsafe abortions account for 13% of maternal mortality worldwide.

In the United States, nearly half of all pregnancies are unintended. Four in 10 of these unintended pregnancies end in abortion, accounting for 22% of all pregnancies, excluding miscarriage. Half of all American women have had an unintended pregnancy, and 35% are estimated to have had an abortion before age 35 years.

Counseling

It is important not to assume that a positive pregnancy test is good news for a patient. Any woman who tests positive for an unplanned pregnancy should be counseled on all options, including abortion, adoption, or parenting the resulting child. The information must be handled sensitively and empathetically, since this decision is personal and may be extremely difficult for a patient. Efforts should be made to ensure that the patient's choice is not coerced. As abortion laws vary from State to State, these restrictions, such as 24-hour waiting periods, spousal notification, and mandatory ultrasound-viewing, must also be considered during counseling.

If the patient elects termination, she must be informed regarding the nature of the procedure and its risks. Legal abortion in the United States is among the safest of medical procedures, with less than 0.3% of abortion patients experiencing a complication requiring hospitalization. Abortion risk increases with gestational age. Based on the most recently published national review of mortality risk from 1988 to1997, mortality risk was determined to be 0.1 per 100000 abortions done at or before 8 weeks, 3.4 in 100000 between 16 weeks and 20 weeks, and 8.9 in 100000 at 21 weeks or more. However, timely access to abortion services may be difficult since 87% of counties in the United States have no abortion providers, and 35% of American women live in those counties. Access to abortion services becomes more difficult with increasing gestational age, since there is a shortage of providers trained to do abortions in later gestations.

Patient History, Physical and Laboratory Tests

A careful history should be taken, which includes documenting the patient's last menstrual period (LMP) and any pregnancy symptoms she may be experiencing. (In this chapter, all gestational ages will refer to menstrual weeks, with the woman's LMP as the reference point.) If the pregnancy has not been confirmed, a urine pregnancy test should be done. On physical exam, assess the size of the uterus and its position (ante- or retroverted, ante- or retroflexed), as well as any tenderness or masses in the

adnexa. A preprocedure ultrasound will confirm the gestational age and help exclude the presence of an ectopic pregnancy or any pathology that may complicate the procedure, such as fibroids, müllerian duct anomalies, or a multiple pregnancy. Since abortions carry a 5% risk of rhesus (Rh) D alloimmunization in susceptible patients, Rh antigen status should also be determined and Rh negative patients treated with D immunoglobulin.

Most procedures are performed under local anesthesia, such as a paracervical block, but this may not be completely effective. Local anesthesia may be augmented with sedation for patient comfort, particularly in later gestational ages. Prophylactic antibiotics are also recommended since a meta-analysis showed that antibiotics reduced the rate of postoperative endometritis by half, including women in low-risk groups.

Methods for First Trimester Abortion

The most common method for first trimester abortion, or abortions performed prior to 13 weeks, is via vacuum aspiration (also known as suction curettage) (**Fig 29.1**). Vacuum aspiration consists of dilating the cervix and inserting a suction cannula that is connected to a vacuum source. Adequate cervical dilatation is achieved through use of serial tapered rods of increasing diameters, known as dilators. The vacuum source can either be from an electric pump or created using a modified 60 cc syringe, known as manual aspiration. Under adequate vacuum, the cannula is rotated to clear the uterus of the products of conception. Another surgical method is dilation and curettage (D&C), in which the cervix is dilated until a curette or forceps of adequate size can be inserted to remove the products. After the procedure, the specimen obtained should be examined immediately to confirm products of conception and the completion of the abortion. If no products of conception are identified, a review of a preprocedure and postprocedure ultrasound and serial beta human chorionic gonadotropin (β-HCG) levels can allow for early diagnosis of an unruptured ectopic pregnancy. In very early gestations (less than 6 weeks) aspiration can miss the pregnancy. The tissue may also be difficult to identify in the specimen or on ultrasound after the procedure. However, careful aspiration can still be attempted with appropiate follow-up.

Prior to 49–63 days of gestation, medical abortion may also be offered (**Table 29.1**, Evidence Box 29.1). Mifepristone is an oral antiprogestin that binds to the progesterone receptor at a greater infinity than progesterone. By blocking progesterone, it alters the lining of the uterus and disrupts the attachment of the embryo. Mifepristone may be administered in combination with misoprostol (a prostaglandin) to induce expulsion of the products of conception. Rather than the single surgical event that occurs

Table 29.1 Patient selection for first trimester abortion method

Medical abortion	Surgical abortion
Able to return for multiple visits and complete entire follow-up	Wants only one visit
Willing to wait several weeks as needed for abortion completion	Prefers to give control of the abortion to the clinician
Able to obtain emergency care as necessary	Desires sedation
Can cope with bleeding and cramping	Desires greater assurance that an abortion is completed
Desires privacy or control over the process	
Realizes that surgical intervention may still be necessary	

with vacuum aspiration, a woman who chooses medical abortion experiences the process as a series of events: taking the medication, feeling symptoms, and experiencing the expulsion. From initiation to completion, medical abortion takes more time than surgical, and involves more observed blood loss. However, women may elect medical abortion because of concerns for the risks of surgical abortion or preferences for privacy and control. Women will experience moderate-to-heavy bleeding and cramping with the expulsion, which may be accompanied by nausea, vomiting, and diarrhea depending on the medication regimen. Eighty-five percent of women will abort within 3 days of misoprostol administration, although for a few patients the process may take up to a few weeks. Completion is most often confirmed by transvaginal ultrasound, although confirmation by clinical exam is also permitted by the US Food and Drug Administration (FDA).

Although the FDA-approved regimen uses oral misoprostol, evidence shows that buccal and vaginal administration is equally if not more effective, with fewer side effects. If medical abortion fails, surgical termination is advised due to the possible risk of fetal anomalies due to misoprostol exposure. Medical abortion should be clearly differentiated from emergency contraception, which does not affect a pregnancy already implanted. Prior to the approval of mifepristone in the United States in 2000, regimens such as methotrexate with misoprostol, or misoprostol alone, were also used to induce medical abortion.

Methods for Second Trimester Abortion

Only 12% of all terminations occur in the second trimester (at or after 13 weeks). Dilation and evacuation (D&E) is considered the safest and preferred method for second trimester termination. The procedure is the same as a vacuum aspiration (dilation of the cervix followed by insertion of a suction cannula), but according to convention, vacuum aspiration refers to procedures done prior to 13 weeks and D&E refers to procedures at or after 13 weeks. However, after 16 weeks, even the large diameter suction cannula is insufficient to empty the uterus. Instead, forceps are used as the primary instrument, with vacuum aspiration as an adjunct.

Although dilators may be used to adequately open the cervix, there is a higher risk of cervical and uterine injury in mechanically opening the cervix to the degree needed for a D&E. Instead, cervical preparation may assist in decreasing this risk. The cervix may be prepared with osmotic dilators, such as laminaria tents, or with a prostaglandin. Laminaria tents, which are narrow rods made of kelp seaweed, are placed in the cervix the day before the scheduled abortion. Overnight, the laminaria absorb fluid from the vagina and cervix and swell to dilate the cervix. Synthetic hygroscopic dilators are also available for this purpose. The number of osmotic dilators needed for a D&E increases with gestational age, with ten or more laminaria achieving the dilatation needed for terminations after 20 weeks (**Fig 29.2**).

The cervix may also be ripened using pharmacologic agents, such as misoprostol. For an early second trimester abortion, misoprostol can be administered buccally or vaginally several hours before the procedure. Compared with abortions following overnight laminaria preparation, procedures following same-day misoprostol ripening were found to be more challenging and took longer to complete. However, misoprostol ripening allows the procedure to be completed in one day, which was preferred

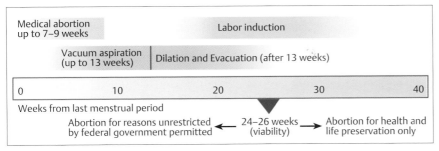

Medical abortion up to 7–9 weeks

Labor induction

Vacuum aspiration (up to 13 weeks)

Dilation and Evacuation (after 13 weeks)

0   10   20   30   40

Weeks from last menstrual period

Abortion for reasons unrestricted by federal government permitted ← 24–26 weeks (viability) → Abortion for health and life preservation only

Fig. 29.1 Timing of medical and surgical methods for termination in the United States.

by patients over the two-day procedure needed for cervical preparation with laminaria.

An advanced variation of the D&E, the intact D&E, was first described in 1995. Also known as dilation and extraction (D&X), this method seeks to widely dilate the cervix, usually with several days of laminaria, and to remove the fetus through the cervix as intact as possible, although decompression of the fetal calvarium may be necessary to complete the procedure. This allows for full pathology evaluation and an opportunity for bonding for patients grieving a medically-compromised but otherwise desired pregnancy. The intact D&E also reduces the risk of the procedure to the patient since less instrumentation is required. However, in 2003 the US Congress passed the "Partial-Birth Abortion Ban," also known as the Federal Abortion Ban, which ostensibly sought to prohibit late-term abortion by intact D&E. However, since the broadly phrased law includes no gestational age limits and reduces the role of physician judgment, it stands to threaten the legality of standard D&Es as well. In contrast with the US Supreme Court's decision in *Roe vs. Wade*, the law has no health exception, making abortions for medical reasons potentially illegal. After multiple challenges to the law, the newly conservative US Supreme Court overturned legal precedence in 2007 with Gonzalez vs. Carhart, and allowed the ban to stand. The repercussions of the law and the ruling on women's health are still being studied.

Another method for second trimester abortion is labor induction. Although D&E is considered a safer and more expeditious procedure, particularly prior to 20 weeks, the shortage of providers trained in safe D&E may limit a patient to labor induction. Pharmacologic agents may be used singly or in combination to achieve a labor pattern adequate to dilate the cervix and expel both fetus and placenta. In the past, regimens included intra-amniotic instillation of agents, such as hypertonic saline, urea, or prostaglandins; systemic prostaglandins; and intravenous high-dose infusion of oxytoxin. More recently, regimens including mifepristone followed by a prostaglandin have come into favor. In a review of two randomized controlled trials comparing D&E to induction by either intra-amniotic prostaglandin F2α or mifepristone with misoprostol, there were more adverse events in the induction group compared to D&E. Although instillation abortion is rarely used now, mifepristone with misoprostol is an effective and acceptable method of medical second trimester abortion if D&E is not a desired or possible option. However, as retained placenta occurs frequently with induction abortion, a vacuum aspiration may still be required to remove the remaining tissue (**Fig 29.2**).

Complications and Long-Term Outcomes

Complications

The overall complication rate of abortion is estimated to be less than 2%. The complications of abortion increase with gestational age. They include infection, incomplete evacuation, excessive bleeding or hemorrhage, failed abortion, and injury to the cervix, uterus and surrounding organs. Of these, infection, bleeding and incomplete evacuation are the most common.

Infection: Postabortal endometritis occurs in 5–20% of women who do not receive prophylactic antibiotics; this rate can be halved if prophylactic antibiotics are given. Symptoms include fever, abdominal pain, and vaginal bleeding heavier than expected, several days to a few weeks after the procedure. An ultrasound will help identify whether the infection is due to retained products of conception. Retained products of conception should be treated with a repeat aspiration. If no retained products are identified, broad-spectrum antibiotics are advised.

Incomplete evacuation: An incomplete evacuation with retained products of conception is usually recognized immediately postprocedure with excessive bleeding. However, patients may present with lower abdominal pain and bleeding at a later point, usually within the first week

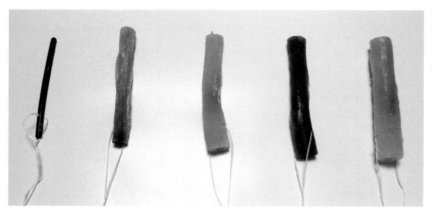

Fig. 29.2 Laminaria tents at 0, 2, 4, 6, and 8 hours of being placed in water. Because laminaria are made of organic material, individual variations in diameter may occur.

of the procedure. Ultrasound may assist with this diagnosis, particularly if a focal mass is identified within the endometrium. Treatment requires a repeat aspiration.

Excessive bleeding/hemorrhage: Immediate excessive bleeding can be a sign of incomplete evacuation or hematometria (uterine distention from blood), uterine atony, abnormal placentation such as placenta accreta, or trauma such as uterine perforation. Bleeding from retained tissue of clot will stop after it is evacuated from the uterus by aspiration. Uterine atony may be treated by pharmacologic measures, such as misoprostol, carboprost, or ergotamines. In later gestations when oxytocin receptors are produced in the uterus, oxytocin may also reduce bleeding from uterine atony. Bleeding from a cervical laceration will cease when the injury is repaired; injuries to the uterus may require repair via laparoscopy or laparotomy. If arteries are lacerated from a perforation, or in cases of abnormal placentation or persistent uterine atony refractory to medications, the patient may require exploratory laparotomy with possible hysterectomy. In recent years, uterine artery embolization has also become a viable uterus-conserving option in hemorrhage.

Failed surgical abortion: A rare complication, failed abortion occurs at about 0.6 per 1000 cases, and more frequently occurs with early rather than late pregnancy terminations. Uterine anomalies, including müllerian duct anomalies or fibroids, increase the risk of this complication, but most failed abortions occur in patients with normal anatomy under the care of experienced physicians. Recognition of failed abortion is usually immediate with the examination of the specimen, but ultrasound and serial β-HCG testing may assist with this diagnosis. Multiple pregnancies may also lead to a failed abortion if only one gestational sac is removed during the procedure.

Cervical injury: The risk of cervical laceration increases with gestational age, particularly when dilators are used. However, if the cervix is prepared with laminaria or misoprostol, the rate of cervical injury in second trimester terminations may be no more than those done in the first trimester.

Uterine perforation: The risk of uterine perforation also increases with gestational age. Perforation can occur during cervical dilation or during instrumentation with the suction cannula or forceps. Exploratory laparoscopy or laparotomy should be done to assess and repair the uterine perforation. Since injuries to the surrounding organs such as bowel and bladder may also occur with perforation, surrounding organs should also be closely inspected for injuries at the time of exploration. This is particularly important in the second trimester, since a uterine perforation at this gestational age may lead to injured bowel requiring resection.

Other Long-Term Outcomes

Studies have been inconclusive regarding any association between abortion and future infertility, miscarriages and low birth weight in subsequent pregnancies. Despite mandatory counseling in some States regarding abortion and breast cancer, the National Cancer Institute has firmly established that there is no association between abortion and breast cancer. Common emotional reactions after an abortion include relief, transient guilt, sadness, and a sense of loss. However, multiple studies from the United States and the United Kingdom have found that abortion does not pose an independent risk for depression.

Key Points

- Therapeutic abortion is the intended interruption of an established pregnancy.
- Therapeutic abortion is an important medical issue worldwide that engenders significant moral debate. Some people believe that abortion should be severely restricted because it interrupts the development of a potential human life. However, the maternal mortality rate decreases significantly wherever and whenever abortion is safe and legal.
- Abortion counseling includes a discussion of all pregnancy options, including abortion, adoption, or parenting, and should be sensitive and empathetic.
- Vacuum aspiration is the most common intervention to terminate a pregnancy up to 13 weeks. After 13 weeks, dilation and evacuation is the preferred method for second trimester termination.
- Up to 63 days of gestation, medical abortion by mifepristone (antiprogestin) and misoprostol (prostaglandin) are effective in causing pregnancy termination.
- Mifepristone and prostaglandins, or prostaglandins alone, can effect non-surgical pregnancy termination in the second trimester by inducing labor.
- Legal therapeutic abortion is extremely safe, with an overall complication rate of less than 2%. Less than 0.3% of abortion patients will experience a complication requiring hospitalization.

Evidence Box 29.1

Medical abortion can be offered as an alternative to vacuum aspiration up to 49–63 days since a patient's last menstrual period. The most commonly used regimen in the United States is mifepristone, followed by a prostaglandin to aid in expulsion of the pregnancy. However, the high cost of mifepristone makes its use somewhat prohibitive in developing countries where medical abortion could otherwise increase the number of safe options for abortion. Prior to the FDA approval of mifepristone in 2000, other medical regimens were used to effect abortion in the United States. These methods may be suitable alternatives to surgical abortion in countries where mifepristone use is not feasible.

Since the "gold standard" for abortion methods is vacuum aspiration, the Cochrane Collaboration sought to gather high-quality randomized controlled trials comparing different methods of medical abortion with vacuum aspiration.

Six high-quality trials were identified that together analyzed four interventions against vacuum aspiration: prostaglandins alone, methotrexate with prostaglandin, mifepristone with prostaglandin, and mifepristone alone (**Table 29.2**). The power to detect differences between vacuum aspiration and the medical regimens were often limited due to small sample sizes, so although efficacy between methods may appear to be very different, statistically these differences may not be significant.

Of these comparisons, only the prostaglandin-only regimen had a statistically significant higher abortion incompletion than surgical abortion (odds ratio of incomplete abortion with medical versus surgical was 2.67, with a 95% confidence interval of 1.06–6.75). However, in communities or societies where medical abortion by prostaglandin alone may be more accessible than surgical abortion, medical abortion by prostaglandins is a reasonable option.

Say L, Kulier R, Gülmezoglu M, Campana A. Medical versus surgical methods for first trimester termination of pregnancy. Cochrane Database Syst Rev 2002 Oct 21;(4) CD003037.

Further Reading

ACOG. Prevention of Rh D alloimmunization. ACOG Practice Bulletin No. 4. Washington DC: American College of Obstetricians and Gynecologists; May 1999

Bartlett LA, Berg CJ, Shulman HB, et al. Risk factors for legal induced abortion-related mortality in the United States. *Obstet Gynecol* 2004;103(4):729–737

Center for Reproductive Rights. The world's abortion laws. May 2008

Durfee SM, Frates MC, Luong A, Benson CB. The sonographic and color Doppler features of retained products of conception. *J Ultrasound Med* 2005;24(9):1181–1186, quiz 1188–1189

Finer LB, Henshaw SK. Disparities in rates of unintended pregnancy in the United States, 1994 and 2001. *Perspect Sex Reprod Health* 2006;38(2):90–96

Gamble SE, Strauss LT, Parker WY, Cook DA, Zane SB, Hamdan S; Center for Disease Control and Prevention (CDC). Abortion surveillance – United States, 2005; 57(SS13); 1–32.

Gilchrist AC, Hannaford PC, Frank P, Kay CR. Termination of pregnancy and psychiatric morbidity. *Br J Psychiatry* 1995;167(2):243–248

Goldberg AB, Drey EA, Whitaker AK, Kang M-S, Meckstroth KR, Darney PD. Misoprostol compared with laminaria before early second-trimester surgical abortion: a randomized trial. *Obstet Gynecol* 2005;106(2):234–241

Grimes DA, Schulz KF. Morbidity and mortality from second-trimester abortions. *J Reprod Med* 1985;30(7):505–514

Guttmacher Institute. An Overview of Abortion in The United States, January 2008

Guttmacher Institute. State Policies in Brief: Counseling and Waiting Periods for Abortion, July 2009

Henshaw SK. Unintended pregnancy and abortion in the USA: Epidemiology and public health impact. In: Paul M, Lichtenberg ES, Borgatta L, Grimes DA, Stubblefield PG, Creinin MD, eds. Management of Unintended and Abnormal Pregnancy, West Sussex: Wiley-Blackwell; 2009: 24–35.

Henshaw SK. Unintended pregnancy in the United States. *Fam Plann Perspect* 1998;30(1):24–29

Joffe, C. Abortion and medicine: A sociopolitical history. In: Paul M, Lichtenberg ES, Borgatta L, Grimes DA, Stubblefield

Table 29.2 Comparison of medical abortion methods

Comparison	RCT studies	Population	Medical regimen	Medical efficacy	Surgical efficacy	OR of incomplete abortion (95% CI)
Prostaglandin alone	Rosen 1984; WHO 1987	≤49 days amenorrhea	9-methylene-PGE2 suppository 50 or 60 mg q6h × 2 doses[a]; PGE2 methyl sulfonamide 0.5 mg i.m. q3h × 3 doses[b]	97.2%[a]; 91%[b]	100%[a];94%[b]	2.67* (1.06, 6.75)
Methotrexate and prostaglandin	Crenin 2000	≤49 days amenorrhea	Methotrexate 50 mg p.o. *5–6 days later:* Misoprostol 800 mcg p.v.	83%	96%	4.57 (0.47, 44.17)
Mifepristone and prostaglandin	Henshaw 1994; Ashok 2002	<63 days[c] or ≤10–13 weeks[d] of amenorrhea	Mifepristone 200 mg[c] or 600 mg[d] p.o. *36–48 hours later:* Misoprostol 800 mcg p.o.[c] or gemeprost 1 mg pessary p.v.[d]	92.6–98%[c]; 94.6%[d]	97.7–98.3%[c]; 97.9%[d]	Not calculated
Mifepristone alone	Legarth 1991	≤43[d]	Mifepristone 600 mg p.o.	76%		3.63 (0.66, 20.11)

[a] Rosen 1984; [b] WHO 1987; [c] Henshaw 1994; [d] Ashok 2002; * statistically significant.
PGE, prostaglandin E, RCT, randomized controlled trial;1` OR, odds ratio; CI, confidence interval.

PG, Creinin MD, eds. Management of Unintended and Abnormal Pregnancy, West Sussex: Wiley-Blackwell; 2009: 1–9

Jones RK, Zolna MR, Henshaw SK, Finer LB. Abortion in the United States: incidence and access to services, 2005. *Perspect Sex Reprod Health* 2008;40(1):6–16

Kapp N and von Hertzen H. Medical methods to induce abortion in the second trimester. In: Paul M, Lichtenberg ES, Borgatta L, Grimes DA, Stubblefield PG, Creinin MD, eds. Management of Unintended and Abnormal Pregnancy, West Sussex: Wiley-Blackwell; 2009: 178–192

Kulier R, Fekih A, Hofmeyr GJ, Campana A. Surgical methods for first trimester termination of pregnancy. *Cochrane Database Syst Rev* 2001; (4):CD002900

Kulier R, Gülmezoglu AM, Hofmeyr GJ, Cheng LN, Campana A. Medical methods for first trimester abortion. *Cochrane Database Syst Rev* 2004; (2):CD002855

Lohr PA, Hayes JL, Gemzell-Danielsson K. Surgical versus medical methods for second trimester induced abortion. Cochrane Database Syst Rev 2008; (1):CD006714

Mekstroth K and Paul M. First trimester aspiration abortion. In:Paul M, Lichtenberg ES, Borgatta L, Grimes DA, Stubblefield PG, Creinin MD, eds. Management of Unintended and Abnormal Pregnancy, West Sussex: Wiley-Blackwell; 2009: 135–156

Middleton T, Schaff E, Fielding SL, et al. Randomized trial of mifepristone and buccal or vaginal misoprostol for abortion through 56 days of last menstrual period. *Contraception* 2005;72(5):328–332

National Cancer Institute. Summary report: early reproductive events and breast cancer workshop. *Issues Law Med* 2005;21(2):161–165

Partial Birth Abortion Ban Act of 2003, S-3. 108th Congress, First session, 2003

Sawaya GF, Grady D, Kerlikowske K, Grimes DA. Antibiotics at the time of induced abortion: the case for universal prophylaxis based on a meta-analysis. *Obstet Gynecol* 1996;87(5 Pt 2):884–890

Say L, Kulier R, Gülmezoglu M, Campana A. Medical versus surgical methods for first trimester termination of pregnancy. Cochrane Database Syst Rev 2002; (4):CD003037

Sedgh G, Henshaw S, Singh S, Åhman E, Shah IH. Induced abortion: estimated rates and trends worldwide. *Lancet* 2007;370(9595):1338–1345

Steinauer JE, Diedrich JT, Wilson MW, Darney PD, Vargas JE, Drey EA. Uterine artery embolization in postabortion hemorrhage. *Obstet Gynecol* 2008;111(4):881–889

Stotland NL. The myth of the abortion trauma syndrome. *JAMA* 1992;268(15):2078–2079

Stubblefield PG, Carr-Ellis S, Borgatta L. Methods for induced abortion. *Obstet Gynecol* 2004;104(1):174–185

WHO. Unsafe abortion: global and regional estimates of incidence of unsafe abortion and associated mortality in 2003. 5th ed. Geneva: World Health Organization; 2007

Winikoff B, Dzuba IG, Creinin MD, et al. Two Distinct Oral Routes of Misoprostol in Mifepristone Medical Abortion: A Randomized Controlled Trial. Obstet Gynecol 2008; 112(6): 1303–1310

Zieman M, Fong SK, Benowitz NL, Banskter D, Darney PD. Absorption kinetics of misoprostol with oral or vaginal administration. *Obstet Gynecol* 1997;90(1):88–92

30 Vaginitis and Vulvitis

Natasha R. Johnson

Vaginitis

Vaginitis is defined as the group of conditions that cause vulvovaginal symptoms such as itching, burning, irritation, and abnormal vaginal discharge. Etiologies of vaginitis can be infectious or noninfectious. The most common causes of infectious vaginitis are bacterial vaginosis (BV), vulvovaginal candidiasis (VVC) and trichomoniasis. Noninfectious etiologies include atrophic vaginitis, allergies, chemical irritation, and various vulvar dermatological conditions. Vaginitis can be associated with sexually transmitted infections, including human immunodeficiency virus (HIV), postsurgical infections, and adverse reproductive outcomes in pregnant women. Vaginitis has a wide differential diagnosis (**Table 30.1**) and successful treatment relies on accurate diagnosis.

Prevalence and Epidemiology

Vaginitis is a common gynecologic problem in the general population, accounting for over 10 million office visits per year. Vaginitis can occur in any age-group (prepubertal, reproductive age, menopausal), with the etiology of vaginitis varying according to estrogen status and individual patient risk factors. Three major types of vaginal infection cause up to 90% of vaginitis cases: BV (22–50%), VVC (17–39%), and trichomoniasis (4–35%).

Pathophysiology / Normal Vaginal Physiology and Flora

In reproductive aged women, physiologic or normal discharge is white or transparent, mostly odorless and pools in the fornices of the vagina. Normal vaginal discharge contains vulvar secretions from sebaceous, sweat, Bartholin and Skene glands, transudate from the vaginal

Table 30.1 Causes of vaginitis

Condition	Causes
Infectious vaginitis	
Bacterial vaginosis	*Gardnerella vaginalis, Mycoplasma hominis, Mobiluncus* species, *Bacteroides* species (other than *Bacteroides fragilis*)
Vulvovaginal candidiasis	*Candida albicans, C. glabrata, C. Tropicalis*
Trichomoniasis	*Trichomonas vaginalis*
Bacterial vaginitis	Group A *Streptococcus*
Desquamative inflammatory vaginitis	Unknown cause, clindamycin and steroid-responsive
Ulcerative vaginitis	*Staphylococcus aureus* and toxic shock syndrome, HIV-associated
Noninfectious vaginitis	
Atrophic vaginitis	Estrogen deficiency (menopausal and postpuerperal)
Chemical irritation	Soaps, perfumes, hygiene products (tampons, pantyliners), latex condoms
Allergic, hypersensitivity vaginitis and contact dermatitis (lichen simplex chronicus)	Sperm, douching, dyes, inhaled allergens, occupational exposures, hygiene products (tampons, pantyliners), latex condoms, diaphragms
Lichen planus (erosive type)	Flat, hyperkeratotic lesions; pruritic or painful; associated with vulvar and oral lesions
Foreign body with or without infection or trauma	Tampons, contraceptive devices, pessary, others

Source: Modified from Owen MK, Clenney TL. Management of vaginitis. Am Fam Physician 2004;70:2125-2132 and Sobel JD. Vaginitis. N Engl J Med 1997;337:1896-1903.

wall, exfoliated vaginal and cervical cells, cervical mucous, endometrial and tubal fluids and normal bacteria and their metabolic products. Normal vaginal discharge typically does not cause symptoms of burning or itching. The quantity and quality of normal vaginal discharge are influenced by the menstrual cycle. The discharge may become more noticeable at times, for example, during pregnancy or at midmenstrual cycle close to the time of ovulation. Age, hormones, sexual activity, contraception, pregnancy, presence of foreign bodies, use of hygienic products, or antibiotics can disrupt the normal flora of the vagina and allow pathogens to grow.

Lactobacilli (Gram-positive rods) are the predominant bacteria in the vagina and the regulator of normal vaginal flora. Lactobacilli make lactic acid and hydrogen peroxide which maintains the normal vaginal pH of 3.8–4.5. This acidic environment inhibits the adherence of bacteria to vaginal epithelium and prevents the growth of pathogens. Estrogen status plays a critical role in determining the normal state of the vagina by enhancing lactobacilli colonization. In prepubertal girls and postmenopausal women who have low levels of estrogen, the vaginal epithelium is thin and the pH of the vaginal secretions is 4.7 or higher. The more basic pH is due to the reduced quantity of lactobacilli. Although lactobacilli are the dominant bacteria in the vagina, other bacteria are also present, such as streptococcal species, *Gardnerella vaginalis*, Gram-negative bacteria and anaerobes. *Candida albicans* can also be found in normal flora in 10–25% of asymptomatic women. Thus, a routine bacterial culture will demonstrate a broad variety of organisms including skin and fecal flora.

Acute vaginitis due to BV reflects a disruption in the normal ecosystem of the vagina from lactobacilli-dominant to mixed flora including *Gardnerella vaginalis*, *Mycoplasma* and anaerobes such as *Peptostreptococci*, *Prevotella* and *Mobiluncus* species. VVC and trichomoniasis result from an overgrowth of candidal species and infection with *Trichomonas vaginalis*, respectively.

Diagnosis

Both the history and physical examination findings are relatively nonspecific. Symptoms such as pruritis and the characteristics of the discharge (e.g., amount and color) do not reliably predict the cause of the acute vaginitis. However, certain features suggest a particular acute vaginitis diagnosis (**Table 30.2**), which can then be confirmed by office analysis (**Table 30.3**). Women frequently diagnose and treat their vulvovaginal symptoms, especially for presumed VVC, with over-the-counter preparations, which may be inappropiate due to inaccurate self-diagnosis. In one study, 95 women who self-diagnosed VVC and purchased over-the-counter antifungal therapy were evaluated and only 34% were found to have VVC on final diagnosis. Although misdiagnosis may have minimal effects on vulvovaginal symptoms, such as itching, odor, or discharge, it may be of greater concern if a patient who self-treats for VVC actually has pelvic inflammatory disease or a urinary tract infection. While tempting to treat empirically, based on symptoms alone, studies have

Table 30.2 Clinical features of vaginitis

Parameter	Normal	Bacterial Vaginosis	Candidiasis	Trichomoniasis
Symptoms	None or physiologic discharge	Malodorous white/gray discharge	Pruritis, soreness, burning, thick, white, "cottage cheese–like" discharge	Malodorous, frothy yellow discharge, dyspareunia, pruritis
Signs	White or clear discharge Normal exam	Thin, white-gray, homogenous adherent discharge No inflammation	Thick, white, curdy discharge Vulvar erythema, edema, fissure	Purulent yellow-green discharge, vulvovaginal erythema, "strawberry" cervix
Vaginal pH	<4.5	>4.5	4.0–4.5	5.0–6.0
Saline microscopy	Normal epithelial cells and lactobacilli	Clue cells (>20%), decreased lactobacilli	Pseudohyphae, budding yeast for nonalbicans candida	Motile trichomonads, PMNs
Potassium hydroxide microscopy	Negative	Negative	Pseudohyphae	Negative
"Whiff"/amine odor	Negative	Positive	Negative	Often positive
Other	–	Culture of no value	Culture if microscopy negative	Culture or rapid antigen/nucleic acid amplification tests if microscopy negative

Table 30.3 Office evaluation of vaginitis

Step 1	History and physical examination
Step 2	Vaginal pH determination
Step 3	Saline and potassium hydroxide microscopy
Step 4	"Whiff" test
Step 5	Vaginal culture for yeast, rapid diagnostic test or culture for Trichomonas if microscopy negative
	Cervical culture or PCR for Chlamydia and Gonorrhea if clinically indicated

shown poor correlation between symptoms and final diagnosis, so this practice should be avoided.

History

Evaluation of women with vaginitis should include a focused history about the vaginal symptoms, including characteristics of the vaginal discharge (color, consistency, and malodor), itching, burning, irritation, swelling, dyspareunia, and dysuria. Directed questions about location of symptoms (vulva, vagina, anus), duration, relation to the menstrual cycle, response to prior treatment including self-treatment with over-the-counter or prescription medications, and recent antibiotic use are important to help determine the etiology. Review of hygienic practices (douching, soaps, detergents, perfumes, powders, sprays, lubricants, daily use of pantyliners) may elicit potential exposure to irritants and allergens and habits detrimental to vulvar skin. Obtaining a sexual history is important as exposure to a new sexual partner increases the risk of acquiring a sexually transmitted infection including Trichomonas or cervicitis related to *Chlamydia trachomatis* and/or *Neisseria gonorrhoeae*. The presence of any associated symptoms should also be ascertained. For example, the presence of associated abdominal/pelvic pain is suggestive of pelvic inflammatory disease and suprapubic pain (especially with dysuria) may indicate cystitis, both uncommon in vaginitis.

Physical Examination

The physical examination should begin with careful evaluation of the vulva, as many patients with vaginitis have vulvar symptoms. Signs of erythema, thickening, fissures, excoriations, plaques, ulcers, thinning, and discharge at the introitus should be noted and can give clues to the etiology. In almost all patients, further assessment will include a speculum examination to inspect the vagina (noting lesions, erythema and characteristics of any discharge

present), the cervix (noting lesions, erythema and "mucopus" or purulent cervical mucous) and to collect specimens for office analysis and microbiology testing. Cervical inflammation is suggestive of cervicitis, not vaginitis, and the cervix typically is erythematous, friable, and with a mucopurulent discharge. A bimanual and abdominal examination should be performed to elicit pelvic and cervical motion tenderness if the patient has abdominal and/or pelvic pain and there is concern for pelvic inflammatory disease.

Office Analysis

Simple office analysis including pH testing, amine-"whiff" test, saline (wet mount) and potassium hydroxide (KOH) microscopy and vaginal/cervical cultures when indicated are important tools in the diagnosis of vaginitis. These tests can be performed by obtaining samples of the vaginal discharge during speculum examination. Vaginal pH should be measured by touching a cotton-tipped swab to the sidewall of the vagina and touching the swab directly to commercially available pH paper (expanded in the pH range 4.0–5.5). The samples should be taken from the lateral vaginal fornix (midway between the introitus and cervix) to avoid false elevations in pH results caused by cervical mucus, blood, semen, or other substances that pool in the posterior fornix. Measurement of vaginal pH is the single most important finding in the diagnostic process and should always be determined. A pH above 4.5 in a premenopausal woman suggests BV or trichomoniasis and can help exclude VVC which typically has a pH in the 4–4.5 range. Premenarchal and postmenopausal women typically have a vaginal pH of 4.7 or higher and pH measurement in these groups is less useful in the evaluation of vaginitis symptoms.

Vaginal discharge can be examined by preparation of a saline and potassium hydroxide (KOH) wet mount. A sample of vaginal discharge is taken from the lateral vaginal fornix using a cotton-tipped swab and placed in one or two drops of 0.9% normal saline solution on one slide and a second sample in 10% KOH solution. Cover slips are placed on the slides and they are examined under a microscope at low and high power. A normal microscopic examination will reveal a predominance of squamous cells and rare polymorphonuclear leukocytes. Clue cells (epithelial cells with borders studded by small bacteria, characteristic of BV), white blood cells, lactobacilli and motile trichomonads are usually identified in the saline specimen. Hyphae or yeast buds of candidal species are more easily seen in the KOH specimen, as KOH lyses cellular elements. An amine odor ("fishy smell") detected immediately after adding 10% KOH to the vaginal discharge sample on the slide is called a positive "whiff" test and suggests BV.

Initial office evaluation (history and physical examination, vaginal pH, wet mount, microscopy, and "whiff" test) has been shown to correctly diagnose 60% of candidal vaginitis, 70% of trichomonad vaginitis, and 90% of BV. In patients with an initial nondiagnostic evaluation, vaginal cultures for yeast and rapid diagnostic tests or culture for Trichomonas (if pH >4.5 and suggestive clinical symptoms) should be performed. If the evaluation excludes the three most common causes of vaginitis (VVC, BV, trichomoniasis), then other causes of vaginitis need to be considered (see **Table 30.1**). Patients considered at risk for sexually transmitted infections—with purulent vaginal or cervical discharge, fever or lower abdominal / pelvic pain—should have a cervical sample obtained for *Chlamydia trachomatis* and *Neisseria gonorrhoeae* testing.

Types of Vaginitis

Vulvovaginal Candidiasis

Approximately one-third of acute vaginitis is due to candidal vulvovaginitis. Most cases of acute VVC are caused by *Candida albicans*, but occasionally are caused by other *Candida* species such as *C. glabrata* and *C. tropicalis*. VVC is common in adults, approximately 75% of women will receive a diagnosis of VVC at least once, and of those, about 50% will have a recurrence. Candidal species can be found in normal flora in 10–25% of healthy asymptomatic women and likely access the vagina via migration from the rectum across the perineum. Symptomatic infection is correlated with a high vaginal fungal load and vaginal infiltration of polymorphonuclear neutrophils. The mechanism by which *Candida* species overgrow and cause symptomatic disease is multifaceted, involving host inflammatory response to invasion and yeast virulence factors. Risk factors for symptomatic infection include antibiotics (inhibit normal bacterial flora), high-estrogen contraceptives (but not low-dose oral contraceptives), pregnancy, diabetes mellitus with poor glycemic control, immunosuppression (e.g., HIV, patients taking corticosteroids), and contraceptive devices (vaginal sponges, diaphragms, intrauterine devices). VVC is not traditionally considered a sexually transmitted disease as it occurs in nonsexually active women and because Candida is considered part of the normal vaginal flora. However, sexual transmission of Candida can occur and VVC is associated with sexual activity. Evidence for this include: 1) an increase in frequency of VVC at the time most women begin regular sexual activity; 2) partners of women infected with VVC are more likely to be colonized with Candida than partners of uninfected women; and 3) VVC episodes may be linked to orogenital and anogenital sex.

Clinical features and diagnosis: Typical symptoms of VVC include vulvar pruritis, burning, vulvar and vaginal soreness, irritation, dysuria (external) and a thick, white vaginal discharge. Physical examination may reveal

vulvar erythema, edema, fissure formation and a thick, white, adherent, "cottage cheese–like" vaginal discharge (**Fig. 30.1**).

Vaginal pH of less than 4.5 and a negative "whiff" test can help distinguish VVC from BV and trichomoniasis. However, diagnosis requires either (1) visualization of blastospores or pseudohyphae on saline or 10% KOH microscopy (**Fig. 30.2**), or (2) a positive culture for yeast in

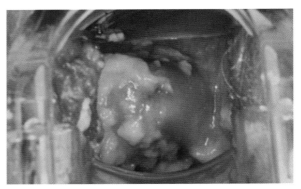

Fig. 30.1   Speculum examination showing characteristic vaginal discharge of vulvovaginal candidiasis is thick, white, curdy, and "cottage cheese"–like. Printed with permission from Seattle STD/ HIV Prevention Training Center, Washington State, Department of Health.

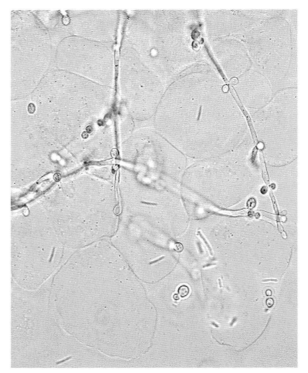

Fig. 30.2   KOH microscopy of candidiasis reveals yeast pseudohyphae, budding yeast and lysed epithelial cells. Printed with permission from Seattle STD/HIV Prevention Training Center, Washington State, Department of Health.

a symptomatic woman. A culture for Candida is indicated by clinical findings if microscopy is negative because microscopy is not sufficiently sensitive to exclude these diagnoses in symptomatic patients. Studies have shown that microscopy can be negative in up to 50% of patients with confirmed VVC. Routine culture is not warranted as an initial diagnostic test for all patients because of its cost, the delay in timely diagnosis, and that it may be positive due to asymptomatic colonization.

Recurrent VVC (four or more documented episodes in one year) occurs in less than 5% of the population. Culture should be performed in women with persistent or recurrent symptoms to confirm the diagnosis, and because many of these women may have non-albicans infections that are resistant to standard therapy. Predisposing factors are identifiable in only a minority of women including diabetics with poor glycemic control and those undergoing immunosuppressive therapy. Other factors that predispose to recurrent VVC are poorly understood and include abnormalities in local vaginal mucosal immunity and genetic susceptibility which is mediated through specific gene polymorphisms.

Treatment: Treatment for VVC is indicated for the relief of symptoms associated with the infection. Women who have asymptomatic colonization do not require treatment. On the basis of clinical presentation, microbiology, host factors and response to therapy, VVC can be classified as complicated or noncomplicated (see **Table 30.4** for criteria). Approximately 90% of infections are uncomplicated and usually respond to treatment within a few days. The remaining 10% are complicated infections, which require a longer course of therapy and may take up to two weeks to resolve completely.

Short-course topical and oral formulations effectively treat **uncomplicated VVC** (see **Table 30.5**). Randomized trials have shown that oral and topical antimycotic medications achieve comparable clinical cure rates of 80–90% for patients who complete the therapy. Topical treatments may cause local burning or irritation, whereas oral medication may occasionally cause gastrointestinal upset, headache, rash, transient liver function test abnormalities, and may interact with other medications. Given similar efficacy between formulations, route of administration is generally individualized to patient factors including patient preference, cost, history of response, or adverse reaction to prior treatments, and contraindications. Patients should be instructed to return for follow-up visits only if symptoms persist or recur within two months of the onset of initial symptoms. Routine treatment of sexual partners is not recommended as VVC is not usually acquired through sexual intercourse.

Women with severe vulvovaginal inflammation or factors suggestive of **complicated VVC infection** (see **Table 30.4**) generally require more aggressive treatment to achieve relief of symptoms. Topical azole treatments are

Table 30.4 Classification of vulvovaginal candidiasis

Variable	Uncomplicated	Complicated
Frequency	Sporadic or infrequent	Recurrent (≥4 per year)
Symptom severity	Mild or moderate	Severe
Organism	*Candida albicans* suspected	Nonalbicans species
Host	Healthy and nonpregnant	Immunocompromised or pregnant

Source: Modified from Sexually transmitted diseases treatment guidelines 2006. Centers for Disease Control and Prevention. MMWR Recomm Rep 2006;55(RR-11):54–56.

Table 30.5 Treatment of uncomplicated vulvovaginal candidiasis

Drug	Formulation	Dosage	Duration
Butoconazole	2% cream [a]	5 g daily	3 days
	2% sustained release cream	5 g daily	1 day
Clotrimazole	1% cream [a]	5 g daily	7–14 days
	100 mg vaginal tablet	100 mg daily	7 days
	100 mg vaginal tablet	200 mg daily	3 days
Miconazole	2% cream [a]	5 g daily	7 days
	100 mg vaginal suppository [a]	100 mg daily	7days
	200 mg vaginal suppository [a]	200 mg daily	3 days
	1200 mg vaginal suppository [a]	1200 mg daily	1 day
Nystatin	100 000-unit vaginal tablet	100 000-unit daily	14 days
Tioconazole	6.5% ointment [a]	5 g daily	1 day
Terconazole	0.4% cream	5 g daily	7 days
	0.8% cream	5 g daily	3 days
	80mg vaginal suppository	80 mg daily	3 days
Fluconazole	150 mg oral tablet	150 mg daily	1 day

[a] Available over the counter.

Source: Modified from Sexually transmitted diseases treatment guidelines 2006. Centers for Disease Control and Prevention. MMWR Recomm Rep 2006;55(RR-11):54–56.

generally required for 7–14 days rather than a 1–3-day course. Fluconazole (150 mg orally) is recommended as two sequential doses 72 hours apart. In a placebo-controlled randomized trial of 556 women with complicated VVC, a second dose of fluconazole 150 mg given 3 days after the first dose increased the cure rate from 67% with a single dose of fluconazole to 80% with the two sequential doses. Non-albicans species (e.g., *Candida glabrata*) are less likely to respond to azole antifungal therapy. Therapy with vaginal boric acid, 600-mg capsules for a minimum of 14 days, has been shown to be effective for azole failures. Treatment of pregnant women is advised for symptom relief. Only topical azole therapies applied for 7 days are recommended for use among pregnant women.

Each individual episode of recurrent VVC responds well to short duration oral or topical azole therapy. However, to minimize recurrences, a longer duration of initial therapy (7–14 days of topical therapy or sequential doses of oral fluconazole) is recommended to induce remission, and then a maintenance antifungal regimen is initiated. Maintenance therapy includes weekly fluconazole (see **Evidence Box 30.1**), topical clotrimazole 200 mg twice weekly, or 500 mg clotrimazole vaginal suppositories once weekly for 6 months. Suppressive regimens are effective in reducing recurrent VVC, but 30–50% of women will have recurrent infections once maintenance therapy is discontinued. Treatment of sexual partners of women with recurrent infection is controversial.

Bacterial Vaginosis

The most common cause of acute vaginitis, BV accounts for 22–50% of cases. BV is a polymicrobial infection characterized by a lack of hydrogen peroxide-producing lactobacilli in the vagina and an overgrowth of other organisms, especially anaerobes. These organisms include *Prevotella*, *Bacteroides* and *Mobiluncus* species, *Gardnerella vaginalis* and *Mycoplasma hominis*. The vaginal pH rises with the loss of lactobacilli, which allows overgrowth of vaginal anaerobes. The anaerobes produce proteolytic enzymes which break down vaginal peptides into amines, which are volatile, malodorous, and associated with the characteristic discharge of BV. The elevated pH also facilitates adherence of *Gardnerella vaginalis* to the epithelial cells, which creates clue cells.

The etiology of the microbial alteration and the role of sexual activity in the pathogenesis of BV are not fully understood. BV is associated with having multiple or new sexual partners, having a female sexual partner, douching, and a lack of vaginal lactobacilli. It is not clear whether or not BV results from acquisition of a sexually transmitted organism. Women who have never been sexually active are rarely affected, and treatment of male sex partners has not been beneficial in preventing the recurrence of BV.

Clinical features and diagnosis: BV is the most prevalent cause of vaginal discharge and malodor; however, more than 50% of women with BV are asymptomatic. When symptomatic, patients may complain of abnormal vaginal discharge and a fishy odor, which is more noticeable after intercourse. Pruritis, burning, dysuria and dyspareunia are uncommon. Besides causing symptoms, BV has been associated with upper genital tract infections including, pelvic inflammatory disease, postprocedural gynecologic infections (after hysterectomy and abortion), endometritis (after cesarean section and vaginal delivery), and acquisition of HIV and other sexually transmitted diseases. Additionally, BV during pregnancy has been associated with spontaneous preterm labor and amniotic fluid infection.

Physical examination typically reveals a thin, gray-white, homogeneous "fishy smelling" vaginal discharge (**Fig 30.3**). The vulva usually appears normal in BV without erythema, edema or fissure formation. The absence of inflammation is the basis of the term "vaginosis" rather than vaginitis.

A clinical diagnosis of BV requires the presence of three of the following four Amsel's criteria: 1) thin homogeneous, gray-white vaginal discharge; 2) vaginal pH higher than 4.5; 3) positive "whiff"-amine test; 4) more than

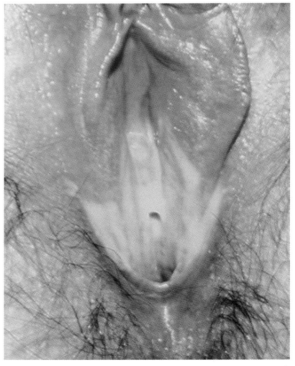

Fig. 30.3 Vaginal introitus with thin, white, homogeneous, "spilt milk" discharge characteristic of bacterial vaginosis. Printed with permission from Seattle STD/HIV Prevention Training Center, Washington State, Department of Health.

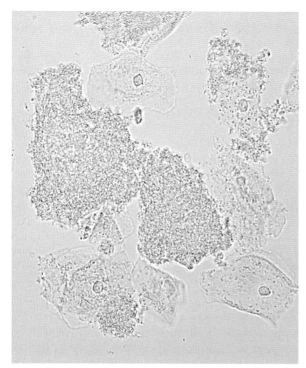

Fig. 30.4   Saline microscopy of bacterial vaginosis reveals clue cells; epithelial cells studded with bacteria, rare leukocytes, and scarce lactobacilli. Printed with permission from Seattle STD/HIV Prevention Training Center, Washington State, Department of Health.

20% clue cells on microscopy (**Fig. 30.4**). A Gram stain of vaginal secretions demonstrating the relative concentration of lactobacilli to other organisms is considered the "gold standard" laboratory method for diagnosing BV, but is used mostly in research settings.

Because the organisms found in BV are part of the normal vaginal flora, the presence of these organisms on a culture does not mean that the patient has BV, and rou-

tine culture is not recommended as a diagnostic tool. Similarly, the Pap test is not reliable for the diagnosis of BV. If a cervical cytology smear suggests BV, women should undergo standard diagnostic testing if applicable (vaginal examination, vaginal pH, "whiff"-amine test, microscopy) and treatment if appropriate. DNA probes for *Gardnerella vaginalis* and diagnostic cards that detect the presence of elevated pH and amines are available for the diagnosis of BV and can be helpful if microscopy is unavailable, but routine use of these tests is limited by cost.

Treatment: BV treatment is indicated for relief of symptoms in women with symptomatic infection and to prevent postoperative infection in asymptomatic women. Treatment for BV before abortion or hysterectomy significantly decreases the risk of postoperative infection complications (cuff cellulitis after hysterectomy and endometritis after abortion). There is limited data to support treatment of BV to decrease acquisition of pelvic infammatory disease, HIV, or other sexually transmitted diseases. Treatment options are shown in **Table 30.6**. Metronidazole or clindamycin administered orally or intravaginally will result in high clinical cure rates of 70–80% at 1 month of follow-up, although metronidazole is the most efficacious. Patients should be advised not to consume alcohol during treatment because of the possibility of a disulfiramlike reaction. It is not necessary to treat sexual partners of affected women, as partner treatment does not affect cure rate or risk of recurrence. Following treatment, approximately 30% of women will have a recurrence of symptoms within 3 months for reasons that are unclear. Recurrences may be treated with prolonged therapy with oral or vaginal metronidazole or clindamycin. Suppressive therapy with maintenance metronidazole gel may be necessary for some women with more than three documented episodes of BV within a year.

Pregnant women with symptomatic BV should be treated with standard therapy (see **Table 30.6**). Neither metronidazole nor clindamycin have known teratogen-

Table 30.6 Treatment of bacterial vaginosis

Drug	Formulation	Dosage	Duration
Metronidazole	500 mg oral[a, b]	Twice daily	7 days
	250 mg oral[b]	Three times daily	7 days
	0.75% intravaginal gel[a]	One applicator (5 g) daily	5 days
Clindamycin	2% cream [a]	One applicator (5 g) at bedtime	7 days
	2% sustained release cream	5 g daily	1 day
	300 mg oral[b]	Twice daily	7 days
	100 g intravaginal ovules	At bedtime	3 days

[a] Recommended regimen.
[b] Recommended regimen in pregnancy.
Source: Modified from Sexually transmitted diseases treatment guidelines 2006. Centers for Disease Control and Prevention. MMWR Recomm Rep 2006;55(RR-11):54–56.

ic effects. Oral therapy is thought to be more effective against potential subclinical upper tract infection. Given that BV is clearly associated with preterm labor and amniotic fluid infection, studies have been conducted to determine whether treating asymptomatic BV in pregnancy will decrease adverse events. Results indicate that treatment of pregnant women who have BV and are at high risk for preterm delivery (prior preterm delivery) may reduce the risk of prematurity. In a recent meta-analysis for the US Preventive Services Task Force, screening and treatment for BV in pregnant women at low or average risk of preterm delivery did not prolong pregnancy. A slight benefit was seen in women at high risk for preterm birth. Thus, evaluation and treatment of pregnant women at high risk for preterm birth with asymptomatic BV is reasonable, but is not beneficial or recommended for pregnant women at low or average risk. The optimal choice of antibiotic and time for initiation of therapy or duration of use remains unclear.

Trichomoniasis

Trichomoniasis accounts for approximately 4–35% of vaginitis diagnosed in symptomatic women, with an estimated annual incidence in the United States of 3–5 million cases. The causative organism is the flagellated protozoan *Trichomonas vaginalis*, which can be found in the vagina, urethra, cervix, Bartholin and Skene glands of infected women. Trichomoniasis is a sexually transmitted infection with a high prevalence of coinfection with other sexually transmitted infections. It is associated with upper genital tract infections such as those described for BV, including infections after delivery, surgery, and abortion as well as pelvic inflammatory disease and preterm delivery.

Clinical features and diagnosis: Symptomatic infected women can have diffuse, malodorous, purulent yellow-green vaginal discharge with associated vulvar burning, pruritis, dysuria, increased urinary frequency and dyspareunia. Some women may have postcoital bleeding, and symptoms may be worse during or immediately after menses. Physical examination can reveal erythema of the vagina and vulva, and green-yellow frothy discharge in 10–30% of infected women. Punctate hemorrhages may be visible on the cervix, which is termed colpitis macularis or "strawberry cervix" in 2–5% cases (**Fig 30.5**).

None of the signs or symptoms is sufficiently sensitive or specific to diagnose trichomoniasis based on clinical features alone. The presence of motile trichomonads on wet mount is diagnostic of infection (**Fig 30.6**), but the sensitivity of microscopy for trichomoniasis is only 50–70%. Other findings include an elevated vaginal pH (>4.5) and an increase of polymorphonuclear leukocytes on sa-

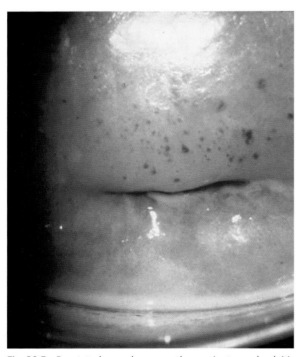

Fig. 30.5 Punctate hemorrhages on the cervix, termed colpitis macularis or "strawberry cervix" seen in trichomoniasis. Printed with permission from Seattle STD/HIV Prevention Training Center, Washington State, Department of Health.

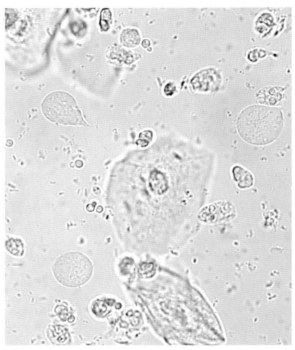

Fig. 30.6 Saline microscopy reveals mobile pear-shaped trichomonads indicative of trichomoniasis. Printed with permission from Seattle STD/HIV Prevention Training Center, Washington State, Department of Health.

line microscopy (see **Table 30.2**). Culture on Diamond medium has a high sensitivity (95%) and high specificity (>95%) and should be considered in patients with suspected trichomoniasis, but not confirmed by microscopy. A point-of-care test for trichomonas antigens, the OSOM Trichomonas Rapid Test which is performed on vaginal secretions, has a sensitivity of 88% and specificity of 98% compared with culture. This test may be a valuable diagnostic tool, especially in settings with a high prevalence of trichomoniasis where microscopy or culture is not available.

Trichomonads are sometimes reported as an incidental finding on Pap tests. The Pap test is an unreliable tool to diagnose trichomoniasis due to its low sensitivity of only 60–70%. Asymptomatic women with trichomonads found on Pap tests should ideally be evaluated by microscopy and/or culture and should not be treated until diagnosis is confirmed. However, liquid-based cytology has been found to have a lower false positive rate (1%) than conventional Pap smears (8%) in a recent study of 203 women in which both liquid-based cytology and culture for *Trichomonas vaginalis* was performed. Thus, it may be reasonable to treat asymptomatic women with trichomonads found on liquid-based cervical cytology.

Treatment: Trichonomiasis treatment is indicated for all symptomatic women and asymptomatic nonpregnant women. Therapy with oral nitroimidazole therapy is highly effective with cure rates reported as high as 90–95% in randomized clinical trials. Regimens include metronidazole or tinidazole as a single oral dose of 2 g (four 500-mg tablets). Single dose regimens are preferable to multiple dose prolonged therapy (e.g., metronidazole 500 mg twice daily for 7 days) as they are equally efficacious, improve compliance and require a shorter period of alcohol abstinence. Oral therapy is preferred to vaginal therapy since systemic administration achieves therapeutic drug levels in the urethra and periurethral glands, which serve as endogenous reservoirs that can increase recurrence rates. Patients should be advised not to consume alcohol during treatment and for 24 hours after completion of metronidazole and 72 hours after tinidazole treatment because of the possibility of a disulfiramlike reaction.

Because *Trichomonas vaginalis* is sexually transmitted, treatment of the patient's partner is essential to maximize cure rates and decrease the risk of recurrence. Sexual partners of infected women should be referred for evaluation of trichomoniasis and concurrent sexually transmitted infections rather than empirically treated. Patients should be instructed to avoid sexual intercourse until they and their sexual partners have completed therapy. In cases of metronidazole allergy, patients may be referred for desensitization and treatment with metronidazole. The prevalence of low-level resistance to metronidazole in patients with trichomonas infection is 2–5%. Prolonged treatment with higher doses of metronidazole

or tinidazole has been successful. It this fails, the Centers for Disease Control and Prevention recommends in vitro culture and drug susceptibility testing.

Metronidazole is considered safe to use in pregnancy for symptomatic women as a single 2-g dose or as a multiple, prolonged dose (500 mg twice daily for 7 days). Data on tinidazole are limited and its safety in pregnant women has not been well evaluated. Like BV, trichomoniasis has been associated with adverse outcomes such as preterm delivery, premature rupture of membranes and low birth weight. However, studies have not shown that metronidazole treatment results in a reduction in perinatal morbidity. One study of treatment for asymptomatic trichomoniasis in pregnant women showed an increased preterm delivery rate in the treated group; however, limitations in the study prevent definitive conclusions regarding risks of treatment. Thus, it is not recommended to treat asymptomatic infections during pregnancy. These patients should be counseled regarding partner treatment and to minimize reinfection of their partners by abstinence or condom use.

Atrophic Vaginitis

Decrease in estrogen levels during perimenopause and menopause can cause vaginal atrophy. Physiologic changes include thinning of the vaginal epithelium and loss of glycogen which leads to changes in the vaginal pH and flora. Patients with symptomatic atrophic vaginitis may have abnormal vaginal discharge, dryness, itching, burning or dyspareunia. Atrophy is diagnosed by the presence of thin, clear vaginal discharge, elevated vaginal pH, and the presence of parabasal cells on microscopy. An amine-"whiff" test will be negative. Treatment consists of vaginal lubricants and moisturizers (eg. Astroglide, Replens) or topical or systemic estrogens.

Vulvitis

Vulvitis refers to inflammation of the vulva that may be due to acute or chronic vaginitis, vulvar skin disorders, or vulvodynia. Vulvar pruritis and pain are the two most common symptoms of vulvar disorders in women. Chronic symptoms can significantly interfere with women's sexual function and sense of wellbeing. Acute vulvar pruritis is typically due to acute vaginitis (e.g., VVC, BV, trichomoniasis), whereas etiologies of chronic pruritis typically include vulvar dermatological disorders, such as lichen sclerosus, lichen simplex chronicus, or psoriasis; neoplasia including vulvar intraepithelial neoplasia, squamous cell carcinoma, and Paget disease of the vulva; or vulvar manifestations of systemic diseases, such as Crohn disease.

Patients presenting with vulvar pain should be evaluated for organic causes, including infections, neoplasias, neurologic disorders, and inflammatory conditions. Vulvodynia, defined as burning, stinging, rawness, or soreness, with or without pruritis, can be generalized or localized depending on site of the pain, and can be spontaneous, provoked or both. Once organic causes are excluded, then the diagnosis of vulvodynia can be made.

Clinical Features and Diagnosis

A careful medical history is important to ascertain the onset, duration, location, and type of vulvar symptoms, precipitating or known risk factors, hygiene practices (e.g., soaps, detergents, douching, topical products), and prior treatments used. Pruritis that is unresponsive to antifungals suggests vulvar dermatitis. Physical examination noting any vulvar lesions, erythema, edema, atrophy, or fissure formation is paramount to the diagnosis. Infectious causes should be excluded with vaginal pH determination, amine-"whiff" test, microscopy using both saline and potassium hydroxide preparations and vaginal culture, if appropriate. Diagnosis of vulvar skin conditions and neoplasia typically requires skin punch biopsy for diagnosis.

Vulvar Dermatoses

Vulvar dermatitis/lichen simplex chronicus: Vulvar dermatitis typically arises from a contact irritant or allergen which can include soaps, bubble baths, body lotions, sanitary or incontinence pads, topical medications, condoms, contraceptive creams, spermicides, semen, antiseptics and laundry detergents. Avoiding allergens and irritants can reduce the occurrence of both contact dermatitis and lichen simplex chronicus. Vulvar dermatitis can also be endogenous, meaning atopic dermatitis or eczema, not related to an irritant or allergen. Women with vulvar dermatitis typically experience chronic irritation and pruritis which causes them to persistently rub and scratch the vulva. Vulvar dermatitis appears as an erythematous, pruritic rash that can be localized or generalized on the vulva. On examination, clinical signs can range from mild erythema, edema and scaling to marked erythema, fissures, skin thickening, erosions and ulcers. Vaginal discharge is usually unremarkable in women with vulvar dermatitis. Evaluation should include vaginal pH, microscopy, and vaginal culture to rule out candidiasis.

Lichen simplex chronicus of the vulva is a chronic eczematous disease characterized by scaling and lichenified plaque with intense and unrelenting pruritis, which may result in sleep disruption. It represents an end-stage response to a variety of processes including environmental factors (e.g., heat, excessive sweating, contact irritants) and dermatological disease (e.g., candidiasis, lichen sclerosus). The skin appears thickened and leathery and can have areas of hyper- or hypopigmentation. Erosions and ulcers can develop from chronic scratching.

Treatment generally consists of identifying and eliminating the causative environmental agent if possible. Topical corticosteroid ointments of low to medium potency (e.g., triamcinolone 0.1 % daily for 2–4 weeks, then taper to twice per week) provide relief of mild symptoms and resolution of the vulvar skin alterations. More severe symptoms may require higher potency topical steroids. If Candida is present, prolonged antifungal treatment is generally required.

Lichen sclerosus: Lichen sclerosus is a chronic inflammatory disorder of the skin that is most commonly seen on the vulva, but extragenital lesions can also be present in women with vulvar disease. It may occur at any age, including prepuberty, but mean age of onset is in the fifth or sixth decade. The exact etiology is unknown, although an autoimmune process or genetic link is probable. Symptoms include pruritis, irritation, burning, pain, dyspareunia and vulvar skin tearing. On examination, the vulvar skin commonly appears white, thinned, and wrinkled (described as "parchment paper" or "cigarette paper"). The vagina is typically spared, but introital narrowing can occur via involvement of the mucocutaneous junctions. Perianal involvement creates the classic "keyhole" or hourglass shape. Loss of vulvar architecture can occur including fusion of the labia minora, phimosis of the clitoral hood and fissures. A biopsy is necessary to exclude other vulvar skin diseases.

The recommended treatment for lichen sclerosus is a high-potency topical corticosteroid ointment which results in symptom relief in 95 % of patients. Steroid regimens generally begin with once-daily application of superpotent topical corticosteroid ointment (e.g. clobetasol propionate 0.05 %) for 4 weeks, then taper to alternate days for 4 weeks, followed by 4 weeks of twice-weekly application. Maintenance therapy (one to three times per week) with topical corticosteroid ointment is often required as symptoms recur in patients who stop therapy. Long-term monitoring is important as there is an association of vulvar lichen sclerosus with squamous cell carcinoma of the vulva, with a 4–5 % risk of malignancy.

Lichen planus: Lichen planus is an uncommon, inflammatory dermatological disorder that affects the skin, nails and mucous membranes. The etiology is unknown, but is most likely related to cell-mediated immunity. Lichen planus can involve the oral mucosa and typically appears as white, reticulate, lacy or fernlike striae (called Wickham striae). Vulvar symptoms include burning, soreness, dyspareunia and increased vaginal discharge. There are three types of lichen planus that can affect the vulva: papulosquamous, hypertrophic, and erosive. The most common and most difficult to treat is the erosive form which involves the vagina in up to 70% of patients. On the vulva, pruritic, purple, shiny papules may be present. Deep, painful, erythematous erosions are found on the posterior vestibule and often extend to the labia minora, resulting in agglutination and loss of the labial architecture. The vaginal epithelium can become erythematous, eroded, acutely inflamed, and denuded of epithelium. Erosive patches if present are extremely friable. Over time, these eroded surfaces may adhere, resulting in scarring and eventually complete obliteration of the vagina. A biopsy is necessary to exclude other vulvar skin diseases. Lichen planus can be very difficult to treat and therapies generally result in only partial relief of symptoms. Treatment options include topical and systemic steroids, and topical and systemic immunosuppressants including cyclosporine, hydroxychloroquine, methotrexate, azathioprine, and cyclophosphamide.

Key Points

- The three most common causes of inflammatory vaginitis are candidiasis, bacterial vaginosis, and trichomoniasis. The characteristics of the vaginal discharge in each condition are: 1) candidiasis—thick, white cottage cheese–like discharge, often with itching; 2) bacterial vaginosis—thin, homogenous discharge with a "fishy" odor; and 3) trichomoniasis—green-yellow purulent discharge.
- Microscopy and pH testing of the vaginal discharge help to make a diagnosis. On microscopy candidiasis is associated with hyphae and buds, bacterial vaginosis with the identification of clue cells (epithelial cells studded with coccobacilli), and trichomoniasis with motile trichomonads. The pH of the normal vaginal epithelium in premenopausal women is less than 4.5. In bacterial vaginosis and trichomoniasis, the pH of the vaginal epithelium is usually greater than 5. In candidiasis the pH is less than 4.5.
- Other causes of vaginitis include atrophy, desquamative inflammatory vaginitis, irritants and allergens.
- Candida is usually treated with an oral or vaginal antimycotic agent. Oral fluconazole as a single dose is a commonly used regimen. Bacterial vaginosis is usually treated with metronidazole. Trichomoniasis is usually treated with metronidazole with evaluation or empiric therapy offered to the patient's sex partner.
- Inflammatory conditions that affect the vulva include dermatitis caused by irritants or allergens, lichen simplex chronicus (a chronic eczemalike disease), lichen sclerosus, or lichen planus.

Evidence Box 30.1

Maintenance fluconazole therapy for recurrent vulvovaginal candidiasis can reduce the rate of recurrence with minimal negative side effects.

A total 387 women with recurrent vulvovaginal candidiasis were each given three 150-mg doses of fluconazole doses at 72-hour intervals to induce clinical remission and then were randomized to receive either oral fluconazole 150 mg or placebo weekly for 6 months, followed by 6 months of observation without therapy. Primary outcome was the percentage of women in clinical remission at the end of the first 6-month period. Secondary efficacy measures were the clinical outcome at 12 months, time to recurrence, and vaginal candidal status.

The proportion of women who remained infection-free was significantly higher in the fluconazole group (91% versus 36% at 6 months, 73% versus 28% at 9 months, and 43% versus 22% at 12 months). The mean time to recurrence in the fluconazole and placebo groups was 10.2 and 4.0 months, respectively. Treatment was discontinued in only one patient because of an adverse event (headache) thought attributable to the fluconazole. Serial liver-function tests were performed during the study; a mild elevation was detected in only one patient during the maintenance phase and the patient did not discontinue therapy. Resistant isolates of *Candida albicans* or superinfection with *C. glabrata* was not observed.

Weekly treatment with fluconazole was effective in preventing symptomatic recurrent vulvovaginal candidiasis as compared to placebo, with minimal side effects. However, long-term cure was not achieved in one-half of the women studied.

Sobel JD, Wiesenfeld HC, Martens M, et al. Maintenance fluconazole therapy for recurrent vulvovaginal candidiasis. N Engl J Med 2004;351:876–883.

Further Reading

ACOG Committee on Practice Bulletins—Gynecology. ACOG Practice Bulletin. Clinical management guidelines for obstetrician-gynecologists, Number 72, May 2006: Vaginitis. *Obstet Gynecol* 2006;107(5):1195–1206

ACOG Committee on Practice Bulletins—Gynecology. ACOG Practice Bulletin No. 93: diagnosis and management of vulvar skin disorders. *Obstet Gynecol* 2008;111(5):1243–1253

Amsel R, Totten PA, Spiegel CA, Chen KC, Eschenbach D, Holmes KK. Nonspecific vaginitis. Diagnostic criteria and microbial and epidemiologic associations. *Am J Med* 1983;74(1):14–22

Anderson MR, Klink K, Cohrssen A. Evaluation of vaginal complaints. *JAMA* 2004;291(11):1368–1379

Bornstein J, Lakovsky Y, Lavi I, Bar-Am A, Abramovici H. The classic approach to diagnosis of vulvovaginitis: a critical analysis. *Infect Dis Obstet Gynecol* 2001;9(2):105–111

Bradshaw CS, Morton AN, Garland SM, Morris MB, Moss LM, Fairley CK. Higher-risk behavioral practices associated with bacterial vaginosis compared with vaginal candidiasis. *Obstet Gynecol* 2005;106(1):105–114

Carr PL, Rothberg MB, Friedman RH, Felsenstein D, Pliskin JS. "Shotgun" versus sequential testing. Cost-effectiveness of diagnostic strategies for vaginitis. *J Gen Intern Med* 2005;20(9):793–799

Crowley T, Low N, Turner A, Harvey I, Bidgood K, Horner P. Antibiotic prophylaxis to prevent post-abortal upper genital tract infection in women with bacterial vaginosis: randomised controlled trial. *BJOG* 2001;108(4):396–402

Eckert LO, Hawes SE, Stevens CE, Koutsky LA, Eschenbach DA, Holmes KK. Vulvovaginal candidiasis: clinical manifestations, risk factors, management algorithm. *Obstet Gynecol* 1998;92(5):757–765

Eckert LO. Clinical practice. Acute vulvovaginitis. *N Engl J Med* 2006;355(12):1244–1252

Ferris DG, Nyirjesy P, Sobel JD, Soper D, Pavletic A, Litaker MS. Over-the-counter antifungal drug misuse associated with patient-diagnosed vulvovaginal candidiasis. *Obstet Gynecol* 2002;99(3):419–425

Fidel PL Jr, Sobel JD. Immunopathogenesis of recurrent vulvovaginal candidiasis. *Clin Microbiol Rev* 1996;9(3):335–348

Fidel PL Jr, Barousse M, Espinosa T, et al. An intravaginal live Candida challenge in humans leads to new hypotheses for the immunopathogenesis of vulvovaginal candidiasis. *Infect Immun* 2004;72(5):2939–2946

Geiger AM, Foxman B. Risk factors for vulvovaginal candidiasis: a case-control study among university students. *Epidemiology* 1996;7(2): 182–187

Giraldo PC, Babula O, Gonçalves AK, et al. Mannose-binding lectin gene polymorphism, vulvovaginal candidiasis, and bacterial vaginosis. *Obstet Gynecol* 2007;109(5):1123–1128

Hauth JC, Goldenberg RL, Andrews WW, DuBard MB, Copper RL. Reduced incidence of preterm delivery with metronidazole and erythromycin in women with bacterial vaginosis. *N Engl J Med* 1995;333(26):1732–1736

Hill GB. The microbiology of bacterial vaginosis. *Am J Obstet Gynecol* 1993;169(2 Pt 2):450–454

Hillier SL, Krohn MA, Cassen E, Easterling TR, Rabe LK, Eschenbach DA. The role of bacterial vaginosis and vaginal bacteria in amniotic fluid infection in women in preterm labor with intact fetal membranes. *Clin Infect Dis* 1995;20(Suppl 2):S276–S278

Kent HL. Epidemiology of vaginitis. *Am J Obstet Gynecol* 1991;165(4 Pt 2):1168–1176

Klebanoff MA, Carey JC, Hauth JC, et al; National Institute of Child Health and Human Development Network of Maternal-Fetal Medicine Units. Failure of metronidazole to prevent preterm delivery among pregnant women with asymptomatic Trichomonas vaginalis infection. *N Engl J Med* 2001;345(7):487–493

Klebanoff MA, Schwebke JR, Zhang J, Nansel TR, Yu KF, Andrews WW. Vulvovaginal symptoms in women with bacterial vaginosis. *Obstet Gynecol* 2004;104(2):267–272

Krieger JN, Tam MR, Stevens CE, et al. Diagnosis of trichomoniasis. Comparison of conventional wet-mount examination with cytologic studies, cultures, and monoclonal antibody staining of direct specimens. *JAMA* 1988;259(8):1223–1227

Landers DV, Wiesenfeld HC, Heine RP, Krohn MA, Hillier SL. Predictive value of the clinical diagnosis of lower genital tract infection in women. *Am J Obstet Gynecol* 2004;190(4):1004–1010

Lara-Torre E, Pinkerton JS. Accuracy of detection of trichomonas vaginalis organisms on a liquid-based papanicolaou smear. *Am J Obstet Gynecol* 2003;188(2):354–356

Larsson PG, Carlsson B. Does pre- and postoperative metronidazole treatment lower vaginal cuff infection rate after abdominal hysterectomy among women with bacterial vaginosis? *Infect Dis Obstet Gynecol* 2002;10(3):133–140

Lynch PJ. Lichen simplex chronicus (atopic/neurodermatitis) of the anogenital region. *Dermatol Ther* 2004;17(1):8–19

Meis PJ, Goldenberg RL, Mercer B, et al; National Institute of Child Health and Human Development Maternal-Fetal Medicine Units Network. The preterm prediction study: significance of vaginal infections. *Am J Obstet Gynecol* 1995;173(4):1231–1235

Morales WJ, Schorr S, Albritton J. Effect of metronidazole in patients with preterm birth in preceding pregnancy and bacterial vaginosis: a placebo-controlled, double-blind study. *Am J Obstet Gynecol* 1994;171(2):345–347, discussion 348–349

Moyal-Barracco M, Edwards L. Diagnosis and therapy of anogenital lichen planus. *Dermatol Ther* 2004;17(1):38–46

Neill SM, Tatnall FM, Cox NH; British Association of Dermatologists. Guidelines for the management of lichen sclerosus. *Br J Dermatol* 2002;147(4):640–649

Nygren P, Fu R, Freeman M, Bougatsos C, Klebanoff M, Guise JM; U.S. Preventive Services Task Force. Evidence on the benefits and harms of screening and treating pregnant women who are asymptomatic for bacterial vaginosis: an update review for the U.S. Preventive Services Task Force. *Ann Intern Med* 2008;148(3):220–233

Reed BD. Risk factors for Candida vulvovaginitis. *Obstet Gynecol Surv* 1992;47(8):551–560

Smith YR, Haefner HK. Vulvar lichen sclerosus : pathophysiology and treatment. *Am J Clin Dermatol* 2004;5(2):105–125

Sobel JD, Chaim W, Nagappan V, et al. Treatment of vaginitis caused by Candida glabrata: use of topical boric acid and flucytosine. *Am J Obstet Gynecol* 2003;189:1297–1300

Sobel JD, Kapernick PS, Zervos M, et al. Treatment of complicated Candida vaginitis: comparison of single and sequential doses of fluconazole. *Am J Obstet Gynecol* 2001;185(2):363–369

Sobel JD, Wiesenfeld HC, Martens M, et al. Maintenance fluconazole therapy for recurrent vulvovaginal candidiasis. *N Engl J Med* 2004;351(9):876–883

Soper D. Trichomoniasis: under control or undercontrolled? *Am J Obstet Gynecol* 2004;190(1):281–290

Soper DE, Bump RC, Hurt WG. Bacterial vaginosis and trichomoniasis vaginitis are risk factors for cuff cellulitis after abdominal hysterectomy. *Am J Obstet Gynecol* 1990;163(3):1016–1021, discussion 1021–1023

Watts DH, Krohn MA, Hillier SL, Eschenbach DA. Bacterial vaginosis as a risk factor for post-cesarean endometritis. *Obstet Gynecol* 1990;75(1):52–58

Workowski KA, Berman SM; Centers for Disease Control and Prevention. Sexually transmitted diseases treatment guidelines, 2006. *MMWR Recomm Rep* 2006; 55(RR-11, RR-11)1–94

31 Sexually Transmitted Diseases

Tanya S. Ghatan

Screening and Risk Factors

Sexually transmitted diseases (STDs) represent a major public health problem, and complications from untreated disease can have serious medical consequences.

A thorough sexual history is important for effective screening. The Centers for Disease Control and Prevention (CDC) recommends the five "P's": Partners, Prevention of pregnancy, Protection from STDs, Practices, and Past history of STDs. It is also important to elicit information about any new sexual partners, history of multiple partners, types of sexual exposure, and condom use. STD screening must be done in a nonjudgmental manner.

Common risk factors for all STDs include young age, African-American race, a new sexual partner, multiple partners, history of prior STD, and illicit substance abuse.

Non-Ulcerative Lesions

Gonorrhea

The causative agent is *Neisseria gonorrhoeae*. Gonococcal infections represent one of the most common sexually transmitted diseases worldwide with approximately 700 000 infections in the United States annually.

Risk factors for acquisition include, but are not limited to, low socioeconomic status, early onset of sexual activity, and substance abuse. There is an unequal transmission rate between sexes, with the male-to-female transmission rate as high as 80–90% compared with 20–25% for female to male.

Infection occurs primarily at the columnar epithelium of the genital tract. The transitional epithelium of the urinary tract is a second location of infection. Symptoms may include cervical purulent discharge, urinary frequency, dysuria, and occasionally rectal discomfort. Many women may have mild to no symptoms. Complications from Gonorrhea may develop regardless of the severity of symptoms. Gonorrhea is a common cause of pelvic inflammatory disease, which in turn can lead to long-lasting pain and infertility.

Currently, DNA probes from either cervical swabs or urine are used to diagnose the infection. Other, less common methods of diagnosis are culture or Gram stain. *Neisseria gonorrhoeae* is a Gram-negative diplococcus described as "paired kidney beans" (**Fig. 31.1**).

Standard treatment is a single dose of ceftriaxone 250 mg intramuscularly. Additionally patients should be treated for Chlamydia if it has not been ruled out secondary to a high incidence of concurrent infection.

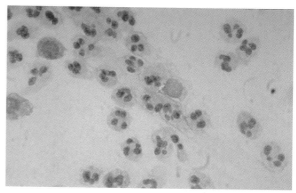

Fig. 31.1 Gonoccocus "Gram-negative diplococcus." Source: University of Washington (Seattle STD/HIV Prevention Training Center).

Chlamydia

The causative agent is *Chlamydia trachomatis*. Chlamydia is the most frequently reported STD in the United States. There is an approximately 2.2% prevalence rate of chlamydial infections with 1 030 911 infections reported to the CDC in 2006. Many women are asymptomatic and therefore do not seek testing or treatment. Risks factors for acquisition are the same as for Gonorrhea and include early onset of sexual activity, multiple sexual partners, a new sexual partner within the previous three months, low socioeconomic status, and a history of a prior STD.

Chlamydia may present as an ocular, respiratory or genital tract infection (**Fig. 31.2**). Chlamydia is primarily acquired through sexual contact although, rarely, vertical transmission may be seen. The organism attaches to columnar epithelial cells in the genital tract. Symptoms usually appear within 1–3 weeks of exposure. Symptoms include mucopurulent cervical discharge, hypertrophic friable cervix, and acute urethral syndrome.

Genetic probes are utilized for diagnosis. Cell culture is the "gold standard" but is difficult and requires at least seven days. Standard treatment is either a single oral dose of azithromycin 1 g or doxycycline 100 mg twice daily for 1 week.

Complications can involve salpingitis leading to infertility, pelvic pain, and ectopic pregnancy. In neonatal infections conjunctivitis and otitis media are common complications.

Annual screening for Chlamydia is recommended for all sexually active women under the age of 25 years. In addition, older women with risk factors and pregnant women should be screened.

Ulcerative Lesions

Syphilis

The spirochete *Treponema pallidum* is the causative agent. Infections are primarily sexually transmitted. The spirochetes enter through abrasions on the skin and mucosal surfaces, where they then replicate (**Fig. 31.3**).

Syphilis may be divided into initial, secondary, and tertiary stages with different symptoms, complications, and treatment for each stage. Syphilis lesions may resolve spontaneously and the patient may remain asymptomatic during any stage of the disease.

The initial lesion or "chancre" is approximately 1 cm in size. It is painless, red and round with raised edges. The chancre appears 3 weeks after exposure, although it may have a 10–60-day incubation period. The chancre will heal without treatment, but the disease will still progress to the secondary stage. The secondary stage may appear 1–3 months after the primary lesion has resolved. It represents a disseminated infection. The typical maculopapular rash occurs on the palms and soles of the feet. The dermatologic lesions may be diverse resulting in syphilis being known as the "great imitator." Malaise, headache and anorexia are also often present.

Syphilis passes into a latent phase upon completion of the secondary stage. This may last for years before tertiary syphilis develops. This allows transmission of syphilis from those who are unaware that they are themselves infected. Tertiary syphilis is rare in the United States. The pathognomic lesions are granulomas or gummas of the

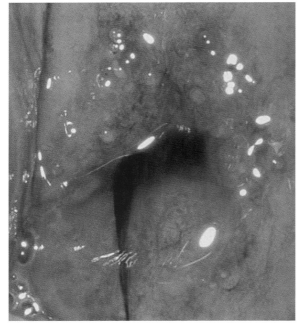

Fig. 31.2 Chlamydial Cervicitis. Source: Conni Cellum and Walter Stamm (Seattle STD/HIV Prevention Training Center).

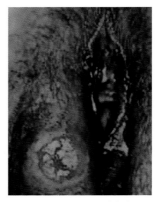

Fig. 31.3 Primary Syphilis lesion

bone and skin representing lesions of necrotic, ulcerative nodules. Other complications of syphilis include neurosyphilis with tabes dorsalis and aortitis.

The spirochetes can be identified utilizing dark-field microscopy, although this is now rarely used for diagnosis. Screening occurs with a nonspecific antibody test. Examples of these are the RPR (rapid plasmin regain) and the VDRL (venereal disease research laboratory) tests. Following a positive screening test infection is confirmed with a specific treponemal test, such as the microhemagglutination assay for *Treponema pallidum* antibodies, or the fluorescent treponemal antibody-absorption technique (FTA). A lumbar puncture is required if neurosyphilis is suspected. There can be up to a 15% false-positive rate with serologic testing. False-positive test results can be seen with autoimmune diseases (e.g., lupus, rheumatoid arthritis), recent viral infections, recent immunizations, chronic liver disease, and pregnancy.

Penicillin is the drug of choice for treatment, with dose and duration dependent on the stage of infection. Early syphilis may be treated with a single, intramuscular dose of penicillin G 2.4 million units. If the infection has been present for at least 1 year or is of unknown duration, weekly injections of penicillin for 3 weeks are required. Neurosyphilis requires intravenous therapy.

Congenital syphilis may result in nonimmune hydrops of the fetus. Other fetal and neonatal complications include thrombocytopenia, profound anemia, hepatosplenomegaly, hutchinson teeth, mulberry molars, saber shins, saddle nose, interstitial keratitis, and 8th cranial nerve deafness.

Herpes Simplex

Genital herpes is a life-long, chronic infection. It is common, with approximately 50 million people in the United States being affected. There are two strains of the herpes simplex virus: HSV-1 and HSV-2. The latter is the more common cause of genital lesions, representing up to 90% of the infections. HSV-1 may be protective against acquiring HSV-2. In the majority of those infected with HSV-2 the disease is undiagnosed, resulting in unintended transmission. Prevention of transmission is an important aspect of managing HSV (Evidence Box 31.1).

HSV is highly contagious, but requires intimate mucocutaneous contact for infection. The primary infection may present with symptoms 3–7 days after exposure. The prodrome may include low-grade fever, malaise, or inguinal lymphadenopathy. Clear, painful, tender vesicles develop on the labia majora, labia minora, or perianal region (**Fig. 31.4**). Asymptomatic lesions may develop in the vagina or on the ectocervix. The vesicles will rupture in 1–7 days resulting in shallow, painful ulcers with raised edges, which heal in 7–10 days without scarring. Some patients may have a severe initial outbreak with significant pain,

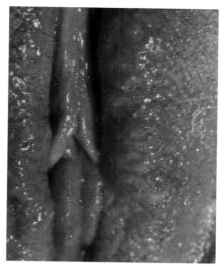

Fig. 31.4 Herpes Outbreak.

dysuria, and urinary retention. Other patients may have a minor outbreak that is relatively asymptomatic, such as to be unaware that they have acquired HSV.

The diagnosis is generally made by a combination of physical exam and diagnostic testing. The traditional Tzanck smear demonstrating multinucleated giant cells is rarely used. Viral culture is the definitive method, although the sensitivity of viral cultures may be low, particularly in a healing lesion. Fluid is cultured from a ruptured vesicle or a debrided ulcer. Serological testing remains difficult to interpret and is an area of ongoing debate in the field.

Treatment includes symptomatic treatment with sitz baths for comfort. Antiviral medications such as acyclovir are given for treatment, with different regimens given for primary versus secondary outbreaks.

Unlike most of the other ulcerative lesions, herpes becomes a chronic disease. It is incurable, with the virus remaining latent in the sensory dorsal nerve-root ganglia. The virus can reactivate and travel back down nerve fibers resulting in secondary outbreaks. These recurrent outbreaks may be rare or frequent. Typically, they are preceded by a prodrome of vulvar burning and pruritus. Such outbreaks are generally shorter than the initial infection and are without systemic findings. Some patients require suppressive therapy as a result of frequent outbreaks (**Table 31.1**).

Viremia in pregnant women with primary herpes increases the risk of poor obstetrical outcomes and of neonatal herpes. There is a 50% rate of neonatal herpes with primary infections. This is significantly reduced in the case of secondary outbreaks to less than 1%. The current recommendations include cesarean delivery for those women with active herpetic lesions at the time of delivery to decrease the risk of neonatal infection. Many physicians will place those patients with a known history of

Table 31.1 Treatment regimens for herpes simplex

First episode	Recurrent episodes	Suppression
Acyclovir 400 mg 3× /day	Acyclovir 400 mg 3× /day	Acyclovir 400 mg 2× /day
Acyclovir 200 mg 5× /day	Acyclovir 800 mg 2× /day	Famcilovir 250 mg 2× /day
Famciclovir 250 mg 3× /day	Famciclovir 125 mg 2× /day	Valacyclovir 500 mg 1× /day
Valacyclovir 1 g 2× /day	Valacyclovir 1 g 1× /day	Valacyclovir 1 g 1× /day
For 7–10 days	For 5 days	

HSV on suppressive therapy with acyclovir at 36-weeks' gestation to decrease the likelihood of their having an active lesion at the time of delivery.

Lymphogranuloma Venereum

Lymphogranuloma venereum (LGV) is caused by the L-serotype of *Chlamydia trachomatis* strains 1, 2, and 3. Unlike Chlamydia, genital ulcers may be seen. Additionally, swelling of the lymph nodes is a prominent feature. LGV must be differentiated from the more common ulcerative lesions of the external genitalia. The exact number of cases of LGV is the United States is unknown. It is thought to be fairly rare, although outbreaks have occurred in the southeastern United States. It is more commonly seen in Africa and Asia. Transmission occurs through direct contact with lesions during intercourse. There is a 6 : 1 ratio of men to women diagnosed with LGV.

LGV can be a difficult diagnosis to make. Other ulcerative STDs are more common. A primary lesion may be a small, genital or rectal lesion that starts to ulcerate. The primary papule is often a shallow ulcer that goes unnoticed. The incubation time from transmission to lesion is wide varying from 3 to 30 days. Additionally, lesions may not be directly visible to the examiner as they are located in the urethra, vagina, or rectum. In the secondary stage there is an enlargement of the lesion and painful inflammation of the inguinal nodes. Fever, malaise and anorexia may develop. If left untreated, severe complications including proctocolitis, rectal strictures, and rectovaginal fistulas may develop.

LGV is primarily a clinical diagnosis. The CDC recommends 3 weeks of doxycycline twice daily as treatment.

Chancroid

Chancroid is an ulcerative lesion caused by *Haemophilus ducreyi*. In the United States, while there are some endemic areas, it is usually seen in outbreaks. There is a male to female ratio of 3 : 1.

Chancroid is characterized by a painful, demarcated but nonindurated ulcer. There can be concomitant painful inguinal lymphadenopathy.

Haemophilus ducreyi is difficult to culture and chancroid is often a clinical diagnosis. The definitive diagnosis requires special culture medium that is not widely available and has a low sensitivity. The diagnosis can be made in the setting of painful genital ulcers, the appearance of the ulcers, the presence of lymphadenopathy, the exclusion of syphilis on serological testing, and negative screening for HSV.

Recommended treatment is a single dose of either ceftriaxone 250 mg intramuscularly or azithromycin 1 g orally (**Table 31.2**).

Table 31.2 Overview of presentation and treatment of ulcerative lesions

	Syphilis	Herpes	Chancroid	LGV
Incubation (average)	7–14 days	3–7 days	4–7 days	3–12 days
Primary lesion	Papule	Vesicle	Papule	Papule/vesicle
No. of lesions	1	Multiple	Few	1
Size	5–15 mm	1–3 mm	2–20 mm	2–10 mm
Pain	No	Yes	Yes	No
Treatment	Penicillin	Acyclovir	Ceftriaxone/azithromycin	Doxycycline

LGV, lymphogranuloma venereum.

Granuloma Inguinale

Donovanosis is an ulcerative disease of the genitalia caused by *Klebsiella granulomatis*. It rarely occurs in the United States, but is endemic in some tropical areas. It is characterized by painless ulcerative lesions in the absence of lymphadenopathy. The lesions are very vascular and bleed easily. It is difficult to culture and is identified only on visualization of the dark-staining Donovan bodies.

Treatment is generally prolonged as the lesions heal inward from the margin and is continued until all the lesions are healed. Azithromycin 1 g is given orally once a week for a minimum of 3 weeks, or ciprofloxacin 750 mg orally twice daily for a minimum of 3 weeks.

Viral Infections

Human Papilloma Virus

Human papilloma virus (HPV) has more the 100 subtypes, many of which infect the genital area. Most are asymptomatic or unrecognized. Condylomata or genital warts may be seen with some of the subtypes (specifically 6 and 11). Others are more strongly associated with cervical neoplasia.

Condyloma is diagnosed by clinical exam. The warts are generally treated by application of trichloroacetic acid (TCA) or podophyllin, which are applied by the provider, or imiquimod cream, which is applied by the patient at home. Resistant or large lesions may require laser therapy, cryotherapy, or surgical excision.

Prophylactic vaccines aimed at the most common HPV subtypes are an effective means of cervical cancer prevention.

Hepatitis B

Hepatitis B is caused by infection with the hepatitis B virus (HBV), which is transmitted via bodily fluids. In the United States vaccination has resulted in a significant decline in the rates of newly acquired hepatitis B.

The incubation time of HBV can be 6 weeks to 6 months. From 50% to 75% of all newly acquired infections may be asymptomatic. In adults, newly acquired HBV leads to acute liver failure and death in approximately 1% of cases. The risk of developing a chronic infection is directly related to age at time of infection. Mother–infant transmissions represent 40% of all chronic HBV infections. Seque-lae of chronic infection include active hepatitis, cirrhosis, and hepatocellular carcinoma.

Human Immunodeficiency Virus

The most common means of acquisition of Human Immunodeficiency Virus (HIV) is sexual transmission. Screening and counseling remain important. The majority of infections in the United States are HIV-1. Diagnosis is done with tests of antibodies to HIV-1, such as rapid screening with enzyme immunoassay, which is confirmed with supplemental testing, such as Western blot analysis.

Key Points

- Sexually transmitted diseases (STDs) are a major public health problem. Consequences of untreated STDs include pelvic inflammatory disease, infertility due to tubal obstruction, endometritis, cervical neoplasia, increased risk of acquiring HIV, pelvic and vulvar pain syndromes.
- The infections most commonly transmitted sexually are Human Papilloma Virus, Herpes Simplex virus types 1 and 2, Chlamydia, Gonorrhea, HIV, hepatitis B, and syphilis.
- Risk factors for acquiring an STD include: age less than 25 years, a new sex partner within 60 days, multiple sex partners, incarceration, contact with sex workers, and use of illicit drugs.
- The risk of acquiring an STD can be significantly decreased by the routine use of male condoms. All men and women should be counseled about the use of condoms. Vaccination for human papillomavirus, hepatitis A and B can reduce the risk of acquiring these STDs.

Evidence Box 31.1

Daily suppressive therapy with valacyclovir has been shown to significantly reduce the risk of transmission of genital herpes in discordant couples.

Genital herpes is a common problem affecting more than 50 million people in the United States. Once acquired, it is a life-long problem with ensuing consequences. Preventing transmission is an important aspect of managing this infection.

In a study of 1484 immunocompetent, heterosexual, monogamous couples who were discordant for HSV-2, patients were randomly assigned to receive either valacyclovir 500 mg once daily or placebo for 8 months. Both partners were counseled regarding safe sex practices and offered condoms at each visit. The susceptible partners were evaluated for herpes monthly. Clinically symptomatic HSV-2 occurred in 4 of 743 susceptible partners in the valacyclovir group compared with 16 of 741 in the placebo group.

Suppressive therapy in the affected partner of a discordant couple is important in having a direct impact on reducing transmission of this life-long infection.

Corey L, Wald A, Patel R, et al. Once-daily valacyclovir to reduce the risk of transmission of genital herpes. N Engl J Med 2004;350(1):11–20.

Further Reading

Cook RL, Hutchison SL, Østergaard L, Braithwaite RS, Ness RB. Systematic review: noninvasive testing for Chlamydia trachomatis and Neisseria gonorrhoeae. *Ann Intern Med* 2005;142(11):914–925

Http://www. cdc. gov/std

Corey L, Wald A, Patel R, et al. Once-daily valacyclovir to reduce the risk of transmission of genital herpes. *N Engl J Med* 2004;350(1):11–20

Kamb ML, Fishbein M, Douglas JM Jr, et al; Project RESPECT Study Group. Efficacy of risk-reduction counseling to prevent human immunodeficiency virus and sexually transmitted diseases: a randomized controlled trial. *JAMA* 1998;280(13):1161–1167

Mao C, Koutsky LA, Ault KA, et al. Efficacy of human papillomavirus-16 vaccine to prevent cervical intraepithelial neoplasia: a randomized controlled trial. *Obstet Gynecol* 2006;107(1):18–27

McNeeley SG Jr. Gonococcal infections in women. *Obstet Gynecol Clin North Am* 1989;16(3):467–478

Pope V. Use of treponemal tests to screen for syphilis. *Infect Med* 2004;21:399–402

Torkko KC, Gershman K, Crane LA, Hamman R, Barón A. Testing for Chlamydia and sexual history taking in adolescent females: results from a statewide survey of Colorado primary care providers. *Pediatrics* 2000;106(3):E32

US Preventive Services Task Force. Guide to clinical preventive services 2005. Recommendations of the U S Preventive Services Task Force. Rockville, Md: Agency for Healthcare Research and Quality; 2005

Workowski KA, Berman SM; Centers for Disease Control and Prevention. Sexually transmitted diseases treatment guidelines, 2006. *MMWR Recomm Rep* 2006; 55(RR-11, RR-11)1–94

32 Pelvic Inflammatory Disease

Tanya S. Ghatan

Definition

Pelvic inflammatory disease (PID) refers to an infection of the upper female genital tract. The infection involves the uterus, fallopian tubes, ovaries, and may evolve into a larger pelvic infection. It may include any combination of endometritis, salpingitis, tubo-ovarian abcess, and peritonitis. Many different organisms are implicated in PID, but the majority are associated with *Neisseria gonorrhoeae* and *Chlamydia trachomatis*.

PID can be a serious complication of sexually transmitted diseases, especially those of gonorrhea and chlamydia. The centers for disease control and prevention (CDC) reports approximately 1 million women in the United States experience an acute episode of PID each year.

Long-term consequences from damage to the fallopian tissues and surrounding tissues include infertility, ectopic pregnancy, pelvic abcesses, and chronic pelvic pain. Over 100 000 women experience infertility annually as a result of PID.

Risk Factors

Risks factors are the same as for any sexually transmitted disease, but a previous episode of PID places a woman at greater risk for developing a second episode. Sexually active women of childbearing age are those at greatest risk, with those under 25 years at the greatest risk. The cervix of teenage girls and young women is not fully developed, which increases the risk of infection. The number of lifetime sexual partners as well as multiple partners increases the risk.

Use of intrauterine devices is associated with an elevated PID risk immediately after insertion compared with women utilizing other methods of contraception; however, this does not persist after placement. This risk is reduced by STD screening and treatment prior to placement.

Signs and Symptoms

PID may present differently, with some women experiencing no symptoms to very mild ones, and others having very severe symptoms. The degree of damage done to the reproductive system does not correlate to the severity of symptoms. Lower abdominal pain, fever, vaginal discharge, painful intercourse, dysuria, and irregular bleeding are common symptoms.

Long-Term Complications

PID can cause significant and permanent damage to the fallopian tubes and reproductive organs of infected patients. Timely treatment can help to prevent complications. Bacteria in the fallopian tubes can cause infection resulting in scar tissue formation and subsequent blockage of the tubes. Approximately 10% of women with PID suffer from infertility, with the risk of infertility increasing with subsequent episodes.

In addition to infertility, scarring damage to the fallopian tubes may result in ectopic pregnancies. Ectoptic pregnancies can be life-threatening if not recognized and treated in a timely fashion.

Long-term chronic pelvic pain is another known complication, which results from scarring in the pelvis involving the fallopian tubes and other structures.

Diagnosis

PID can be a subtle infection that is difficult to diagnose. It is frequently missed due to mild or subtle symptoms. There is no single test for PID. Diagnosis is usually clinical and occurs in the office or emergency room. For this reason, a low-threshold diagnosis should be maintained.

Physical exam remains at the core of diagnosis: if cervical motion tenderness, uterine tenderness, or adnexal tenderness is present, treatment should be initiated. Additional criteria that have been used to increase specificity are listed in **Table 32.1**. Pelvic ultrasound imaging and laparoscopy are occasionally used to provide additional confirmation of diagnosis, generally in cases where other diagnoses are possible, such as appendicitis.

Treatment

Outpatient

Empiric treatment in sexually-active young women and those at risk should be initiated if they are experiencing pelvic or lower abdominal pain, no other cause can be identified, and if cervical motion tenderess, uterine tenderness, or adnexal tenderness are present.

PID treatment is based on broad-spectrum coverage of the most likely causal organisms (**Table 32.2**). All treatment regimens should be effective against *Neisseria gonorrhoeae* and *Chlamydia trachomatis*. Prompt treatment should be initiated as soon as the diagnosis is made to prevent long-term sequelae.

Patients being treated with outpatient therapy must be re-evaluated within 72 hours of initiating outpatient therapy. Clinical improvement needs to be demonstrated otherwise admission for in-patient therapy is required (Evidence Box 32.1).

In-patient

Hospitalization is required for treatment if any of the following conditions is present:
- severe illness (nausea, vomiting, high fever)
- pregnancy
- unresponsive to, or unable to tolerate, oral medication
- tubo-ovarian abscess
- other surgical emergencies have not been ruled out (e.g., appendicitis)

There has been significant debate as to whether to hospitalize adolescents with PID for treatment; however, there is no long-term evidence suggesting benefit from hospitalization.

There are several different recommendations for parenteral antibiotics (**Table 32.3**). Intravenous (IV) therapy may be discontinued after 24 hours of clinical improvement, and doxycycline continued for 14 days of total therapy. Other regimens including levofloxacin and metronidazole have been recommended by the CDC.

Table 32.1 Criteria relevant to diagnosis of pelvic inflammatory disease

Oral temperature >38.3 °C (>101 °F)
Mucopurulent cervical or vaginal discharge
Large number of white blood cells on wet prep.
Elevated erythrocyte sedimentation rate
Elevated C-reactive protein
Laboratory documentation of *N. gonorrhoeae* or *C. trachomatis*

Table 32.2 Treatment regimens for pelvic inflammatory disease

Regimen A	
Levofloxacin 500 mg orally for 14 days *or* **Oflaxacin** 400 mg orally twice a day for 14 days with or without **Metranidazole** 500 mg orally twice a day for 14 days	
Regimen B*	
Ceftriaxone 250 mg IM and **Doxycycline** 100 mg orally twice a day for 14 days	**Cefoxitin** 2 g IM with probenicid 1 g orally and **Doxycycline** 100 mg orally twice a day for 14 days

* Metronidazole 500 mg orally twice a day for 14 days may be added for anaerobic coverage.

Table 32.3 Parenteral antibiotics regimens

Regimen A	Regimen B
Cefotetan 2 g IV every 12 hours *or* **Cefoxitin** 2 g IV every 6 hours and **Doxycycline** 100 mg orally or IV every 12 hours	**Clindamycin** 900 mg IV every 8 hours and **Gentamicin** IV (weight based) single or divided dose regimens

Tubo-Ovarian Abscess

If a patient is unresponsive to therapy for PID, further investigation is warranted to rule out tubo-ovarian abscess (TOA). The diagnosis can be made clinically in the setting of PID with the appreciation of adnexal or posterior cul-de-sac fullness. However, radiologic imaging in the form of ultrasonography or computed tomography is generally utilized.

Patients diagnosed with TOA must be hospitalized for broad-spectrum antibiotic therapy. If they remain unresponsive to antibiotics or show evidence of rupture, surgical intervention may be necessary. Interventional radiology may be utilized for drainage of the abscess. Depending on the location and size of the abcesses, surgery may include unilateral or bilaterally salpingo-oophorectomy or total abdominal hysterectomy.

Key Points

- Pelvic inflammatory disease (PID) is defined as the infection of the female upper genital tract and is manifested by one or more of the following syndromes: salpingitis, pelvic peritonitis, endometritis, oophoritis, and/or perihepatitis.
- The most common consequences of untreated PID are tubal occlusion and scarring, tubal infertility, tubo-ovarian abscess, and chronic pelvic pain.
- The risk of infertility following PID is increased by multiple episodes of PID, the severity of the infection(s), presence of chlamydia, and delay in diagnosis and treatment.
- A common in-hospital regimen used to treat PID is intravenous cefoxitin plus oral doxycycline, or clindamycin plus gentamicin. A common outpatient regimen used to treat PID is intramuscular ceftriaxone plus oral doxycycline. Oral metronidazole may be added to the regimen if anaerobic infection is suspected.

Evidence Box 32.1

In mild-to-moderate pelvic inflammatory disease there is no difference in overall reproductive outcomes between in-patient and outpatient therapy of either mild or moderate disease.

Pelvic inflammatory disease (PID) can have serious long-term sequelae impacting on a patient's long-term fertility. In the United States, most PID is managed on an outpatient basis. In 2002 the Pelvic Inflammatory Disease Evaluation and Clinical Health (PEACH) study found no difference between in-patient and outpatient treatment groups.

In the PEACH clinical trial 831 women with clinical signs and symptoms of mild-to-moderate PID were randomized to in-patient treatment (IV cefoxitin and doxycycline) or outpatient therapy (oral doxycycline and one IM injection of cefoxitin). The study compared the two groups over a mean of 84 months of follow-up for primary outcomes of first pregnancy, first live-birth or ectopic pregnancy, time to first pregnancy, and infertility and demonstrated no difference in outcomes between the two groups. This study reinforces that there is no basis for the older recommendation of hospitalizing nulligravid women and teenagers for the treatment of PID, unless there are clinical factors such as the inability to take or tolerate oral medications due to nausea and vomiting.

The PEACH study and its subsequent follow-up demonstrate that outpatient therapy does not negatively impact reproductive outcomes in patients with mild-to-moderate PID.

Ness RB, Trautmann G, Richter H, et al. Effectiveness of treatment strategies of some women with pelvic inflammatory disease: a randomized trial. Obstet Gynecol 2005;106(3):573–580.

Further Reading

Gaitán H, Angel E, Diaz R, Parada A, Sanchez L, Vargas C. Accuracy of five different diagnostic techniques in mild-to-moderate pelvic inflammatory disease. *Infect Dis Obstet Gynecol* 2002;10(4):171–180

Http://www.cdc.gov/std

Ness RB, Soper DE, Holley RL, et al. Effectiveness of inpatient and outpatient treatment strategies for women with pelvic inflammatory disease: results from the Pelvic Inflammatory Disease Evaluation and Clinical Health (PEACH) Randomized Trial. *Am J Obstet Gynecol* 2002;186(5):929–937

Workowski KA, Berman SM; Centers for Disease Control and Prevention. Sexually transmitted diseases treatment guidelines, 2006. *MMWR Recomm Rep* 2006; 55(RR-11, RR-11)1–94

US Preventive Services Task Force. Guide to clinical preventive services 2005. Recommendations of the US Preventive Services Task Force. Rockville, Md: Agency for Healthcare Research and Quality; 2005

33 Endometriosis and Adenomyosis

Robert L. Barbieri

Endometriosis

Definition

Endometriosis is the presence of endometrial glands and/ or stroma outside of the uterus. Women with endometriosis typically present for medical care with one or more of the following three problems:

1. Pelvic pain that impacts daily function
2. Infertility
3. A complex adnexal mass due to an ovarian cyst of endometriosis (endometrioma)

Prevalence and Epidemiology

Approximately 5% of women between the ages of 15 and 45 years have endometriosis. The peak incidence appears to occur between 20 and 30 years of age (**Fig. 33.1**). In sharp contrast, the peak incidence of uterine leiomyomas (fibroids) occurs between 35 and 45 years of age. Many reproductive exposures influence the risk of developing endometriosis. Reproductive factors that increase the risk of developing endometriosis include early menarche, short menstrual cycles of less than 26 days, prolonged menstrual flow lasting more than 7 days, nulliparity, and low circulating androgen levels. Reproductive factors that decrease the risk of developing endometriosis include multiple births, long intervals of lactation, oligo- or amenorrhea, and late menarche.

Etiology

Many mechanisms may contribute to the development of endometriosis including:

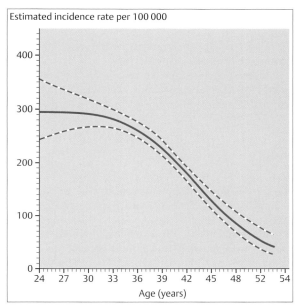

Fig. 33.1 Age-specific incidence of laparoscopically confirmed endometriosis among premenopausal women with no past infertility history in the Nurses' Health Study II (1989–1999). Dashed and dotted lines, 95% confidence intervals.

- *retrograde menstruation* of small viable pieces of endometrial glands and stroma through the fallopian tubes into the peritoneal cavity
- *metaplasia of the pelvic peritoneal lining* into endometrial glands and stroma caused by irritation of the peritoneum from retrograde transported menstrual blood
- *immune system dysfunction* that prevents the removal of retrograde menstruated endometrium from the peritoneal cavity
- *excess hormonal stimulation by estrogen* and decreased exposure to androgens
- *somatic genetic mutations* that result in the monoclonal expansion of precursor cells into endometriosis ovarian cysts

Historically, retrograde menstruation has been the most commonly cited theory for the development of endometriosis. In humans and nonhuman primates, cervical stenosis—an anatomical abnormality that results in an increase in the volume of retrograde menstruated endometrium—uniformly results in the development of endometriosis if estrogen is present.

Hormonal factors play a key role in the development of endometriosis. Estrogen stimulates the growth of endometriosis. Physiological levels of progesterone also support the growth of endometriosis. Androgens decrease the growth of endometrial glands and stroma. Women with high levels of estrogen and low levels of androgen are at increased risk for developing endometriosis. Women with low levels of estrogen (amenorrhea, menopause) and high levels of androgens (polcystic ovary syndrome) are at low risk of developing endometriosis. Pharmacologic doses of androgenic progestins (norgestrel) decrease the growth of endometriosis tissue.

Endometriosis requires estrogen for its continued growth. Bilateral oophorectomy is uniformly effective in the treatment of endometriosis.

History

The most common symptoms reported by women with endometriosis are dysmenorrhea, dyspareunia, and pain with bowel movements (dyschezia). Based on the history, it is often difficult to distinguish the dysmenorrhea associated with endometriosis from that caused by primary dysmenorrhea (dysmenorrhea caused by prostaglandin stimulation of the uterine muscle). However, women with endometriosis and dysmenorrhea often report that the pelvic pain is not well relieved by nonsteroidal anti-inflammatory agents. Most women with endometriosis are nulliparous. Unlike women with primary dysmenorrhea, many women with dysmenorrhea and endometriosis present with severe pain to emergency rooms or have frequent doctor visits for pelvic pain. Women with pelvic pain that is impacting their daily life function and is not relieved by ibuprofen or cyclic oral contraceptives should be counseled regarding the option of laparoscopic surgery to diagnose endometriosis.

Physical Examination

About 40% of women with endometriosis and pelvic pain have a significant physical finding on pelvic examination. The most common physical findings associated with endometriosis are:
- uterosacral ligament thickening or nodularity (due to endometriosis within or on the uterosacral ligament)

- lateral displacement of the cervix (endometriosis may inflame and shorten one uterosacral ligament pulling the cervix to one side of the vagina; **Fig. 33.2**)
- Cervical stenosis

Women with advanced endometriosis often have ovarian cysts and these may be palpable on bimanual examination. Extensive training in pelvic examination techniques, such as a residency in gynecology, is necessary to reliably recognize uterosacral ligament thickening or nodularity. However, lateral cervical displacement and cervical stenosis can be diagnosed with less extensive training. Lateral cervical displacement is present when the outer border of the cervix is lateral to the axial midline. For the majority of women, the cervix is reliably within the axial midline. For about 25% of women with endometriosis, the outer border of the cervix is lateral to the axial midline. Cervical stenosis is likely present if the diameter of the cervical os is less than 4 mm. The common cotton-tipped applicator used in medicine has a maximal diameter of approximately 4.5 mm. If the cotton-tipped applicator cannot fit into the cervical os, the clinician should be alert that cervical stenosis may be present. About 5% of women with endometriosis have cervical stenosis.

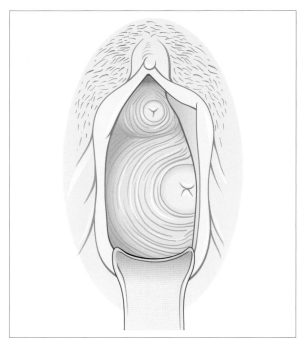

Fig. 33.2 In normal women, the body of the cervix is inside the axial midline. In some women with endometriosis, shortening of one uterosacral ligament because of scarring has pulled the cervix to the ipsilateral side of the vagina, resulting in lateral displacement of the cervix. In lateral displacement of the cervix, the body of the cervix is lateral to the axial midline.

Diagnosis

The "gold standard" for the diagnosis of endometriosis is surgical visual diagnosis, typically performed by laparoscopy. Laparoscopy is an ambulatory surgery procedure that is typically performed under general anesthesia. *An advantage of surgical diagnosis of endometriosis is that therapeutic excision or ablation of the endometriosis implants can occur at the same time as the diagnostic surgery.* At the time of laparoscopy, a systematic and comprehensive assessment of the pelvis and lower abdomen permits the detection of even very small implants (1 mm in diameter) of endometriosis. The most common locations of endometriosis are:

- left and right ovaries
- uterosacral ligaments and the cul-de-sac of Douglas
- anterior bladder peritoneum
- other pelvic peritoneal surfaces such as the broad ligament
- appendix and bowel

Endometriosis may also occur outside the pelvis on the pleural lining causing catamenial hemothorax.

Alternative approaches to the diagnosis of endometriosis have been proposed, but are not uniformly accepted. For example, some authorities have recommended that in a woman with a classic history and physical exam findings of endometriosis—such as progressive, severe dysmenorrhea and physical exam findings of uterosacral ligament nodularity—a presumptive *clinical diagnosis* of endometriosis can be made and treated with hormones. No nonsurgical imaging methodology is effective in diagnosing endometriosis.

Investigators have tried to identify serum markers for the presence of endometriosis. The best available serum marker of advanced endometriosis is CA-125. Approximately 70% of women with moderate and severe endometriosis have elevated serum levels of CA-125. However, the majority of women with minimal and mild endometriosis have normal levels of CA-125. Also, gynecologic diseases such as fibroids and pelvic inflammatory disease can sometimes cause elevations of CA-125, reducing the specificity of this test for the diagnosis of endometriosis.

The **differential diagnosis** of endometriosis includes adenomyosis, pelvic inflammatory disease, chronic appendicitis, uterine leiomyomas, diverticulitis, and ovarian neoplasms.

Staging

At the time of laparoscopy, the extent of the endometriosis lesions should be assessed to surgically stage the disease. The American Society of Reproductive Medicine recognizes four stages to the disease process. Minimal disease (stage I) involves a few small peritoneal lesions of endometriosis. Mild disease (stage II) involves the presence of many small peritoneal lesions of endometriosis. Moderate disease (stage III) typically involves the presence of peritoneal lesions of endometriosis, plus ovarian cysts containing endometriosis tissue (endometriomas) and minor pelvic adhesions. Severe disease (stage IV) typically involves ovarian cysts of endometriosis and major pelvic adhesions and scarring (**Fig. 33.3**). For the purposes of planning treatment, stages I and II can be combined as "early-stage endometriosis" and stages III and IV can be combined as "advanced endometriosis." In a review of 100 consecutive cases of endometriosis, the distribution of stages was: stage I 41%, stage II 32%, stage III 15%, and stage IV 12%.

Treatment

Most women with endometriosis typically present with one or more of the following three complaints:

1. Pelvic pain that impacts daily function
2. Infertility
3. A complex adnexal mass due to an ovarian cyst of endometriosis (endometrioma)

Treatment is focused on the specific complaint of the patient.

Endometriomas

Endometriomas are ovarian cysts containing endometriosis tissue. Evidence suggests that endometriomas are monoclonal tumors that arise from a somatic mutation in a precursor cell. In general, endometriomas do not regress spontaneously. Hormone treatment may cause the endometrioma to shrink in size, but they return to their pretreatment size after hormone treatment is discontinued. Endometriomas are complex ovarian cysts because ultrasound typically demonstrates the presence of complex echoes within the cyst.

Generally, persistent, complex ovarian cysts need to be surgically removed to achieve a definitive diagnosis. Some complex ovarian cysts are caused by ovarian cancer. Surgical removal and pathological analysis are required to determine the cause of a complex ovarian cyst. Some clinicians will expectantly manage small, nongrowing complex cysts (<4 cm in diameter) that are thought to be endometriomas. This approach may spare the patient a sur-

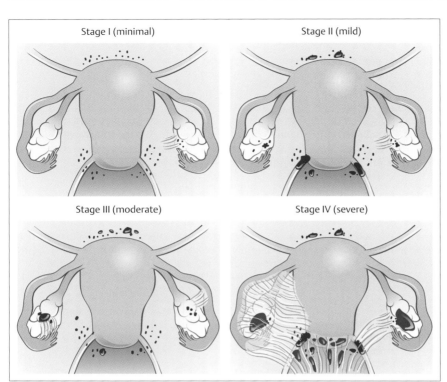

Stage I (minimal)

Stage II (mild)

Stage III (moderate)

Stage IV (severe)

Fig. 33.3 Visual examples of the four stages of endometriosis.

gical procedure where some normal ovarian tissue will be removed and scar tissue might arise postoperatively.

Infertility

Seventy-five percent of cases of infertility are caused by:
- anovulation or poor oocyte quality
- abnormal semen parameters such as poor sperm motility
- blocked fallopian tubes

About 25 % of cases of infertility are not associated with these three problems. Among these 25 % of cases, approximately 40 % of the female partners (8 % of all infertility couples) have endometriosis. Many authorities recommend that female partners of infertile couples should have a laparoscopy to look for endometriosis if the initial infertility evaluation (detection of ovulation, semen analysis, hysterosalpingogram) is normal. At the time of initial diagnostic laparoscopy, the endometriosis lesions can be excised.

For infertile couples with infertility due to endometriosis, a stepwise approach to treatment is warranted (**Table 33.1**).

One large, well-designed randomized study has reported that surgical treatment of endometriosis is effective in improving fertility in couples where the woman has minimal or mild endometriosis (see Evidence Box 33.1).

Pelvic Pain That Impacts Function

Treatment of women with pelvic pain caused by endometriosis typically involves a stepwise approach that begins with inexpensive treatments with few side effects and progresses to expensive treatments with many side effects. Hormonal treatment of endometriosis is based on the following facts:
- Estrogen stimulates the growth of endometriosis.
- Androgens inhibit the growth of endometriosis.
- High doses of androgenic progestins (such as norgestrel, norethindrone, or norethindrone acetate) inhibit the growth of endometriosis.

Surgical treatment of endometriosis is based on two concepts:
1. Surgical removal of endometriosis lesions can reduce the pain associated with the disease.
2. Surgical removal of both ovaries permanently stops 95 % of the endogenous production of estrogen, which will cure the disease, but will cause surgical menopause.

Cyclic estrogen–progestin contraceptives plus non-steroidal anti-inflammatory agent: The most commonly used hormonal treatment of pain caused by endometriosis is a combination cyclic estrogen–progestin contraceptive plus a nonsteroidal anti-inflammatory agent. The estrogen–progestin contraceptive is often effective because most preparations are "progestin-dominant," contain androgenic progestins, and prevent the growth of endometrial

Table 33.1 Approach to the treatment of infertility-associated endometriosis

Step 1	Identify and treat other causes of infertility: anovulation, tubal occlusion, abnormal semen analysis
Step 2	Use laparoscopic surgery to excise or ablate endometriosis implants. Allow 9 months to achieve pregnancy
Step 3	If the fallopian tubes are open and there are no dense ovarian adhesions, consider clomiphene plus intrauterine insemination (IUI):
	Treat the female partner with clomiphene to cause double ovulation
	Just before ovulation, harvest a high concentration of sperm from an ejaculated semen specimen using centrifugation and then use a catheter to place the sperm in the uterus
Step 4	If the fallopian tubes are open and there are no dense ovarian adhesions, consider FSH injections plus IUI:
	Treat the female partner with FSH injections followed by HCG injection to cause double or triple ovulation
	Perform IUI just before ovulation
	Warning: this step can result in twin and triplet pregnancy. Some couples may prefer to skip this step.
Step 5	In vitro fertilization treatment

FSH, follicular stimulating hormone; HGH, human chorionic gonadotropin

tissue. The physiology of the endometrium requires an interval of estrogen alone followed by estrogen and progesterone to promote maximal growth. In the contraceptive, the presence of a synthetic progestin with the first pill blocks endometrial growth in most women. In addition, many synthetic progestins are synthesized from a testosterone precursor and retain significant androgenic properties. Androgens block the growth of the endometrium.

Noncyclic estrogen–progestin contraceptives: If women prefer to avoid menses and the worry about developing pain with menses, a noncyclic treatment regimen with continuous estrogen–progestin contraceptive may be warranted. The typical cyclic estrogen–progestin contraceptive has 21 active hormone pills and seven "placebo" pills. Some new cyclic estrogen–progestin contraceptives have 24 active hormone pills and seven "placebo" pills. An alternative to monthly cyclic therapy is to prescribe 84 active hormone pills in a row and then seven "placebo" pills. This will reduce the amount of menstrual bleeding experienced by most women.

Progestin-only treatment: Endometriosis lesions require estrogen to grow. An alternative to an estrogen–progestin contraceptive treatment is to treat the patient with "high doses" of a progestin as a single agent. High doses of progestins cause endometriosis lesions to stop growing both by a direct inhibitory action on the lesions and "indirectly" by suppressing luteinizing hormone (LH) and follicular stimulating hormone (FSH) secretion, resulting in a decrease in ovarian estrogen production. Suppression of ovarian estrogen production can result in amenorrhea and regression of endometriosis lesions. Progestin-only treatments can be associated with significant adverse side effects, including weight gain, daily breakthrough menstrual bleeding, and "blue" moods or depression. Typical regimens of progestin-only treatment are listed in **Table 33.2**.

In one clinical trial, 274 women with pelvic pain due endometriosis were randomized to receive either medroxyprogesterone depot 104 mg SC every 12 weeks or leuprolide acetate depot 11.25 mg IM every 12 weeks for 24 weeks of treatment. After completing hormone therapy, the women were followed up for 52 weeks. Both treatments were very effective in relieving pelvic pain. More subjects discontinued the medroxyprogesterone than the leuprolide therapy. During treatment, leuprolide resulted in more bone loss and more hot flushes. Medroxyprogesterone caused more breakthrough bleeding. Both treatments are very effective for the treatment of pelvic pain caused by endometriosis. Medroxyprogesterone acetate is significantly less expensive than leuprolide.

The progestin (levonorgestrel) releasing intrauterine device system has been demonstrated to be effective in relieving pelvic pain associated with endometriosis in small studies without a placebo control group.

Analogues of gonadotropin releasing hormone: Gonadotropin releasing hormone (GnRH) is a native hypothalamic decapeptide that is released in a pulsatile manner and stimulates the pituitary to secrete LH and FSH. In turn, LH and FSH cause ovarian follicle development, ovulation, and corpus luteum development. The estradiol secreted from the ovarian follicle and the estradiol and progesterone secreted from the corpus luteum cause endometrial growth. In the absence of an implanted embryo secreting human chorionic gonadotropin, the corpus luteum under-

Table 33.2 Progestins that are effective in the treatment of endometriosis when utilized as a single agent

Progestin	Dose
Norethindrone acetate	5 mg daily, orally
Medroxyprogesterone acetate	50 mg daily, orally
Medroxyprogesterone acetate	104 mg SC every 90 days
Norgestrel	0.075 mg daily, orally

goes involution and estradiol and progesterone secretion cease, causing the sloughing of the endometrium (menstruation). The entire menstrual system is controlled by the pulsatile release of hypothalamic GnRH.

Synthetic changes in the GnRH decapeptide can create agonist analogues with a long half-life. Paradoxically, the chronic administration of these analogues results in an initial stimulation of LH and FSH release, followed by a marked suppression of both LH and FSH secretion, resulting in amenorrhea. It is thought that the long half-life of the agonist analogues blocks the ability of the pituitary to recognize pulses of GnRH, resulting in a paradoxical "downregulation" and "desensitization" of pituitary gonadtrope function. The administration of agonist GnRH analogues (leuprolide, nafarelin, goserelin) reliably causes cessation of ovarian estrogen and progesterone production and amenorrhea (**Table 33.3**). In the opinion of this author, the GnRH analogues are the most effective and reliable treatment of pelvic pain caused by endometriosis. However, GnRH analogues are associated with many hypoestrogenic side effects including vasomotor symptoms, insomnia caused by hot flushes, vaginal dryness, and bone loss (osteopenia).

To try to prevent the hypoestrogenic side effects of the GnRH analogues, low-dose estrogen or high-dose progestin "add-back" have been used. The idea of add-back is that the GnRH analogue is used to treat the endometriosis, and the add-back is used to treat the side effects of the GnRH analogue. When used as a single agent, the GnRH analogues are approved by the Food and Drug Administration (FDA) for 6 months of treatment. When used with add-back, the GnRH analogues are approved for up to 12 months of treatment. Clinicians have reported using GnRH agonist plus add-back treatment for up to 10 years without significant complications. The commonly used GnRH analogues and add-back regimens are listed in **Table 33.4**.

For women with severe pain who have excellent relief of pain with a GnRH analogue, treatment for up to fiive years has been successful with few side effects. If treatment with GnRH analogues is planned to extend past 12 months, a bone mineral density measurement should be obtained to assess whether the patient has osteoporosis. In most women, when the GnRH analogue is discontinued, the bone density increases, returning to the normal range.

Danazol: Estrogens cause endometriosis lesions to grow. Androgens cause endometriosis lesions to regress. Danazol is an oral androgen approved by the FDA for the treatment of endometriosis at doses in the range of 200–800 mg daily. Doses as low as 50 mg daily may effectively relieve pelvic pain. Danazol treatment at doses of 200–800 mg daily typically results in amenorrhea, because it is an androgen that causes the native endometrium to regress. In addition, danazol blocks LH and FSH secretion, resulting in a decrease in ovarian secretion of estradiol. As an androgen, danazol is associated with weight gain, increased muscle mass, and deepening of the voice. Owing to these androgenic side effects, danazol is seldom prescribed in North America.

Aromatase Inhibitors: Endometriosis lesions require estrogen for growth. Some endometriosis lesions are capable of locally transforming androgen precursors into estrogen, thereby locally manufacturing their own steroid growth factor. Pilot studies indicate that aromatase inhibitors may be useful as an adjunctive agent in combination with another hormonal agent such as a GnRH analogue or an estrogen–progestin contraceptive. This use of the aromatase inhibitors is not FDA approved. Osteoporosis is a side effect associated with aromatase inhibitor treatment.

Table 33.3 Gonadotropin releasing hormone (GnRH) agonists approved for the treatment of endometriosis

GnRH agonist	Dose
Leuprolide acetate depot	3.75 mg IM every 4 weeks or 11.25 mg IM every 12 weeks
Goserelin acetate	3.6 mg SC implant every 4 weeks
Nafarelin	200 µg twice daily as a nasal spray

Table 33.4 Steroid hormone regimens that have been documented to be effective in the treatment of pelvic pain caused by endometriosis [a]

Hormone regimen	Comments	Reference
Transdermal estradiol patch 25 µg daily plus medroxyprogesterone acetate 2.5 mg daily	This regimen does not completely prevent bone loss. The estradiol concentration achieved is around 30 pg/mL	Howell 1995
Norethindrone acetate 5 mg daily	This high dose of progestin and may be associated with symptoms such as bloating and mood changes	Hornstein 1998
Conjugated equine estrogen 0.625 mg daily plus norethindrone 5 mg daily	This regimen preserves bone density and markedly reduces vasomotor symptoms	Hornstein 1998

[a] Gonadotropin releasing hormone (GnRH) agonist treatment combined with low-dose steroid "add-back" causes atrophy in endometriosis lesions, improves pelvic pain, and minimizes vasomotor symptoms and bone loss associated with the hypoestrogenism caused by the GnRH agonist.

Laparoscopic and definitive surgery: For the surgical removal of endometriosis implants, a laparoscopy is typically performed. Treatment of the implants may involve the use of electrosurgery or laser energy to destroy the implants, or surgical removal of the implants with scissors or scalpel (Harmonic scalpel). Randomized prospective studies have reported that surgical destruction of endometriosis implants in women with pelvic pain caused by endometriosis results in significantly superior pain relief than diagnostic surgery where no implants are destroyed (see Evidence Box 32.2)

Definitive surgery of endometriosis involves bilateral salpingo-oophorectomy and often hysterectomy. The removal of both ovaries results in a 95 % reduction in endogenous estrogen production (the remaining 5 % of estrogen production arises from aromatization of adrenal androgens in fat and muscle). The removal of 95 % of estradiol secretion reliably causes regression of the endometriosis lesions. Bilateral salpingo-oophorectomy results in sterility and is only an option for women who are sure that they have had all the children they desire. In addition, bilateral salpingo-oophorectomy usually results in severe menopausal symptoms, including hot flushes, insomnia, and bone loss. Luckily, most women can receive low-dose estrogen replacement, such as conjugated estrogens 0.625 mg daily, with no return of their endometriosis or pain symptoms.

Combined surgical and hormonal therapy: Randomized trials indicate that combining laparoscopic removal of endometriosis implants plus postoperative hormone therapy produces pain relief that is superior to surgery alone. Many women with disabling pelvic pain caused by endometriosis will receive a combination of surgical and hormonal treatment.

Presacral neurectomy: Transection of the nerves between the pelvis and sacrum may reduce the perception of pelvic pain in some women. In one clinical trial, 71 women with moderate-to-severe endometriosis and functionally significant midline pelvic pain were randomized to treatment with resection of endometriosis lesions with or without a presacral neurectomy. The addition of a presacral neurectomy to resection of endometriosis lesions resulted in a decrease in midline pelvic pain, but no improvement on dysmenorrhea or overall pelvic pain scores. Side effects of the presacral neurectomy included the development of constipation and urinary urgency.

Presacral neurectomy should be reserved for women who have not had improvement of their pain with hormonal or other surgical procedures.

Menopause: From a biological perspective, menopause occurs when all the functional follicles in the ovary have been depleted. At menopause, estradiol secretion decreases by 95 %. Menopause is usually associated with complete regression of endometriosis lesions and resolution of pain symptoms. In a small number of women with endometriosis, treatment with estrogen hormone replacement therapy after the onset of menopause may cause a recurrence of the endometriosis lesions and pelvic pain. However, the vast majority of women with a history of endometriosis can receive low-dose estrogen hormone therapy for the treatment of menopausal symptoms without having a recurrence of endometriosis.

Adenomyosis

Definition

Adenomyosis is the presence of endometrial glands and stroma in the myometrium. It is often associated with myometrial hypertrophy. There are no accepted noninvasive techniques for diagnosing adenomyosis. The diagnosis is typically made on pathological analysis of hysterectomy specimens. Consequently, it is difficult to precisely define the prevalence and epidemiology of this disease.

Etiology and Epidemiology

The cause of adenomyosis is unknown. The most commonly cited hypothesis is that the baso-endometrium invades the myometrium to give rise to foci of endometrial glands and stroma in the myometrium. Factors that may increase the risk of endometrial invasion of the myometrium include chronically increased intrauterine pressure and uterine trauma, for example, at the time of delivery or surgical curettage. Most women diagnosed with adenomyosis (which requires removal of the uterus) are aged between 35 and 50 years. Uterine myomata coexist in about 50 % of cases of adenomyosis.

History and Physical Examination

The clinical diagnosis of adenomyosis should be suspected if the triad of menorrhagia, dysmenorrhea, and a slightly enlarged, "boggy" uterus is present on bimanual examination. On physical examination, most adenomyotic uteri are similar in size to a gravid uterus between 8 and 12 weeks of pregnancy.

Diagnosis

Adenomyosis is only a pathological diagnosis. It is defined as the presence of endometrial glands and stroma in the myometrium 2–3 mm below the endomyometrial junction. The pathological diagnosis of adenomyosis is highly dependent on the histological sections processed from the uterine specimen. For example, in one study of 200 consecutive hysterectomy specimens, the diagnosis of adenomyosis was made in 31% of the cases if three sections were analyzed, and in 62% of the cases if six sections were analyzed. Autopsy studies report that about 50% of women of reproductive age have adenomyosis. Most adenomyotic uteri weigh between 100 and 200 g (normal uterus weighs about 80 g).

The **differential diagnosis** of adenomyosis includes endometriosis and uterine myoma.

Attempts have been made to develop imaging tests that can identify adenomyosis. Transvaginal ultrasound can be used to look at the endometrial–myometrial junction and to attempt to identify heterogeneity in the myometrium, asymmetric thickening of the myometrium, and myometrial cysts, all consistent with adenomyosis. However, the sensitivity and specificity of ultrasound for the detection of adenomyosis are about 68% and 65%, respectively. For a disease with high prevalence, this sensitivity and specificity of transvaginal ultrasound are too low for it to be used as a definitive test. Magnetic resonance imaging (MRI) of the uterus is the most useful imaging test and has a sensitivity of 70% and specificity of 86%. T2-weighted MRI sequences are helpful in differentiating adenomyosis and uterine myomata. A junction zone greater than 12 mm on MRI suggests the presence of adenomyosis. Attempts have been made to develop hysteroscopic biopsy techniques to diagnosis adenomyosis. These methods tend to have high specificity but low sensitivity. Because the disease is so "patchy," it is easy to miss on a nondirected biopsy.

Treatment

Hysterectomy is the most commonly used treatment of adenomyosis. Some pilot studies suggest that hormonal treatments that are effective for uterine myoma are also effective for adenomyosis (see Chapter 49, Uterine Leiomyomas). For example, GnRH analogues have been reported to improve the menorrhagia and dysmenorrhea associated with adenomyosis. In pilot studies, uterine artery embolization may be effective for the treatment of the menorrhagia and pelvic pain caused by adenomyosis.

Key Points

- Endometriosis is the presence of endometrial glands and/or stroma outside of the uterus. Women with endometriosis typically present for medical care with one of the following problems: 1) pelvic pain, 2) infertility, or 3) a complex adnexal mass.
- Approximately 5% of women between the ages of 15 and 45 years have endometriosis. The peak incidence is between 20 and 30 years of age. This differs from uterine leiomyomas which have a peak incidence between 35 and 45 years of age.
- Endometriosis lesions are stimulated to grow by physiological concentrations of estradiol. In a severely hypoestrogenic state, endometriosis lesions undergo atrophy.
- The diagnosis of endometriosis is made by direct surgical visualization of lesions, usually at the time of laparoscopy.
- Pelvic pain caused by endometriosis can be treated with surgical resection of lesions or by hormonal therapy including the suppression of ovarian estrogen production.
- Adenomyosis is the presence of endometrial glands and stoma in the wall of the myometrium. Women with adenomyosis often report pelvic pain and heavy menses. The diagnosis of adenomyosis is often suspected clinically but is definitively made only after histological analysis of a hysterectomy specimen.

Evidence Box 33.1

Laparoscopic surgical removal of endometriosis implants appears to improve fertility in infertile women with early-stage endometriosis.

A total of 341 women with infertility and early stage (stages I and II) endometriosis were randomly assigned to a diagnostic laparoscopy combined with surgical excision or ablation of endometriosis lesions or a diagnostic laparoscopy only. During 36 weeks of postoperative follow-up, 31% of the women in the active treatment group and 18% of the women in the diagnostic laparoscopy only group became pregnant (*P* = 0.006). There was a significantly higher calculated monthly pregnancy rate in the active treatment group: 4.7% versus 2.4% per cycle pregnancy rate. Pregnancy losses occurred in approximately 20% of women who became pregnant, with no difference between the groups. This study indicates that laparoscopic surgical removal of endometriosis implants appears to improve fertility in infertile women with early-stage endometriosis. This study also suggests that there is a cause–effect relationship between early stage endometriosis and infertility.

From a clinical perspective it should be noted that treatment of these same couples with *one cycle of in vitro fertilization* could be expected to be associated with a pregnancy rate in the range of 35–45%.

Marcoux S, Maheux R, Berube S. Laparoscopic surgery in infertile women with minimal or mild endometriosis. Canadian Collaborative Group on Endometriosis. N Engl J Med 1997;337:217–222.

Evidence Box 33.2

Laproscopy and surgical excision of endometriosis lesions reduces pelvic pain in the majority of female patients, but some report no pain relief of their symptoms.

Fifty-one women with pelvic pain were randomized to have a laparoscopy with no treatment interventions (diagnostic-only) or a laparoscopy with surgical excision of endometriosis lesions. Thirteen women were excluded from the study because three became pregnant, three withdrew their consent, and seven did not have endometriosis at the time of surgery (three had pelvic inflammatory disease, one had endosalpingiosis, and three had no detected pathology). Of the remaining 39 women, 19 had the diagnostic-only procedure and 20 had the diagnosis plus excision of implants procedure. Six months after the procedure, improvement in pain was reported by 80% of the women in the group with excision of endometriosis lesions and 30% of the group that had only diagnostic laparoscopy ($P = 0.002$). Of interest is that the diagnostic procedure did appear to have a moderate "placebo" effect, with 30% of the group reporting improvement in pain. A clinically important finding is that 20% of the women who had excision of their endometriosis lesions did not have improvement in their pain symptoms. This is an important fact to relate to patients with pelvic pain considering laparoscopic surgery. The women in the diagnostic-only group had a follow-up laparoscopy 6 months after their initial surgery. Of note, 45% of the women had worsening of their endometriosis during the 6-month interval.

Abbott J, Hawe J, Hunter D, Holmes M, Finn P, Garry R. Laparoscopic excision of endometriosis: a randomized, placebo-controlled trail. Fertil Steril 2004;82:878–884.

Further Reading

Abbott J, Hawe J, Hunter D, Holmes M, Finn P, Garry R. Laparoscopic excision of endometriosis: a randomized, placebo-controlled trial. *Fertil Steril* 2004;82(4):878–884

American Fertility Society. Revised American Fertility Society classification of endometriosis: 1985. *Fertil Steril* 1985;43(3):351–352

Attar E, Bulun SE. Aromatase inhibitors: the next generation of therapeutics for endometriosis? *Fertil Steril* 2006;85(5):1307–1318

Barbieri RL, Niloff JM, Bast RC Jr, Scaetzl E, Kistner RW, Knapp RC. Elevated serum concentrations of CA-125 in patients with advanced endometriosis. *Fertil Steril* 1986;45(5):630–634

Barbieri RL. Stenosis of the external cervical os: an association with endometriosis in women with chronic pelvic pain. *Fertil Steril* 1998;70(3):571–573

Candiani GB, Fedele L, Vercellini P, Bianchi S, Di Nola G. Presacral neurectomy for the treatment of pelvic pain associated with endometriosis: a controlled study. *Am J Obstet Gynecol* 1992;167(1):100–103

Hornstein MD, Hemmings R, Yuzpe AA, Heinrichs WL. Use of nafarelin versus placebo after reductive laparoscopic surgery for endometriosis. *Fertil Steril* 1997;68(5):860–864

Hornstein MD, Surrey ES, Weisberg GW, Casino LA; Lupron Add-Back Study Group. Leuprolide acetate depot and hormonal add-back in endometriosis: a 12-month study. *Obstet Gynecol* 1998;91(1):16–24

Howell R, Edmonds DK, Dowsett M, et al. Gonadotropin releasing hormone analogue plus hormone replacement therapy for the treatment of endometriosis: A randomized trial. *Fertil Steril* 1995; 64: 474–81.

Kitamura Y, Allison SJ, Jha RC, Spies JB, Flick PA, Ascher SM. MRI of adenomyosis: changes with uterine artery embolization. *AJR Am J Roentgenol* 2006;186(3):855–864

Marcoux S, Maheux R, Bérubé S; Canadian Collaborative Group on Endometriosis. Laparoscopic surgery in infertile women with minimal or mild endometriosis. *N Engl J Med* 1997;337(4):217–222

Missmer SA, Hankinson SE, Spiegelman D, et al. Reproductive history and endometriosis among premenopausal women. *Obstet Gynecol* 2004;104(5 Pt 1):965–974

Missmer SA, Hankinson SE, Spiegelman D, Barbieri RL, Marshall LM, Hunter DJ. Incidence of laparoscopically confirmed endometriosis by demographic, anthropometric, and lifestyle factors. *Am J Epidemiol* 2004;160(8):784–796

Propst AM, Storti K, Barbieri RL. Lateral cervical displacement is associated with endometriosis. *Fertil Steril* 1998;70(3):568–570

Schlaff WD, Carson SA, Luciano A, Ross D, Bergqvist A. Subcutaneous injection of depot medroxyprogesterone acetate compared with leuprolide acetate in the treatment of endometriosis-associated pain. *Fertil Steril* 2006;85(2):314–325

Sutton CJ, Ewen SP, Whitelaw N, Haines P. Prospective, randomized, double-blind, controlled trial of laser laparoscopy in the treatment of pelvic pain associated with minimal, mild, and moderate endometriosis. *Fertil Steril* 1994;62(4):696–700

34 Chronic Pelvic Pain

Robert L. Barbieri

Definition

Chronic pelvic pain refers to menstrual or nonmenstrual pain of at least 6 months duration occurring below the umbilicus. Common gynecologic symptoms associated with chronic pelvic pain include dysmenorrhea (pain with menses), dyspareunia (pain with sexual intercourse), dyschezia (pain associated with bowel movements), and pain not associated with menses or intercourse. Vulvar and vaginal introitus pain occasionally occurs in combination with pelvic pain. Chronic pelvic pain is commonly associated with bladder and bowel symptoms including frequent and/or painful urination, diarrhea, constipation, and bloating.

Diagnosis

Chronic pelvic pain is a symptom, not a specific disease diagnosis. Chronic pelvic pain may be caused by gynecologic causes such as pelvic inflammatory disease, endometriosis, adenomyosis and uterine fibroids (**Table 34.1**). Nongynecologic causes of chronic pelvic pain include irritable bowel syndrome, bladder pain syndrome (interstitial cystitis), diverticulitis, and fibromyalgia. Mental health issues such as depression, anxiety, somatization, narcotic dependency, and a history of physical, psychological, or sexual abuse may contribute to the onset and severity of chronic pelvic pain. The gynecologic causes of chronic pelvic pain are reviewed in their individual chapters. The most common nongynecologic causes of chronic pelvic pain are reviewed below.

Table 34.1 Causes of chronic pelvic pain

Gynecologic causes	Endometriosis
	Pelvic inflammatory disease and adhesions
	Adenomyosis
	Fibroids (leiomyoma)
	Ovarian cancer
	Primary and secondary dysmenorrhea
Urinary tract causes	Interstitial cystitis/painful bladder syndrome
	Chronic urethral syndrome
	Bladder neoplasia
Gastrointestinal causes	Irritable bowel syndrome
	Inflammatory bowel disease
	Diverticular colitis
	Colon cancer
	Chronic intestinal pseudo-obstruction
	Constipation
	Celiac disease
Musculoskeletal causes	Fibromyalgia
	Pelvic floor muscle spasm
Mental health issues related to chronic pain	Substance abuse
	Sexual and physical abuse
	Depression and anxiety
	Somatization

Irritable Bowel Syndrome

A diagnosis of irritable bowel syndrome is likely in patients who have abdominal or pelvic pain with two or more associated symptoms such as: pain relieved by defecation; pain associated with looser or more frequent stools; abdominal distention; mucus in the stool; or feeling of incomplete evacuation. About 35% of women with chronic pelvic pain also have irritable bowel syndrome.

Bladder Pain Syndrome (Interstitial Cystitis)

This syndrome is characterized by bladder pain of variable severity that persists over a prolonged period. It is diagnosed by the presence of chronic pain related to the urinary bladder accompanied by at least one additional urinary symptom such as daytime and nighttime urinary frequency, with exclusion of other causes such as urinary tract infection.

Musculoskeletal Causes

Fibromyalgia is a chronic pain condition that presents with diffuse musculoskeletal pain. Excessive tenderness in 11 or more of 18 musculoskeletal areas is considered diagnostic. Myofascial pain syndromes are a musculoskeletal cause of chronic pain that is confined to one anatomical region. Palpation of a trigger point produces a characteristic and reproducible pain pattern. About 15% of women with chronic pelvic pain meet the criteria for myofascial pain syndrome.

Prevalence and Epidemiology

In a survey of the medical records of 284000 female patients, from 12 to 70 years of age in the United Kingdom, 3.8% had a diagnosis of chronic pelvic pain. Chronic pelvic pain accounts for about 10% of all referrals to gynecologists, 15% of all hysterectomy procedures, and 40% of gynecological laparoscopy procedures.

Three common symptoms associated with chronic pelvic pain are dysmenorrhea, dyspareunia, and noncyclic pelvic pain. In a systematic review of 121 epidemiologic studies of chronic pelvic pain the following risk factors were identified for each of these symptoms. For noncyclic pelvic pain, the main risk factors were heavy menses, evidence of pelvic pathology, drug or alcohol abuse, pel-

vic inflammatory disease, a history of sexual abuse, psychologic comorbidity, and a history of prior cesarean delivery. For dyspareunia, the main risk factors were hypoestrogenism, pelvic inflammatory disease, sexual abuse, and a history of anxiety or depression. For dysmenorrhea, the main risk factors were early menarche, heavy and frequent menses, a history of cigarette smoking, premenstrual syndrome, sexual abuse, and anxiety or depression. Dysmenorrhea was reported less frequently by women who exercised and used oral contraceptives.

Etiology

The central nervous system perception of chronic pelvic pain often arises from both nociceptive and neuropathic pain pathways. Nociceptive pain is the pain caused by direct tissue damage and inflammation. Nociceptive pain can be somatic or visceral. Somatic pain is well localized and variable in description: sharp, crushing, etc. Visceral pain is poorly localized and often deep, dull and cramping. Women with chronic pelvic pain often have both somatic and visceral components to their symptoms.

Neuropathic pain arises from abnormal neural activity that originally was caused by a disease or injury, but it persists regardless of the disease activity. Central neuropathic pain is caused by abnormal nervous system activation in the absence of an active disease stimulus such as that observed with phantom limb pain or poststroke pain. Nonsympathetic neuropathic pain is due to damage to a peripheral nerve without autonomic changes, such as seen with post-herpetic neuralgia. Neuropathic pain often contributes to the chronic pelvic pain syndrome. Chronic pelvic pain can often be best treated by multimodal therapy that impacts both nociceptive and neuropathic causes of pain.

History

An effective approach to the woman with chronic pelvic pain is characterized by an empathic clinical attitude that explicitly recognizes the patient's pain symptoms and the adverse effect they have on the patient's life and functional level. Direct or indirect comments that suggest "the pain is in your head" undermine the patient's trust in the clinician and reduces the effectiveness of treatment. Patients with chronic pelvic pain want to be: 1) understood and taken seriously; 2) have an individualized approach to their problem; 3) receive a clear explanation of what is causing their problem; and 4) be given reassurance that treatment may help to relieve their symptoms.

The history is the most important step in the evaluation of a woman with chronic pelvic pain. A template for obtaining a thorough history and physical examination for women with pelvic pain is available at the International Pelvic Pain Society website (www.pelvicpain.org). Many authorities recommend using a written questionnaire for obtaining a systematic history in these patients. The history should focus on the characteristics and severity of the pain (**Fig. 34.1**) and symptoms related to the following systems: gynecologic, gastrointestinal, urinary tract, musculoskeletal, psychological, neurologic, and prior tests and treatments. It is important to assess the patient for comorbid mental health disease such as depression, anxiety, and a history of sexual or physical abuse.

Physical Examination and Laboratory Studies

Authorities in the field of chronic pelvic pain recommend a comprehensive physical exam with specific components of the exam performed in the standing, supine, and lithotomy positions. The standing position is especially useful to identify hernias and postural abnormalities. In the supine position, maneuvers such as active leg flexion and obturator and psoas sign testing may be performed. The supine position is also useful for examining the abdomen, symphysis, and inguinal areas. The classical lithotomy position is used for the gynecologic examination. Many experts use a single-finger pelvic exam to try to identify specific areas of tenderness along the pelvic floor muscles such as the levator ani, piriformis, and obturator muscles.

Carnett's test is used to assess abdominal wall and myofascial tenderness during muscle contraction. In the supine position, the patient tenses her abdominal muscles by raising her head or by raising both legs off the table. At the same time an examining finger is kept on the previously identified painful abdominal wall site. If the pain increases during the tensing of abdominal wall muscles, it may have a myofascial or abdominal wall component. If the pain is unchanged or decreases, it is not likely due to an abdominal wall component.

Standard laboratory testing for chronic pelvic pain includes: 1) a complete blood count with differential and erythrocyte sedimentation rate or C-reactive protein assay to look for chronic inflammation or infection; 2) a urinalysis to look for infection or inflammation; 3) testing for chlamydial and gonorrheal infections; and 4) pelvic ultrasound imaging to look for ovarian cysts, hydrosalpinges or uterine abnormalities that could not be detected on physical examination. In a select subset of patients with chronic pelvic pain, laparoscopy may be helpful to assess for the presence of endometriosis, pelvic adhesions, and pelvic inflammatory disease.

Treatment

If a disease has been identified as causing the pain syndrome, treatment of the disease is the optimal approach. Treatments of the following diseases are discussed in other chapters: endometriosis and adenomyosis (Chapter 33), uterine fibroids (Chapter 50), vulvar and vaginal pain

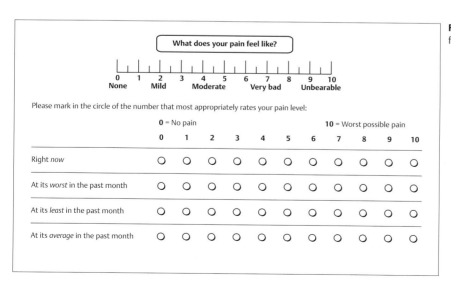

Fig. 34.1 An example of a pain scale for gauging chronic pelvic pain.

(Chapter 30), chronic pelvic inflammatory disease (Chapters 36 and 37).

Gabapentin and Amitriptyline

Treatment focused on neuropathic pain pathways may be helpful for the treatment of chronic pelvic pain. Gabapentin and amitriptyline are two medications commonly used to treat neuropathic pain conditions. In one clinical trial, 56 women with chronic pelvic pain were randomized to treatment with gabapentin (maximum dose 3600 mg daily) or amitriptyline (maximum dose 150 mg daily) or both. All three treatments resulted in improvement in pain symptoms. Gabapentin was slightly superior to amitriptyline. Combination therapy was not better than gabapentin alone. Amitriptyline therapy is much less expensive than gabapentin therapy, but is associated with more side effects such as drowsiness. Amitriptyline in doses as low as 10 mg nightly may be a helpful adjuvant in the treatment of pelvic pain.

Hysterectomy

There are no randomized clinical trials evaluating the effectiveness of hysterectomy versus other approaches in the treatment of chronic pelvic pain. Large prospective cohort studies have reported that most women undergoing hysterectomy for chronic pelvic pain have significant improvement in their pain symptoms and quality of life after hysterectomy (Evidence Box 34.1)

Pelvic Nerve Transection Procedures

Transection of the nerves in the uterosacral ligaments reduces chronic pain manifesting as dysmenorrhea, but does not reliably improve other chronic pelvic pain symptoms. Dysmenorrhea is usually very responsive to medical treatment. Therefore, the use of uterosacral nerve transection in the management of pelvic pain has a very limited role. Presacral neurectomy is an extensive surgical procedure that results in the transection of the superior hypogastric nerve plexus, which is on the anterior surface of the sacrum. It is typically reserved for women who have not responded to standard medical and surgical procedures, and who have predominantly midline, infra-umbilical pain. In women with chronic pelvic pain due to endometriosis, the combination of presacral neurectomy plus resection of endometriosis lesions has been reported to result in more pain relief than resection of endometriosis lesions alone. Major complications following presacral

neurectomy include constipation and urinary urgency, occurring in 5–20% of patients.

Interdisciplinary Pain Practice

Interdisciplinary pain practices are an important resource in the management of chronic pelvic pain. These practices commonly provide the following services: comprehensive history and physical examination; psychological assessment and counseling; behavioral and relaxation feedback therapies; acupuncture; transcutaneous electric nerve stimulation; and implantable nerve stimulation units. Clinicians in pain practices often try to guide patients to reduce their use of narcotic pain medications because of the problems of tolerance and dependence on opioids.

Key Points

- Chronic pelvic pain (CPP) refers to menstrual or nonmenstrual pain of at least 6 months duration occurring below the umbilicus. It is a symptom associated with many different diseases.
- Gynecologic causes of CPP include pelvic inflammatory disease, endometriosis, adenomyosis, and uterine leiomyomas. Nongynecologic causes of CPP include irritable bowel syndrome, bladder pain syndrome (also known as interstitial cystitis), diverticulitis, and fibromyalgia. Mental health issues such as depression, anxiety, somatization, narcotic dependency, and a history of sexual assault or abuse may contribute to the symptoms.
- About 4% of women report symptoms consistent with CPP.
- Treatment of CPP may be improved by involvement of a multispecialty pain practice that combines medical, surgical, and mental health treatment.

Evidence Box 34.1

Hysterectomy is effective for the treatment of chronic pelvic pain.
There are no randomized trials comparing hysterectomy to other treatment modalities for women with chronic pelvic pain. However, prospective studies of large cohorts of women have reported that hysterectomy is effective for the treatment of chronic pelvic pain. In one study, approximately 400 women undergoing a hysterectomy with a history of pelvic pain were followed postoperatively for 24 months. The women were approximately 41 years old, 68% were Caucasian and 31% Black, and approximately 50% were college graduates. Following hysterectomy there was a reduction in the reported pain symptoms and an improvement in activity level and social functioning. Prior to surgery approximately 95% of the women reported that their pelvic pain was a "big problem" or a "medium problem." At 24 months after surgery approximately 15% of the women reported that their pelvic pain was a "big problem" or a

"medium problem." Prior to surgery approximately 50% of the women reported pain during sex, whereas 24 months after surgery approximately 10% of the women reported pain during sex.

Hartmann KE, Ma C, Lamvu GM, Langenberg PW, Steege JF, Kjerulff KH. Quality of life and sexual function after hysterectomy in women with preoperative pain and depression. Obstet Gynecol 2004;104:701–709.

Further Reading

Carlson KJ, Miller BA, Fowler FJ Jr. The Maine Women's Health Study: I. Outcomes of hysterectomy. *Obstet Gynecol* 1994;83(4):556–565

Carnett JB. Intercostal neuralgia as a cause of abdominal pain and tenderness. *Surg Gynecol Obstet* 1926;42:625–632

Hartmann KE, Ma C, Lamvu GM, Langenberg PW, Steege JF, Kjerulff KH. Quality of life and sexual function after hysterectomy in women with preoperative pain and depression. *Obstet Gynecol* 2004;104(4):701–709

Johnson NP, Farquhar CM, Crossley S, et al. A double-blind randomised controlled trial of laparoscopic uterine nerve ablation for women with chronic pelvic pain. *BJOG* 2004;111(9):950–959

Latthe PL, Mignini L, Gray R, Hills R, Khan K. Factors predisposing women to chronic pelvic pain: systematic review. *BMJ* 2006;332(7544):749–755

Price J, Farmer G, Harris J, Hope T, Kennedy S, Mayou R. Attitudes of women with chronic pelvic pain to the gynaecological consultation: a qualitative study. *BJOG* 2006;113(4):446–452

Sator-Katzenschlager SM, Scharbert G, Kress HG, et al. Chronic pelvic pain treated with gabapentin and amitriptyline: a randomized controlled pilot study. *Wien Klin Wochenschr* 2005;117(21-22):761–768

Williams RE, Hartmann KE, Sandler RS, Miller WC, Savitz LA, Steege JF. Recognition and treatment of irritable bowel syndrome among women with chronic pelvic pain. *Am J Obstet Gynecol* 2005;192(3):761–767

Zondervan KT, Yudkin PL, Vessey MP, Dawes MG, Barlow DH, Kennedy SH. Prevalence and incidence of chronic pelvic pain in primary care: evidence from a national general practice database. *Br J Obstet Gynaecol* 1999;106(11):1149–1155

Zullo F, Palomba S, Zupi E, et al. Effectiveness of presacral neurectomy in women with severe dysmenorrhea caused by endometriosis who were treated with laparoscopic conservative surgery: a 1-year prospective randomized double-blind controlled trial. *Am J Obstet Gynecol* 2003;189(1):5–10

35 Pelvic Relaxation, Urinary Incontinence, and Urinary Tract Infection

Jon I. Einarsson

Pelvic Relaxation

Incidence

Pelvic relaxation or pelvic organ prolapse is a common condition, with a recent study finding the prevalence of stage 2 and greater pelvic organ prolapse to be 37% in a population of 1004 women seeking care at a gynecologic clinic. While some of these women are asymptomatic, genital prolapse remains one of the most common reasons for gynecologic surgery in women after the fertile period.

Subtypes and Anatomy

Pelvic organ prolapse is often divided into three main subtypes, depending on where the prolapse is located (**Fig. 35.1**). In anterior prolapse (cystocele), the urinary bladder protrudes into the vagina. In posterior prolapse (rectocele), the rectum and/or the rectosigmoid protrudes into the vagina. Apical prolapse occurs when the cervix or the vaginal apex (following a hysterectomy) falls down through the vagina. Anterior and posterior prolapse are usually defects in the endopelvic fascia, which is a thick layer of connective tissue in the vagina, that is, the muscularis layer of the vaginal wall. This connective tissue can become detached from the normal attachments to the pelvic sidewall and/or become weakened or torn during childbirth or through wear and tear such as with chronic cough or constipation. Apical prolapse is more commonly associated with detachment or tearing of the uterosacral ligaments and the cardinal ligaments that connect to the pericervical ring to maintain the vaginal apex in a normal anatomic position.

Symptoms

Pelvic organ prolapse causes pelvic pressure, pain, painful intercourse and significantly impacts the quality of life of those who suffer from it. A cystocele can cause frequent urination or urinary retention, and a rectocele can cause difficulty in emptying the rectum during bowel movements.

Etiology

Several etiologic factors that contribute to pelvic organ prolapse have been identified such as higher age, increased parity, obesity, and heritability.Recent evidence also suggests that women with pelvic organ prolapse have smaller amounts of collagen in the fibrous connective tissue of the endopelvic fascia.

Diagnosis

Diagnosis is made during a detailed pelvic exam. It is important to distinguish between prolapse in different vaginal compartments, since surgical treatment varies. A standardized system to evaluate and report pelvic organ prolapse, called the POP-Q system, is widely used in research and clinical practice. Some consider this to be too complex and prefer a simpler system, such as the Baden–Walken halfway system. In this system, 1st degree prolapse extends halfway to the introitus, 2nd degree prolapse extends to the introitus, 3rd degree prolapse extends halfway outside the introitus and 4th degree prolapse means that there is complete eversion of the pelvic organs (procidentia).

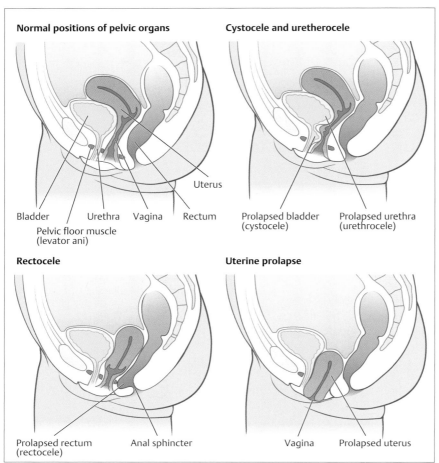

Normal positions of pelvic organs

Uterus

Bladder   Urethra   Vagina   Rectum
Pelvic floor muscle
(levator ani)

Cystocele and uretherocele

Prolapsed bladder   Prolapsed urethra
(cystocele)   (urethrocele)

Rectocele

Prolapsed rectum   Anal sphincter
(rectocele)

Uterine prolapse

Vagina   Prolapsed uterus

Fig. 35.1 Anatomy of the most common types of pelvic organ prolapse.

Treatment

It is important to point out that asymptomatic pelvic organ prolapse usually does not require any therapy. Since conservative measures such as Kegel exercises or physical therapy do not seem to be effective, the main therapeutic option for symptomatic pelvic organ prolapse is reconstructive surgery, where defects in the endopelvic fascia are identified and repaired. While these surgical therapies can be effective, relapse rates of up to 50–60% have been reported. In order to reduce relapse rates, synthetic polypropylene mesh has been used to improve long-term success. While effective, synthetic mesh is costly and can cause erosions and, rarely, pelvic infections. The anterior and posterior compartment are usually repaired by re-approximating the endopelvic fascia with or without a mesh overlay. The "gold standard" treatment for apical prolapse is abdominal sacrocolpopexy with mesh (**Fig. 35.2**). Less invasive vaginal approaches such as the sacrospinous ligament fixation are especially applicable to older or less active patients. Recently, laparoscopic apical repairs have become more commonplace, thereby combining long-term durability and low morbidity.

These are especially applicable to younger active women, since sacrocolpopexy is associated with a lower rate of dyspareunia than the vaginal repairs.

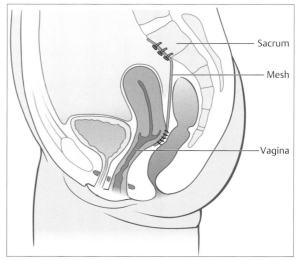

Sacrum

Mesh

Vagina

Fig. 35.2 Sacrocolpopexy involves attaching the vaginal apex to the promontory of the sacrum.

Urinary Incontinence

Incidence and Subtypes

Urinary incontinence, or involuntary leakage of urine, affects about 25% of premenopausal women and 40% of postmenopausal women.

The two most common types of urinary incontinence are stress incontinence and urge incontinence. Women who leak urine during coughing, sneezing, laughing, or lifting are considered to have stress urinary incontinence, and women who leak urine immediately following a strong urge to urinate have urge incontinence. Urge incontinence is also associated with frequent urination (more than 12 times during the day) and nocturia (urinating more than once at night). Some women have mixed urinary incontinence, with components of both stress and urge incontinence.

Overflow incontinence is a rare type of urinary incontinence, where women do not have normal bladder sensation or are unable to adequately empty the bladder. This leads to frequent urination, urinary leakage, and frequent urinary tract infections because urine stays in the urinary bladder at all times.

Pathogenesis

If the urethral sphincter is weak, this can result in a subtype of stress urinary incontinence called intrinsic sphincter deficiency. The more common type is caused by too much mobility of the urethra (urethral hypermobility). The urethra is supported by connective tissue that can be weakened during childbirth, due to genetic defects in collagen or other connective tissue building blocks, or due to chronic cough or constipation. When the support of the urethra is weak or soft, the urethra sinks into the weakened connective tissue with increased intra-abdominal pressure, such as during cough or exercise. The pressure inside the bladder then becomes more than the pressure in the urethra leading to leakage of urine. This is similar to trying to stop a flow of water through a rubber hose by stepping on it. If the rubber hose is lying on soft grass, it is difficult to stop the flow of water by stepping on the hose, since the hose sinks into the grass and mud beneath it. However, if the hose is sitting on a hard surface, such as a sidewalk, it is much easier to stop the flow of water.

The causes of urge incontinence are more complex and often no specific cause is found. The most common cause is overactivity of the detrusor muscle of the bladder. The detrusor muscle is designed to be relaxed during bladder filling and only contract during bladder emptying. However, for a variety of reasons that are not fully understood, the bladder muscle sometimes becomes overactive, which leads to a strong urge to urinate. If the muscle contractions are very strong, this can lead to a sudden leakage of urine. Sometimes triggers can cause this, such as the sound of running water, but this may be completely unprovoked. The contractions of the bladder muscle are controlled by the autonomic nervous system. Therefore, women who have sustained an injury to the spine or have neurologic disorders such as multiple sclerosis and diabetes often have symptoms of urge incontinence.

Diagnosis

A detailed history is the first step in diagnosing urinary incontinence, inquiring about duration of symptoms, medications, fluid intake, when the leaking occurs and how much this affects quality of life. A urinary diary can be helpful both for the patient and the physician. The patient notes freqency and amount of urination as well as frequency and amount of fluid intake. She will also be asked to note any urine leakage, if there was a strong sense of urgency prior to the leak and what she was doing when it happened. A simple, validated three-item questionnaire can also be useful to discern between urge and stress incontinence in clinical practice (**Fig. 35.3**).

Simple urodynamics can be performed in the doctor's office with minimal equipment. The patient first produces a urine sample to check for an infection. The post-void residual can then be measured by using ultrasonography or by inserting a narrow catheter into the bladder. Normally, the bladder should empty completely during urination, but a post-void residual greater than 100 mL is generally considered abnormal.

Next, the bladder is filled with water through the catheter to determine whether the bladder distends normally. Most women will feel that their bladder is filling with urine at 100–150 mL. When the bladder is filled up to about 300 mL, most women would go to the bathroom if socially convenient. The maximum capacity of the bladder is normally about 400–450 mL, which is associated with an extreme urgency. If the bladder starts to contract during the filling process, this is an indication of an overactive detrusor muscle. After filling the bladder with about 300 mL the catheter is removed and the patient is asked to stand up and cough or jump to see if there is any leakage, which would indicate a diagnosis of stress incontinence.

A more sophisticated way to measure the function of the urinary bladder is with so called multichannel urodynamics. During this test, narrow catheters are placed into the bladder and the vagina. Additionally, small electrodes are placed on the inner thigh to measure the contractions of the pelvic muscles. The bladder is slowly filled with water, but here the amount of water is more accurately measured and the results are automatically drawn on a strip of

1. During the past 3 months, have you leaked urine (even a small amount)?

☐ Yes   ☐ No
                  │
                  ▼
          Questionnaire completed

2. During the past 3 months, did you leak urine (check all that apply):

☐ a. When you were performing some physical activity, such as coughing, sneezing , lifting, or exercise?

☐ b. When you had the urge or feeling that you needed to empty your bladder, but you could not get to the toilet fast enough?

☐ c. Without physical activity and without a sense of urgency?

3. During the past 3 months, did you leak urine most often (check only one):

☐ a. When you were performing some physical activity. such as coughing, sneezing , lifting, or exercise?

☐ b. When you had the urge or feeling that you needed to empty your bladder, but you could not get to the toilet fast enough?

☐ c. Without physical activity and without a sense of urgency?

☐ d. About equally as often with physical activity as with sense of urgency?

Definitions of types of urinary incontinence are based on responses to question 3:

Response to question 3	Type of incontinence
a. Most often with physical activity	a. Stress-only or stress-predominant
b. Most often with the urge to empty the bladder	b. Urge-only or urge-predominant
c. Without physical activity or sense of urgency	c. Other-cause-only or other-cause-predominant
d. About equally with physical activity and sense of urgency	d. Mixed

Fig. 35.3 The simple 3-IQ questionnaire to distinguish between stress and urge urinary incontinence.

paper or fed into a computer. The vaginal pressure is approximately the same as inside the abdomen and is used as a point of reference. For example, when the patient moves, the pressor sensor in the bladder may indicate increased activity in the bladder; however, since the same measurement is shown from the vagina, the investigators know that this was not a real change in bladder pressure. In fact, the computer automatically deducts the abdominal pressure from the bladder pressure to give a measurement of true bladder pressure. Multichannel urodynamics are used to diagnose stress, urge, and overflow incontinence. Unfortunately, 50% of women with urge incontinence will have a normal urodynamic test. This is because stress and unfamiliar surroundings can strongly influence bladder function. About 20% of women with stress incontinence will not leak during the test for the same reason.

Cystoscopy may be indicated to examine the bladder and urethra, especially with concurrent symptoms of bladder pain or hematuria. The cystoscope is similar to the hysteroscope and consists of a long narrow lens with an attached camera and light source. Cystoscopy can be performed easily in the office with minimum discomfort. The cystoscope is gently advanced through the urethra and into the bladder. Water is used to distend the bladder to allow for a complete and thorough examination. The ureteral openings can be clearly seen and the bladder can be examined for bladder stones, inflammation, or cancer.

Treatment of Stress Urinary Incontinence

Nonsurgical Therapy

Women with stress urinary incontinence should initially try nonsurgical therapy. Over 50% of women with stress urinary incontinence improve considerably following 6–8 weeks of daily kegel exercises. Kegel exercises are basically regular contractions of the pelvic muscles. These are the same muscles that help to stop the flow of urine or the passage of gas. The pelvic floor muscles envelope the urethra, vagina and rectum and help women to stay continent. These muscles become stronger and bulkier with exercise, which puts pressure on the urethra and helps to prevent leakage of urine. Kegel exercises therefore should be performed regularly by women of all ages. It is important to do Kegel exercises continuously since recurrences are common. One recommended routine includes three bouts of 10 contractions every day. It is helpful to associate the exercises with a daily activity, such as when stopping at a red light or brushing teeth. Some women also practice their pelvic muscles during intercourse. It is important not to do kegel exercises during urination, since this can lead to abnormal urination patterns. A referral to a physical therapist that specializes in pelvic muscle treatments can be very helpful for women who have a difficult time learning how to perform kegel excercises effectively.

Surgical Therapy

Until recently, the "gold standard" for surgical treatment of stress urinary incontinence was the Burch procedure, which was developed in the 1950s. This is performed through a pfannenstiel incision under general anesthesia and is associated with hospital stay of two to three days and a relatively prolonged recovery. The Burch procedure is still being performed, but mostly in the setting of a concurrent abdominal surgery. However, since the vaginal slings are more simple to perform and are associated with quicker recovery they have become the standard of care, especially since they have been shown to have similar efficacy when compared with the Burch procedure in clinical trials. **Figure 35.4** shows the most common surgical treatment options for stress urinary incontinence.

The suburethral sling is a very effective treatment option for women with stress urinary incontinence. The sling consists of a polypropylene mesh that is placed under the mid-urethra through a small incision in the vagina. The mesh is slipped loosely under the urethra so that it doesn't compress it too much, since this may lead to urinary retention. During a cough or other activities that cause increased abdominal pressure the mesh provides urethral support, thereby preventing urinary leakage. The procedure is often performed under local anesthesia and intravenous sedation. Recovery is usually rapid with many patients back to normal activities in 3–4 days. The mesh is guided in place with needles that travel either up under the pubic bone (tension-free vaginal tape, TVT) or out laterally through the obturator foramen (transobturator tape, TOT). The TOT is a more recent variant of the TVT and has the advantage of less risk of injury to the urinary bladder and internal organs. Since the tape or mesh that is slipped under the urethra is made out of artificial material, this is usually a permanent solution, and long-term results have been favorable with 85–90% of women still being continent at 5 to 10 years after surgery.

Yet another option for the treatment of stress urinary incontinence is injection of a bulking material such as collagen or carbon particles next to the urethra in order to create more pressure around the urethra and thereby decreasing urinary incontinence. Periurethral injection of autologous myoblasts and fibroblasts appears to show some promise (Evidence Box 35.1).

Treatment of Urge Incontinence

Women with urge incontinence should initially consider kegel exercises and bladder training. Bladder training involves training the bladder to gradually expand, thereby allowing the woman to go to the bathroom with longer intervals. For example, if a patient goes to the bathroom every hour, she should try to refrain for 1 hour and 15 minutes for 1 week and increase this interval by 15 minutes in subsequent weeks. The goal is to have at least 3 hours between bathroom visits. This can be very effective, but demands a lot of effort and dedication.

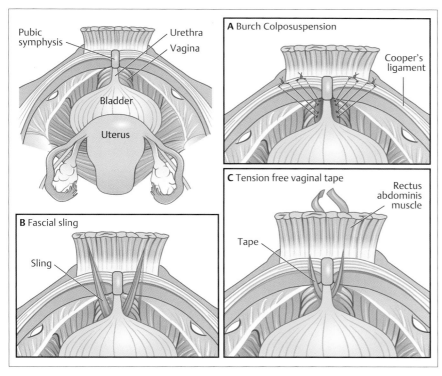

Fig. 35.4 Surgical procedures for stress urinary incontinence.
A Non-absorbable sutures are placed through Cooper's ligament and at the mid-urethra and the bladder neck.
B The fascial sling is passed under the bladder neck and fastened to the abdominal fascia.
C The tension free vaginal tape is passed under the midurethra, through the space of Retzius and through the anterior abdominal wall.

Pubic symphysis — Urethra — Vagina — Bladder — Uterus

A Burch Colposuspension — Cooper's ligament

B Fascial sling — Sling

C Tension free vaginal tape — Rectus abdominis muscle — Tape

Simple life-style changes can be very effective as well. If the problem is mostly frequent urination at night, simply stopping all fluid intake after 7 p.m. can be helpful. Women who have edema or leg swelling often experience frequent urination at night. A simple remedy is to lie almost flat (helps to have legs elevated) in the late afternoon, such as while watching or listening to the evening news. This helps to mobilize some of the extra fluid that is outside the vascular system into the blood stream. This leads to more urine production and in turn may result in more frequent urination during the evening hours, but not during the night. Women should also limit their intake of drinks that contain caffeine, such as coffee, tea, soda, and ice-tea. Caffeine irritates the bladder and can increase urgency symptoms.

If conservative methods fail, the next step is to try anticholinergic medication. There are several options available, but they all block cholinergic receptors in the detrusor muscle, resulting in less contractility of the muscle and thereby relieving the urgency symptoms in many cases. The main side effects of these medications are due to the anticholinergic effects on other organs, such as constipation, dry mouth, and blurred vision. Some patients are not able to take these medications because of these side effects and they are contraindicated in patients with narrow angle glaucoma. Recently, intravesicular botox injections and neuromodulation with stimulation of the sacral nerves have been added to the treatment armamentarium for urge incontinence, but long-term efficacy of these therapies has not been well established.

Urinary Tract Infection

Incidence

Urinary tract infections in women are very common with as many as 10% of women experiencing one episode per year, and with 60% of women having one episode during their lifetime. As many as 5% of women experience recurrent episodes.

Etiology

Escherichia coli, which most likely originates from the rectum, is the most common pathogen and accounts for about 80% of urinary tract infections. The main risk factor associated with urinary tract infections in women of reproductive age is sexual activity, and it is unusal for young women who are not sexually active to develop urinary tract infections. In postmenopausal women, the main risk factors include diabetes, incontinence, incomplete bladder emptying and history of urinary tract infections at a younger age.

Diagnosis

The most common symptoms include urinary frequency, dysuria, urgency, and lower abdominal pain. Hematuria or new onset of urinary incontinence are other, less common symptoms. Microbiologic diagnosis is usually defined as greater than 10^3 colony-forming units per milliliter of urine; however, empiric treatment can be started prior to getting back the results of the urinary culture, since women with the typical symptoms described above have a very high chance of having a urinary tract infection. It is nevertheless important to obtain a culture, especially in the setting of recurrent urinary tract infections, since some organisms are resistant to the most commonly used antibiotics.

Treatment

The most commonly used antimicrobials include nitrofurantoin, trimethoprim–sulfamethoxazole, fluoroquinolones, amoxicillin, and cephalosporins. The initial choice depends on the patient population and the setting of the infection, but trimethoprim–sulfamethoxazole (Bactrim) is a common first choice for patients who are not pregnant. Nitrofurantoin is the usual first choice in pregnant patients, since it appears to be safe to take during pregnancy. Three-day regimens have been shown to be equally as effective as longer duration regimens, although pregnant patients and patients with recurrent infections may benefit from a seven-day course of antibiotics.

Prevention

Preventive therapy may be considered for patients with recurrent infections. One antibiotic dose may be taken every night, or every other night, or directly after intercourse. High fluid intake, especially with cranberry or lingonberry juice, may also be of benefit.

Key Points

- Pelvic organ prolapse refers to a hernia in one of the pelvic organs, uterus, vagina, bladder or bowel/rectum. The most common symptoms of prolapse are a sense of pressure or heaviness in the pelvis or vagina and visual protrusion of tissue from the vagina. Prolapse may be associated with urinary incontinence.

- Urinary incontinence is defined as the involuntary loss of urine. In population surveys, weekly loss of urine is reported by about 10% of women. Many women with urinary incontinence will not report their symptoms unless specifically questioned by a clinician.
- There are two major types of incontinence. Stress incontinence occurs when an increase in intra-abdominal pressure, such as with laughing or coughing, overcomes sphincter closure in the absence of a bladder muscle contraction, resulting in the involuntary loss of urine. Urge incontinence, also known as detrusor overactivity, occurs when spontaneous bladder muscle contractions cause the loss of urine.
- Urinary incontinence can be treated with behavioral training, antimuscarinic medications, or surgery.
- Women with urinary tract infections typically present with symptoms of urinary frequency, pain on urination, urgency or blood in the urine. The most common cause of urinary tract infections is bowel bacteria. For adult women with no medical problems, a short-course treatment, 1–3 days, is often indicated. A common regimen is trimethoprim–sulfamethoxazole 160/800 mg twice daily for 3 days. For women with associated medical issues such as pregnancy, indwelling urinary catheters, or immunosuppression, antibiotic treatment should last at least 7 days.

Evidence Box 35.1

Injection of autologous myoblasts and fibroblasts shows promise for treatment of stress urinary incontinence in women.

Injection of a bulking material is one treatment option for patients with urinary incontinence caused by intrinsic sphincter deficiency. By adding volume to the internal sphincter, there is more support at the bladder neck, which can help to prevent urinary leakage. In this trial, the researchers randomly assigned 42 women to receive injections of autologous myoblasts and fibroblasts and 21 women were assigned to receive conventional transvaginal collagen injections. The researchers then followed up these women for 1 year and checked their incontinence status and measured the thickness and contractility of the urinary sphincter.

After 1 year of follow-up 38 of the 42 women injected with autologous cells were completely continent, compared with 2 of the 21 patients given conventional treatment with collagen. The mean thickness and contractility of the urinary sphincter were also significantly greater in women who received the autologous cells. No adverse effects were recorded in any of the 63 patients.

Injection of autologous cells into the urinary sphincter is a novel treatment for urinary incontinence. More rigorous trials with longer follow-up are needed before this becomes a part of the standard treatment armamentarium.

Strasser H, Marksteiner R, Margreiter E, et al. Autologous myoblasts and fibroblasts versus collagen for treatment of stress urinary incontinence in women: a randomized controlled trial. Lancet 2007;369:2179–2186.

Further Reading

Baden WF, Walker TA. Statistical evaluation of vaginal relaxation. *Clin Obstet Gynecol* 1972;15(4):1070–1072

Brown JS, Bradley CS, Subak LL, et al; Diagnostic Aspects of Incontinence Study (DAISy) Research Group. The sensitivity and specificity of a simple test to distinguish between urge and stress urinary incontinence. *Ann Intern Med* 2006;144(10):715–723

Bump RC, Mattiasson A, Bø K, et al. The standardization of terminology of female pelvic organ prolapse and pelvic floor dysfunction. *Am J Obstet Gynecol* 1996;175(1):10–17

Hay-Smith EJ, Dumoulin C. Pelvic floor muscle training versus no treatment, or inactive control treatments, for urinary incontinence in women. *Cochrane Database Syst Rev* 2006;(1):CD005654

Hirata H, Matsuyama H, Yamakawa G, et al. Does surgical repair of pelvic prolapse improve patients' quality of life? *Eur Urol* 2004;45(2):213–218

Holroyd-Leduc JM, Tannenbaum C, Thorpe KE, Straus SE. What type of urinary incontinence does this woman have? *JAMA* 2008;299(12):1446–1456

Maher C, Baessler K, Glazener CM, Adams EJ, Hagen S. Surgical management of pelvic organ prolapse in women. *Cochrane Database Syst Rev* 2007;(3):CD004014

Nicolle LE. Uncomplicated urinary tract infection in adults including uncomplicated pyelonephritis. *Urol Clin North Am* 2008;35(1):1–12, v

Novara G, Ficarra V, Boscolo-Berto R, Secco S, Cavalleri S, Artibani W. Tension-free midurethral slings in the treatment of female stress urinary incontinence: a systematic review and meta-analysis of randomized controlled trials of effectiveness. *Eur Urol* 2007;52(3):663–678

Nygaard IE, Heit M. Stress urinary incontinence. *Obstet Gynecol* 2004;104(3):607–620

Progetto Menopausa Italia Study Group. Risk factors for genital prolapse in non-hysterectomized women around menopause. Results from a large cross-sectional study in menopausal clinics in Italy. *Eur J Obstet Gynecol Reprod Biol* 2000;93(2):135–140

Söderberg MW, Falconer C, Byström B, Malmström A, Ekman G. Young women with genital prolapse have a low collagen concentration. *Acta Obstet Gynecol Scand* 2004;83(12):1193–1198

Swift S, Woodman P, O'Boyle A, et al. Pelvic Organ Support Study (POSST): the distribution, clinical definition, and epidemiologic condition of pelvic organ support defects. *Am J Obstet Gynecol* 2005;192(3):795–806

Whiteside JL, Weber AM, Meyn LA, Walters MD. Risk factors for prolapse recurrence after vaginal repair. *Am J Obstet Gynecol* 2004;191(5):1533–1538

Section II Breasts

36 The Breast and Benign Breast Disease

Robert L. Barbieri

Breast Structure and Function

The breast overlies the chest wall from the second to the sixth rib. The medial border is the sternum, the lateral border is the latissimus dorsi, the superior border the clavicle, and the inferior border is the costal margin and the upper rectus sheath. The breast contains glandular adipose and connective tissues. The glandular tissues of the breast are arranged in 15 to 20 lobes (**Fig. 36.1**). Each lobe consists of a branching arrangement of lobules and acini. The acini are lined by a layer of milk-secreting epithelial cells. Each acinus is surrounded by a criss-crossing array of contractile myoepithelial cells. The lumens of the acini connect to collecting intralobular ducts which empty into the main collecting system of the lobe. Each lobe drains into the nipple. The nipple consists of a pigmented areola. The sebaceous glands that are located on the perimeter of the areola are the glands of Montgomery. The glandular tissue of the lobules and acini are embedded in adipose tissue which accounts for most of the breast volume. The lobules are separated by Cooper ligaments, which are connective tissue sheets that run from the subcutaneous tissue to the chest wall.

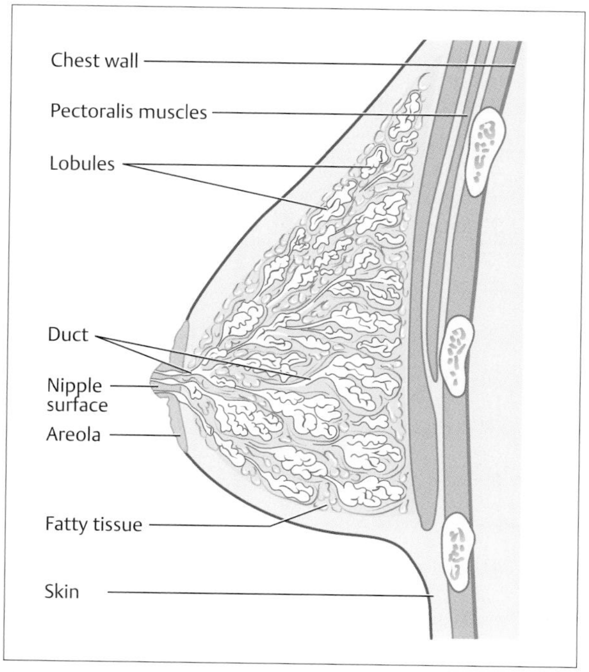

The main function of the breast is secretion of milk. Breast milk contains the milk proteins casein and lactalbumin, free fatty acids, and the milk sugar lactose. Lactose is a disaccharide of glucose and galactose. The breast is sensitive to the sex steroids, estradiol, progesterone, and testosterone, and to reproductive protein hormones including prolactin and oxytocin. During puberty and pregnancy these hormones stimulate the breast to grow. Estradiol stimulates the ductal system and progesterone stimulates the growth of the acini and the stromal tissues. In eu-estrogenic environments, androgens inhibit breast growth.

Breast Examination

In premenopausal women, the breast examination is best timed after menses but before ovulation. For postmenopausal women, the breast examination can be performed at any time. The examination begins with inspection of the breast with the patient in both upright and supine positions to look for asymmetry, skin changes such as erythema or dimpling, and nipple inversion, retraction, or discharge. The regional lymph nodes, especially those in the axilla, clavicular area and neck should be palpated for enlargement. A bimanual examination of the breast should be performed with the patient in the sitting and supine positions with the arm extended above the head. In the sitting position the breast can be supported by one hand while palpating it with the finger pads, not the fin-

Fig. 36.1 Anatomy of the breast.

Chest wall

Pectoralis muscles

Lobules

Duct

Nipple surface

Areola

Fatty tissue

Skin

ger tips, of the other hand. Palpation of the breast usually is performed in concentric circles starting from the nipple and moving outward, or in vertical strips starting laterally and moving toward the sternum. Using light pressure, the finger pads can be used to exam the breast tissue immediately under the skin. Using firmer pressure the finger pads can be used to exam the breast tissue deep to the skin. Gentle, but firm, pressure around the areolar area can be performed to check for breast secretion. Breast self-examination can be reviewed at the completion of the examination.

Lactation

During pregnancy the breast is exposed to high levels of lactogenic hormones, including prolactin, human placental lactogen and placental growth hormone, a variant of pituitary growth hormone. In the nonpregnant woman, prolactin concentration is about 15 ng/mL. During the third trimester of pregnancy, prolactin concentration is about 300 pg/mL. Serum human placental lactogen concentration is 6 000 000 pg/mL during the third trimester. These lactogenic and growth factors stimulate the alveoli to grow and prepare for lactation. During pregnancy, the very high serum concentrations of progesterone block lactogenesis. After delivery of the placenta, the rapid decrease in estradiol and progesterone releases the block to lactogenesis and results in an increase in the production of the milk proteins, fatty acids, and sugar that occurs over 3–5 days.

During suckling, neural signals from the nipple travel through thoracic nerves 4, 5 and 6 to the paraventricular and supraoptic nuclei and stimulate the release of oxytocin from the hypothalamus–posterior pituitary. Oxytocin causes contraction of the myoepithelial cells causing the flow of milk through the ducts to the nipple. Visual and auditory stimuli can also cause the release of oxytocin. Suckling stimulates the pituitary to release prolactin, which maintains lactogenesis by stimulating gene transcription in the alveolar epithelial cells, increasing the production of the milk proteins, fatty acids, and sugar.

Breast-Feeding

The best food for a newborn and infant is breast milk. Breast milk is recommended as the exclusive or main nutrient source of food during the first 6 months of life. From 6 months to 1 year of age, breast milk should be combined with solid food. Human breast milk has immediate and long-term health benefits for the newborn and infant. Breast milk provides benefits to gastrointestinal action, defense against infections, and possibly a reduced risk of developing obesity as an adult.

Hormones in breast milk, including epidermal growth factor and nerve growth factor, help the immature gastrointestinal mucosa of the newborn to grow and mature an epithelial barrier that helps protect against infections acquired through the gastrointestinal tract. In addition milk contains the secretory immunoglobulin IgA and IgG, interleukins, lysozyme, and immune cells that likely reduce the risk of infection. In developing countries, neonatal morbidity and mortality are reduced by breast-feeding compared with bottle feeding. In developed countries, the rate of neonatal hospitalization is less among breast-fed infants. In one population-based survey among approximately 16 000 infants living in the United Kingdom, exclusive breast-feeding reduced the risk of hospitalization for diarrhea by 60 % compared with never-breast-fed infants. Similarly the risk of hospitalization for respiratory infection was reduced by about 50 % by breast-feeding. Breast-feeding may also reduce the risk of otitis media by about 50 %. Breast-feeding during infancy may also reduce the risk of obesity, diabetes, and myocardial infarction in later life.

In developed countries there are no major contraindications to breast-feeding except for active maternal infection with HIV, because of the risk of maternal-to-infant infection; and maternal consumption of certain drugs, such as cyclophosphamide and amiodarone, which may affect the newborn and infant. If the newborn is affected by galactosemia—an inherited inborn error metabolism that prevents the proper metabolism of galactose—no exposure to lactose should occur. In developing countries, women infected with HIV may need to breast-feed because of lack of formula supplements. For these women, treatment with an antiretroviral agent such as nevirapine, or the combination of nevirapine plus zidovudine, reduces the risk of transmission of HIV to the infant by about 50 %.

Mastitis, Breast Abscess, and Galactocele

Mastitis is a common infection of the breast, typically with *Staphylococcus aureus* or *Streptococcus*, which presents as a firm, erythematosus, swollen and tender quadrant or localized area of the breast. Most women with mastitis present with a high temperature, greater than 38.3 °C. Treatment of mastitis includes continued breast-feeding, to move milk through the ducts, an antipyretic agent such as ibuprofen, and an antibiotic such as dicloxacillin 500 mg taken orally, four times daily for 10–14 days.

A breast abscess is an uncommon problem in breast-feeding women, which may be preceded by untreated or incompletely treated mastitis. As with most abscesses, treatment involves drainage of the abscess by needle aspiration or incision-drainage, and antibiotic treatment. About 1 % of healthy women are carriers of methicillin-resistant *Staphylococcus aureus* (MRSA). There is a developing trend that up to 50 % of cases of breast abscess are caused by MRSA, necessitating the use of active surveillance and broad-spectrum antibiotics such as vancomycin. Theoretically, maternal treatment with vancomycin could cause diarrhea in newborns.

A galactocele is a cystic collection of milk caused by an obstructed duct. Needle aspiration reveals milk as demonstrated by the presence of milk fats.

Breast-Feeding and Amenorrhea

Suckling activates multiple neuroendocrine systems that inhibit gonadotropin-releasing hormone (GnRH) secretion and the pituitary secretion of luteinizing hormone and follicular stimulating hormone, which inhibits ovulation. The degree to which breast-feeding suppresses GnRH secretion and inhibits ovulation is influenced by the intensity of the breast-feeding, the nutritional status of the mother and the body mass and body composition of the mother. Lactation is a major metabolic challenge for the mother, especially if she is undernourished. When nutrition is adequate and the body mass and composition are normal, breast-feeding is less likely to cause prolonged anovulation. During exclusive breast-feeding about 40 % of women will remain anovulatory at 6 months postpartum. Lactating women who remain anovulatory may have higher serum prolactin levels than those who become ovulatory during lactation.

Breast-Feeding and Contraception

High doses of estrogen, progestin, and androgens suppress lactation. Steroid contraceptive hormones, especially those that contain both estrogen and progestin, significantly alter the volume of breast milk and its composition. Standard estrogen–progestin oral contraceptives reduce breast milk volume by about 40 %. In contrast, a progestin-only contraceptive reduces daily breast milk volume by about 10 %. Standard estrogen–progestin

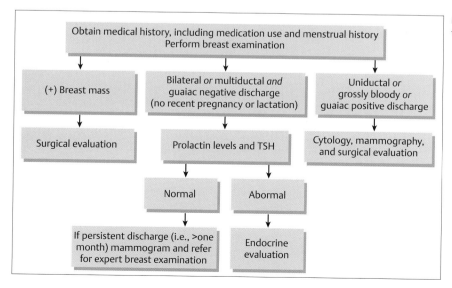

Fig. 36.2 Algorithm for the evaluation of nipple discharge.

oral contraceptives also reduce the breast milk concentration of lactalbumin, lactoferrin, and lactose, but these reductions are very modest and within the lower part of the normal range. The neurocognitive development and weight gain of exclusively breast-fed infants whose mothers took steroid contraceptives appear to be normal. However, if exclusive breast-feeding is planned, it is probably best to use a progestin-only contraceptive or an intrauterine device.

Nipple Discharge

Nipple discharge is common among women. An simplified algorithm for the evaluation of nipple discharge is presented in **Fig. 36.2**. Nipple discharges can be milky, clear, bloody, or purulent. Galactorrhea is a milky nipple discharge that occurs when a woman is not breast-feeding and is more than 6 months from her last breast-feeding. The unique characteristic of galactorrhea is the presence of milk fat. Galactorrhea can be caused by elevated serum prolactin, breast stimulation, chest wounds or chest inflammation, for example, shingles. If a woman with galactorrhea is ovulating normally, the discharge is probably caused by excessive sensitivity of the breast to normal levels of prolactin. If a woman has galactorrhea and is anovulatory, it is likely that serum prolactin is elevated. Causes of hyperprolactinemia include pregnancy, pituitary tumor, primary hypothyroidism, renal failure, and psychotropic medications that block the action of dopamine, such as phenothiazines. Dopamine agonists, such as bromocriptine or cabergoline, suppress prolactin secretion and can be used to treat bothersome galactorrhea.

In 5% of women, a nipple discharge is associated with breast cancer. For a woman with a nipple discharge, the likelihood of cancer as the cause is increased if the discharge is unilateral, bloody, associated with a breast mass, or if the woman is greater than 40 years of age. Unilateral nipple discharge is more likely to be associated with a breast mass (50% of cases) and ductal carcinoma in situ (10% of cases) or invasive cancer (1% of cases). The most common breast mass associated with unilateral discharge is a papilloma, a tumor growing form the lining of the breast duct. Up to 30% of women with a bloody discharge have intraductal carcinoma that is either in situ or invasive. All women with a unilateral discharge or a bloody discharge should have a complete breast examination, mammography, and ultrasound scan if indicated and cytological analysis of the discharge (**Fig. 36.2**). If a breast mass is detected during the evaluation, surgical consultation is necessary for biopsy or excision.

Breast Pain

Breast pain, or mastalgia, is a common cause of patient-initiated visits to a physician for breast problems. Mastalgia that is bilateral, associated with the luteal and menses phases of the menstrual cycle in a woman of less than 35 years of age, is almost always benign and needs no further evaluation except for a physical examination to detect a breast mass. These women may be offered reassurance, well-fitted breast support, and analgesics. If the pain is refractory to this treatment, tamoxifen, danazol, and bromocriptine have all been demonstrated to reduce mastalgia in clinical trials.

In women over 35 years of age with mastalgia, or in women where the breast pain is unilateral, evaluation should include physical examination, mammography and/or ultrasound scanning of the breast. If the findings are normal, treatment as described above may be recommended. If a suspicious lesion is identified, referral to a breast surgeon for biopsy or excision is recommended. About 2% of women with breast pain have an underlying breast cancer as the cause of the symptom.

Breast Problems in Children and Adolescents

In newborns, breast and chest exam should include assessment of breast size, nipple position, presence of accessory nipples, and nipple discharge. In children and adolescents an annual breast exam may be warranted. The onset of breast growth in girls, thelarche, typically begins between 8 and 13 years of age, with a median of 10 years and a standard deviation of about 1 year. Adolescent breast development is described using the Tanner staging system (**Fig. 36.3**).

Accessory breast tissue, including accessory nipples, is present in about 1% of newborns. Accessory nipples may be present anywhere along the milk line, with the most common site being just below the normally situated breast. The lower axilla is the most common site for accessory glandular breast tissue. Breast asymmetry is common among adolescents in Tanner stages 2, 3, and 4. Some cases of asymmetry resolve by age 18 years or achievement of Tanner stage 5. About 20% of adolescents have persistent breast asymmetry. A padded brassiere, or a brassiere that is padded on the side that supports the smaller breast, helps to mask the asymmetry.

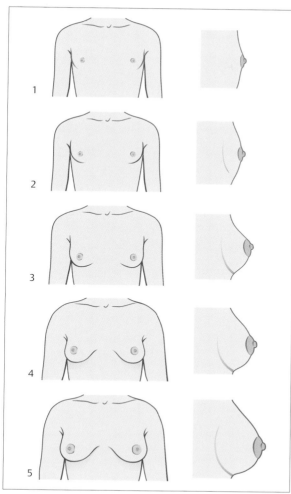

Fig. 36.3 Tanner staging of breast development. Stage 1: prepubertal stage. Stage 2:breast bud stage with elevation of breast and enlargement of areola. Stage 3: further enlargement of breast and areola; no separation of the contour between breast and areola. Stage 4: areola and papilla form a secondary mound above the level of the breast. Stage 5: projection of papilla only, with recession of areola. From Marshall WA, Tanner JM. Arch Dis Child 1970; 45:13. Copyright BMJ Publishing Group.

Approach to the Palpable Breast Mass

Among women 40–70 years of age, about 10% will present to a physician for evaluation of a breast lump or mass. About 10% of women who present with a breast lump have breast cancer as the cause of the lump. The timing and method of detection of the lump, change in size of the lump, and a family history of breast cancer should be elicited from the patient. A physical examination should be performed including an assessment of the presence of nipple discharge. All women presenting with a breast

lump should have an imaging study. Some authorities recommend that if a premenopausal woman reports a breast lump, and the physician can detect no breast mass, that the woman should return for a follow-up examination immediately after the next menstrual period. We prefer to perform an imaging study in all women who self-detect a breast lump. If the woman is over 35 years of age a mammogram and/or ultrasound scan is recommended. If the woman is less than 35 years old, an ultrasound scan may be initially recommended. In women younger than 35 years, breast density limits the usefulness of mammography.

Biopsy is often warranted if mammography demonstrates an area of increased density, irregular margins, speculation and/or irregularly clustered microcalcifications. If a suspicious mass is detected on mammography or ultrasonography, a core needle biopsy will provide tissue for histological analysis. This step will help with surgical planning if a malignancy is detected.

If ultrasound scanning demonstrates a simple cyst, no biopsy is necessary. Needle aspiration of the cyst may reduce its size. If the cyst fluid is clear at needle aspiration, it need not be sent for cytology. If the cyst fluid is bloody it should be sent for cytology. If ultrasound scanning demonstrates a complicated cyst, including lesions with internal echoes, fluid and debris levels, and thin septations, the cyst should be aspirated and the fluid sent for cytology. If ultrasound scanning demonstrates a complex cyst including solid components, a core needle biopsy is warranted.

Benign Breast Cysts and Masses

Following the seminal work of Dupont and Page in 1985 (see Further Reading), benign breast lesions are often classified into three categories based on their level of proliferation and atypia: 1) nonproliferative cysts and masses; 2) proliferative lesions without atypia; and 3) proliferative lesions with atypia. Of all breast biopsies that are not cancerous, 67% are nonproliferative, 29% are proliferative without atypia, and 4% are proliferative with atypia. Nonproliferative lesions are not associated with a marked increase in the risk of breast cancer. Women with proliferative lesions without atypia have about a 1.6 to 1.9-fold increased risk of developing breast cancer. Women with proliferative lesions with atypia have a 3.7 to 4.24-fold risk of developing breast cancer (Evidence Box 36.1).

Nonproliferative Lesions

Breast Cysts

As noted above, breast cysts can be classified by their ultrasound characteristics into three classes: simple, complicated, and complex. Simple breast cysts are never associated with breast cancer. Complex breast cysts, where ultrasonography demonstrates a solid component, may be associated with breast cancer. Due to this risk, complex breast cysts require biopsy for pathological diagnosis.

Fibrocystic Changes

Women with fibrocystic changes, also called fibrocystic breast disease or chronic cystic mastitis, usually present with breast pain or discomfort that increases in intensity during the luteal phase or the first days of menses. Women with fibrocystic changes may also present with tender, palpable nodules. On biopsy, fibrocystic changes are characterized by microcysts and macrocysts with interlobular fibrosis. Almost all women with fibrocystic changes are premenopausal. Ovarian estradiol and progesterone secreted during the luteal phase probably stimulate breast glands to swell causing the mastalgia. On physical examination a dominant breast mass is not present, but multiple millimeter-sized lumps that are often clustered in the outer upper quadrant of the breast are detected. Fibrocystic changes are usually multifocal and bilateral. Treatment usually involves analgesics for pain. Some authorities believe that avoiding caffeine is helpful. Estrogen–progestin contraceptives may help to reduce the severity of the symptoms.

Proliferative Breast Masses Without Atypia

Fibroadenoma

Fibroadenomas are the most common lesion of the breast. They are characterized by a proliferation of epithelial and mesenchymal cells. Stromal cells proliferate around tubular glands or compressed ducts. Most women present with a firm, nontender, mobile breast mass. In 80% of cases they present as a unifocal lesion. In 20% they present with two or more lesions in the same breast or lesions in both breasts. Fibroadenomas grow under stimulus by estrogen and regress in postmenopause. A core biopsy is required to make the diagnosis. The use of estrogen–progestin contraception appears to reduce the risk of developing a fibroadenoma.

Phyllodes Tumor

Phyllodes tumor is a rare fibroepithelial tumor that resembles fibroadenoma and is capable of a diverse range of biological behavior. Phyllodes tumors typically present as a large, bulky mass greater than 4 cm in diameter with a smooth surface in women 40–45 years of age. Most phyllodes tumors are benign and have a clinical course similar to that of a fibroadenoma, but occasionally the tumor is capable of metastasizing. There is a high rate of

recurrence after simple excision, and a tumor-free border greater than 1 cm is recommended at surgery.

Ductal Lesions

The normal breast duct has two layers of cuboidal cells with a specialized luminal border and basal contractile myoepithelial cells. An increase in the number of cell layers in the duct is ductal epithelial hyperplasia. In usual ductal hyperplasia, there is no cellular atypia. These lesions do not require treatment.

Papilloma

Papilloma is a benign tumor of the epithelium of the mammary ducts. Women with papilloma often present with bloody or blood-tinged nipple discharge. Papillomatosis is the presence of five or more separate papillomas within a segment of the breast. Papillomatosis is more likely to be associated with breast cancer and requires thorough imaging and wide excisional biopsy.

Adenosis

Adenosis is characterized by an increased number and size of lobular acini, forming crowded glandlike structures. Sclerosing adenosis and microglandular adenosis are two types that have been studied in the greatest detail. Sclerosing adenosis presents as a palpable mass or suspicious mammogram finding. It is histologically characterized by disordered acinar and myoepithelial elements, which on first viewing has features similar to infiltrating carcinoma. Microglandular adenosis often lacks the outer myoepithelial layer seen in other types of adenosis. This lesion can be mistaken for tubular carcinoma. The demonstration of an intact basal lamina with laminin or type IV collage immunostaining helps to differentiate this lesion from tubular carcinoma.

Radial Scars

These lesions are usually incidental histological findings on breast tissue biopsied for another reason. They are characterized by a fibroelastic core with entrapped ducts surrounded by radiating ducts and lobules. Treatment of these lesions involves complete excision.

Proliferative Lesions With Atypia

Atypical Hyperplasia

Atypical hyperplasia lesions may affect either the ducts or the lobules. In these lesions there is marked cellular proliferation with loss of architectural organization in apical–basal cell orientation. When these lesions are detected on core biopsy they require surgical excision to confirm the diagnosis. As noted above, women with these lesions have about a 4-fold increased risk of developing breast cancer, and the risk appears to be life-long. For these women a formal quantitative assessment of breast cancer using the Gail model is warranted. Risk reduction strategies include dedication to annual breast cancer screening, avoiding the use of estrogen during the postmenopause, avoid more than one alcohol drink per day, and use of risk-reducing hormone treatment with a selective estrogen receptor modulator such as tamoxifen or raloxifene. (see Chapter 37, Breast Cancer)

Epithelial Hyperplasia

Flat epithelial atypia usually presents with calcifications on mammography, resulting in a biopsy. Excision of the entire lesion is recommended, because in about 30% of cases, more advanced lesions will be detected on histology of the excisional biopsy.

Lobular-Type Epithelial Proliferation and Lobular Carcinoma in Situ

Lobular-type epithelial proliferation and lobular carcinoma in situ (LCIS) have similar features, consisting of lobular type epithelial proliferation with the main difference being the extent of proliferation. LCIS does not directly cause abnormalities on physical examination and mammography. The disease is usually diagnosed incidentally during a breast biopsy for another reason. LCIS is diagnosed in about 0.5% of breast biopsies. LCIS is not thought to be a direct precursor to breast cancer, but is a marker for increased breast cancer risk, both in the affected and the contralateral breast. Most women with LCIS never develop breast cancer. Risk reduction strategies include dedication to annual breast cancer screening, avoiding the use of estrogen during the postmenopause, avoiding more than one alcohol drink per day, and use of risk-reducing hormone treatment with a selective estrogen receptor modulator such as tamoxifen or raloxifene.

Ductal Carcinoma in Situ

Ductal carcinoma in situ is a proliferative disorder confined to the smaller and larger ducts with heterogeneous malignant potential. Unlike LCIS, ductal carcinoma in situ is a direct precursor to breast cancer and is reviewed in Chapter 37, Breast Cancer.

Miscellaneous Lesions

Lipoma

Most human lipomas are caused by a somatic mutation that involves the rearrangement of chromosomal material on the long arms of chromosomes 12 and 14. This rearrangement results in an increase in the expression of a high-mobility group gene, *hmgA2,* the product of which is an embryonic–fetal histone protein that participates in the regulation of cell growth. Lipomas of the breast are usually solitary benign tumors of adult adipocytes. They are usually soft, smooth, mobile, and nontender. Excisional biopsy is often recommended to both diagnose and treat these lesions in one step.

Fat Necrosis

Following breast trauma or breast surgery, the breast may develop a localized area of scarring that is palpable as a lump on breast exam, and has characteristics of cancer on mammography and/or ultrasonography. Core needle biopsy or excisional biopsy is useful to provide a definitive diagnosis (**Fig. 36.4a, b**)

Adenoma

Adenomas are benign epithelial tumors of the breast that are usually smooth and mobile with lobules. Unlike fibroadenomas they contain very little stromal tissue. Adenomas commonly occur during pregnancy and the puerperium. They are often managed by surgical excision.

Inflammatory Masses

Inflammatory masses of the breast include acute mastitis (see above), granulomatous mastitis and foreign body reactions. Granulomatous mastitis can be caused by sarcoidosis, Wegener granulomatosis, tuberculosis, a foreign material, or it may be idiopathic. Idiopathic granulomatous mastitis (IGM) presents as an inflammatory breast mass that often has inflammation in the overlying skin. On physical examination, a firm breast mass, nipple retraction, *peau d'orange* changes, and axillary adenopathy may be present raising the suspicion of cancer. Imaging studies usually are worrisome and a biopsy is necessary to make the diagnosis. If IGM is caused by an autoimmune disorder, glucocorticoid treatment may be beneficial. Excisional biopsy is often recommended. Foreign materials such as silicone may cause a granulomatous reaction in the breast. Fibrosis and contractions may lead to firm nodules that may be tender.

The screening, prevention, diagnosis, and treatment of breast cancer are discussed in Chapter 37.

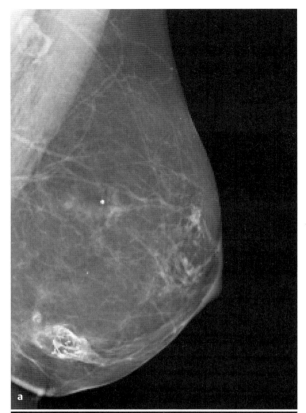

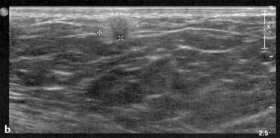

Fig. 36.4a, b   This 40-year-old patient had a 2-cm palpable lump in the left breast without axillary adenopathy.

a Mammogram of left breast demonstrating a circumscribed area of bright contrast.

b Ultrasound scan demonstrating a noncystic left breast lesion. Core needle biopsy demonstrated fat necrosis with acute and chronic inflammation. The patient had previously had a left breast reduction procedure.

Key Points

- The best food for a newborn and infant is breast milk. Breast milk is recommended as the exclusive or main nutrient source of food during the first 6 months of life. From 6 months to 1 year of age, breast milk should be combined with solid food. Breast milk provides benefits to gastrointestinal action, defense against infection, and may reduce the risk of obesity as an adult.

- Mastitis is a common infection of the breast. Usual organisms are *Staphylococcus aureus* and *Streptococcus*. Methicillin-resistant *Staphylococcus aureus* may increase the likelihood that mastitis will progress to a breast abscess. Mastitis presents with fever and a firm erythematosus swollen and tender quadrant of the breast. The treatment is continued breast-feeding to move milk through the breast ducts, an antipyretic agent, and an antibiotic such as dicloxacillin 500 mg taken orally, four times daily for 10–14 days.

- All women presenting with a breast lump should have an imaging study done. If the woman is less than 35 years old, ultrasonography is the usual first study. If the woman is over 35 years old a mammogram and ultrasound scan may be indicated. If the ultrasound scan demonstrates a simple cyst, it can be needle-aspirated. If the cyst fluid is clear it can be discarded. If the cyst fluid is bloody it should be sent for cytology. If imaging demonstrates a complex cyst or a suspicious mass a core needle biopsy should be obtained.

- Benign breast lesions are often classified as: 1) nonproliferative lesions (simple cysts, fibrocystic changes); 2) proliferative lesions without atypia (fibroadenoma, papilloma, adenosis, radial scars); and 3) proliferative lesions with atypia (atypical hyperplasia, epithelial hyperplasia, lobular-type epithelial proliferation, lobular carcinoma in situ). Women with proliferative lesions without atypia have a twofold increased life-long risk of breast cancer. Women with proliferative lesions without atypia have a 4-fold increased life-long risk of developing breast cancer.

Evidence Box 36.1.

Young women with a breast biopsy demonstrating atypical hyperplasia should undergo consultation for interventions that might reduce their risk of developing breast cancer.

In a study to investigate the correlation of the histology of various benign breast lesions with the risk of breast cancer, Hartmann et al. (2005) followed 9087 patients with a breast biopsy showing benign disease for a median of 15 years. At the initial biopsy, 66% had nonproliferative disease, 29% had a proliferative lesion without atypia, and 4% had atypical hyperplasia. After a median of 15 years of follow-up, breast cancer had been diagnosed in 6% of the women with nonproliferative disease, 10% of the women with a proliferative lesion without atypia, and 19% of the women with atypical hyperplasia. The risk of developing breast cancer after a biopsy for benign breast disease was 1.27 for non-proliferative disease, 1.88 proliferative disease without atypia and 4.24 for atypical hyperplasia. In women less than 45 years of age, a breast biopsy showing atypical hyperplasia was associated with a 7-fold increased risk of a later diagnosis of breast cancer. Similar results have been reported by other investigators (London et al. 1992).

Hartmann LC, Sellers TA, Frost MH, et al. Benign breast disease and the risk of breast cancer. N Engl J Med 2005;353:229–237.

London SJ, Connolly JL, Schnitt SJ, Colditz GA. A prospective study of benign breast disease and the risk of breast cancer. JAMA 1992;267:941–944.

Further Reading

Dupont WD, Page DL. Risk factors for breast cancer in women with proliferative breast disease. *N Engl J Med* 1985;312(3):146–151

Guray M, Sahin AA. Benign breast diseases: classification, diagnosis, and management. *Oncologist* 2006;11(5):435–449

Harder T, Bergmann R, Kallischnigg G, Plagemann A. Duration of breastfeeding and risk of overweight: a meta-analysis. *Am J Epidemiol* 2005;162(5):397–403

Hartmann LC, Sellers TA, Frost MH, et al. Benign breast disease and the risk of breast cancer. *N Engl J Med* 2005;353(3):229–237

Kumwenda NI, Hoover DR, Mofenson LM, et al. Extended antiretroviral prophylaxis to reduce breast-milk HIV-1 transmission. *N Engl J Med* 2008;359(2):119–129

London SJ, Connolly JL, Schnitt SJ, Colditz GA. A prospective study of benign breast disease and the risk of breast cancer. *JAMA* 1992;267(7):941–944

Quigley MA, Kelly YJ, Sacker A. Breastfeeding and hospitalization for diarrheal and respiratory infection in the United Kingdom Millennium Cohort Study. *Pediatrics* 2007;119(4):e837–e842

Srivastava A, Mansel RE, Arvind N, Prasad K, Dhar A, Chabra A. Evidence-based management of Mastalgia: a meta-analysis of randomised trials. *Breast* 2007;16(5):503–512

Stafford I, Hernandez J, Laibl V, Sheffield J, Roberts S, Wendel G Jr. Community-acquired methicillin-resistant Staphylococcus aureus among patients with puerperal mastitis requiring hospitalization. *Obstet Gynecol* 2008;112(3):533–537

Stuebe AM, Rich-Edwards JW, Willett WC, Manson JE, Michels KB. Duration of lactation and incidence of type 2 diabetes. *JAMA* 2005;294(20):2601–2610

Vessey M, Yeates D. Oral contraceptives and benign breast disease: an update of findings in a large cohort study. *Contraception* 2007;76(6):418–424

37 Breast Cancer: Prevention, Screening, Diagnosis, and Treatment

Robert L. Barbieri

Breast cancer is the most common cancer of women in developed countries. After lung cancer, it is the second most common cause of cancer death in women. Through to 90 years of age, the lifetime risk of breast cancer is about 12%. Ninety-five percent of all invasive breast cancers are diagnosed in women greater than 45 years of age. For women with a family history of breast cancer, the personal risk for breast cancer is approximately doubled.

Epidemiology

The rate of breast cancer is highest in developed countries and lowest in developing countries. Breast cancer rates tend to be negatively correlated with cervical cancer rates. In other words, the higher the rate of breast cancer in a geographic region, the lower the rate of cervical cancer. Breast cancer occurs about 100 times more frequently in women than men, indicating the importance of estrogen in the etiology of breast cancer. In postmenopausal women, obesity is associated with a modest increase in the risk of breast cancer, possibly through excessive extra-ovarian aromatization of androgens to estrogen and increased circulating peptide growth factors such as IGF-I. Regular physical activity is associated with a modest reduction in the risk of developing breast cancer. Alcohol consumption of two or more glasses per day increases the risk of breast cancer. Family history is an important risk factor for breast cancer. For women with one first-degree relative with breast cancer, the increase in risk is about twofold. With two affected first-degree relatives, the increase in risk is about threefold. Exposure to chest irradiation, especially before age 45 years, is a strong risk factor for breast cancer.

Reproductive Risk Factors

Younger age at menarche and later age at menopause are both associated with an increased risk of breast cancer. Bilateral oophorectomy before 40 years of age reduces the risk of breast cancer by 50%. Nulliparous women are at a 50% increased risk of developing breast cancer. Women who give birth at a young age are at decreased risk of breast cancer. Immediately following pregnancy there is a slight increased risk of breast cancer, but in the 10 years following pregnancy there is a reduced risk of developing breast cancer. Breast-feeding is strongly associated with a reduction in the risk of breast cancer. Abortion is not associated with breast cancer risk.

Changes in reproductive patterns may account, in part, for the increased risk of breast cancer in developed countries. In past centuries, the average woman had six births during her lifetime and breast-fed for 24 months per child. Currently, the average woman has two births and breast-feeds for 3 months per child. It is estimated that if women in developed countries reverted to the birth and breast-feeding patterns of previous centuries, the rate of breast cancer in the population would be reduced by at least 50%.

Reproductive Hormones

Many studies report that endogenous estrogen concentration in postmenopausal women is associated with breast cancer risk (Evidence Box 37.1). The greater the serum level of estradiol and two precursors to estradiol, estrone sulfate and dehydroepiandrosterone sulfate, the greater the risk of estrogen and progesterone receptor-positive breast cancer. Reproductive steroids do not impact the risk of estrogen and progesterone receptor-negative negative breast cancer. In premenopausal women it is difficult to assess the relationship between reproductive steroids and breast cancer risk because of the constantly changing levels of hormones throughout the cycle. The best current data does suggest that in premenopausal women increased estrogen levels are associated with an increased risk of breast cancer.

Oral Contraceptives

The best available current data indicates that estrogen–progestin contraceptives are not associated with an increased risk of breast cancer.

Postmenopausal Hormone Therapy

There is widespread concern that estrogen–progestin hormone therapy in postmenopausal women may be associated with an increased risk of cancer. In the Women's Health Initiative, treatment with conjugated equine estrogen 0.625 mg plus medroxyprogesterone actetate 2.5 mg daily was associated with a hazard ratio of 1.2 for breast cancer compared with placebo. In contrast, in the same study, treatment with conjugated estrogen 0.625 mg alone and without a progestin was not associated with an increased risk of breast cancer. These results, plus previous observational findings, suggest that it is the combination of both estrogen plus progestin that is associated with the greatest increase in the risk of breast cancer in postmenopausal women.

Breast Cancer Genetics

Mutations in many genes, including *BRCA1, BRCA2, p53, PTEN,* and *STK11,* are associated with a very high risk of breast cancer. The biological mechanisms that link mutations of *BRCA1* and *BRCA2* with breast and ovarian cancer are discussed in Chapter 45. Among women with a critical BRCA1 mutation, about 50% will develop breast cancer. In families with a high penetrance of breast cancer, the risk of developing breast cancer is greater than 80% by age 70 years.

Tests to screen for BRCA mutations are commercially available. These tests are very expensive because there are many mutations in the *BRCA* genes that may cause cancer. The population that should be tested has not been definitively defined. Testing should only be performed if the results will aid in the medical or surgical treatment of affected individuals and their family members. Criteria for testing include: 1) two first-degree relatives with breast cancer, one of whom was diagnosed at age 50 years or less; 2) three or more first- or second-degree relatives with breast cancer with no reference to the age of diagno-

sis; 3) in first- or second-degree relatives, a combination of both breast and ovarian cancer or a single relative with both ovarian and breast cancer, or two or more relatives with ovarian cancer; 4) a first-degree relative with bilateral breast cancer; 5) history of breast cancer in a male relative.

Prevention

Quantitative Assessment of Risk

Quantitative tools for predicting the risk of breast cancer include the Gail model, Breast Cancer Risk Assessment, Claus, and Tyrer–Cuzick tools. The Gail model is the most widely utilized and uses seven factors to predict risk: current age, age at menarche, age at first live birth, number of first-degree relatives with breast cancer, number of prior breast biopsies, the presence of atypical hyperplasia on biopsy, and race. The calculator is available at: http://www.cancer.gov/bcrisktool/ Using the Gail model, for women 35–59 years of age, a 5-year risk of at least 1.66% is considered to be "at increased risk" and such women are considered suitable for hormonal chemoprevention (see below). A similar calculator, the Breast Cancer Risk Assessment (BCRA) tool, is based on the Gail model but contains more recently available population data. This model is suitable for use by women of different races and ethnicities. This calculator is available at: http://bcra.nci.nih.gov/brc/q1.htm As new breast cancer risk factors are identified, such as breast density at mammography, available risk calculators are being constantly updated and refined.

Hormone Prevention

Numerous clinical trials have demonstrated that treatment with a selective estrogen receptor modulator such as tamoxifen or raloxifene reduces the risk of invasive and noninvasive breast cancer in women at increased risk.

In the National Surgical Adjuvant Breast and Bowel Project (NSABP) the entry criteria were: 1) women 60 years of age or older; 2) women between 35 and 59 years of age with a 5-year risk for breast cancer of at least 1.66% as predicted by the Gail model; or 3) women greater than 35 years of age and a personal history of lobular carcinoma in situ (LCIS) (see Chapter 36, The Breast and Benign Breast Disease). Women (N = 13 388) meeting these entry criteria were randomized to tamoxifen 20 mg daily orally or placebo. The study was discontinued after a median of 48 months of treatment, but many women who were randomized to tamoxifen continued to take the treatment. The cumulative incidence of invasive breast cancer was 4.3% in the placebo group and 2.5% in the tamoxifen group. In the women who entered the study with LCIS, 1.2% in the placebo group and 0.6% in the tamoxifen group developed invasive cancer. All of the risk reduction was due to a decrease in the number of estrogen receptor-positive tumors. The risk reduction was 36% for women <50 years old and 51% for women ≥60 years. Tamoxifen treatment did not have an impact on survival. The risks associated with tamoxifen therapy included endometrial cancer (risk ratio 3.3), pulmonary emboli (risk ratio 1.5), and stroke (risk ratio 2.2). During the study 53 cases of endometrial cancer were diagnosed in the tamoxifen group and 17 cases in the placebo group. Raloxifene is also approved for hormonal chemoprevention of breast cancer. It has different properties from tamoxifen as outlined in Evidence Box 37.2. The aromatase inhibitors anastrozole and letrozole are under active study to assess their utility in the prevention of breast cancer.

Risk-Reducing Bilateral Mastectomy

For women carrying a mutation in the BRCA1 or BRCA2 genes, prophylactic bilateral total mastectomy is associated with a 90% reduction in the risk of developing breast cancer. The significant impact of bilateral mastectomy on quality of life has limited the widespread acceptance of this approach to risk reduction.

Risk-Reducing Bilateral Salpingo-oophorectomy

In carriers of mutations in the BRCA1 or BRCA2 genes prophylactic bilateral salpingo-oophorectomy (BSO) reduces the risk of both breast and ovarian cancers. In one retrospective study BSO was associated with a 95% reduction in the risk of ovarian cancer and a 50% reduction in the risk of breast cancer. BSO is typically planned for a woman at a time after completion of her family, but before the youngest age of onset of breast and ovarian cancer in her family.

Screening

Screening refers to the wide-scale diagnostic testing of a population at average risk of a disease. For a population at very high risk of a disease, "early disease detection" is probably a better term for the diagnostic tests that are performed. Screening is inherently associated with significant costs, many false-positive tests, and may induce anxiety in the population being screened. The costs of screening must be balanced against the potential benefits.

Breast Self-Examination

There is very little evidence that teaching patients to perform breast self-examination significantly impacts the rate of breast cancer death. However, women who perform a very thorough breast self-examination may detect breast tumors at an earlier stage than women who do not perform self-examination or only perform a cursory self-examination.

Physical Examination by a Clinician

Breast physical examination by a clinician can detect about 50% of breast cancers. Mammography detects about 90% of breast cancers. In some instances a breast cancer not detected at mammography can be palpated on clinical examination. In countries where it is widely available, mammography plays a more important role than physical examination for the detection of breast cancer. In developing countries where mammography is not widely available, clinical breast examination is of significant value in screening for breast cancer.

Mammography

Screening mammography is recommended annually for all women greater than 40 years of age. In one comprehensive meta-analysis of clinical trials, annual mammography reduced the risk of breast cancer mortality by 22% in women ≥50 years and 15% in women 40–50 years of age. For healthy women, evidence supports annual screening mammography to at least 80 years of age.

Mammograms are typically reviewed by two imaging specialists and assigned to one of the Breast Imaging Report and Data System (BIRADS) categories (**Fig. 37.1**). These seven categories are:

1. BIRADS 0—incomplete study; additional imaging required;
2. BIRADS 1—normal; normal interval follow-up recommended;
3. BIRADS —very likely benign; normal interval follow-up;

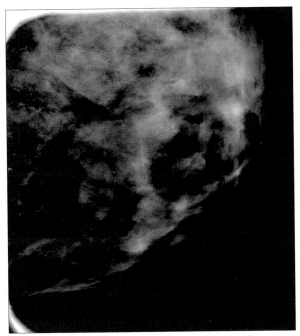

Fig. 37.1 Mammogram, BIRADS 4c with invasive breast cancer localized by a 7 mm focus of pleiomorphic calcifications.

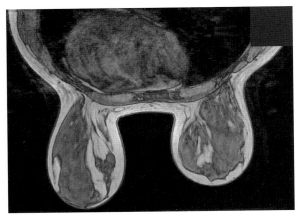

Fig. 37.2 Magnetic resonance imaging of the breast.

Magnetic Resonance Imaging

Magnetic resonance imaging (MRI) is an important new modality in the detection of early-stage breast cancer (**Fig. 37.2**). Currently, MRI is more sensitive and less specific for the diagnosis of breast cancer than mammography. Given the reduced specificity of MRI compared with mammography, it is not recommended for screening of average-risk populations. MRI is only recommended for the early detection of disease in women known to be carriers for BRCA1 or BRCA2, or women with a history of chest irradiation. MRI may also be warranted for women with a personal history of breast cancer to detect disease in residual breast tissue. MRI imaging requires the injection of a contrast agent such as gadolinium. Gadolinium may cause nephrogenic systemic fibrosis, a serious renal disease. The technology for MRI imaging of the breast is rapidly evolving and the specificity of the technique will improve. It is likely that the role of MRI in the diagnosis of breast disease will increase in the coming years.

4. BIRADS 3—probably benign; a short interval follow-up is recommended: follow-up mammogram in 4 months for masses and 6 months for microcalcifications;
5. BIRADS 4—suspicious abnormality; biopsy recommended;
6. BIRADS 5—highly suggestive of malignancy; biopsy should be performed;
7. BIRADS 6—malignancy known to be present by pathology: imaging is performed for planning treatment.

The rates of malignancy with BIRADS 3 and 5 readings are 2% and 95%, respectively. BIRADS 4 is a broad category and is divided into three subcategories: BIRADS 4a, 4b, and 4c which represent low, intermediate, and moderate–high risk, respectively. For women with a BIRADS 4c or 5 reading, if the initial biopsy demonstrates benign histology, repeat biopsy or excisional biopsy is warranted because the presence of cancer is so likely.

If the mammogram shows a mass lesion, an ultrasound scan is ordinarily performed to determine whether the mass is a simple, complicated or complex cyst, or entirely solid.

Diagnosis

The diagnosis of breast cancer is usually made by a core biopsy or surgical excision of a lesion. In countries where mammography is available, 90% of breast cancers will be detected by mammography. Many of the lesions detected by mammography are not palpable. In general, a first step following a BIRADS 4 or 5 mammogram is an image-guided (stereotactic mammography or ultrasonography) core biopsy. Alternatively a mammogram can be performed and a needle placed into the lesion. The patient is then transferred to the operating room where an excisional biopsy can be performed. In general, a surgical excisional biopsy is not used as the first step in obtaining tissue for diagnosis. Image-guided core biopsy or palpation-guided core biopsy are preferred as initial steps because they allow for better planning of further surgical and adjuvant treatment. Following a core biopsy, a surgical microclip is placed at the site of the biopsy for identification of the biopsy site during future imaging studies and surgery. If a breast mass is palpable and the mammogram is normal, the mass should be biopsied or excised unless it is a simple cyst as demonstrated by ultrasonography. Simple cysts may be aspirated as the first step in management. If the mammogram demonstrates a BIRADS 4c or 5 result, physical examination and ultrasound scanning of the axilla may help to determine whether the lymph nodes are involved.

If the core biopsy or needle-guided excisional biopsy demonstrates a breast cancer, further surgical staging and treatment planning should be undertaken by a multidisciplinary team focused on breast cancer treatment. After diagnosis of invasive breast cancer by core biopsy, surgical staging requires surgical management of the tumor site and sampling of local and regional lymph nodes and a clinical assessment of metastasis to distant organs. At a minimum, clinical assessment includes a thorough physical exam, a complete blood count, liver function tests, and chest imaging.

Treatment

Many factors influence the treatment of breast cancer including lymph node involvement, tumor size, histological type, the presence of estrogen and progesterone receptors, HER2 overexpression, patient age, myocardial function, and menopausal status (**Table 37.1**). A Web-based tool, "Adjuvant!" provides guidance about the relative utility of chemotherapy, hormone, and HER2 therapy for individual patients. This calculator is available online at: http://www.adjuvantonline.com/index.jsp.

Table 37.1 Breast cancer 5-year survival rate based on tumor size and number of lymph nodes involved with metastatic cancer

Tumor size (cm)	No. of lymph nodes with metastatic cancer		
	0 nodes with cancer	1 to 3 nodes with cancer	≥4 nodes with cancer
<2	96%	87%	66%
2–5	89%	80%	59%
>5	82%	73%	46%

Source: Adapted from Fitzgibbons PL, Page DL, Weaver D, et al. Prognostic factors in breast cancer. College of American Pathologists Consensus Statement 1999. Arch Pathol Lab Med 2000;124:966–978.

Local Therapy to Control the Tumor

Initial Surgical Treatment

Surgical treatment is needed by all women with breast cancer. Breast conserving surgery is as effective as mastectomy, but is less disfiguring than mastectomy. Breast conserving surgery, also known as lumpectomy, plus radiation therapy involves removing the cancer in its entirety, with wide margins, and simultaneously attempts to preserve as much breast tissue as possible. Absolute contraindications to breast conserving surgery are few, but include a history of prior radiotherapy to the chest wall (which precludes further radiotherapy), widespread, multicentric breast cancer, and the inability to obtain disease-free resection margins.

Initial surgical treatment of breast cancer must also include sampling of local and regional lymph nodes. Cancer involvement in local and regional lymph nodes significantly increases the risk of disease recurrence and metastasis, necessitating more aggressive adjuvant therapy. Two current approaches are axillary lymph node dissection and sentinel lymph node (SLN) biopsy (**Fig. 37.3**). SLN biopsy is performed by injecting a dye or radioiso-

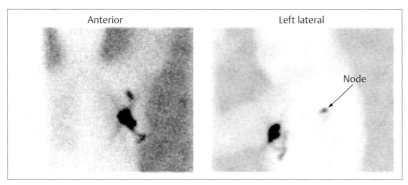

Anterior   Left lateral

Node

Fig. 37.3 Sentinel node detected by lymphoscintigraphy. A dose of 400 µCi of technetium-99 was injected in four intradermal locations and one deep location in the breast. An axillary sentinel node was detected by the technetium injection.

tope into the area near the breast tumor. The dye or radioisotope may be locally concentrated in active local and regional nodes. This can guide the surgeon to resect fewer lymph nodes with a higher yield for potentially positive nodes. If the SLN biopsy reveals a positive lymph node, axillary dissection must be performed.

Radiotherapy

Radiotherapy is almost always performed after breast conserving surgery to reduce the risk of local recurrence, and may also be needed following mastectomy. Older women, greater than 70 years of age, with good-prognosis breast cancer (estrogen receptor-positive) may not need radiotherapy. Recent trials have indicated that it may be possible to reduce the dose and number of days needed to complete effective radiotherapy to as few as 22 days with a total dose of 43 Gy. Radiotherapy and chemotherapy are not typically given simultaneously because of increased side-effects. They are usually administered sequentially.

Adjuvant Systemic Therapy to Reduce the Risk of Recurrence and Death

For many women with breast cancer, adjuvant systemic therapy with chemotherapy, hormone therapy, or trastunzumab reduces the risk of breast cancer recurrence and death from breast cancer. Adjuvant therapy benefits most women with breast cancer, but the clinical impact is greatest for women with cancer involvement of the local and regional lymph nodes. In general all women with node-positive cancer and women with breast cancer lesions greater than 1 cm should be offered adjuvant therapy. A Web-based tool, "Adjuvant!" provides guidance about the relative utility of chemotherapy, hormone, and HER2 therapy for individual patients. This calculator is available online at: http://www.adjuvantonline.com/index.jsp

Chemotherapy

For women over the age of 70 the benefits of chemotherapy are uncertain. For younger women who are eligible for adjuvant therapy, chemotherapy increases survival. Chemotherapy is the standard adjuvant therapy for women with estrogen receptor-negative tumors. For women with lymph node negative and estrogen receptor-positive tumors, a 21-gene assay that may predict the risk of recurrence may help to determine whether chemotherapy is warranted. For women with early-stage disease one of the most commonly administered chemotherapy regimens is doxorubicin plus cyclophosphamide plus paclitaxel or docetaxel.

Hormone Therapy

Hormone therapy benefits women with estrogen and/or progesterone receptor-positive breast cancer, but not those with estrogen or progesterone receptor-negative tumors. Standard hormone therapy regimens typically involve the use of both a selective estrogen receptor modulator (tamoxifen or raloxifene) plus an aromatase inhibitor (anastrozole or letrozole). For example, one common regimen is to prescribe tamoxifen 20 mg daily for 5 years followed by an aromatase inhibitor. Alternatively, tamoxifen 20 mg daily can be prescribed for 2 years followed by an aromatase inhibitor for 3 years to complete 5 years of therapy.

Trastuzumab: Human epidermal growth factor receptor 2 (HER2) is a transmembrane tyrosine kinase involved in cell replication. In about 20% of breast tumors, HER2 is overexpressed and plays a role in tumor growth. Trastuzumab is a humanized monoclonal antibody directed against HER2 that interferes with HER2 function and decreases the rate of breast cancer growth. For women with HER2 positive cancers the addition of trastunzumab as monotherapy or in addition to chemotherapy improves survival. The combination of trastunzumab plus doxorubicin appears to increase the risk of cardiotoxicity.

Locally Advanced Breast Cancer

Locally advanced breast cancer is diagnosed when the initial tumor is very large (>5 cm), there is extensive lymph node involvement, or the chest wall or skin is directly involved by the tumor. For these lesions, multimodal therapy including surgery, radiotherapy, and chemotherapy is standard. For these patients, chemotherapy is often given before surgery to increase the success of breast preserving surgery.

Medical Care for Breast Cancer Survivors

Fertility

Following therapy for breast cancer many women become menopausal because chemotherapy, especially cyclophosphamide, is cytotoxic to ovarian follicles. For women interested in preserving future fertility, a quick cycle of ovarian stimulation with oocyte retrieval and cryopreservation of oocytes or embryos prior to initiating chemotherapy is sometimes an option. Another experimental option is to perform laparoscopy and excise a strip of ovarian cortex containing follicles and oocytes for cryopreservation prior to starting chemotherapy. Alternative approaches involve the use of donor oocytes to achieve a pregnancy at a future date.

Pregnancy

Most observational studies report that pregnancy in breast cancer survivors does not have a detrimental effect on breast cancer recurrence or survival. Most of these studies have a sample size of 50 women or less, limiting their generalizeability. In order to minimize the likelihood of a recurrence of breast cancer during a pregnancy, most authorities recommend that breast cancer survivors wait at least two to three years after completing their initial treatment before becoming pregnant. This will reduce the risk that women destined to have a recurrence of breast cancer shortly after primary treatment will attempt to become pregnant.

Hormone Therapy

Many women with breast cancer have menopausal symptoms such as hot flushes and insomnia. Many oncologists are concerned that treating breast cancer survivors with estrogen or estrogen–progestin will increase the risk of cancer recurrence. Many gynecologists believe that low doses of hormone therapy for short periods are unlikely to have significant adverse effects on cancer outcome and may significantly improve disabling symptoms.

Few randomized trials are available to guide treatment decisions for this problem. In one clinical trial, 434 breast cancer survivors with menopausal symptoms were randomized to receive 2 years of hormone therapy or no hormone therapy. Hormone therapy consisted of estrogen-alone for hysterectomized women and estrogen–progestin for women with a uterus. After a median follow up of 4 years, 39 women in the hormone group and 17 in the no-hormone group had a recurrence of breast cancer. The cumulative incidence of a breast cancer recurrence at 5 years was calculated to be 22 % in the hormone group and 8 % in the placebo group.

In survivors of breast cancer, menopausal symptoms are best treated without estrogen or progestin, using agents such as selective serotonin receptor uptake inhibitors.

Bone Density

Many survivors of breast cancer have osteoporosis. This is commonly caused by estrogen deficiency associated with premature ovarian failure following chemotherapy and the use of aromatase inhibitors that reduce estrogen to very low levels. Breast cancer survivors should have a baseline bone density measured, and if osteoporosis is present they should be treated with an oral or intravenous bisphosphonate. In women with bone metastases, treatment with bisphosphonates can reduce the rate of growth and spread of bone metastases.

Key Points

- Breast cancer is the most common cancer of women in developed countries. It is the second most common cause of death in women, after lung cancer.
- Breast cancer rates tend to be negatively correlated with cervical cancer rates. The higher the rate of breast cancer in a geographic region, the lower the rate of cervical cancer.
- Risk factors for breast cancer are: young age at menarche, late age of menopause, nulliparity, late age of first birth, breast biopsy demonstrating proliferative benign breast lesions and family history of breast cancer.
- Critical mutations in *BRCA1* and *BRCA2* genes are associated with a marked increase in the risk of breast cancer.
- Screening mammography is recommended annually for all women aged 40 years or more. Annual screening mammorgraphy reduces the risk of breast cancer mortality by 20 % in women over 50 years old and by 10 % in women 40–50 years old.
- In postmenopausal women, estrogen–progestin treatment for more than 5 years increases the risk of breast cancer.
- In women at increased risk of breast cancer, treatment with selective estrogen receptor modulators, such as raloxifene or tamoxifen, reduces the risk of developing breast cancer by about 50 %.

Evidence Box 37.1

Endogenous levels of estradiol are an important risk factor for breast cancer in postmenopausal women.

In 1989 and 1990, blood was collected from 32 826 healthy nurses who were free of breast cancer. Through to June 1998, 264 new cases of invasive cancer and 41 cases of in situ breast cancer were diagnosed in this cohort. For each woman with breast cancer, two women without breast cancer were selected as controls. When the analysis was restricted to women with estrogen and progesterone receptor-positive cancers, the women with highest estradiol levels had a 3.3 increased relative risk (95 % confidence interval, 2.0 to 5.4) of developing breast cancer compared with the women with lowest estradiol levels. Similar associations were observed for androgens that are substrates for aromatization and precursors for estradiol synthesis. There was no association between progesterone or sex hormone-binding globulin concentrations and the risk of developing breast cancer. Given the relationship between endogenous levels of estradiol and the risk of breast cancer, it is not surprising that antiestrogens such as tamoxifen and raloxifene decrease the risk of developing breast cancer.

Missmer SA, Eliassen AH, Barbieri RL, Hankinson SE. Endogenous estrogen, androgen and progesterone concentrations and breast cancer risk among postmenopausal women. J Natl Cancer Inst 2004;96:1856–1865.

Evidence Box 37.2

Tamoxifen and raloxifene reduce the risk of breast cancer by about 50% in women with an increased risk of developing the disease.

In the STAR trial 19 747 women >35 years of age with an estimated risk of developing breast cancer >1.66% over the next 5 years (using the Gail model) were randomized to receive either tamoxifen 20 mg daily or raloxifene 60 mg daily for 5 years. Raloxifene is a selective estrogen receptor modulator with less estrogen agonist activity in the endometrium than tamoxifen. One hypothesis of the study was that raloxifene would cause fewer cases of endometrial cancer than tamoxifen.

Data from 19 471 women were available for analysis at 4 years. The average 5-year risk for developing breast cancer in the study population was 4%. This indicates that the group was at high risk for breast cancer. The cumulative incidence rate of invasive breast cancer in the raloxifene and tamoxifen groups was similar 2.48% and 2.51%, respectively. The estimated reduction in the rate of breast cancer in both groups was about 50%. Interestingly, tamoxifen, but not raloxifene, decreased the risk of developing ductal carcinoma in situ and lobular carcinoma in situ in this study. Of the women who had a uterus, raloxifene was associated with a 38% reduced risk of developing endometrial cancer compared with tamoxifen. In the raloxifene group the risk of developing deep venous thrombosis or pulmonary emboli was reduced by 25% and 35%, respectively, compared with the tamoxifen group. In the raloxifene group 21% fewer cataracts were reported compared to the tamoxifen group. Patient-reported quality of life was similar in the two groups. The authors conclude that both tamoxifen and raloxifene are effective in reducing the risk of developing invasive breast cancer in women at high risk for the disease. Raloxifene is associated with fewer adverse events than tamoxifen.

Vogel VG, Costantino JP, Wickerham DL, et al. Effects of tamoxifen versus raloxifene on the risk of developing invasive breast cancer and other disease outcomes. JAMA 2006;295:2727–2741.

Further Reading

Chlebowski RT, Hendrix SL, Langer RD, et al; WHI Investigators. Influence of estrogen plus progestin on breast cancer and mammography in healthy postmenopausal women: the Women's Health Initiative Randomized Trial. *JAMA* 2003;289(24):3243–3253

Collaborative Group on Hormonal Factors in Breast Cancer. Breast cancer and breastfeeding: collaborative reanalysis of individual data from 47 epidemiological studies in 30 countries, including 50 302 women with breast cancer and 96 973 women without the disease. *Lancet* 2002;360(9328):187–195

Collaborative Group on Hormonal Factors in Breast Cancer. Familial breast cancer: collaborative reanalysis of individual data from 52 epidemiological studies including 58,209 women with breast cancer and 101,986 women without the disease. *Lancet* 2001;358(9291):1389–1399

Clarke M, Collins R, Darby S, et al; Early Breast Cancer Trialists' Collaborative Group (EBCTCG). Effects of radiotherapy and of differences in the extent of surgery for early breast cancer on local recurrence and 15-year survival: an overview of the randomised trials. *Lancet* 2005;366(9503):2087–2106

Eliassen AH, Missmer SA, Tworoger SS, et al. Endogenous steroid hormone concentrations and risk of breast cancer among premenopausal women. *J Natl Cancer Inst* 2006;98(19):1406–1415

Fisher B, Costantino JP, Wickerham DL, et al. Tamoxifen for the prevention of breast cancer: current status of the National Surgical Adjuvant Breast and Bowel Project P-1 study. *J Natl Cancer Inst* 2005;97(22):1652–1662

Fitzgibbons PL, Page DL, Weaver D, et al. Prognostic factors in breast cancer. College of American Pathologists Consensus Statement 1999. *Arch Pathol Lab Med* 2000;124(7):966–978

Harris L, Fritsche H, Mennel R, et al; American Society of Clinical Oncology. American Society of Clinical Oncology 2007 update of recommendations for the use of tumor markers in breast cancer. *J Clin Oncol* 2007;25(33):5287–5312

Holmberg L, Iversen OE, Rudenstam CM, et al; HABITS Study Group. Increased risk of recurrence after hormone replacement therapy in breast cancer survivors. *J Natl Cancer Inst* 2008;100(7):475–482

Humphrey LL, Helfand M, Chan BK, Woolf SH. Breast cancer screening: a summary of the evidence for the U.S. Preventive Services Task Force. *Ann Intern Med* 2002;137(5 Part 1):347–360

Lee SJ, Schover LR, Partridge AH, et al; American Society of Clinical Oncology. American Society of Clinical Oncology recommendations on fertility preservation in cancer patients. *J Clin Oncol* 2006;24(18):2917–2931

Marchbanks PA, McDonald JA, Wilson HG, et al. Oral contraceptives and the risk of breast cancer. *N Engl J Med* 2002;346(26):2025–2032

Meijers-Heijboer H, van Geel B, van Putten WL, et al. Breast cancer after prophylactic bilateral mastectomy in women with a BRCA1 or BRCA2 mutation. *N Engl J Med* 2001;345(3):159–164

Missmer SA, Eliassen AH, Barbieri RL, Hankinson SE. Endogenous estrogen, androgen, and progesterone concentrations and breast cancer risk among postmenopausal women. *J Natl Cancer Inst* 2004;96(24):1856–1865

Newcomb PA, Weiss NS, Storer BE, Scholes D, Young BE, Voigt LF. Breast self-examination in relation to the occurrence of advanced breast cancer. *J Natl Cancer Inst* 1991;83(4):260–265

Rebbeck TR, Lynch HT, Neuhausen SL, et al; Prevention and Observation of Surgical End Points Study Group. Prophylactic oophorectomy in carriers of BRCA1 or BRCA2 mutations. *N Engl J Med* 2002;346(21):1616–1622

Stefanick ML, Anderson GL, Margolis KL, et al; WHI Investigators. Effects of conjugated equine estrogens on breast cancer and mammography screening in postmenopausal women with hysterectomy. *JAMA* 2006;295(14):1647–1657

Thomas DB, Gao DL, Ray RM, et al. Randomized trial of breast self-examination in Shanghai: final results. *J Natl Cancer Inst* 2002;94(19):1445–1457

U.S. Preventive Services Task Force. Genetic risk assessment and BRCA mutation testing for breast and ovarian cancer susceptibility: recommendation statement. *Ann Intern Med* 2005;143(5):355–361

Vogel VG, Costantino JP, Wickerham DL, et al; National Surgical Adjuvant Breast and Bowel Project (NSABP). Effects of tamoxifen vs raloxifene on the risk of developing invasive breast cancer and other disease outcomes: the NSABP Study of Tamoxifen and Raloxifene (STAR) P-2 trial. *JAMA* 2006;295(23):2727–2741

von Schoultz E, Johansson H, Wilking N, Rutqvist LE. Influence of prior and subsequent pregnancy on breast cancer prognosis. *J Clin Oncol* 1995;13(2):430–434

Section III   Procedures

38 Surgical Procedures in Gynecology

Jon Ivar Einarsson

Gynecologic surgery can be divided into four main categories based on the mode of surgical access: vaginal surgery, abdominal surgery via a laparotomy, abdominal surgery via laparoscopy, and hysteroscopic surgery. The vaginal and hysteroscopic approaches are unique to gynecologic surgery, whereas surgeons of other specialties also perform surgical procedures via laparotomy and laparoscopy. This chapter offers an overview of these surgical procedures as well as an introduction to appropriate preoperative patient selection. We will also discuss simple gynecologic procedures that can be safely performed in the office setting.

Historical Perspective

Gynecologic surgery has come a long way since the first planned vaginal hysterectomy performed in 1813 by Dr. Conrad Langenbeck in Germany. At this time there was no knowledge of antisepsis or anesthesia. Cervical amputation was sometimes performed as a treatment for severe uterine prolapse, but no one had attempted a complete removal of the uterus prior to this. Dr. Langenbeck had summoned a colleague to help him, but since the other doctor was suddenly incapacitated by an episode of severe gout, Dr. Langenbeck had to perform the surgery by himself. The surgery was difficult and he had to use his teeth at one point to tie suture, but nevertheless the patient survived despite "considerable hemorrhage."

Charles Clay in England performed the first abdominal hysterectomy in 1843, where an unexpected finding of a fibroid uterus prompted the hysterectomy. Unfortunately, the patient died from a "great hemorrhage." In those days an exploratory laparotomy was occasionally performed for the removal of a large adnexal mass. Dr. Burnham from Lowell, Massachusetts, performed the first successful (i.e., the patient survived) abdominal hysterectomy in 1853. Despite apparent success, this prompted the following statement from the *London Medico-Chirurgical Review* in 1853: "We consider extirpation of the uterus, not previously protruded or inverted, one of the most cruel and unfeasible operations that ever was projected or executed by the head or hand of man."

Much has changed since then, with hysterectomy currently being the second most commonly performed major surgical procedure (after a cesarean section) in the United States. A more recent revolution is the advent of laparoscopic surgery and other minimally invasive surgical techniques. The first laparoscopic hysterectomy was performed in 1988 and since then rapid advances have been made in technology, equipment, and surgical techniques. Undoubtedly, this rapid evolution will continue in the near future.

Vaginal Surgery

The vaginal approach offers a minimally invasive option for performing an abdominal incision, and has been shown to offer patients faster and less painful postoperative recovery than that experienced after a laparotomy. Some of the more common procedures performed vaginally include:

- cystocele repair
- rectocele repair
- hysterectomy
- sling placement for stress urinary incontinence

Vaginal surgery is an excellent option under the above-mentioned circumstances, although it is not always appropriate. Vaginal surgery sometimes does not allow for adequate visualization of the whole pelvic cavity or the upper abdomen. When a more thorough evaluation of the abdomen is needed, either a laparotomy or laparoscopy is indicated. Common relative contraindications to vaginal surgery include:

- large uterus (uterus extends to above the pelvis or >280 g)
- nulliparity

- narrow pubic arch (>90 °)
- previous cesarean section or other pelvic surgery
- history of pelvic pain and/or endometriosis
- adnexal mass

Abdominal Surgery

Abdominal surgery is performed through a laparotomy, which essentially is a large abdominal incision. The most common type of an abdominal incision used in gynecology is called a Pfannenstiel incision. The reported benefits of this type of incision include better cosmetic outcome and decreased risk of incisional hernias and fascial defects compared with a vertical incision. However, a recent case–control study found no significant difference in fascial defects between a vertical incision and a Pfannenstiel incision. The disadvantages of a Pfannenstiel incision include limited exposure to the upper abdomen, limited extensibility, and potentially longer surgical time.

A midline incision is usually made along the linea alba and can be extended above the umbilicus. The advantages of a midline incision include excellent exposure of the entire abdomen, allowance of a rapid entry into the abdomen, and extensibility. A midline incision should be strongly considered in cases such as a hysterectomy for the very large uterus (>18–20 weeks of pregnancy), gynecologic cancer and extensive peritoneal infection.

Laparoscopy

Laparoscopy is essentially abdominal surgery through very small incisions. In order to maintain a safe and adequate exposure, the abdominal cavity is insufflated (expanded) using inert carbon dioxide gas (no risk of explosion or chemical reaction to the process of surgery). This creates enough space inside the abdomen to allow the surgeon to perform the operation in a safe and effective manner. Patients are often placed in the Trendelenburg position following induction of anesthesia to allow for more exposure, since this makes the bowel fall away from the surgical field in the pelvis. Following induction of anesthesia a 5–10 mm incision is made in the umbilicus. The belly button provides the shortest distance from the skin to the inside of the abdominal cavity. Additionally, it is relatively easy to hide the incision inside the belly button. A Veres needle is commonly inserted through the incision into the abdominal cavity to begin insufflation. Some physicians prefer to do an open approach, where

the abdominal cavity is entered bluntly following sharp dissection down to the level of the peritoneum. This can be especially useful in women with previous surgeries where bowel and omentum can be attached to the underside of the umbilicus. Following insufflation of carbon dioxide gas up to a pressure of 15–25 mmHg, a 5–12-mm trocar is placed through the incision and the laparoscope advanced through the trocar and into the abdominal cavity. (The trocar is essentially a sleeve that allows frequent instrument changes through the abdominal incision without losing intra-abdominal pressure.) A number of ancillary trocars can then be placed depending on the nature of the surgical procedure. Commonly, two to four incisions are used during laparoscopic gynecologic surgery. A video camera is attached to the end of the laparoscope and allows the surgeons and other staff to observe the procedure at all times. Since the surgeons are working in a three-dimensional field, depth perception is reduced while observing the procedure on a two-dimensional screen. Also, the ends of the instruments do not allow as much rotation and movement as the human wrist, which can sometimes make fine or complicated maneuvers, such as suturing, difficult. As a result of these challenges, gynecologic surgeons often need additional training to learn how to compensate for these limitations of laparoscopy. The main advantages of laparoscopy are listed in **Table 38.1** and a schematic illustration of the basic laparoscopy setup is depicted in **Fig. 38.1**.

It is well documented that laparoscopic surgery is superior to abdominal surgery when it comes to postoperative pain levels, recovery time, and time to resumption of normal activities. It has also been associated with reduced bleeding, wound infection rate, and intraperitoneal adhesion formation. However, these cases usually take longer to perform than open surgery and initially certain complications are more common. A large cohort study found that ureteral injuries were more common during laparoscopic hysterectomy than abdominal hysterectomy.

Table 38.1 Advantages of laparoscopy

For patients	Faster recovery
	Less pain
	Smaller incisions
	Early return to normal activities
	Shorter hospital stay
For physicians	Excellent visibility
	Magnification of the lens
	Finer dissection
	All members of the surgical team can follow the progress of the surgical procedure

However after the completion of the first 30 cases, the complication rate decreased dramatically.

The whole operating room team is more important in laparoscopy than during traditional laparotomy because the equipment used is more complex and requires more expertise. The surgeons cooperate closely with the nurses, who often handle the equipment, and the scrub techs who hand the proper instruments to the surgeons during the case. In addition, the Trendelenburg position requires some modification in anesthesia techniques.

The anesthesiologist is critical when it comes to management of the patient during and after surgery. Many of the medications that are used during and after surgery have a strong effect on the outcome and general well-being in the hours immediately after surgery. Some of these effects include nausea and vomiting, paralysis of the intestines causing bloating and a "gassy feeling," constipation, drowsiness, and pain. By optimizing the medications used during and after surgery, all these effects can be minimized effectively .

Hysteroscopy

A hysteroscope has a similar structure to a laparoscope with a long lens, a camera and a light source. However, the hysteroscope is thinner to enable it to pass through the cervical canal. The hysteroscope is passed through the vagina and then the cervix, allowing the physician to view the uterus from the inside (**Fig. 38.2**). This is especially useful in cases where there is abnormal uterine bleeding, uterine fibroids or polyps, or during an infertility work-up. Because the hysteroscope is very thin (only 3–4 mm), it can pass almost painlessly through the cervix, allowing the procedure to be done in the office with no requirement for anesthesia. The average pain level during office hysteroscopy is only 2 to 3 on a 10-point scale, where 0 is no pain and 10 is worst pain ever. A clear view of the uterine cavity allows for an accurate diagnosis and treatment of smaller issues. Additionally, hysteroscopic sterilization is now routinely performed in the office. More complicated cases are still performed in the operating room under general or spinal anesthesia, since these cases take longer and the instruments used are larger, requiring dilation of the cervix. Extensive dilation of the cervix can be very painful and is therefore better suited for the operating room. The uterine cavity is expanded during hysteroscopy using water which runs through the hysteroscope and into the uterine cavity under some pressure. Therefore, the physician is essentially examining the uterine cavity "under water" during hysteroscopy. For diagnostic purposes physicians normally use a sterile saline solution. Saline has similar salt proportion to human blood, making it less likely to cause thinning of the blood should it

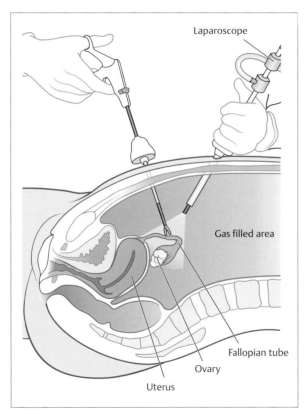

Fig. 38.1 Laparoscopy setup. The laparoscope is inserted through a trocar in the umbilicus and instruments are passed through ancillary trocars as needed. The abdomen is insufflated with carbon dioxide gas, providing the surgeon with adequate room to effectively accomplish the surgery. A camera and a light source are attached to the laparoscope to provide excellent lighting and visualization of the pelvic organs.

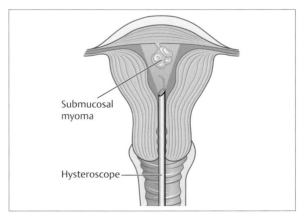

Fig. 38.2 Hysteroscopy principles. The hysteroscope is passed through the vagina and cervix into the uterine cavity. The uterine cavity is expanded with a liquid medium and a camera and a light source are attached to the hysteroscope to provide excellent lighting and visualization of the uterine cavity.

get into the blood stream. If there is thinning of the blood and thus proportionately more water than electrolytes (such as sodium and potassium), this can have potentially devestating effects on the heart physiology causing arrythmias, and in severe cases it can cause hyponatremia with brain edema, confusion, lethargy, agitation, headache, seizures, and even death.

Sometimes it is neccessary to use other liquid media during hystereoscopy. Since there are no free ions in these media, it is possible to use monopolar energy without the dissipation of energy into the fluid as would occur when using normal saline. These media usually have a slightly lower concentration of salts (hypo-osmolar) than the blood. Therefore, if a large amount enters the blood stream, this can result in thinning of the blood and potential electrolyte imbalances. To reduce this risk, modern operating rooms now have special pumps that measure the fluid deficit by constantly measuring the amount of fluid that goes into and out of the uterus. Most hospitals have set rules as to when to stop a case, and the most common stopping point is when the fluid deficit has reached 1000 mL. A high fluid deficit is more common in the following scenarios: lengthy surgery; removal of large fibroids; abnormal connections betweens arteries and veins in the uterus; high water pressure used by the surgeon during the case. Surgeons can minimize the fluid deficit by utilizing the following measures: use the lowest water pressure that allows for a clear view; inject vasopressin intracervically (causes arterial constriction thereby reducing blood flow to the uterus and fibroids); complete the case as quickly as possible.

Using current monitoring guidelines, the risk of complications is reduced. However, women need to be aware of the possibility that the operation may not be completed safely because of excessive water deficit, and that additional surgery might be required at a later date.

Common Gynecologic Procedures

Hysterectomy

Each year approximately 600 000 hysterectomies are performed in the United States, that is, a little more than one uterus is removed during every minute of each year. The vast majority (90%) is performed for noncancerous conditions, such as fibroids, abnormal uterine bleeding, and prolapse of the pelvic organs, with fibroids being the most common indication (30–35%). This incredible number of surgeries means that approximately one-third of American women will have had a hysterectomy by the age of 60 years. Surprisingly, 60% of hysterectomies in the United States are performed via a laparotomy. This is

despite convincing scientific evidence that clearly shows that an abdominal hysterectomy is associated with more pain, more blood loss, longer hospital stay, and longer recovery period than the minimally invasive alternatives: laparoscopic hysterectomy and vaginal hysterectomy. There are probably several reasons for this, including inadequate training, low reimbursement rates, and insufficient surgical volume to develop minimally invasive surgical skills.

Alternatives to Hysterectomy

There are several alternatives that can be attempted prior to proceeding with a hysterectomy. Simply placing a hormonal intrauterine device can significantly reduce menstrual bleeding and allow some women to avoid having a hysterectomy. Uterine fibroid embolization or a myomectomy can be attempted in women with uterine fibroids. However, there are cases where other options are not appropriate or a woman might have had enough of her excessive bleeding and is not willing to accept a 10–15% chance that her initial treatment will not be successful. A hysterectomy is a permanent solution for uterine fibroids, abnormal uterine bleeding, and adenomyosis. It is also often helpful for women with endometriosis, although this is not always the case. Hysterectomies have traditionally been performed in many women with pelvic organ prolapse, but physicians have recently come to understand that the uterus is really just an "innocent bystander" and probably has nothing to do with the prolapse itself, since this is due to torn ligaments and worn-out connective tissue. Hysterectomies are also commonly performed for cancer of the uterus and cervix. However, when these cancers are more advanced, it is better to leave the uterus in place, since the uterus will help to shield other pelvic organs, such as the urinary bladder and the rectum, during the ensuing radiotherapy.

Approaches to Performing a Hysterectomy

There are three main approaches to performing a hysterectomy: abdominal (through a laparotomy incision), laparoscopic, and vaginal. **Table 38.2** lists appropriate surgical candidates for each approach.

Abdominal Hysterectomy

Abdominal hysterectomy is performed through a laparotomy incision. A Pfannenstiel incision is commonly used for smaller uteri for cosmetic reasons; however, a vertical incision is needed for uteri larger than 18–20 weeks in size. Once inside the abdomen, the bowel is pushed away using laparotomy sponges and a retractor is put into the incision to maintain visibility. The round ligaments are

Table 38.2 Mode of access for hysterectomy

Mode of access	Surgical candidates
Vaginal hysterectomy	Small mobile uterus (<12 weeks in size)
	No previous abdominal surgeries
	No previous history of endometriosis
Laparoscopic hysterectomy	Narrow introitus
	Minimal or no uterine descent
	History of multiple abdominal surgeries
	History of endometriosis
	Intent to remove adnexa
Abdominal hysterectomy	Very large uterus (>16–20 weeks)
	Extensive pelvic adhesive disease
	Intraoperative injury
	Hysterectomy for a malignancy in a uterus that will not fit through the vagina

usually clamped, cut and tied first. Next the utero-ovarian ligament or the infundibulopelvic ligaments are clamped, cut and tied, depending on whether or not the ovaries are being removed. The broad ligament is then dissected and cut down to the level of the uterine arteries bilaterally. A bladder flap is then created by cutting the vesicouterine peritoneum and gently moving the urinary bladder off the lower uterine segment. The uterine arteries are then skeletonized, clamped, cut and tied bilaterally. Finally, the uterus is either cut from the cervix (supracervical hysterectomy, SCH) or the vagina is cut around the cervix (total abdominal hysterectomy, TAH) and the uterus is removed through the abdominal incision. The top of the vagina is sutured with absorbable sutures. Once hemostasis has been assured, all instruments and sponges are removed from the abdomen and the abdominal incision is closed in a few layers. The basic steps of an abdominal hysterectomy are depicted in **Fig. 38.3**.

There has been some controversy around the issue of whether or not to remove the cervix during a hysterectomy. Proponents of TAH argue that this is a complete procedure since the cervix is really just an extension of the uterus. In addition, by leaving the cervix in place there might be a higher risk of cervical cancer in the future. Women who have a hysterectomy and keep their cervix also have a 5–20% risk of having continued vaginal spotting. This is usually not a large amount of bleeding, but it can be a nuisance, especially since it is often sporadic. Proponents of SCH argue that healthy tissue should not be removed. In addition, some have argued the cervix is important for sexual function and by keeping it in place there might be less risk of damage to the bladder, rectum,

or ureters since there is less dissection involved. Finally, as long as a woman goes for her regular check up and has a Pap smear, her risk for developing cervical cancer is very small. Recently, there have been three randomized clinical trials comparing TAH and SCH. The investigators did not find a significant difference in sexual, urinary, or bowel function, except that one of the studies found that patients in the TAH group had a significantly lower risk of developing urinary incontinence following the procedure. Similarly, there were no significant differences in other outcomes, postoperative pain or recovery times, except that one of the studies found that hospital stay in the SCH group was significantly shorter than in the TAH group. Women in the SCH group did have a significantly higher rate of vaginal spotting after the hysterectomy (Evidence Box 38.1).

Based on this evidence, there does not seem to be much benefit to keeping the cervix; however, if a woman would like to keep her cervix she can safely do so, as long as she realizes that she may have some continued vaginal spotting afterward. Women who have a history of abnormal Pap smears in the past should probably have a total hysterectomy, because of the potential risk of developing cervical dysplasia in the future. Also, one study that followed 70 patients for 5 years after a supracervical hysterectomy found that 23% of them needed to have the cervix removed during this time period because of symptoms of either pain or bleeding. Most of the patients with continued symptoms had a history of endometriosis and it is possible that some of the endometriosis may have been present in the cervix, leading to persistent pelvic pain. Based on this, women who are having a hysterectomy because of endometriosis or pelvic pain should strongly consider having the cervix removed at the time of their surgery.

Vaginal Hysterectomy

Vaginal hysterectomies performed today are a little more sophisticated than the first vaginal hysterectomy that was performed in 1813, but the basic principles are the same. A vaginal hysterectomy is essentially an abdominal hysterectomy in reverse order. The patient lies supine with the feet held up in the air by specially designed stirrups. The surgeon grasps the cervix and makes a circular incision around it. The bladder and rectum are then gently dissected from the cervix and uterus using sharp and blunt dissection. Next, clamps are placed on the uterosacral ligaments and uterine arteries and they are clamped, cut, and tied. The broad ligament, round ligament and either utero-ovarian or infundibulopelvic ligaments are then serially clamped, cut, and tied to free the uterus, which is subsequently removed through the vagina and the top of the vagina is sutured with absorbable suture. The basic steps of a vaginal hysterectomy are depicted in **Fig. 38.4**.

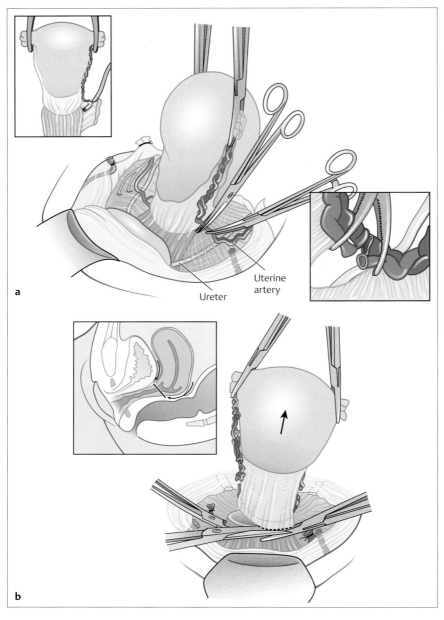

Uterine artery

Ureter

a

b

Fig. 38.3a,b Steps during abdominal hysterectomy. An abdominal hysterectomy starts with division of the round ligaments, followed by the division of the utero-ovarian ligament or the infundibulopelvic ligaments, depending on whether or not the ovaries are being removed. The broad ligament is dissected to the level of the uterine arteries and moving the urinary bladder off the lower uterine segment creates a bladder flap. The uterine arteries are then skeletonized, clamped, cut, and tied bilaterally. Finally, the uterus is either cut from the cervix (supracervical hysterectomy) or the vagina is cut around the cervix (total abdominal hysterectomy) and the uterus is removed through the abdominal incision. The top of the vagina is closed with absorbable sutures. **a** Ligation of the uterine artery. Clamp placement is perpendicular to the uterine vasculature. **b** Resection of the uterus.

Vaginal hysterectomy has several advantages. It is minimally invasive and recovery time is shorter than that following an abdominal surgery. It requires only a few simple instruments, which means that it is less expensive to perform than a laparoscopic hysterectomy, where more specialized equipment is needed. It is especially applicable in women with pelvic organ prolapse, since there is easy access to perform concomitant procedures. The main disadvantage of the vaginal approach is decreased intra-abdominal visibility. It is also more technically difficult to perform in patients with extensive adhesions and endometriosis. Also, it is not well suited when there are ovarian masses that need to be removed, since vaginal oo-

phorectomy is not possible in 10% of cases. A narrow pelvic arch might also make the procedure technically difficult to complete.

Because vaginal hysterectomy is the least expensive method, and a minimally invasive method with similar recovery times as a laparoscopic hysterectomy, it should be the first choice in women with a relatively small uterus who have delivered their children vaginally, have no history of previous surgery in the pelvis or of endometriosis, and who do not have any ovarian masses or cysts present.

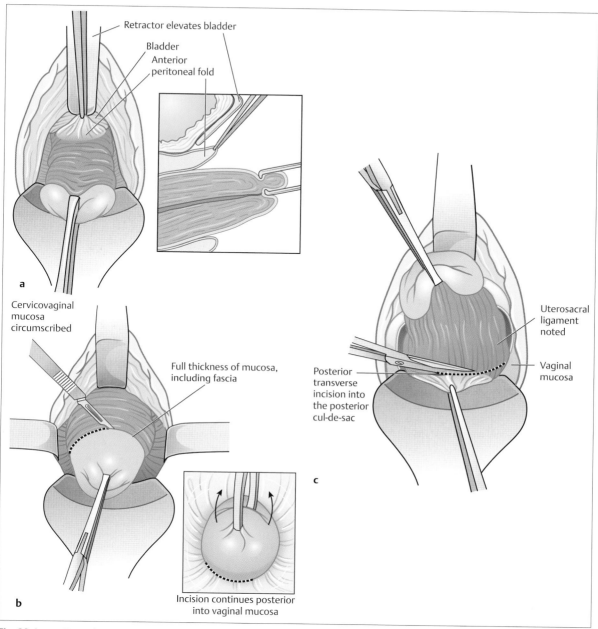

Fig. 38.4a–c Steps during vaginal hysterectomy. A vaginal hysterectomy begins with a circular incision around the cervix. The posterior cul-de-sac is then entered sharply and the uterosacral ligaments are divided. The bladder and rectum are then gently dissected from the cervix and uterus using sharp and blunt dissection, and the peritoneum is entered between the uterus and the urinary bladder. Next, the uterine arteries are divided. The broad ligament, round ligament, and either utero-ovarian or infundibulopelvic ligaments are then serially divided to free the uterus, which is removed and the top of the vagina is closed using absorbable suture. **a** Identification of the anterior peritoneal reflection. **b** Incision into the anterior vaginal mucosa. This is performed at the level of the cervicovaginal mucosa. **c** Incising the posterior cul-de-sac. Scissors are used to enter the vagina through the posterior cul-de-sac.

Laparoscopic Hysterectomy

Laparoscopic hysterectomy is intended to replace abdominal hysterectomy. It has several advantages over abdominal hysterectomy. It has been well established that patients who have a laparoscopic hysterectomy have less pain, less bleeding, less risk of infection, and are quicker to return to work and normal activities than women who have had an abdominal hysterectomy. Therefore, it should be the first option in women who are not good candidates for a vaginal hysterectomy as outlined previously. The laparoscopic approach gives the surgeon superior visibility inside the pelvis than during vaginal surgery, and even better visibility than during abdominal surgery. This is in part because of the possibility to magnify the image on the screen and because the lighting is much better during laparoscopy.

Following insertion of laparoscopic trocars, the procedure is carried out in a similar manner to the abdominal hysterectomy. Instead of using a clamp and sutures, most surgeons now use thermal energy to seal and cut the blood vessels, since this saves significant time over the traditional suturing technique. This adaptation was necessary, since clamps used during open surgery are not as well suited for laparoscopic surgery. Once the uterus is completely freed it is either delivered through the vagina or through an electronic morcellator (see section on uterine fibroids). The top of the vagina is sutured either laparoscopically or through the vagina using absorbable sutures.

The average time to resumption of normal activities after a laparoscopic or a vaginal hysterectomy is approximately 3 weeks. Some women are up and running in less than a week, but most women take a little longer than that. This is a big difference compared with the 6–8 weeks it takes to get back to normal after an abdominal hysterectomy.

With advancements in anesthesia and surgical techniques, many patients are able to go home the same day after a laparoscopic or a vaginal hysterectomy, which is an added benefit to those patients who do not want to spend the night in a hospital. Many patients elect to stay overnight and a few require a longer hospital stay, especially if there are any complications.

Complications of Hysterectomy

It is important to remember, regardless of the method used, that a hysterectomy is a major surgical procedure and can lead to serious complications. Fortunately, these complications are rare, especially in the hands of an experienced surgeon. The most common complications following a hysterectomy are infection and bleeding. Infection usually occurs either in the skin incision or in the vaginal cuff. Most often these infections respond to antibiotic therapy, but occasionally additional surgery is needed. The average blood loss during a vaginal and a laparoscopic hysterectomy is approximately 80–100 mL, which is equal to the amount of blood lost during three normal menstrual cycles. Occasionally, significant bleeding can be encountered and therefore adequate preoperative counseling of the use of blood products is needed. This is especially important in women who are already anemic because of long-standing menorrhagia. Damage to other pelvic organs is also a potential risk, such as injury to the urinary bladder, bowel, or the ureters.

Fortunately, the risk of these major complications is less than 1%. However, they can be very serious and

in some cases fatal. They become especially dangerous when they are not recognized during surgery, as may be the case with injuries to the bowel, where severe infection can develop rapidly following a bowel injury that is not corrected during surgery. Every attempt is therefore made to recognize these injuries during surgery. Occasionally, surgeons will cut into these organs on purpose, such as in the case of endometriosis or cancer, so experienced gynecologic surgeons are used to dealing with these complications.

Finally, women should always be aware that any time a hysterectomy is attempted laparoscopically or vaginally, there is a small risk that it will be necessary to make a larger incision to safely complete the procedure. How often this happens depends on the experience of the surgeon, the difficulty of the surgery and the appropriateness of patient selection, but overall this should not happen more than 5% of the time.

Myomectomy

Uterine fibroids are benign tumors that arise from the myometrium. The uterus is mostly made out of smooth muscle cells, designed to expand with the growing pregnancy and to help with vaginal delivery by contracting forcefully at the end of pregnancy. Uterine fibroids can grow underneath the endometrium (submucosal), in the myometrium (intramural), or underneath the uterine serosa (subserosal). **Figure 38.5** gives a schematic presentation of common locations of uterine fibroids.

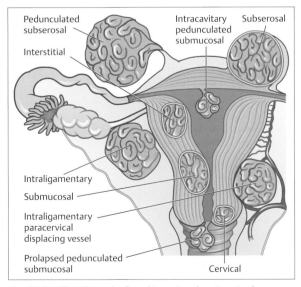

Fig. 38.5 Fibroids can be found in various locations in the uterus. The figure shows a classification of uterine myomas by location. Reproduced courtesy of Dr. William J. Mann, Jr.

Uterine fibroids are very common and are found in about 25 % of women between the ages of 18 and 45 years. When examining surgically removed uteri from women of all ages, up to 80 % of women are found to have some fibroids present. African-American women have a higher risk of developing uterine fibroids compared with Caucasian women.

Diagnosis

Large fibroids can usually be identified during a regular physical exam. Ultrasound scanning can identify most fibroids and is easily performed in a doctor's office. The addition of saline infusion sonohysterography can help to identify fibroids that are inside the uterine cavity. Office hysteroscopy is also a helpful tool for the detection of uterine fibroids inside the uterine cavity. Magnetic resonance imaging (MRI) provides excellent information in regard to the exact location and size of the fibroids. It is a very useful tool to determine appropriate treatment options, such as removal of the uterine fibroids (myomectomy), embolization or focused ultrasound. MRI can also be helpful in determining whether there is something else in the uterus that is causing the symptoms, such as adenomyosis or a leiomyosarcoma. It is, however, the most expensive diagnostic option and should be used selectively.

Treatment for Uterine Fibroids

It is important to note that since fibroids are not cancerous, no treatment at all is probably the best option for women who are asymptomatic. The main indications for a myomectomy are listed in **Table 38.3.** The traditional treatment for uterine fibroids is via a laparotomy with either removal of the uterus (hysterectomy) or removal of the fibroids (myomectomy). Hysterectomy has usually been recommended for women who are not planning to have any more children, since there is a 15–20 % recurrence of symptoms following a myomectomy that requires additional surgery. However, some women want to conserve their uterus, even though they are not going to have any more children. It is important to respect their wishes as long as they fully understand the risks and benefits associated with their decision.

Table 38.3 Indications for a myomectomy

Abnormal uterine bleeding
Pelvic pain or pressure
Urinary frequency and/or hydronephrosis
Infertility
Recurrent pregnancy loss

As mentioned previously, myomectomy is commonly performed in women who want to retain their fertility. It is possible to remove most fibroids laparoscopically or hysteroscopically, however there are certain limitations such as size and location, which we will discuss. It depends largely on the surgeon's skill and experience as to what cases can be performed laparoscopically. In general, fibroids larger than 10 cm that are inside the uterine muscle (intramural) can be difficult to remove. Also, if there are many fibroids (>5) it can be difficult to complete the surgery laparoscopically. Fibroids that are located next to large blood vessels or in the cervix can also be challenging to remove laparoscopically. A main limiting factor is laparoscopic suturing. Suturing laparoscopically is a very advanced skill and many gynecologists do not have the capability to do this properly. It is critical to close the uterine incision adequately, to minimize the risk of uterine rupture during a subsequent pregnancy.

Procedure: A myomectomy is usually performed in the following manner. An incision is made into the uterine serosa and carried all the way into the fibroid. The fibroid is then freed from the uterus by pulling and cutting away its attachments. Once the fibroid is removed the uterine incision is closed in layers, usually three to four, depending on the depth of the uterine incision. **Figure 38.6** presents a schematic depiction of the basic surgical steps during a myomectomy.

The fibroid itself is removed via the abdominal incision, or by using a morcellator if this performed laparoscopically. A laparoscopic morcellator is a long hollow cylinder with a sharp circular blade at one end. A grasper is put through the morcellator and the tissue is pulled toward the circular blade. The blade is activated by pressing a button or a pedal, resulting in rapid circulatory blade motion. By pulling the tissue into the blade, the fibroid can be removed from the abdomen in long strips of tissue, similar to apple cores. Using this techniqe, large amounts of tissue can be removed through a 1.2–1.5 cm wide opening.

Because suturing is the most challenging part during a laparoscopic myomectomy, some modifications have been developed. One is called a laparoscopically assisted myomectomy (LAM). During this technique the fibroid is released laparoscopically as previously described and then a small laparotomy incision (5–6 cm) is made above the pubic hairline. The fibroid is removed through this incision and the uterus is sutured through it as well. This technique is well suited when dealing with a large number of fibroids or when physicians are not proficient in laparoscopic suturing. It is not well suited for fibroids that are located on the back of the uterus, since it is difficult to reach this area through a small incision.

Another alternative is using the da Vinci robot for the myomectomy. The da Vinci robot consists of three to four mechanical arms that are controlled by the surgeon from

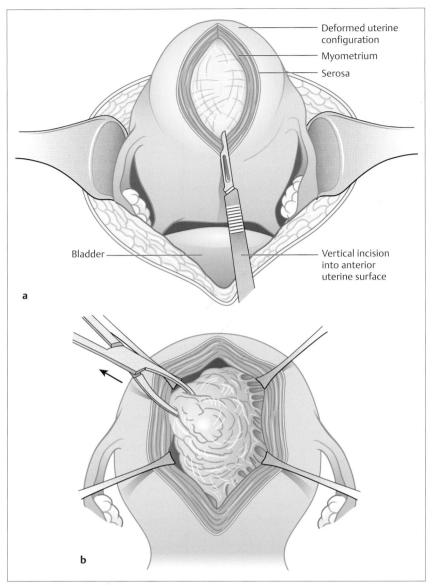

Deformed uterine configuration

Myometrium

Serosa

Bladder

Vertical incision into anterior uterine surface

a

b

Fig. 38.6a, b Steps during a myomectomy. A myomectomy starts with an incision into the uterine serosa. This is followed by an extraction of the fibroid using traction and careful dissection. Finally, the uterine wall is closed in layers (endometrium, myometrium, serosa).
a Abdominal myomectomy. Initial vertical incision into the anterior uterine surface.
b Towel clamp placed on myoma for traction to aid in dissection. Reproduced courtesy of Dr. William J. Mann, Jr.

a separate control unit (console). The arms of the robot can carry various instruments and the instruments can move freely at the tip, allowing much more freedom of movement than with traditional laparoscopy. In addition, the surgeon has three dimensional vision of his environment through the control unit. This greatly facilitates laparoscopic suturing and allows more surgeons to be able to complete these cases laparoscopically. However, the robot has some disadvantages, including lack of tactile sensation, long set-up times and significantly increased cost.

Oophorectomy

Gynecologists have become more conservative when it comes to removing the ovaries in the last few years, especially in women who have not yet entered menopause. A bilateral oophorectomy can result in significant postmenopausal symptoms, such as hot flushes, night sweats, insomnia, irritability and vaginal dryness. Recent evidence also suggests that women who had their ovaries removed have a lower life expectancy than women with intact ovaries.

The main indications for an oophorectomy are:
- malignancy
- prophylaxis due to breast cancer or hereditary conditions (e.g., BRCA 1 and 2 mutations)
- pelvic pain
- endometriosis

Oophorectomy secondary to malignancy will be covered in Chapter 51. Briefly, oophorectomy has been shown to reduce the incidence of breast cancer and ovarian cancer in women with the BRCA 1 and 2 mutations. In addition, it reduces the risk of recurrence in women diagnosed with breast cancer.

Pelvic pain localized to either the right or left side of the pelvis can sometimes be relieved with a unilateral oophorectomy. Conservative measures and a search for alternative sources of pelvic pain should precede this step.

Women with severe pelvic pain associated with endometriosis sometimes benefit from a bilateral oophorectomy. Again, this should be a last ditch effort. Retrospective studies have demonstrated that women who have a bilateral oophorectomy in conjunction with endometriosis surgery have a significantly decreased risk of having repeat surgery for pelvic pain.

Technique

The ovary descends to the pelvis from the abdomen during fetal development. The ovary receives its blood supply from the infundibulopelvic ligament and the utero-ovarian ligament. The infundibulopelvic ligament contains the ovarian artery and vein. The ovarian arteries arise from the abdominal aorta and the ovarian veins end up in the vena cava (right ovarian vein) and the renal vein (left ovarian vein). It is easy to remember which goes where by imagining that the liver pushes everything on the right side downward, so that the right ovarian vein does not reach the renal vein.

Care must be taken during transection of the infundibulopelvic ligament, since the ureter crosses over the pelvic brim and into the pelvis in close vicinity to the ovary and the infundibulopelvic ligament. Identification of the ureter is therefore the first step of an oophorectomy, followed by a transection of the infundibulopelvic ligament. The ovary is subsequently released from its filmy attachments to the mesosalpinx and finally from the uterus by transecting the utero-ovarian ligament. With a normal sized ovary and no pelvic adhesive disease or endometriosis, an oophorectomy is a relatively simple procedure. However, an oophorectomy can be a very challenging procedure given the above-mentioned conditions, often requiring extensive adhesiolysis and ureterolysis. In addition, postmenopausal women often have very small ovaries that can be difficult to identify, especially in the context of severe pelvic adhesive disease.

Ovarian Cystectomy

It is not uncommon for ovarian cysts to occur, in fact this happens every month in most women of reproductive age. However, persistent ovarian cysts that are abnormal in nature (see Chapter 51) need to be surgically removed. This can be accomplished laparoscopically or via a laparotomy. The laparoscopic approach is preferable due to lower postoperative morbidity if the cyst is relatively small (<10 cm) and of low malignant potential. During this procedure the ovarian cortex is incised and peeled off the underlying ovarian cyst. This is essentially like peeling a balloon off an underlying balloon filled with water. It is important to get a clear tissue plane started initially in the event that the cyst ruptures, since it is more difficult to find the correct plane following cyst rupture. The basic surgical steps of an ovarian cystectomy are shown in **Fig. 38.7**.

Every effort is made to avoid spillage of the ovarian cyst content. However, it depends on the nature of the cyst as to how easy it is to remove it intact. For example, endometriomas are very difficult to remove without rupture, since there is often no clear surgical plane present. Smaller dermoid cysts are much easier to peel from the ovary, but nevertheless rupture and spillage of contents can occur, especially with larger cysts. This is usually of no consequence, provided that the peritoneal cavity is thoroughly irrigated with saline following spillage. Once the cyst is peeled off the ovary it is placed in a bag and removed through one of the trocar sites. The ovary usually does not need to be sutured back together; however, meticulous hemostasis should be assured. The procedure is essentially the same when performed via a laparotomy, except that the extraction of the mass is much simpler.

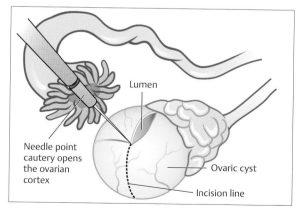

Fig. 38.7 Steps during a laparoscopic ovarian cystectomy. The ovarian cortex is incised in the direction of the ovarian axis, followed by a careful dissection of the cyst wall from the overlying ovary. The cyst is then removed through a bag to avoid spillage of contents into the peritoneal cavity. . Reproduced courtesy of Dr. William J. Mann, Jr.

If there is a suspicion of malignancy, peritoneal washings should be obtained at the beginning of the procedure, the mass should be sent for a frozen section and surgical staging should be completed in the event of malignancy. The effects of intraoperative spillage on prognosis are uncertain, with some studies showing no effect on recurrence or survival and others showing increased rates of recurrence with intraoperative spillage. Most experts agree that spillage should be avoided when dealing with a suspicious adnexal mass; if intraoperative spillage occurs, full surgical staging should be undertaken followed by a course of prophylactic chemotherapy.

Dilation and Curettage

This time honored procedure has been largely replaced by office-based evaluation of the endometrial cavity; that is, office endometrial biopsy, ultrasound imaging, and office hysteroscopy. It has been relatively well established that dilation and curettage alone is a relatively poor therapeutic and diagnostic option, since it misses up to 60% of intrauterine abnormalities subsequently found at hysterectomy. Therefore, hysteroscopy should be performed concurrently with dilation and curettage to improve the diagnostic accuracy of this procedure.

Dilation and curettage can be performed in the office with paracervical block or in the operating room under general anesthesia. A speculum is placed in the vagina and the cervix grasped with a tenaculum. A uterine sound is placed through the cervix to evaluate the size of the endometrial cavity, followed by a gradual dilation of the cervix if needed. A sharp curette is then passed through the cervix into the endometrial cavity and the endometrial lining is systematically sampled and the tissue withdrawn through the cervix and sent for pathology.

Potential complications of include uterine perforation, cervical laceration, infection and formation of intrauterine adhesions (Asherman syndrome). Perforation most commonly occurs during dilatation of the cervix. If the perforation is in the fundal area and was made with a blunt dilator the patient will usually only require 1 week of postoperative antibiotic therapy. However, if the perforation is performed with a sharp object, or if the perforation occurs in the lateral and more vascular segments of the uterus, more careful evaluation is needed, such as an immediate laparoscopy to evaluate any internal bleeding or damage to internal organs.

Robotic Surgery

As a relatively recent development, robotic surgery holds much promise as an improvement to some of the limitations of operative laparoscopy. This includes the ability for wristlike movements at the tip of the instrument, three-dimensional vision, and comfortable work environment for the surgeon. These features enhance the surgeon's capabilities to perform complex laparoscopic suturing and meticulous dissections. However, there are some limitations as well. The robot does not allow any tactile sensation for the surgeon who must rely on visual cues to guide in tying sutures and pulling on tissue. The robot is bulky and requires a relatively long setup time and a larger operating room. It is also difficult to effectively use a uterine manipulator owing to the bulk of the robot. That being said, the robot is currently being used for lymph node dissections, laparoscopic radical hysterectomies, laparoscopic tubal re-anastomosis, and laparoscopic myomectomies. Other applications are in development. It is very likely that, with time, robotic surgery will become more streamlined and will be appropriately incorporated into the armamentarium of minimally invasive surgical techniques.

Office Procedures

Endometrial Biopsy

An endometrial biopsy is most commonly used to evaluate the endometrium in women who present with abnormal uterine bleeding. This is mainly to rule out endometrial hyperplasia or endometrial cancer. An endometrial biopsy using a Pipelle seems to be at least as effective as a dilation and curettage for the diagnosis of endometrial malignancies with a detection rate of 99.6% and 91% in postmenopausal and premenopausal women, respectively.

Procedure

An endometrial biopsy involves placing a narrow (3–4 mm) plastic tube (Pipelle) through the cervix into the uterus to sample the endometrium. A speculum is placed in the vagina, the cervix is visualized and the plastic tube is passed through the cervix and into the uterus. Occasionally the cervix needs to be grasped with a tenaculum for counter-traction; however, this should not be done routinely as it can be relatively painful. The endometrial biopsy catheter has a small opening at the distal end and inside the hollow tube is a small plunger that can be withdrawn for gentle suction. The tube is twisted inside the uterine cavity, thereby gently scraping cells from the endometrium which are in turn suctioned into the catheter by withdrawing the plunger. This part usually takes less than a minute.

The average pain level during an endometrial biopsy is 3 to 5 on a 10-point scale; however, some women are not able to tolerate this procedure in the office, often due to cervical stenosis or anatomical distortion caused by uterine fibroids. The endometrial sample is placed in formaldehyde and sent to the pathology lab for evaluation.

Saline Infusion Sonohysterography

This is an extension of the pelvic ultrasound exam. A narrow plastic catheter is placed into the uterus and during the ultrasound exam 10–15 mL of water are injected into the uterine cavity. The water briefly expands the uterine cavity and acts as a contrast medium during ultrasonography. This allows for a more precise visualization of the endometrium, especially if there is suspicion of uterine polyps or submucous fibroids.

Office Hysteroscopy

The hysteroscope is passed through the vagina and then the cervix, allowing the physician to view the uterus from the inside. This is especially useful for the evaluation of abnormal uterine bleeding, uterine fibroids or polyps, or during an infertility work-up. Because the hysteroscope is very thin (only 3–4 mm), it can pass almost painlessly through the cervix, allowing the physician to perform the procedure in the office with no required anesthesia. The average pain level that women feel during office hysteroscopy is only 2 to 3 on a 10-point scale. Some prefer the vaginoscopic approach, where the hysteroscope is placed into the vagina without a speculum or a tenaculum on the cervix. The hysteroscope is then advanced through the cervix and into the uterus. The vaginoscopic approach has been associated with slightly less pain and discomfort when compared with traditional hysteroscopy; however, this is not always possible especially in case of cervical stenosis when dilation of the cervix is required. Office hysteroscopy allows for accurate diagnosis and treatment for smaller issues, such as endometrial polyps, removal of an intrauterine device, or treatment of intrauterine adhesions. In addition, it is more convenient for the physician and the patient, since the procedure can be accomplished in less than 5 minutes.

Key Points

- Hysterectomy is one of the most common surgical procedures.
- Hysterectomy can be performed using three main approaches: laparoscopy, abdominal laparotomy, or vaginal surgery.
- Evidence indicates that vaginal hysterectomy is the best option if it is technically feasible. Vaginal hysterectomy is associated with fewer complications than laparoscopic or abdominal hysterectomy.
- Compared with abdominal hysterectomy, laparoscopic hysterectomy uses more operating room time, but is associated with faster patient recovery.
- For all hysterectomy procedures thromboprophylaxis and pre-incision antibiotics to reduce infectious morbidity are recommended.
- The continuous development of advanced surgical equipment is permitting most gynecologic procedures that were historically performed through an abdominal laparotomy incision to be replaced by procedures performed through the laparoscope. Laparoscopic surgery is associated with more rapid patient recovery and return to full function than abdominal laparotomy surgery.

Evidence Box 38.1

Cervix removal at hysterectomy has minimal effect on perioperative and postoperative morbidity.

A total of 279 women scheduled to undergo an abdominal hysterectomy for benign indications were randomized to have either a supracervical hysterectomy or a total abdominal hysterectomy. The primary end-point of the study was the incidence of stress urinary incontinence following hysterectomy with one-year of follow-up. Other outcome measures included bowel function, sexual function, and incidence of postoperative complications.

There were no statistically significant differences in urinary, bowel, or sexual function between the two groups. There was an improvement in nocturia and stress urinary incontinence following surgery in both groups. Women in the supracervical hysterectomy group had a shorter hospital stay (5.2 days vs. 6.0 days) and a lower rate of fever (6% vs. 19%). However, 7% of women in the supracervical hysterectomy group experienced cyclical bleeding and 2% had cervical prolapse.

This was the first, well-designed prospective randomized trial comparing clinical outcomes following supracervical and total hysterectomy. Subsequent clinical trials have noted similar results. This indicates that cervix removal at the time of hysterectomy is not an important factor for postoperative bowel, bladder, or sexual function. Patients can elect to retain the cervix following appropriate counseling with their physician, provided there is not a strong indication for cervix removal, such as severe cervical dysplasia

Thakar R, Ayers S, Clarkson P, Stanton S, Manyonda I. Outcomes after total versus subtotal abdominal hysterectomy. N Engl J Med 2002;347(17):1318–1325.

Further Reading

Advincula AP, Song A, Burke W, Reynolds RK. Preliminary experience with robot-assisted laparoscopic myomectomy. *J Am Assoc Gynecol Laparosc* 2004;11(4):511–518

Berridge DL, Winter TC. Saline infusion sonohysterography: technique, indications, and imaging findings. *J Ultrasound Med* 2004;23(1):97–112, quiz 114–115

Bettocchi S, Ceci O, Vicino M, Marello F, Impedovo L, Selvaggi L. Diagnostic inadequacy of dilatation and curettage. *Fertil Steril* 2001;75(4):803–805

Byrne H, Ball E, Davis C. The role of magnetic resonance imaging in minimal access surgery. *Curr Opin Obstet Gynecol* 2006;18(4):369–373

Dembo AJ, Davy M, Stenwig AE, Berle EJ, Bush RS, Kjorstad K. Prognostic factors in patients with stage I epithelial ovarian cancer. *Obstet Gynecol* 1990;75(2):263–273

Dijkhuizen FP, Mol BW, Brölmann HA, Heintz AP. The accuracy of endometrial sampling in the diagnosis of patients with endometrial carcinoma and hyperplasia: a meta-analysis. *Cancer* 2000;89(8):1765–1772

Domchek SM, Friebel TM, Neuhausen SL, et al. Mortality after bilateral salpingo-oophorectomy in BRCA1 and BRCA2 mutation carriers: a prospective cohort study. *Lancet Oncol* 2006;7(3):223–229

Einarsson JI, Henao G, Young AE. Topical analgesia for endometrial biopsy: a randomized controlled trial. *Obstet Gynecol* 2005;106(1):128–130

Gerges FJ, Kanazi GE, Jabbour-Khoury SI. Anesthesia for laparoscopy: a review. *J Clin Anesth* 2006;18(1):67–78

Gimbel H, Zobbe V, Andersen BJ, et al. Lower urinary tract symptoms after total and subtotal hysterectomy: results of a randomized controlled trial. *Int Urogynecol J Pelvic Floor Dysfunct* 2005;16(4):257–262

Guida M, Di Spiezio Sardo A, Acunzo G, et al. Vaginoscopic versus traditional office hysteroscopy: a randomized controlled study. *Hum Reprod* 2006;21(12):3253–3257

Hendrix SL, Schimp V, Martin J, Singh A, Kruger M, McNeeley SG. The legendary superior strength of the Pfannenstiel incision: a myth? *Am J Obstet Gynecol* 2000;182(6):1446–1451

Johnson N, Barlow D, Lethaby A, Tavender E, Curr E, Garry R. Surgical approach to hysterectomy for benign gynaecological disease. *Cochrane Database Syst Rev* 2006;19(2):CD003677

Kozak LJ, Owings MF, Hall MJ; National Center for Health Statistics. National Hospital Discharge Survey: 2002 annual summary with detailed diagnosis and procedure data. *Vital Health Stat 13* 2005;158(158):1–199

Learman LA, Summitt RL Jr, Varner RE, et al; Total or Supracervical Hysterectomy (TOSH) Research Group. A randomized comparison of total or supracervical hysterectomy: surgical complications and clinical outcomes. *Obstet Gynecol* 2003;102(3):453–462

Leodolter S. The transvaginal surgical school in Austria. Retrospect-present-future . [Article in German] *Gynakol Geburtshilfliche Rundsch* 1995;35(3):142–148

Lethaby A, Ivanova V, Johnson NP. Total versus subtotal hysterectomy for benign gynaecological conditions. *Cochrane Database Syst Rev* 2006;19(2):CD004993

Lethaby AE, Cooke I, Rees M. Progesterone or progestogen-releasing intrauterine systems for heavy menstrual bleeding. *Cochrane Database Syst Rev* 2005;18(4):CD002126

Mäkinen J, Johansson J, Tomás C, et al. Morbidity of 10110 hysterectomies by type of approach. *Hum Reprod* 2001;16(7):1473–1478

Namnoum AB, Hickman TN, Goodman SB, Gehlbach DL, Rock JA. Incidence of symptom recurrence after hysterectomy for endometriosis. *Fertil Steril* 1995;64(5):898–902

Okaro EO, Jones KD, Sutton C. Long term outcome following laparoscopic supracervical hysterectomy. *BJOG* 2001;108(10):1017–1020

Paparella P, Sizzi O, Rossetti A, De Benedittis F, Paparella R. Vaginal hysterectomy in generally considered contraindications to vaginal surgery. *Arch Gynecol Obstet* 2004;270(2):104–109

Parker WH, Broder MS, Liu Z, Shoupe D, Farquhar C, Berek JS. Ovarian conservation at the time of hysterectomy for benign disease. *Obstet Gynecol* 2005;106(2):219–226

Practice Committee of the American Society for Reproductive Medicine. Myomas and reproductive function. *Fertil Steril* 2006; 86(5, Suppl)S194–S199

Reich H, DeCaprio J, McGlynn F. Laparoscopic hysterectomy. *J Gynecol Surg* 1989;5:213–216

Sainz de la Cuesta R, Goff BA, Fuller AF Jr, Nikrui N, Eichhorn JH, Rice LW. Prognostic importance of intraoperative rupture of malignant ovarian epithelial neoplasms. *Obstet Gynecol* 1994;84(1):1–7

Subramanian S, Clark MA, Isaacson K. Outcome and resource use associated with myomectomy. *Obstet Gynecol* 2001;98(4):583–587

Sutton C. Hysterectomy: a historical perspective. *Baillieres Clin Obstet Gynaecol* 1997;11(1):1–22

Sutton C. Hysteroscopic surgery. *Best Pract Res Clin Obstet Gynaecol* 2006;20(1):105–137

Taniguchi F, Harada T, Iwabe T, Yoshida S, Mitsunari M, Terakawa N. Use of the LAP DISK (abdominal wall sealing device) in laparoscopically assisted myomectomy. *Fertil Steril* 2004;81(4):1120–1124

Thakar R, Ayers S, Clarkson P, Stanton S, Manyonda I. Outcomes after total versus subtotal abdominal hysterectomy. *N Engl J Med* 2002;347(17):1318–1325

van Sprundel TC, Schmidt MK, Rookus MA, et al. Risk reduction of contralateral breast cancer and survival after contralateral prophylactic mastectomy in BRCA1 or BRCA2 mutation carriers. *Br J Cancer* 2005;93(3):287–292

Part IV Reproductive Endocrinology, Infertility, and Related Topics

39 Amenorrhea and Dysfunctional Uterine Bleeding

Robert L. Barbieri

Amenorrhea

The menstrual cycle is orchestrated through the interaction of the hypothalamus, pituitary gland, ovaries, and uterus (**Table 39.1**). The conductor of the system is the hypothalamus that sets the beat by secreting gonadotropin-releasing hormone (GnRH) in a pulsatile fashion into the portal circulation. In turn, pulses of GnRH stimulate the pituitary to secrete luteinizing hormone (LH) and follicle-stimulating hormone (FSH), which cause the development of an ovarian follicle.

When the follicle reaches a size commensurate with the capacity to ovulate, the follicle secretes sufficient estradiol to trigger a surge of LH secretion from the pituitary. The LH surge causes the follicle to undergo rupture (ovulation) and the oocyte contained in the follicle matures and prepares for fertilization by proceeding through the final steps in meiosis I. If fertilization occurs, the embryo may implant in the endometrium about 6 days after ovulation. If no fertilization occurs, the corpus luteum is programmed to undergo apoptosis and cease secretion of estradiol and progesterone, causing the onset of menses and the beginning of a new cycle. At the endometrial level, in the uterus, the menstrual cycle has three key phases: 1) estradiol stimulates endometrial growth (from about 3 mm to 14 mm in depth); 2) progesterone induces differentiation of the endometrium in preparation for embryo implantation; and 3) the withdrawal of estradiol and progesterone results in sloughing of the endometrium and menstrual bleeding.

Diseases and physiological processes that affect any of the four components of this orchestrated system can result in the absence of menstruation—amenorrhea. A girl may not start to menstruate when she reaches puberty (primary amenorrhea), or a woman who has been menstruating may have her cycles cease (secondary amenorrhea).

Secondary Amenorrhea

Secondary amenorrhea, or adult-onset amenorrhea, is present when a woman who had been menstruating has no menses for longer than three of her previous cycles, or 6 months.

The most common causes of secondary amenorrhea are:
- pregnancy
- polycystic ovary syndrome (see Chapter 40)

Table 39.1 The normal ovulatory menstrual cycle is an orchestrated performance led by the hypothalamus

Organ	Key hormonal product(s)	Hormones that stimulate secretion	Hormones that inhibit secretion
Hypothalamus	Pulsatile GnRH	Kisspeptin, GPR54	Prolactin, opioids
Pituitary	LH and FSH	GnRH	Combination of estrogen and progesterone. Inhibins
Ovary	Estradiol and progesterone	LH, FSH, IGF-I, insulin	Antimüllerian hormone
Uterine endometrium	Prostaglandins		

FSH, follicle-stimulating hormone; GnRH, gonadotropin-releasing hormone; GPR54, ??? IGF-1, insulinlike growth factor 1; LH, luteinizing hormone.

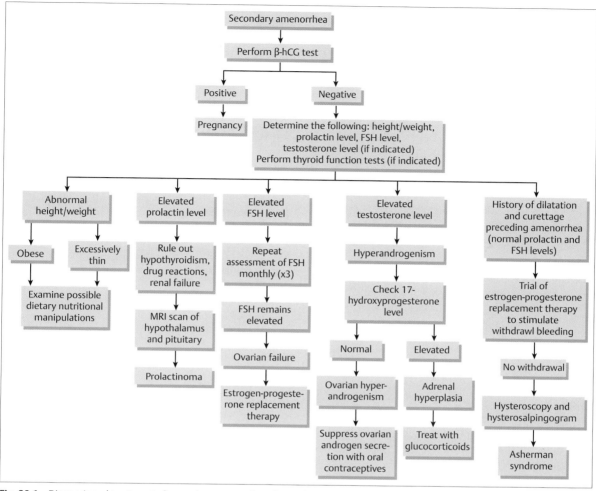

Fig. 39.1 Diagnosis and treatment of secondary amenorrhea. β-HCG, human chorionic gonadotropin; FSH, follicle-stimulating hormone.

- functional causes of decreased GnRH secretion such as low body mass index (BMI), eating disorders, strenuous exercise, and psychological stress
- prolactin-secreting pituitary tumor
- primary ovarian failure
- intrauterine adhesions (Asherman syndrome) (**Table 39.2**).

Secondary amenorrhea affects less than 1% of the adult female population, if pregnancy is excluded as a cause.

Determining the cause of secondary amenorrhea begins with a focused history (past menstrual pattern, evidence for eating disorder, psychological stress, strenuous exercise), physical examination (calculated BMI, presence of hirsutism or virilization, galactorrhea), and measurement of serum human chorionic gonadotropin (HCG), prolactin, FSH, and testosterone. Based on this data, use of an algorithm can help direct diagnosis and care (**Fig. 39.1**).

Hypothalamic Dysfunction

Low BMI, vigorous exercise, psychosocial stress, and nutritional abnormalities decrease GnRH production. This reduces LH and FSH secretion, stops ovarian follicle growth and secretion of estradiol and progesterone, and causes amenorrhea.

Diagnosis: The patient typically has a history of regular vigorous exercise, psychosocial stress, reduced caloric intake and/or an eating disorder. On physical examination, the BMI may be less than 20 kg/m². Serum FSH, prolactin and testosterone levels are usually in the normal range. Rarely, hypothalamic dysfunction caused by infiltrative processes or tumors, such as sarcoidosis, histiocytosis, and hypothalamic cysts may cause amenorrhea.

A progestin withdrawal test may help to assess the severity of the hypoestrogenism. In a patient with a hypothalamic cause of secondary amenorrhea, and no uterine bleeding after a progestin withdrawal test, the circulating

Table 39.2 The most common causes of secondary amenorrhea in women who are not pregnant.

Organ	Cause	Relative frequency
Hypothalamus	Abnormalities of height/ weight and nutrition	15%
	Strenuous exercise	10%
	Psychological stress	10%
	Tumors of the hypothalamus including sarcoidosis, histiocytosis, craniopharyngioma)	<0.1%
Pituitary	Prolactin-secreting pituitary tumor	17%
	Empty sella syndrome	1%
	Sheehan syndrome	<1%
	ACTH-secreting tumor (Cushing disease)	<1%
	GH-secreting tumor (acromegaly)	<1%
Ovary	Polycystic ovary syndrome	30%
	Primary ovarian failure	10%
Uterus	Asherman syndrome (intrauterine adhesions)	5%
Other	Nonclassical adrenal hyperplasia	<1%
	Thyroid disease	1%
	Ovarian tumors	<1%

ACTH, adenocorticotropin; GH, growth hormone.

estrogen levels are likely to be very low, and osteoporosis and vaginal atrophy may be present or develop. Women with nutritional causes of secondary amenorrhea may have triiodothyronine levels less than 70 ng/dL, reverse triiodothyronine levels more than 40 ng/dL, and elevated levels of urinary free cortisol (as observed in depressed women or women under significant stress).

Treatment: Reversing the underlying cause of hypothalamic dysfunction often results in resumption of ovulatory menses. For example, for women with low BMI, nutritional counseling and supportive physician guidance may be associated with weight gain and resumption of ovulatory menses. Many women with amenorrhea and low GnRH secretion prefer to maintain the exercise and nutritional regimens that caused the amenorrhea. These women may be best treated with hormone therapy to prevent osteoporosis and vaginal atrophy. Cyclic or continuous hormone therapy may be used. Low doses of

hormone therapy, such as that used to treat menopausal women; or standard doses of an estrogen–progestin contraceptive may be used for hormone therapy. Vitamin D (800 IU/day) and calcium (1200–1500 mg/day) should be advised to slow the rate of decline in bone mineral density associated with low estrogen levels.

Pituitary Dysfunction

The most common pituitary diseases that cause secondary amenorrhea are prolactin-secreting pituitary tumors (prolactinomas), the empty sella syndrome, Sheehan syndrome, and other pituitary tumors.

Prolactin-Secreting Pituitary Tumors

Most pituitary tumors are monoclonal, which indicates that they arise from a somatic mutation in a single progenitor cell. In general, pituitary tumors do not metastasize and are slow growing.

Diagnosis: The most common causes of an elevation in the serum prolactin level are, in order of decreasing frequency:
- pregnancy
- the use of psychotropic medications that are dopamine agonists, such as haloperidol
- prolactin-secreting pituitary tumors
- hypothyroidism
- renal failure

If the prolactin is elevated and the HCG, thyroid-stimulating hormone and creatinine levels are normal, a magnetic resonance imaging (MRI) scan of the hypothalamus and pituitary should be performed to determine whether a pituitary tumor is detectable, and whether it is less than 10 mm in size (microadenoma) or greater than 10 mm (macroadenoma); this difference has clinical implications for treatment. If the MRI shows a pituitary tumor, it is important to measure serum insulinlike growth factor 1 (IGF-1) levels to assess if there is co-secretion of both prolactin and excessive quantities of growth hormone (GH).

Treatment: Microprolactinomas (<10 mm in diameter) have a generally benign course and can be managed by a primary care physician or endocrinologist. Observational studies indicate that over an interval of 10 years, 95% of microproalctinomas do not increase in size. The initial treatment of microprolactinomas should be a dopamine agonist such as bromocriptine or cabergoline. When treated with a dopamine agonist, most women with a prolactinoma will have normalization of their prolactin levels, shrinkage of their pituitary tumor, and resumption of ovulatory menses. If the patient prefers, she may be safely treated with an estrogen–progestin contraceptive, instead of a dopamine agonist. Estrogen–progestin treatment will prevent problems associated with hypoestrogenism, such as osteoporosis, but it will not lower the elevated levels of prolactin. In most cases, estrogen–progestin treatment does not cause the prolactinoma to grow.

Macroprolactinomas (>10 mm in diameter) may be associated with significant complications including headaches, visual field loss due to compression of the optic chiasm, or pituitary apoplexy. Management of macroprolactinomas should be led by an endocrinologist. The initial treatment of a macroprolactinoma is a dopamine agonist, but radiotherapy or surgery may be indicated in selected cases.

Women with a prolactinoma who wish to become pregnant should receive treatment with a dopamine agonist to induce ovulation. Dopamine agonists directly suppress prolactin production by the tumor, which allows for an increase in GnRH secretion, which stimulates, LH, FSH, estradiol, and progesterone secretion. Dopamine agonists normalize prolactin levels in about 80% of women with a prolactinoma. The main side effects with dopamine agonist treatment are nausea, vomiting, and orthostatic hypotension.

Empty Sella Syndrome

The roof of the pituitary gland (the diaphragm of the sella) is perforated by the pituitary stalk, which connects the hypothalamic median eminence to the pituitary. If the perforation in the diaphragm sella is excessively large, the pia mater and accompanying cerebrospinal fluid can herniate into the pituitary fossa. Herniation of this fluid, which is under pressure, can produce compression atrophy of the pituitary gland resulting in hypopituitarism and amenorrhea. The syndrome can be diagnosed by MRI. Therapy is directed to the replacement of documented hormonal deficiencies.

Sheehan Syndrome

Sheehan syndrome is the onset of hypothalamic and pituitary dysfunction after severe obstetric hemorrhage and maternal hypotension at delivery. During pregnancy, the pituitary volume increased by approximately 100%. The increase in pituitary size and the low-flow, low-pressure nature of the portal circulation may make the pituitary and parts of the hypothalamus susceptible to ischemic injury brought on by obstetric hemorrhage and hypotension. Sheehan syndrome seldom occurs in developed countries, but is common in countries that do not have easily available blood banking and obstetric surgical services. Worldwide, Sheehan syndrome is the most common cause of hypopituitarism.

Every possible pattern of pituitary hormone deficiency has been reported in Sheehan syndrome, but growth hormone and prolactin deficiency are the most common presentation . Consequently, many women with Sheehan syndrome will first present postpartum with a failure to have the onset of lactation. Measurement of thyroxine, prolactin, IGF-1, and cortisol after stimulation with adrenocorticotropin (ACTH) are laboratory tests that help to define the pattern of hormone deficiency. Treatment of Sheehan syndrome involves the specific replacement of those hormones that are deficient.

Ovarian Dysfunction

Primary Ovarian Failure

Primary ovarian failure occurs when all functional ovarian follicles have been lost. Ovarian failure in patients younger than age 40 years is termed premature ovarian failure. The causes of premature ovarian failure include genetic abnormalities involving the X chromosome, autoimmune processes (such as polyglandular autoimmune disease or myasthenia gravis), chemotherapy (especially with alkylating agents), and pelvic radiotherapy (>500 cGy to the ovaries).

Diagnosis: Loss of all ovarian follicles causes a decrease in estradiol and inhibin B negative feedback on pituitary FSH secretion, resulting in a marked increase in serum FSH levels. Complete ovarian failure is typically associated with serum FSH levels greater than 25 IU/L. In women with incipient ovarian failure, FSH levels are often between 15 and 25 IU/L and may fluctuate from cycle to cycle. Clinically, women with premature ovarian failure may report vasomotor symptoms (hot flushes) or vaginal dryness.

Treatment: There are no treatments to reverse the loss of all ovarian follicles. Women with premature ovarian failure are at high risk for the development of osteoporosis, and they should be treated with estrogen–progestin therapy. For women with ovarian failure who desire fertility, oocyte donation is effective.

Polycystic Ovary Syndrome

(See Chapter 40.)

Uterine Dysfunction

Asherman Syndrome (Intrauterine Adhesions)

Asherman syndrome is the presence of intrauterine scar tissue that interferes with normal endometrial growth and shedding. The condition typically develops after intrauterine surgery, such as a vigorous endometrial curettage or hysteroscopic surgery. The presence of infection at the time of the intrauterine surgery increases the risk of developing Asherman syndrome postoperatively. A history of intrauterine surgery proceeding the onset of amenorrhea suggests that Asherman syndrome may have occurred. For patients whose history is suggestive, a common approach to assessing uterine endometrial function is to administer conjugated equine estrogens, 2.5 mg for 35 days, plus medroxyprogesterone acetate for days 26–35. The estrogen and progestin are then discontinued. Absence of withdrawal bleeding strongly suggests Asherman syndrome. The diagnosis can be confirmed by an imaging test such as a hysterosalpingogram, or by direct visualization of the scar tissue with hysteroscopy. The treatment of Asherman syndrome involves surgical lysis of the intrauterine adhesions by operative hysteroscopy followed by stimulation of endometrial growth with estrogen. An intrauterine device is often placed to prevent coaptation of the two sides of the endometrium during healing. Women who become pregnant after treatment of Asherman syndrome are at increased risk for defects of placentation, such as placenta accreta. This is due to the disruption of the function of the endometrial stroma by the disease and treatment.

Primary Amenorrhea

Primary amenorrhea is present when the first menses has not occurred by the time a girl reaches 16 years of age. Average age of onset of the first menses is about 12 to 13 years, with a standard deviation of about 1.5 years. Consequently, girls who have reached 16 years of age without experiencing their first menses are more than 2 standard deviations away from the mean onset of menarche. Girls who reach age 14 years and have no breast development are likely to develop primary amenorrhea. Average age of onset of breast development is about age 10 years with a standard deviation of about 1.5 years. The most common causes of primary amenorrhea are: genetic abnormalities of the sex chromosomes, physiological delay of puberty, müllerian agenesis, transverse vagina septum or imperforate hymen, absence of hypothalamic production of GnRH, anorexia nervosa, and hypopituitarism . Less common causes of primary amenorrhea include hyper-

prolactinemia, hypothyroidism, pituitary tumors, Cushing disease, and craniopharyngioma (**Table 39.3**).

Primary amenorrhea is evaluated by focusing on the serum FSH level; the status of breast development, and the presence of the cervix and uterus as determined by an imaging study (**Fig. 39.2**).

If the FSH level is elevated, a diagnosis of gonadal dysgenesis can be made in most cases. A karyotype should be obtained in such cases to determine whether a Y chromosome is present. Girls with gonadal dysgenesis and a fragment or entire Y chromosome have a high rate of malignant transformation of the gonad to a dysgerminoma or gonadoblastoma. In these cases, the gonads need to be surgically removed.

Turner Syndrome

Turner syndrome is caused by the loss of all, or part of, an X chromosome. The most common karyotypes associated with the syndrome are 45,X and 45,X/46,XX. Turner syndrome is the most common sex-chromosome abnormality in female conceptions, but most pregnancies with this abnormality miscarry before birth. About 1:2000 to 1:5000 births of girls are affected with Turner syndrome.

Most girls with Turner syndrome are short and stocky and have a square shaped chest. Turner syndrome is associated with the premature depletion of the ovarian fol-

Table 39.3 The most common causes of primary amenorrhea.

Cause/disease	Rate of occurrence
Abnormalities of sex chromosomes causes gonadal failure (e.g., 45,X—Turner syndrome)	45%
Physiological delay of puberty (functional and temporary decrease in GnRH secretion)	20%
Müllerian agenesis (Mayer–Rokitansky–Kuster–Hauser syndrome)	15%
Transverse vaginal septum or imperforate hymen	5%
Absence of GnRH secretion	5%
Anorexia nervosa	2%
Hypopituitarism	2%
Androgen insensitivity	1%
Hyperprolactinemia	1%
Adrenal hyperplasia	1%
Hypothyroidism	1%
Pituitary tumors	1%
Craniopharyngioma	1%

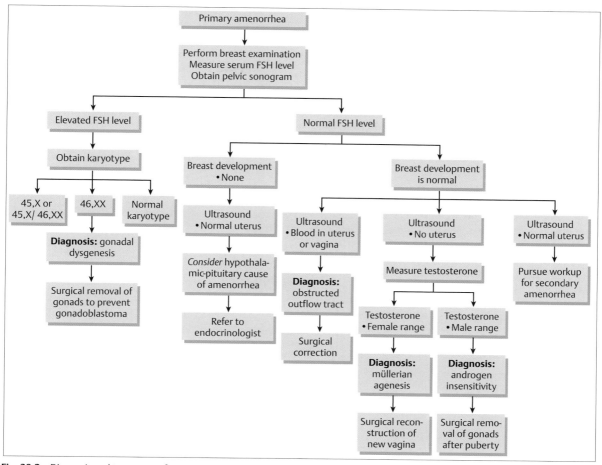

Fig. 39.2 Diagnosis and treatment of primary amenorrhea. FSH, follicle-stimulating hormone.

licle pool, resulting in the loss of all or almost all ovarian follicles before puberty. In the absence of functional ovarian follicles at puberty, no estrogen or progesterone is secreted from the ovary and breast development and menses cannot occur (primary amenorrhea). Women with Turner syndrome are hypoestrogenic. Estrogen treatment may begin as early as age 12 years with no adverse impact on the achievement of adult height. In the initial phase of estrogen treatment, low-doses, comparable to those given menopausal women are utilized. The dose of estrogen can be increased to standard estrogen doses in combination estrogen–progestin contraceptives over two to to four years. Progestins may be initiated within two years after starting estrogen, or when breakthrough bleeding occurs.

Most women with Turner syndrome, who have not been treated with GH, are less than 152 cm (60 in) tall. In order to increase adult height, girls with Turner syndrome have been treated with GH to accelerate linear growth. Heights in the range of 163 cm (64 in) tall are commonly achieved after GH therapy. GH treatment may begin as early as 1 year of age. Girls with Turner syndrome are at

increased risk for vascular anomalies including elongated transverse arch, anomalous pulmonary connection, and persistent left superior vena cava. In the presence of hypertension, women with Turner syndrome are at increased risk for aortic dilatation and dissection. MRI of the chest and echocardiography may be useful in detecting these anomalies. Learning and psychosocial problems are common in girls with Turner syndrome and a learning and psychological evaluation are recommended at the time of entry into school.

If the FSH level is normal, then breast development should be assessed and an imaging study should be used to determine whether a uterus and a cervix are present. If breast development is absent and a uterus is present, the differential diagnosis includes hypothalamic and pituitary causes of amenorrhea; the patient should be referred to an endocrinologist. If breast development is normal and a uterus is present, the differential diagnosis is the same as for secondary amenorrhea (see above). However, if the pelvic ultrasound exam shows that the patient has a uterus, but the uterus or vagina is dilated by blood, the diagnosis is a blocked reproductive outflow tract (transverse vaginal septum or imperforate hymen). Surgical relief of the outflow tract is necessary to prevent the development of hematocolpos, hematometria, and endometriosis.

If breast development is present and no uterus is observed on an imaging study, then the serum testosterone should be assessed. If the testosterone is in the normal range for a girl the likely diagnosis is müllerian agenesis. Treatment of müllerian agenesis involves the use of vaginal dilators to expand the caliber and length of the nascent vagina or surgery to create a neovagina. These interventions can be scheduled for the time when the patient is expected to be having sexual relations.

In a patient with breast development, no uterus, and a testosterone level in the male range, the likely diagnosis is androgen insensitivity. Females with androgen insensitivity usually do not have pubic or axillary hair. Breast development is usually normal, because in the absence of a tissue androgen receptor, low levels of estrogen have a stimulatory effect on breast growth. The karyotype in these patients is 46,XY and their gonads are intra-abdominal. These patients are at increased risk for developing a gonadoblastoma, but typically not until after puberty is completed. Consequently, surgical removal of the gonads is scheduled for after the completion of puberty to take advantage of the estrogen and estrogen precursors (testosterone and androstenedione) secreted by the gonads, which will help stimulate puberty.

Dysfunctional Uterine Bleeding

In women with normal ovulatory menstrual cycles, cycle length varies between 24 and 34 days. Menstrual flow normally lasts between 2 and 7 days and total blood loss is less than 80 mL, with an average loss of 35 mL. Before age 20 years and after age 45 years menstrual cycle length tends to be more variable, in association with anovulatory cycles.

Terminology

Menorrhagia refers to excessive or prolonged menstrual bleeding, greater than 80 mL per cycle or a menses that lasts longer than 7 days. In ovulatory women menorrhagia is typically caused by a uterine anatomical problem such as fibroids or endometrial pathology. Polymenorrhea refers to menses that occur more frequently than every 24 days. Metrorrhagia is light bleeding from the uterus at irregular intervals. Menometrorrhagia refers to heavy bleeding from the uterus at irregular intervals.

The term dysfunctional uterine bleeding is typically reserved for cases where there is excessive bleeding in the absence of a uterine or endometrial abnormality. Typically this occurs in anovulatory women. In anovulatory cycles, estrogen secretion from the follicle causes endometrial growth. The absence of ovulation prevents progesterone secretion and the endometrium cannot develop secretory changes and prostaglandin synthesis in an orderly manner, preventing the occurrence of a normal pattern of menstrual bleeding. Estrogen stimulation of the endometrium in the absence of progesterone will almost always result in heavy bleeding at irregular intervals that is the hallmark result in dysfunctional uterine bleeding. Dysfunctional uterine bleeding is a diagnosis of exclusion, because other causes of heavy bleeding such as endometrial cancer and fibroids need to be excluded.

Diagnosis

The initial approach to a woman with dysfunctional uterine bleeding is to rule out other causes of the bleeding including pregnancy, uterine or endometrial pathology, and if anemia is present to rule out systemic problems such as a coagulopathy. The diagnostic approach to dysfunctional bleeding should include: 1) serum hCG testing to rule out pregnancy; 2) pelvic ultrasound exam to assess the presence of uterine fibroids or endometrial pathology such as endometrial polyps; and 3) endometrial biopsy to rule out endometrial hyperplasia or cancer and to assess for secretory endometrium (a sign of ovulation). A hemoglobin concentration should be assessed to check for anemia. The presence of anemia corroborates that very significant uterine blood loss is occurring, and/or that the patient is seriously iron deficient. If the hemoglobin concentration is less than 10 g/dL, there is an increased likelihood that the patient has a coagulopathy, and a platelet count, prothrombin time, partial thromboplastin time, and von Willebrand screen should be obtained.

Treatment

Treatment of dysfunctional uterine bleeding differs for women who are hemodynamically stable compared to those who are not. For women who are not hemodynamically stable, and have severe uterine bleeding, treatment options include:

- Placement of a Foley catheter balloon into the uterine cavity and inflating the balloon to tamponade the uterus.
- Use of intravenous estrogen; for example, conjugated equine estrogen 25 mg intravenously for up to 6

doses, to rapidly stimulate endometrial regrowth and stabilize uterine and endometrial blood vessels.

- Dilation and curettage, which may sometimes reduce uterine bleeding.
- Uterine artery embolization using interventional radiology techniques, which may decrease blood flow to the uterus and endometrium.
- Hysterectomy, as a last treatment option for uncontrollable dysfunctional uterine bleeding in a hemodynamically unstable women.

For women who are hemodynamically stable, the treatment options include:

- Estrogen–progestin contraceptives; for example, 35 µg ethinyl estradiol plus 1 mg norethindrone, given orally as a dose of one pill four times daily until bleeding is controlled. This is followed by a taper of the estrogen–progestin contraceptive to one pill daily. Anti-nausea medicine is often required to prevent vomiting of the estrogen–progestin contraceptive, owing to the high-dose estrogen.
- Progestin-only therapy; for example, medroxyprogesterone acetate 10–60 mg daily for 14 days is often effective in the treatment of abnormal uterine bleeding. Alternative progestin regimens include norethindrone acetate 5 mg daily for 14 days or megestrol acetate 20–120 mg daily for 14 days. In a randomized, head-to-head trial of estrogen–progestin contraceptive versus progestin-only treatment, both treatments demonstrated similar efficacy in reducing uterine blood loss (see Evidence Box 39.1)
- If the patient does not desire future fertility, endometrial ablation is often effective in resolving the bleeding.

Key Points

- Secondary amenorrhea, also known as adult-onset amenorrhea, is diagnosed when a women who had been menstruating has no menses for longer than three of her previous cycle lengths, or 6 months. The most common causes of secondary amenorrhea are: pregnancy, polycystic ovary syndrome, low body mass index, low body fat, strenuous exercise, psychological stress, prolactin producing tumors, primary ovarian failure, and intrauterine adhesions (Asherman syndrome).
- Examination and laboratory testing for secondary amenorrhea includes measurement of body mass index, assessment for hirsutism and virilization, pelvic exam to assess the uterus for pregnancy, serum follicle-stimulating hormone (FSH), prolactin, and thyroid-stimulating hormone. A progestin withdrawal test is performed to establish the function of the endometrium and the patency of the distal reproductive tract.
- Primary amenorrhea is present when the first menses has not occurred by the time a girl reaches 16 years of age. Girls who reach age 14 years and have no breast development are likely to develop primary amenorrhea and a diagnostic evaluation may be initiated in these cases. The most common causes of primary amenorrhea are genetic abnormalities of the sex chromosomes (45,X—Turner syndrome), physiological delay

of puberty, müllerian agenesis, transverse vaginal septum, imperforate hymen, anorexia, and hypopituitarism.

- Examination and laboratory tests performed for girls with primary amenorrhea include: physical examination of breast developmental stage (Turner stage); serum FSH; and an imaging study of uterus, cervix, and vagina. If the FSH level is elevated, a karyotype should be obtained.
- Dysfunctional uterine bleeding is defined as the presence of heavy menses or irregular menses in the absence of structural abnormalities of the uterus or histologic abnormalities of the endometrium. The condition is usually associated with oligo-ovulation or anovulation. The relatively excessive overproduction of estrogen in relation to progesterone causes the abnormal bleeding. First-line treatment of dysfunctional uterine bleeding includes estrogen–progestin or progestin medications.

Evidence Box 39.1

Estrogen-progestin contraceptive and medroxyprogesterone acetate have similar efficacy in the treatment of dysfunctional uterine bleeding.

Dysfunctional uterine bleeding is diagnosed when there is excessive bleeding in the absence of a uterine or endometrial abnormality. In a trial of hormonal treatment of dysfunctional uterine bleeding, 40 women with acute uterine bleeding were randomized to treatment with three times daily medroxyprogesterone acetate (MPA) 20 mg or ethinyl estradiol (EE) 35 µg plus 1 mg norethindrone. After one week of treatment doses were reduced to MPA 20 mg daily and EE-norethindrone one pill daily for 3 additional weeks. Inclusion criteria included a hemoglobin >8 g/dL, no current pregnancy, and a normal uterus by physical examination or pelvic ultrasound.

After 14 days of treatment, 33 women remained in the trial. At the 14 day visit 88% of the women in EE-norethindrone group and 76% of the women in the MPA group reported cessation of bleeding. The median time to cessation of bleeding was 3 days in both groups. Patient satisfaction was similar in both groups. Both regimens can be recommended for the treatment of acute dysfunctional uterine bleeding.

Munro MG, Mainor N, Basu R, Brisinger M, Barreda L. Oral medroxyprogesterone acetate and combination oral contraceptives for acute uterine bleeding. Obstet Gynecol 2006; 108: 924–9.

Further Reading

Corenblum B, Donovan L. The safety of physiological estrogen plus progestin replacement therapy and with oral contraceptive therapy in women with pathological hyperprolactinemia. *Fertil Steril* 1993;59(3):671–673

Dijkhuizen FP, Mol BW, Brölmann HA, Heintz AP. The accuracy of endometrial sampling in the diagnosis of patients with endometrial carcinoma and hyperplasia: a meta-analysis. *Cancer* 2000;89(8):1765–1772

Fraser IS, Critchley HO, Munro MG, Broder M; Writing Group for this Menstrual Agreement Process. A process designed to lead to international agreement on terminologies and definitions used to describe abnormalities of menstrual bleeding. *Fertil Steril* 2007;87(3):466–476

Jialal I, Naidoo C, Norman RJ, Rajput MC, Omar MA, Joubert SM. Pituitary function in Sheehan's syndrome. *Obstet Gynecol* 1984;63(1):15–19

Kouides PA, Conard J, Peyvandi F, Lukes A, Kadir R. Hemostasis and menstruation: appropriate investigation for underlying disorders of hemostasis in women with excessive menstrual bleeding. *Fertil Steril* 2005;84(5):1345–1351

Lee PA, Guo SS, Kulin HE. Age of puberty: data from the United States of America. *APMIS* 2001;109(2):81–88

Munro MG, Mainor N, Basu R, Brisinger M, Barreda L. Oral medroxyprogesterone acetate and combination oral contraceptives for acute uterine bleeding: a randomized controlled trial. *Obstet Gynecol* 2006;108(4):924–929

Reindollar RH, Byrd JR, McDonough PG. Delayed sexual development: a study of 252 patients. *Am J Obstet Gynecol* 1981;140(4):371–380

Reindollar RH, Novak M, Tho SP, McDonough PG. Adult-onset amenorrhea: a study of 262 patients. *Am J Obstet Gynecol* 1986;155(3):531–543

Schlechte J, Dolan K, Sherman B, Chapler F, Luciano A. The natural history of untreated hyperprolactinemia: a prospective analysis. *J Clin Endocrinol Metab* 1989;68(2):412–418

Touraine P, Plu-Bureau G, Beji C, Mauvais-Jarvis P, Kuttenn F. Long-term follow-up of 246 hyperprolactinemic patients. *Acta Obstet Gynecol Scand* 2001;80(2):162–168

Valdes C, Malini S, Malinak LR. Ultrasound evaluation of female genital tract anomalies: a review of 64 cases. *Am J Obstet Gynecol* 1984;149(3):285–292

Webster J, Piscitelli G, Polli A, Ferrari CI, Ismail I, Scanlon MF; Cabergoline Comparative Study Group. A comparison of cabergoline and bromocriptine in the treatment of hyperprolactinemic amenorrhea. *N Engl J Med* 1994;331(14):904–909

40 Polycystic Ovary Syndrome, Hirsutism, and Virilization

Robert L. Barbieri

Polycystic ovary syndrome (PCOS) is a common gynecologic endocrine disorder that is characterized by both *reproductive abnormalities*, including excess ovarian secretion of androgens and oligo-ovulation, and *metabolic abnormalities* such as insulin resistance, the metabolic syndrome, and an increased risk for diabetes mellitus. The key to understanding PCOS is to recognize the dual defects in reproductive and metabolic function associated with the syndrome.

Definition and Diagnosis

Two major approaches to the definition of PCOS are in clinical use (**Table 40.1**). According to the National Institutes of Health (NIH) definition, *hyperandrogenism plus oligo-ovulation* must both be present to diagnose the condition. Hyperandrogenism can be diagnosed by clinical examination, based on the presence of significant hirsutism, or by laboratory testing with the demonstration of elevated levels of serum testosterone, androstenedione, and/or dehydroepiandrosterone sulfate (DHEAS). Oligo-ovulation can usually be diagnosed by history based on the report of menstrual cycles greater than 35 days. Most women with PCOS report fewer than six menses per year. In addition, the NIH definition suggests that other diseases which cause hyperandrogenism should be excluded, such as nonclassical adrenal hyperplasia due to 21-hydroxylase deficiency. Exclusion of the latter disease is best accomplished by demonstrating that the serum 17-hydroxyprogesterone level is less than 2 ng/mL in the early morning during the follicular phase of the menstrual cycle.

In 2003, the European Society of Human Reproduction and Embryology (ESHRE) and the American Society for Reproductive Medicine (ASRM) jointly proposed a new approach to the definition of PCOS. In this new approach, two of the following three criteria must be present to diagnose PCOS: 1) hyperandrogenism, 2) oligo-ovulation or

Table 40.1 The two most widely used definitions for diagnosis of polycystic ovary syndrome are the National Institutes of Health (NIH) diagnostic criteria and the European Society of Human Reproduction and Embryology / American Society for Reproductive Medicine (ESHRE/ASRM) diagnostic criteria*

NIH criteria	ESHRE/ASRM criteria **
1. Hyperandrogenism as evidenced by clinical findings, such as hirsutism, and/ or laboratory findings such as elevated serum testosterone, androstenedione, or DHEAS *plus*	1. Hyperandrogenism
2. Oligomenorrhea or amenorrhea *and*	2. Oligomenorrhea or amenorrhea
3. Rule out other causes of hyperandrogenism such as nonclassical adrenal hyperplasia due to 21-hydroxylase deficiency by demonstrating a normal 17-hydroxyprogesterone level (<2 ng/mL)	3. Multifollicluar ovary demonstrated by high-resolution transvaginal ultrasonography. More than 12 small follicles 2–9 mm in diameter in each ovary. An alternative ultrasonographic criterion is an ovarian volume >10 mL

DHEAS, dihydroepiandrosterone sulfate.
*The author prefers the NIH criteria for diagnosing polycystic ovary syndrome.
**The diagnosis is made when *two* of the three listed conditions are present.

anovulation, 3) transvaginal ultrasound demonstration of the presence of more than 12 small follicles in each ovary (**Fig. 40.1**).

The strength of the NIH definition is that diagnosis can largely be made using clinical history (oligomenorrhea) and physical examination (hirsutism). The ESHRE/ASRM definition requires transvaginal ultrasound examination of the ovary, a resource-intensive test. The ESHRE/ARMS definition also permits the diagnosis of PCOS if no hyperandrogenism is present, but the patient has both oligo-ovulation and a multifollicluar ovary on ultrasound examination. *Many authorities believe that hyperandrogenism is the key feature of PCOS and the diagnosis should not be made unless hyperandrogenism is present.* TheESHRE/ASRM definition would increase the prevalence of PCOS by about 50%, with many women being diagnosed with very mild forms of the syndrome.

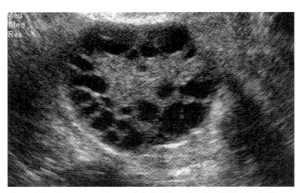

Fig. 40.1   A commonly used definition of a "multi-follicular" ovary is the presence of 12 or more small follicles with diameters of 2–9 mm in each ovary. Image obtained by transvaginal ultrasound scan of one ovary: more than 20 small follicles are demonstrated, clearly indicating that this is a multifollicular ovary.

Prevalence and Epidemiology

PCOS is a common gynecologic endocrine problem. Approximately 6–8% of women of reproductive age (15–45 years) have PCOS as defined by the NIH criteria.

Etiology and Pathophysiology

The etiology of PCOS remains a mystery. PCOS is characterized by defects in both the reproductive and metabolic systems. Most women with PCOS have abnormally increased gonadotropin-releasing hormone (GnRH) pulse frequency, suggesting that a hypothalamic neuroendocrine abnor-

mality is a key cause of the syndrome . The cause of the increased GnRH pulse frequency is not known. Increased GnRH pulse frequency results in increased pituitary secretion of luteinizing hormone (LH) which, in turn, stimulates the ovarian theca and stroma to over-secrete androstenedione and testosterone. Increased LH secretion results in increased ovarian androgen production which, in turn, causes hirsutism by stimulating the growth of the pilosebaceous unit in androgen dependent areas such as the face. Increased LH and ovarian androgen secretion causes stunted growth of ovarian follicles, resulting in the accumulation of small follicles, 2–9 mm in diameter. In the absence of the growth of a large follicle (20–25 mm in diameter), the LH surge does not occur and ovulation is not triggered. In the absence of ovulation, the menstrual pattern is oligomenorrhea or amenorrhea. The stunted growth of the ovarian follicles results in the accumulation of many small follicles 2–9 mm in diameter that can be detected by transvaginal ultrasonography. The ESRHE/ASRM definition of PCOS requires that more than 12 small follicles, 2–9 mm in diameter, be detected in each ovary by sonography.

Many women with PCOS also have excessive adrenal secretion of the androgen precursors, androstenedione, and DHEAS. These androgen precursors can be converted to the potent androgens, testosterone (**Fig. 40.2**) and dihydrotestosterone.

The metabolic abnormalities of PCOS include:
- insulin resistance and a compensatory hyperinsulinemia
- the metabolic syndrome (**Table 40.2**) characterized by centripetal obesity, increased visceral fat, dyslipidemia, and mild hypertension
- increased risk for developing diabetes mellitus
- dyslipidemia
- elevated serum concentrations of markers of endothelial inflammation, such as C-reactive protein, interleukin-6, interleukin-18, and endothelin-1

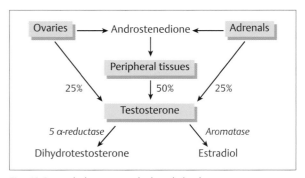

Fig. 40.2   Both the ovary and adrenal glands secrete testosterone and androstenedione. In turn, androstenedione can be converted to testosterone in peripheral tissues. In the pilosebaceous unit, testosterone is converted to the potent androgen, dihydrotestosterone.

Table 40.2 Criteria for diagnosing the metabolic syndrome, which is defined as the presence of 3 of the 5 factors below*

Findings from physical examination
1 Abdominal obesity. Waist circumference greater than 88 cm (35 in) in women and 102 cm (40 in) in men
2 Elevated blood pressure. Blood pressure greater than 130/85 mmHg or drug treatment for elevated blood pressure
Findings from laboratory testing
3 Elevated blood glucose. Fasting plasma glucose higher than 100 mg/dL or drug treatment for elevated blood glucose
4 Elevated triglycerides. Fasting serum triglycerides 150 mg/dl or higher or drug treatment for elevated triglycerides
5 Low level of high-density lipoprotein–cholesterol (HDL-C). Fasting serum HDL-C ≤50 mg/dL for women and ≤40 mg/dL for men, or drug treatment for low HDL-C

*Approximately 40% of women with PCOS have the metabolic syndrome, which increases the risk for developing diabetes mellitus and cardiovascular disease.
Source: Grundy SM, Cleeman JL, Daniels SR, et al. Diagnosis and management of the metabolic syndrome: an American Heart Association/National Heart Lung and Blood Institute Scientific Statement. Circulation 2005;112:2735–2752.

Recently, women with PCOS have also been documented to be at increased risk for sleep apnea and nonalcoholic steatohepatitis.

For women with insulin resistance and adequate pancreatic beta-cell function, a glucose load (or other mixed meal) results in a marked increase in insulin secretion and circulating insulin in an attempt to overcome the peripheral resistance to insulin action. Both lean (**Fig. 40.3**) and obese women with PCOS often have insulin resistance. In general, obese women with PCOS have more severe insulin resistance than obese normally-ovulating women or lean women with PCOS.

History

Menstrual Dysfunction

Women with PCOS typically have fewer than six menses per year. In most women with PCOS, the menstrual dysfunction begins during the teen years. The differential diagnosis of oligomenorrhea is extensive. Other causes of oligomenorrhea include pregnancy, stress or exercise-induced oligomenorrhea (hypothalamic amenorrhea), eating disorders including anorexia or bulimia, abnormally reduced body fat with a normal body mass index (BMI), premature ovarian failure, hyperprolactinemia, and non-classical adrenal hyperplasia.

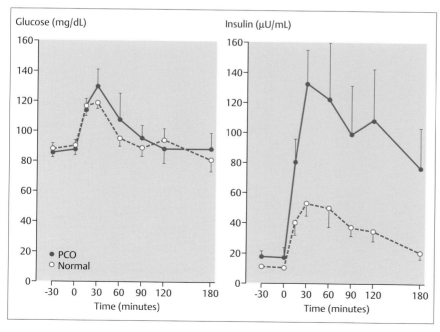

Fig. 40.3 Many women with polycystic ovary syndrome (PCOS) are insulin resistant. In an insulin-resistant woman the ingestion of glucose results in the excess secretion of insulin in an attempt to overcome the peripheral insulin resistance. In this study normally cycling women (open circles) and lean women with PCOS (closed circles) were given an oral glucose load. Glucose and insulin were frequently sampled for 2 hours. The lean PCOS women had markedly increased serum insulin levels compared with the normally cycling women. Given the normal levels of glucose in both groups, this indicates peripheral insulin resistance in the lean women with PCOS. Source: Chang RJ, Nakamura RM, Judd HL, Kaplan SA. Insulin resistance in non-obese patients with polycystic ovary syndrome. *J Clin Endocrinol Metab.* 1983;57:356–9.

Oligo-ovulation

Moliminal symptoms such as dysmenorrhea, breast tenderness, and abdominal bloating typically occur in association with ovulatory cycles. Due to anovulation, women with PCOS may report fewer moliminal symptoms with their menses.

Physical Examination

Hyperandrogenism

Women with PCOS typically have signs of hyperandrogenism, the most frequent of which are hirsutism and acne. Hirsutism is often quantitatively assessed using the Ferriman–Gallwey scoring system. Nine different body areas are graded 0 (no hirsutism) to 4 (marked hirsutism), and the individual score for each body part is summed for a total score (**Fig. 40.4**). Approximately 5% of the female population has a total score greater than or equal to 8.

Severe hyperandrogenism can lead to signs of virilization including male pattern hair loss, severe hirsutism, increased upper body muscle mass, deepening of the voice, and clitoromegaly.

Obesity and Insulin Resistance

Approximately 50% of women with PCOS have a BMI greater than 30 kg/m² and/or a waist circumference greater than 88 cm (35 in). Women with severe insulin resistance may have acanthosis nigricans or an increased number of skin tags (achrochordons). Both acanthosis nigricans and skin tags typically occur more frequently in body folds, such as the nape of the neck, the axilla, and the inner thighs.

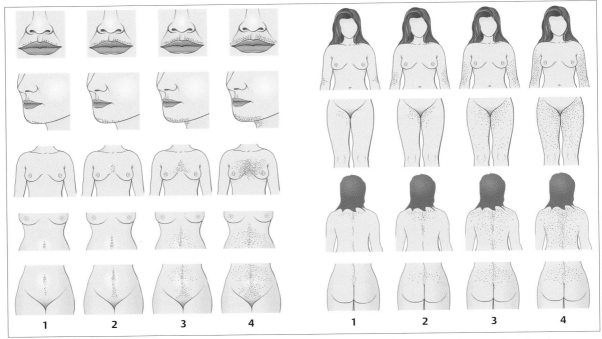

Fig. 40.4   The modified Ferriman–Gallwey scoring system for quantitatively assessing the severity of hirsutism. Nine discrete areas are independently scored from 0 to 4 based on the severity of hirsutism. If no hirsutism is present in an area, the score is zero. If marked hirsutism is present, the score is 4. The scores for each of the nine areas are summed to arrive at a total hirsutism score. A hirsutism score of 8 or greater is present in about 5% of the population. Hirsutism varies by ethnic and racial group. Source: Hatch R, Rosenfield RS, Kim MH, Tredway D. Hirsutism: Implications, etiology and management. *Am J Obstet Gynecol* 1981;140:815–30.

Laboratory Tests

Increased Serum Androgens

Most women with PCOS have an abnormally increased serum concentration of an androgen such as testosterone, androstenedione, and/or DHEAS. Testosterone is extremely difficult to measure accurately and many clinical assays have been developed to separate male levels of serum testosterone (7 ng/mL) from normal female levels of testosterone (0.4 ng/mL), but are unable to reliably detect the modest increase in serum testosterone observed in most women with PCOS (0.7–0.9 ng/mL). The laboratory measurements of androstenedione and DHEAS are more straightforward and have greater reliability.

Decreased Serum Sex Hormone Binding Globulin

In PCOS, increased androgens and insulin resistance result in decreased liver production and serum levels of sex hormone binding globulin (SHBG), resulting in increased free testosterone.

Women with marked oligomenorrhea or amenorrhea should have measurement of human chorionic gonadotropin (to rule out pregnancy), prolactin, follicle-stimulating hormone (FSH), and thyroid-stimulating hormone, to rule out other causes of secondary amenorrhea.

Increased Serum Luteinizing Hormone

LH levels are raised in most women with PCOS. However, serum LH is secreted in a pulsatile manner (high peaks and low valleys). The pulsatile nature of LH secretion makes it difficult to measure accurately. In addition, serum LH is influenced by BMI, with higher BMI associated with lower LH levels in both normal ovulatory women and women with PCOS. A single LH measurement should be interpreted in light of the patient's BMI, but nomograms adjusting LH for BMI are not widely available. The LH to FSH ratio may partially correct for some of these measurement problems. An LH to FSH ratio of ≥2 is suggestive of increased LH secretion, and PCOS.

Abnormal Glucose Level

In women with PCOS, an oral glucose challenge is more sensitive in detecting abnormal glucose dynamics than a fasting glucose determination. Approximately 3 % of women with PCOS have a fasting glucose level greater than or equal to 126 mg/dL, which defines the cutoff for diagnosing diabetes mellitus. If a 75 gm oral glucose challenge is used, 7.5 % of women with PCOS have a 2-hour glucose value greater than 200 mg/dL, which defines the cutoff for diagnosing diabetes mellitus. Using the oral glucose challenge, 35 % of women with PCOS have a 2-hour glucose value between 140 and 200 mg/dL, which defines the prediabetes syndrome of "impaired glucose tolerance." Many authorities recommend that all women with PCOS have an oral glucose challenge to screen for diabetes mellitus.

Insulin Resistance

It is difficult to assess insulin resistance with available clinical laboratory assays for insulin. Instead, authorities recommend screening for the metabolic syndrome (see **Table 40.2**).

Dyslipidemia

Many women with PCOS have increased LDL–cholesterol (>130 mg/dL) decreased HDL–cholesterol (<50 mg/dL) and increased fasting triglycerides (>150 mg/dL). More than 50 % of women with PCOS have dyslipidemia.

Pelvic Ultrasound Exam

Transvaginal ultrasonography is required to observe the multifollicular ovary present in most women with PCOS.

Treatment

Women with PCOS typically present for medical care with one or more of the following chief complaints:

- oligomenorrhea
- hirsutism
- anovulatory infertility
- excessive weight gain
- irregular uterine bleeding (**Table 40.3**)

Table 40.3 The most common chief complaints of patients with polycystic ovary disease and their first-line hormonal therapy and alternative treatments

Chief complaint	First-line hormonal therapy	Alternative treatments
Oligomenorrhea or amenorrhea	Estrogen–progestin contraceptive, cyclic	Cyclic progestin withdrawal or metformin
Hirsutism	Estrogen–progestin contraceptive plus an anti-androgen such as spironolactone	Vaniqa topical cream, mechanical methods of hair removal, electrolysis, laser treatment of excess hair.
Infertility	Clomiphene	Metformin
Excess weight gain	Life style changes: exercise plus diet	Weight loss medications, including metformin
Irregular uterine bleeding	High dose continuous progestin therapy	Hysterectomy if endometrial cancer is present

Oligomenorrhea

In women with oligomenorrhea caused by PCOS, estrogen–progestin contraceptives (oral or vaginal ring) have many beneficial effects, including resumption of cyclic uterine withdrawal bleeding. The beneficial effects of estrogen–progestin contraceptives include:

- marked suppression of pituitary LH secretion resulting in a significant reduction in ovarian androgen production
- decrease in circulating testosterone
- increase in liver production of SHBG reducing the circulating free testosterone concentration
- decrease in adrenal androgen production (mechanism unknown)
- prevention of endometrial hyperplasia
- induction of regular uterine withdrawal bleeding
- improvement in hirsutism

The multitude of benefits makes estrogen–progestin therapy the mainstay for treatment of PCOS in women who are not actively trying to become pregnant. Estrogen-progestin treatment can be continued for many years, until the woman desires to become pregnant.

Hirsutism

(See below.)

Anovulatory Infertility

Anovulatory infertility caused by PCOS is one of the most frequent reasons a patient consults a fertility specialist. The standard infertility evaluation includes: documentation of the ovulatory status of menstrual cycles, a semen analysis, and a hysterosalpingogram. For the treatment of anovulatory infertility in women with PCOS, a stepwise approach should be used, beginning with less resource-intensive treatments and advancing to more expensive treatments if earlier interventions are unsuccessful (**Table 40.4**).

For infertile women with PCOS who are overweight, weight loss will often result in resumption of ovulatory menses and pregnancy. If weight loss cannot be achieved, or is not effective, the first-line hormonal agent for ovulation induction is clomiphene. Clomiphene is a mixed estrogen antagonist–agonist (similar to tamoxifen) with more marked antagonist effects in the hypothalamus and pituitary. For severely oligo-ovulatory women, a uterine withdrawal bleed is induced with a 5-day course of a synthetic progestin, such as medroxyprogesterone acetate 10 mg daily. Withdrawal bleeding will often start after the 5-day course of the synthetic progestin. Counting the first day of bleeding as cycle day 1, clomiphene is prescribed at a dose of 50 mg daily for cycle days 5 to 9 (or alternatively cycle days 3 to 7). The LH surge which occurs about 40 hours before ovulation can be monitored by testing for a surge in urine LH concentration using an over-the-counter home LH assay kit. Ovulation typically occurs between cycle days 14 to 21. The Food and Drug Administration (FDA) has approved clomiphene treatment with doses as high as 100 mg daily for 5 days (Evidence Box 40.1).

If both weight loss and clomiphene are ineffective in inducing ovulation, metformin, an insulin sensitizer, may be effective. Metformin at a dose between 1500 mg and

Table 40.4 Ovulation induction in infertile women with polycystic ovary syndrome (PCOS) should be approached with a stepwise plan. The initial steps require fewer medical resources and are associated with a low frequency of serious adverse effects

Step	Treatment	Resource intensity	Comments
1	Weight loss	Modest	Weight loss of 10% of body mass is often associated with ovulation. Many overweight women find it difficult to lose weight
2	Clomiphene	Inexpensive	The mainstay of hormonal treatment of infertility caused by PCOS
3	Metformin	Inexpensive	May take 3–6 months of daily therapy to result in regular ovulatory menses
4	Letrozole or anastrozole	Inexpensive	Not approved by the FDA for ovulation induction
5	Short course glucocorticoid therapy with or without clomiphene	Inexpensive	May be especially useful in women with elevated serum DHEAS level
6	FSH injections	Expensive and requires intensive monitoring	Increased risk of twin and triplet pregnancy
7	Ovarian surgery to reduce follicle number and thecal cell over-production of androgens	Requires surgery and general anesthesia	Patient begins to ovulate without hormones. Low risk of twin pregnancy
8	In vitro fertilization	A very resource-intensive process. In vitro fertilization requires administration of expensive medications (FSH), intensive monitoring and two procedures (oocytes retrieval and embryo transfer)	Very high success rate. Increased risk of twin and triplet pregnancy.

DHEAS, dihydroepiandrosterone sulfate; FSH, follicle-stimulating hormone.

2550 mg daily reduces insulin secretion and enhances target tissue response to insulin. For many women with PCOS, this will result in resumption of ovulation. It may take 3–6 months of daily metformin therapy to induce ovulation in women with PCOS. Recently, aromatase inhibitors have been demonstrated to be effective in the induction of ovulation in women with PCOS. Aromatase inhibitors, such as letrozole or anastrozole, decrease hypothalamic-pituitary concentrations of estradiol, resulting in an increase in pituitary FSH secretion which, in turn, stimulates follicular growth. Commonly utilized regimens include letrozole 2.5 mg daily or anastrozole 1 mg daily for cycle days 5 to 9. Aromatase inhibitors are not FDA-approved for ovulation induction, and the teratogenicity of these agents in humans has not been studied in great detail.

If weight loss, clomiphene, metformin, anastrozole, and glucocorticoids are ineffective, resource-intensive treatments such as FSH injections, ovarian surgery, or in vitro fertilization are extremely effective infertility treatments (**Table 40.4**). FSH injections and in vitro fertilization are associated with increased risk of twin and triplet pregnancies, which are associated with increased risk of poor obstetric and newborn outcomes due to premature birth.

Excess Weight Gain

One of the most difficult problems in women with PCOS is excess weight gain. Approximately 50% of women with PCOS are obese, defined as a BMI greater than 30 kg/m². The cause of the increased weight gain in women with PCOS is not clear. Along with the neuroendocrine abnormality in GnRH secretion, women with PCOS may also have hypothalamic abnormalities in mechanisms governing eating and metabolism. Life style modifications, including calorie restriction and increased exercise, are clearly the first step for the treatment of excess weight gain . Setting a goal of 150 minutes of exercise per week, plus a 10% reduction in weight, has been demonstrated to help reduce the risk of developing diabetes mellitus in patients with prediabetes. The addition of metformin 1700 mg daily to life style changes may slightly improve the weight loss caused by life style changes alone.

When morbid obesity is present, defined as a BMI greater than 40 kg/m², and life style changes are not effective in producing weight loss, bariatric surgery can be considered. In morbidly-obese women with PCOS, bariatric surgery has been demonstrated to result in weight loss and improve menstrual cyclicity and reduce circulating androgens.

Irregular Uterine Bleeding

Most women with PCOS have infrequent menses. Some women with PCOS have menses more than once per month and a few develop heavy uterine bleeding. The evaluation of these women includes endometrial biopsy, because women with PCOS and heavy or frequent menses are at increased risk for endometrial hyperplasia or cancer. The treatment of endometrial cancer is typically hysterectomy. The treatment of endometrial hyperplasia is most often high-dose, continuous progestin therapy, such as megestrol acetate 60–240 mg daily or norethindrone acetate 5 mg daily, followed by repeat biopsy to assess the efficacy of treatment. If the endometrial biopsy shows follicular or menstrual endometrium (no hyperplasia or cancer), there are many options for treatment including estrogen–progestin contraceptives, levonorgestrel-releasing intrauterine system, and GnRH agonists such as leuprolide acetate

Hirsutism

Hirsutism is the presence of an excess quantity of dark and thick "terminal hairs" in sites that are androgen dependent, such as the face, chest, and abdomen. In these sites, stimulation of the pilosebaceous unit by the potent androgens, testosterone and dihydrotestosterone, can stimulate the linear growth and thickness of the hair fiber, along with increasing the amount of pigment incorporated in the hair. Hirsutism can be quantitatively assessed on physical examination using the modified Ferriman–Gallwey scoring system (**Fig. 40.4**). Ferriman-Gallwey scores greater than or equal to 8 are considered abnormal and indicative of hirsutism.

Hirsutism is best treated by a combined approach that includes both hormonal therapy and an adjuvant therapy such as topical eflornithine, electrolysis, laser treatment, or mechanical removal of excess hair. The best hormonal treatment for hirsutism is a combination of an estrogen–progestin contraceptive plus an anti-androgen such as spironolactone 100 mg daily . Spironolactone is both an anti-mineralocorticoid (effective as an antihypertensive agent) and an anti-androgen. Spironolactone has a chemical structure that is similar to testosterone (**Fig. 40.5**). The estrogen–progestin contraceptive reduces the excess secretion of pituitary LH and ovarian androgens, which will improve hirsutism. The addition of an anti-androgen helps to block androgen action in the pilosebaceous unit, which will further enhance the effectiveness of the hormonal therapy. In cases of marked hirsutism, clinical trials have demonstrated the importance

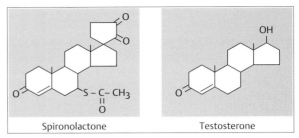

Fig.40.5 The chemical structure of spironolactone (an antimineralocorticoid and anti-androgen) and testosterone (a potent androgen). Spironolactone shares structural similarities with testosterone and can bind to the androgen receptor, blocking its action to increase transcription of androgen-regulated genes.

of therapy with an anti-androgen. In Europe, the anti-androgens flutamide (androgen receptor blocker) and finasteride (5α-reductase inhibitor, which blocks dihydrotestosterone synthesis) are commonly used to treat hirsutism. However, in the United States these drugs are only approved to treat prostate disorders and are not approved for use by women.

Virilization

Severe hyperandrogenism can lead to signs of virilization including male pattern hair loss, severe hirsutism, increased upper body muscle mass, deepening of the voice, and clitoromegaly. Women with virilization typically have markedly elevated serum testosterone levels, often exceeding 2 ng/mL. Since testosterone levels decrease with age, serum testosterone levels greater than 1.5 ng/mL are very concerning in women over 40 years of age.

The most common causes of virilization are: 1) ovarian hyperthecosis; 2) an ovarian androgen-secreting tumor, such as Sertoli–Leydig cell tumor; and 3) an adrenal androgen secreting tumor such as adrenal adenoma.

Ovarian hyperthecosis typically occurs in association with severe insulin resistance: acanthosis nigricans and glucose intolerance are typically present. This condition is unlikely to be associated with metastatic disease. The ovaries often need to be removed to correct the condition.

A Sertoli–Leydig cell tumor is typically unilateral and can be detected by pelvic ultrasound exam as a solid ovarian mass. In one series, the average age of women with this tumor was 25 years. The primary approach to a Sertoli–Leydig cell tumor is surgery, usually total abdominal hysterectomy with bilateral salpingo-oophorectomy, for definitive diagnosis, staging, and treatment. Survival is related to the stage and degree of differentiation, with an overall 5-year survival of 70–90%.

An adrenal adenoma or adrenal carcinoma causing virilization can usually be detected by magnetic resonance imaging of the adrenal glands, along with measurement of adrenal androgens such as DHEA, DHEAS, and androstenedione.

Key Points

- The polycystic ovary syndrome (PCOS) is diagnosed when both hyperandrogenism and oligo-ovulation or anovulation are present. Hyperandrogenism is usually manifested by hirsutism and/or acne. Oligo-ovulation or anovulation is usually manifested by oligomenorrhea or amenorrhea.
- PCOS is a disease of both reproduction and metabolism. Most women with PCOS have elevated pituitary secretion of lureinizing hormone (LH), which stimulates the ovarian theca and stroma to secrete androgens such as androstenedione and testosterone. Many women with PCOS have insulin resistance and compensatory hyperinsulinemia. Hyperinsulinemia works in concert with LH to stimulate ovarian androgen production.
- Women with PCOS typically present with one or more of the following problems: irregular menses, hirsutism, anovulatory infertility, or obesity.
- Irregular menses and hirsutism are often treated with an estrogen–progestin, which decreases pituitary LH secretion and ovarian androgen production. Hirsutism may also be treated with estrogen–progestin plus an anti-androgen such as spironolactone.
- Anovulatory infertility is treated with clomiphene, which is a mixed estrogen antagonist–agonist.
- Obesity is best treated with life style changes such as calorie restriction and exercise. In obese women with PCOS, weight reduction often results in regular ovulatory cycles, regular menses, and return of fertility. Women with PCOS and a body mass index >40 kg/m^2 who have not been able to lose weight through life style changes may be offered bariatric surgery.

Evidence Box 40.1

Clomiphene is superior to metformin for ovulation induction in women with polycystic ovarian syndrome.

A total of 626 women with polycystic ovarian syndrome (PCOS) and anovulatory infertility were randomized to one of three treatments: 1) clomiphene 50 mg daily for 5 days from cycle day 3 to 7; 2) metformin 1000 mg twice daily; or 3) a combination of the two, for up to 6 months. Note that clomiphene was only taken for 5 days each month, and metformin was taken daily throughout the entire study. The average age of the study participants was 28 years, the average body mass index (BMI) was 35 kg/m^2, and the average waist circumference was 102 cm. Ninety-two percent of the women had a multifollicular ovary consistent with PCOS.

The ovulation rate per month (number of ovulations / number of months in the study) was 49 % with clomiphene, 29 % with metformin, and 60 % with the combination. The live-birth rate (number of live births / number of patients in the group) was 22.5 % in the clomiphene group, 7.2 % in the metformin group, and 26.8 % in the clomiphene plus metformin group. The live-birth rates were two times greater in the women with a BMI <30 kg/m^2 compared with the women with a BMI >35 kg/m^2. The rate of multiple pregnancy was 6 % with clomiphene, 0 % with metformin, and 3.1 % with clomiphene plus metformin. Gastrointestinal side effects such as nausea and diarrhea were more frequent in the metformin group. Vasomotor symptoms were more frequent in the clomiphene group. During the study, the group assigned to metformin therapy lost a modest amount of weight.

These results demonstrate that for most patients clomiphene is superior to metformin first-line monotherapy for the treatment of anovulatory infertility caused by PCOS. In addition, the study demonstrates the importance of reducing BMI prior to inducing ovulation in women with PCOS.

Legro RS, Barnhart KH, Schlaff WD, et al. Clomiphene, metformin or both for infertility in the polycystic ovary syndrome. N Engl J Med 2007;356:551–566.

Further Reading

Apridonidze T, Essah PA, Iuorno MJ, Nestler JE. Prevalence and characteristics of the metabolic syndrome in women with polycystic ovary syndrome. *J Clin Endocrinol Metab* 2005;90(4):1929–1935

Bayar U, Basaran M, Kiran S, Coskun A, Gezer S. Use of an aromatase inhibitor in patients with polycystic ovary syndrome: a prospective randomized trial. *Fertil Steril* 2006;86(5):1447–1451

Bayer SR, DeCherney AH. Clinical manifestations and treatment of dysfunctional uterine bleeding. *JAMA* 1993;269(14):1823–1828

Casper RF, Mitwally MF. Review: aromatase inhibitors for ovulation induction. *J Clin Endocrinol Metab* 2006;91(3):760–771

Costello MF, Shrestha B, Eden J, Johnson NP, Sjoblom P. Metformin versus oral contraceptive pill in polycystic ovary syndrome: a Cochrane review. Human Reprod 2007; e pub. Jan 29

Diamanti-Kandarakis E, Spina G, Kouli C, Migdalis I. Increased endothelin-1 levels in women with polycystic ovary syndrome and the beneficial effect of metformin therapy. *J Clin Endocrinol Metab* 2001;86(10):4666–4673

Ehrmann DA. Polycystic ovary syndrome. *N Engl J Med* 2005;352(12):1223–1236

Escobar-Morreale HF, Botella-Carretero JI, Alvarez-Blasco F, Sancho J, San Millán JL. The polycystic ovary syndrome associated with morbid obesity may resolve after weight loss induced by bariatric surgery. *J Clin Endocrinol Metab* 2005;90(12):6364–6369

Farquhar CM, Williamson K, Gudex G, Johnson NP, Garland J, Sadler L. A randomized controlled trial of laparoscopic ovarian diathermy versus gonadotropin therapy for women with clomiphene citrate-resistant polycystic ovary syndrome. *Fertil Steril* 2002;78(2):404–411

Ferriman D, Gallwey JD. Clinical assessment of body hair growth in women. *J Clin Endocrinol Metab* 1961;21:1440–1447

Grundy SM, Cleeman JI, Daniels SR, et al; American Heart Association; National Heart, Lung, and Blood Institute. Diagnosis and management of the metabolic syndrome: an American Heart Association/National Heart, Lung, and Blood Institute Scientific Statement. *Circulation* 2005;112(17):2735–2752

Guzick DS. Polycystic ovary syndrome. *Obstet Gynecol* 2004;103(1):181–193

Hatch R, Rosenfield RL, Kim MH, Tredway D. Hirsutism: implications, etiology, and management. *Am J Obstet Gynecol* 1981;140(7):815–830

Hoeger KM, Kochman L, Wixom N, Craig K, Miller RK, Guzick DS. A randomized, 48-week, placebo-controlled trial of intensive lifestyle modification and/or metformin therapy in overweight women with polycystic ovary syndrome: a pilot study. *Fertil Steril* 2004;82(2):421–429

Inal MM, Yildirim Y, Taner CE. Comparison of the clinical efficacy of flutamide and spironolactone plus Diane 35 in the treatment of idiopathic hirsutism: a randomized controlled study. *Fertil Steril* 2005;84(6):1693–1697

Knochenhauer ES, Key TJ, Kahsar-Miller M, Waggoner W, Boots LR, Azziz R. Prevalence of the polycystic ovary syndrome in unselected black and white women of the southeastern United States: a prospective study. *J Clin Endocrinol Metab* 1998;83(9):3078–3082

Legro RS, Barnhart HX, Schlaff WD, et al; Cooperative Multicenter Reproductive Medicine Network. Clomiphene, metformin, or both for infertility in the polycystic ovary syndrome. *N Engl J Med* 2007;356(6):551–566

Legro RS, Kunselman AR, Dodson WC, Dunaif A. Prevalence and predictors of risk for type 2 diabetes mellitus and impaired glucose tolerance in polycystic ovary syndrome: a prospective, controlled study in 254 affected women. *J Clin Endocrinol Metab* 1999;84(1):165–169

Legro RS, Kunselman AR, Dunaif A. Prevalence and predictors of dyslipidemia in women with polycystic ovary syndrome. *Am J Med* 2001;111(8):607–613

Pagán YL, Srouji SS, Jimenez Y, Emerson A, Gill S, Hall JE. Inverse relationship between luteinizing hormone and body mass index in polycystic ovarian syndrome: investigation of hypothalamic and pituitary contributions. *J Clin Endocrinol Metab* 2006;91(4):1309–1316

Setji TL, Holland ND, Sanders LL, Pereira KC, Diehl AM, Brown AJ. Nonalcoholic steatohepatitis and nonalcoholic Fatty liver disease in young women with polycystic ovary syndrome. *J Clin Endocrinol Metab* 2006;91(5):1741–1747

Shaw RJ, Lamia KA, Vasquez D, et al. The kinase LKB1 mediates glucose homeostasis in liver and therapeutic effects of metformin. *Science* 2005;310(5754):1642–1646

Solomon CG, Hu FB, Dunaif A, et al. Long or highly irregular menstrual cycles as a marker for risk of type 2 diabetes mellitus. *JAMA* 2001;286(19):2421–2426

Tarkun I, Arslan BC, Cantürk Z, Türemen E, Sahin T, Duman C. Endothelial dysfunction in young women with polycystic ovary syndrome: relationship with insulin resistance and low-grade chronic inflammation. *J Clin Endocrinol Metab* 2004;89(11):5592–5596

Tasali E, Van Cauter E, Ehrmann DA. Relationships between sleep disordered breathing and glucose metabolism in polycystic ovary syndrome. *J Clin Endocrinol Metab* 2006;91(1):36–42

The Rotterdam ESHRE/ASRM-Sponsored PCOS consensus workshop group. Revised 2003 consensus on diagnostic criteria and long-term health risks related to polycystic ovary syndrome (PCOS). *Hum Reprod* 2004;19(1):41–47

Waldstreicher J, Santoro NF, Hall JE, Filicori M, Crowley WF Jr. Hyperfunction of the hypothalamic-pituitary axis in women with polycystic ovarian disease: indirect evidence for partial gonadotroph desensitization. *J Clin Endocrinol Metab* 1988;66(1):165–172

Young RH, Scully RE. Ovarian Sertoli-Leydig cell tumors. A clinicopathological analysis of 207 cases. *Am J Surg Pathol* 1985;9(8):543–569

Zawadzki JK, Dunaif A. Diagnostic criteria for polycystic ovary syndrome. Polycystic ovary Syndrome. In: Dunaif A, Givens JR, Haseltine FP, et al., eds. Current Issues in Endocrinology and Metabolism. Boston, Mass: Blackwell Scientific Publications; 1992:377–384.

41 Dysmenorrhea: Painful Menstruation

Robert L. Barbieri

Definition

For clinical purposes, dysmenorrhea, or painful menstruation, is divided into two major categories: primary and secondary. Primary dysmenorrhea is the presence of recurrent, crampy pelvic pain in the lower abdomen that occurs just before and/or during menstruation in the absence of suspected or proven pelvic pathology. Secondary dysmenorrhea is painful menstruation in the presence of a disease that causes the recurrent, cyclic pain symptoms, such as endometriosis, adenomyosis, or uterine leiomyomata.

Diagnosis

The diagnosis of primary dysmenorrhea is made in women with painful menstruation who do not have evidence of pelvic pathology such as endometriosis, adenomyosis, or uterine leiomyomata. In women with severe dysmenorrhea, imaging studies such as sonography may be helpful in detecting major pelvic pathology such as uterine leiomyomata, adenomyosis, or ovarian endometriosis. In women with severe dysmenorrhea who do not respond to standard treatment with nonsteroidal anti-inflammatory drugs (NSAIDs) and/or estrogen–progestin contraceptives, laparoscopy may be indicated to diagnose and treat endometriosis.

Prevalence and Epidemiology

The average age of onset of menses is 12 years and 13 years of age in African-American and Caucasian girls, respectively. In the first 2 years after menarche, about 50% of menstrual cycles are anovulatory. Eventually, for most adolescents, ovulation occurs monthly and menstrual cycle length stabilizes between 24 and 35 days. Painful menstruation is most likely to occur in association with an ovulatory menstrual cycle (**Table 41.1**).

In a population-based sample of 25% of the 19-year-old women living in Gothenburg, Sweden, 72% of subjects reported dysmenorrhea, of which 15% reported that menstruation associated pelvic pain limited their ability to go to school, or to work effectively. In a study of 1546 Canadian women ≥18 years, 60% reported dysmenorrhea and 17% reported that the painful menstruation adversely impacted their school or work performance.

Table 41.1 Time interval from menarche (first menses) to onset of dysmenorrhea in adolescents

Years between first menses and onset of dysmenorrhea	Percentage of adolescents
Within 1 year	38%
1–2 years	21%
2–3 years	20%
3–4 years	10%
4–5 years	8%
5–6 years	3%

Source: Adapted from Andersch B, Milson I. An epidemiologic study of young women with dysmenorrhea. Am J Obstet Gynecol 1982;144:655–660.

Etiology

Dysmenorrhea is caused by frequent and prolonged uterine contractions, where the uterine pressure is greater than mean arterial pressure, resulting in relative ischemia and triggering of pain nerve fibers in the uterus. From one perspective, dysmenorrhea represents uterine "angina." Pain nerve fibers in the uterus may also be sensitized or triggered by chemicals secreted by the sloughing endometrium, including prostaglandins and cytokines.

The biochemical sequence that results in frequent and prolonged uterine contractions includes the following. 1) During the menstrual cycle, the sequential stimulation of the endometrium by estradiol during the ovarian follicular phase (endometrial proliferative phase) followed by estradiol plus progesterone during the ovarian luteal phase (endometrial secretory phase) produces an increase of endometrial stores of arachidonic acid, a precursor to prostaglandin production. 2) Just before the onset of menses and during menses, the arachidonic acid stores are converted to prostaglandin $F_{2\alpha}$, prostaglandin E_2 and leukotrienes, which induce uterine contractions. In women with dysmenorrhea, uterine pressures can reach 180 mmHg with resting pressures as great as 80 mmHg. In addition the uterine contractions can be prolonged. 3) Frequent and prolonged uterine contractions that decrease blood flow to the uterus cause uterine ischemia and trigger pain nerve fibers. During uterine ischemia, anaerobic metabolites can accumulate in the uterus and stimulate small type-C pain neurons. From an evolutionary point of view, forceful uterine myometrial contractions during menstruation is probably a physiological adaptation that results in the constriction of uterine blood vessels and limits the magnitude of menstrual blood loss.

Evidence that uterine and endometrial prostaglandins play a central role in causing dysmenorrhea includes the reports that endometrial concentrations of prostaglandins E_2 and $F_2\,\alpha$ correlate with the severity of the dysmenorrhea, that cyclooxygenase inhibitors decrease menstrual fluid prostaglandin levels and reported menstrual pain, and that painful uterine contractions can be caused by administering prostaglandins to pregnant women.

In women with primary dysmenorrhea and increased prostaglandin E_2 and $F_2\,\alpha$ production, the large and small bowel may be hypersensitive to mechanical stimuli. In some women, pain from the bowel may contribute to the visceral pain of dysmenorrhea.

History

Historical features that may be helpful to assess include:
- age of menarche
- date of onset of last two menses
- relationship between onset of symptoms and number of days of symptoms, first and last day of menstrual flow
- location and severity of symptoms
- presence of associated symptoms such as nausea, diarrhea, and back pain
- efficacy of NSAIDs in treating symptoms

In addition to abdominal and pelvic pain, many women with dysmenorrhea report, nausea, diarrhea, and back pain.

For women with dysmenorrhea, the history can be focused on attempting to determine if a primary or secondary form of the disorder is present. The more severe the symptoms and the greater their functional impact, the more likely that a secondary form of the disorder is present. Women with severe dysmenorrhea who have a negligible response to NSAIDs are also at increased risk for having pelvic pathology that is causing the pain. **Table 41.2**

Table 41.2 Assessment of severity of dysmenorrhea using a verbal multidimensional scoring system. This scoring system correlates well with assessment of pain using a linear analogue scale (0–10 cm)

Grade	Description of dysmenorrhea	Impact of dysmenorrhea on work life	Systemic symptoms	Use and efficacy of nonsteroidal anti-inflammatory analgesics
0	No dysmenorrhea	None	None	None needed
1	Pain is present during menses, but life activities not significantly impacted	Minimal to none	None	Rarely needed, and effective when taken
2	Moderate pain, daily activities are affected	Moderate	Few	Medications needed and often effective
3	Severe menstrual pain, major impact on life	Severe	Prevalent	Medications needed, but seldom effective enough to return patient to full function

Source: Adapted from Andersch B, Milson I. An epidemiologic study of young women with dysmenorrhea. Am J Obstet Gynecol 1982;144:655–660.

provides a simple approach for assigning women with dysmenorrhea to one of three grades of severity. Women with dysmenorrhea in grade 3 should be suspected of having secondary dysmenorrhea.

Physical Examination and Laboratory Studies

Women with primary dysmenorrhea have a normal pelvic exam. For young, nonsexually active adolescents with mild dysmenorrhea, the pelvic exam can be deferred. Women with secondary dysmenorrhea caused by endometriosis, adenomyosis, and uterine leiomyomata may also have a normal pelvic exam. In many cases, women with uterine leiomyomata have an enlarged, irregularly shaped, multilobular uterus. Women with adenomyosis may have a uterus that is at the upper limits of normal in size and tender on palpation. Women with endometriosis may have a number of physical findings including: 1) cervical stenosis, as demonstrated by a cervical os diameter of less than 4 mm; 2) nodular or indurated uterosacral ligaments due to endometriosis lesions on those ligaments; 3) displacement of the cervix to a lateral vaginal fornix due to asymmetric shortening of one uterosacral ligament, cardinal ligament complex (**Fig. 41.1**). Some women with endometriosis affecting the ovary have enlarged adnexa on pelvic exam. Endometriosis commonly

produces inflammation that causes the pelvic tissues to become indurated and "woody," with fixed and nonmobile pelvic structures.

Laboratory tests and imaging studies do not typically help with the evaluation of primary dysmenorrhea, but may be helpful to identify pelvic pathology in women with grade 3 dysmenorrhea who have a secondary cause. Pelvic ultrasonography is useful for detecting uterine leiomyomata, which are ovarian cysts caused by endometriosis and adenomyosis. Magnetic resonance imaging is more sensitive than ultrasonography for the diagnosis of adenomyosis. The level of serum cancer antigen CA-125 is often elevated in women with advanced endometriosis and in some women with uterine leiomyomata or chronic pelvic inflammatory disease. The sensitivity and specificity of CA-125 for diagnosing advanced endometriosis is in the range of 0.54 and 0.96, respectively, limiting its clinical utility.

Treatment

Primary dysmenorrhea is thought to be caused by excessive prostaglandin stimulation of uterine myometrial contractions, resulting in uterine ischemia and pain. Pharmacologic agents that inhibit prostaglandin synthesis and/or action (e.g., NSAIDs), and agents that directly inhibit uterine contractions (e.g., calcium channel block-

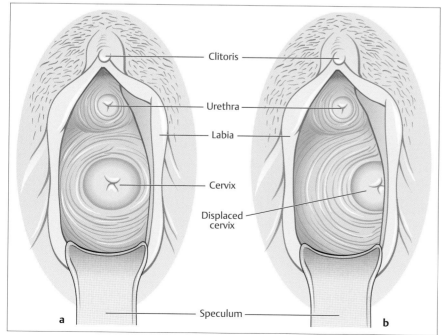

Fig. 41.1a,b The presence of a cervix displaced to one side of the vagina in a woman with severe dysmenorrhea should raise the suspicion of endometriosis, or other pelvic pathology. Some women with endometriosis have asymmetric shortening of one uterosacral ligament. This can result in the cervix being pulled to one side of the vagina.
a Normally placed cervix with the cervical os in the midline (same line as mid clitoris and urethral opening.
b Lateral displacement of the cervix to the left side of the vagina due to shortening of the left uterosacral ligament caused by endometriosis.

Clitoris
Urethra
Labia
Cervix
Displaced cervix
Speculum

ers) have been demonstrated to be effective therapy for dysmenorrhea. As will be discussed in more detail below, placebo treatment reduces reported menstrual pain in a substantial number of women. Consequently, to assess properly the relative effectiveness of active treatment versus placebo, controlled trials are necessary.

Nonpharmacologic treatment

Continuous Heat Therapy

Application of a heat wrap to the lower abdomen/pelvis appears to be effective treatment for dysmenorrhea. In one clinical trial 81 women were randomized to one of four groups:
1. A nonheated abdominal patch plus placebo
2. An abdominal heat patch plus placebo
3. A non-heated abdominal patch plus ibuprofen 400 mg three times daily for 2 days
4. An abdominal heat patch plus ibuprofen 400 mg three times daily for 2 days.

All three active treatment groups demonstrated a similar improvement in menstrual pain compared with the nonheated abdominal patch plus placebo. The investigators concluded that continuous low-level heat therapy was as effective as ibuprofen for the treatment of primary dysmenorrhea.

Other Nonpharmacologic Interventions

Clinical trials have reported that the following interventions may be effective in the treatment of dysmenorrhea:
- aerobic exercise
- a low-fat vegetarian diet
- vitamin B_1, 100 mg daily
- vitamin B_6, 200 mg daily
- vitamin E, 500 units daily
- fish oil supplements
- magnesium supplements
- Asian herbal remedies

We do not recommend these interventions as first-line treatment, because their clinical efficacy versus standard nonsteroidal anti-inflammatory therapy has not been determined.

Nonsteroidal Anti-Inflammatory Drugs

NSAIDs are first-line therapy for the treatment of primary dysmenorrhea. Over 50 clinical trials have reported that NSAIDs cause more symptom improvement than placebo in women with dysmenorrhea. A representative estimate over multiple menstrual cycles of treatment is that significant symptom improvement is reported by about 15% of women treated with placebo versus 70% of women treated with a NSAID. An important methodological issue is that in the treatment of primary dysmenorrhea a "placebo effect" is most prominent in the first cycle of treatment but, as a trial is extended over many cycles, the placebo effect wanes. For example, in one study the effectiveness of placebo treatment was found to deteriorate over four cycles of therapy, with symptom improvement reported in 84%, 29%, 16%, and 10% over the first, second, third, and fourth placebo treatment cycles, respectively. In contrast, in this study the beneficial effects of NSAIDs persisted over multiple cycles. This important observation indicates that high-quality clinical trials need to assess the efficacy of an intervention over multiple menstrual cycles.

Many NSAIDs are effective for the treatment of dysmenorrhea (**Table 41.3**). There is no consistent evidence from large clinical trials that one NSAID is better than another for the treatment of dysmenorrhea. Consequently, side effect profile and cost should guide treatment decisions. A commonly used regimen is ibuprofen 400–800 mg three to four times daily (maximal dose 3200 mg daily) starting 1 day before the expected onset of menses, or the day of menses and continued for 2–4 days. Cyclo-oxygenase 2 (COX-2) inhibitors (e.g., rofecoxib and diclofenac) and fenamate (e.g., mefanamic acid) NSAIDs are effective in the treatment of dysmenorrhea, but are more expensive than phenylproprionic acid NSAIDs such as ibuprofen and naproxen.

Table 41.3 Nonsteroidal anti-inflammatory drugs commonly used for the treatment of primary dysmenorrhea

Agent	Initial dose	Common dose regimen
Ibuprofen	400 mg	400–800 mg, 3 to 4 times daily
Naproxen	500 mg	250 mg, 3 to 4 times daily
Naproxen sodium	550 mg	275 mg, 3 to 4 times daily

Estrogen–Progestin Contraceptives

No high-quality randomized trials compare directly the efficacy of estrogen–progestin contraceptives versus NSAIDs for the treatment of dysmenorrhea. A few clinical trials have reported that estrogen–progestin contraceptives are superior to placebo for the treatment of dysmenorrhea (Evidence Box 41.1). Estrogen–progestin contraceptives reduce endometrial growth and the endometrial production of arachidonic acid and its prostaglandin metabolites, resulting in reduced intensity of uterine contractions during menses, and improvement in symptoms of dysmenorrhea. For women with dysmenorrhea who desire contraception, estrogen–progestin contraceptives may be particularly beneficial. These agents may be prescribed as monthly cycles (21 active pills, 7 days off; or 24 active pills, 4 days off) or extended cycles, where active agents are taken continuously (365 days a year of active pill use) or in long cycles (84 active pills, 7 days off). Extended cycles may be associated with less menstrual pain than regular monthly cycles. The most common adverse effect of extended cycle therapy is breakthrough uterine bleeding.

For patients with endometriosis and dysmenorrhea, estrogen–progestin contraceptives have been demonstrated to be superior to placebo for pain relief. Since some women diagnosed with primary dysmenorrhea have undiagnosed endometriosis, estrogen–progestin contraceptives may provide effective treatment for women with either condition.

Inhibitors of Uterine Myometrial Contraction

Nifedipine, a calcium channel blocker that inhibits uterine smooth muscle contraction, has been reported to decrease menstrual pain when administered in single doses of 20–40 mg. The side effects of nifedipine include facial flushing, tachycardia, and headache. Many women with primary dysmenorrhea also report headaches during menses, and nifedipine may worsen the headache symptoms.

Acupuncture

In one large clinical trial, women with dysmenorrhea were randomized to treatment with 3 months of acupuncture (needle acupuncture with manual manipulation of needles) versus no acupuncture. Subjects assigned to the no-acupuncture group had a 15% decrease in menstrual pain score. Subjects in the acupuncture group reported a 50% decrease in menstrual pain score . Sham acupuncture, which is known to be a "strong" placebo, was not used in this study as the control. In addition, acupuncture was not tested against NSAIDs, which are known to be effective and less expensive than acupuncture.

Levonorgestrel-Releasing Intrauterine System

The levonorgestrel-releasing intrauterine system produces decreased menstrual flow in over 50% of women using the device. The system releases levonorgestrel, a potent progestin, directly into the uterine cavity, which inhibits the growth of endometrium and the synthesis of prostaglandins. Consequently, many women with dysmenorrhea who are treated with the levonorgestrel intrauterine system report a decrease in menstrual pain. No large-scale clinical trials of this device versus placebo or a standard agent, such as ibuprofen or oral contraceptives, have been reported. It should be noted that intrauterine devices with copper have been reported to be associated with increased menstrual pain.

Transcutaneous Electrical Nerve Stimulation

Transcutaneous electrical nerve stimulation (TENS) decreases menstrual pain by blocking spinal transmission of signals from pain fibers to the brain. High frequency TENS has been demonstrated to be superior to placebo for the treatment of dysmenorrhea. However, TENS alone and TENS plus ibuprofen have not been demonstrated to be superior to ibuprofen alone for the treatment of dysmenorrhea.

Unproven Therapies

Spinal Manipulation

Four trials of spinal manipulation for the treatment of primary and secondary dysmenorrhea have been reported. Active spinal manipulation was no more effective than sham spinal manipulation in these trials.

Laparoscopic Uterine Nerve Ablation

Clinical trials have not clearly demonstrated that laparoscopic uterine nerve ablation provides long-term effective treatment of dysmenorrhea. Given the need for anesthesia and major surgery to perform this operation, and the absence of strong evidence to support its use, it is not recommended for the treatment of primary dysmenorrhea.

Treatment Failure

For women thought to have primary dysmenorrhea who do not respond to NSAIDs, estrogen–progestin contraceptives, and dietary/life style interventions, the possibility of the presence of pelvic pathology such as endometriosis, fibroids, and adenomyosis should be considered. In one study of women with severe dysmenorrhea who did not respond to NSAIDs, laparoscopy demonstrated minimal or mild endometriosis in the majority of the women.

Key Points

- Dysmenorrhea, or painful menstruation, is divided into two major categories: primary and secondary. Primary dysmenorrhea is the presence of recurrent, crampy pelvic pain in the lower abdomen that occurs just before and/or during menstruation in the absence of suspected or proven pelvic pathology. Secondary dysmenorrhea is painful menstruation in the presence of a disease that causes pelvic pain such as endometriosis, adenomyosis, or uterine leiomyomas.
- Dysmenorrhea is probably caused by prostaglandins released from the sloughing endometrium, which induces prolonged uterine contractions and a relative uterine ischemia, thereby triggering pain neurons.
- First-line treatment of dysmenorrhea is nonsteroidal anti-inflammatory agents that block prostaglandin action.
- Estrogen–progestin treatment reduces endometrial prostaglandin production, thereby improving symptoms of dysmenorrhea.
- Nonpharmacologic approaches that may help relieve the pain of menstruation include: heat therapy, aerobic exercise, a low-fat vegetarian diet, vitamin B_1, vitamin B_6, vitamin E, fish oil supplements, magnesium supplements, and herbal remedies.

Evidence Box 41.1

Low-dose estrogen–progestin contraceptives are effective for the treatment of primary dysmenorrhea.

Along with nonsteroidal anti-inflammatory drugs (NSAIDs), estrogen–progestin contraceptives are first-line agents for the treatment of primary dysmenorrhea. However, many more clinical trials document the efficacy of NSAIDs compared to estrogen–progestins for dysmenorrhea. In one clinical trial, 76 adolescents with moderate to severe dysmenorrhea were randomly assigned to 3 months of treatment with a placebo pill or an estrogen–progestin contraceptive used in a cycle of 21 active pills, 7 inactive pills. The low-dose, estrogen–progestin contraceptive used in this trial contained 20 µg of ethinyl estradiol and 100 µg of levonorgestrel in the active pills. Using the Moos Menstrual Distress Questionnaire, placebo treatment was associated with an approximately 50% reduction in pain score and estrogen–progestin treatment was associated with to a decrease in self-reported pain, 61% of the women in the estrogen–progestin group discontinued their use of NSAIDs compared with 36% in the placebo group.

Davis AR, Westhoff C, O'Connell K, Gallagher N. Oral contraceptives for dysmenorrhea in adolescent girls. Obstet Gynecol 2005;106:97–104.

Further Reading

Akin MD, Weingand KW, Hengehold DA, Goodale MB, Hinkle RT, Smith RP. Continuous low-level topical heat in the treatment of dysmenorrhea. *Obstet Gynecol* 2001;97(3):343–349

Andersch B, Milsom I. An epidemiologic study of young women with dysmenorrhea. *Am J Obstet Gynecol* 1982;144(6):655–660

Barbieri RL, Niloff JM, Bast RC Jr, Scaetzl E, Kistner RW, Knapp RC. Elevated serum concentrations of CA-125 in patients with advanced endometriosis. *Fertil Steril* 1986;45(5):630–634

Brinkert W, Dimcevski G, Arendt-Nielsen L, Drewes AM, Wilder-Smith OH. Dysmenorrhoea is associated with hypersensitivity in the sigmoid colon and rectum. *Pain* 2007;132(Suppl 1):S46–S51

Burnett MA, Antao V, Black A, et al. Prevalence of primary dysmenorrhea in Canada. *J Obstet Gynaecol Can* 2005;27(8):765–770

Davis AR, Westhoff C, O'Connell K, Gallagher N. Oral contraceptives for dysmenorrhea in adolescent girls: a randomized trial. *Obstet Gynecol* 2005;106(1):97–104

Dawood MY, Ramos J. Transcutaneous electrical nerve stimulation (TENS) for the treatment of primary dysmenorrhea: a randomized crossover comparison with placebo TENS and ibuprofen. *Obstet Gynecol* 1990;75(4):656–660

Dawood MY. Primary dysmenorrhea: advances in pathogenesis and management. *Obstet Gynecol* 2006;108(2):428–441

Fedele L, Marchini M, Acaia B, Garagiola U, Tiengo M. Dynamics and significance of placebo response in primary dysmenorrhea. *Pain* 1989;36(1):43–47

Harada T, Momoeda M, Taketani Y, Hoshiai H, Terakawa N. Low-dose oral contraceptive pill for dysmenorrhea associated with endometriosis: a placebo-controlled, double-blind, randomized trial. *Fertil Steril* 2008;90(5):1583–1588

Herman-Giddens ME, Slora EJ, Wasserman RC, et al. Secondary sexual characteristics and menses in young girls seen in office practice: a study from the Pediatric Research in Office Settings network. *Pediatrics* 1997;99(4):505–512

Kissler S, Zangos S, Kohl J, et al. Duration of dysmenorrhoea and extent of adenomyosis visualised by magnetic resonance imaging. *Eur J Obstet Gynecol Reprod Biol* 2008;137(2):204–209

Legro RS, Pauli JG, Kunselman AR, et al. Effects of continuous versus cyclical oral contraception: a randomized controlled trial. *J Clin Endocrinol Metab* 2008;93(2):420–429

Ling FW; Pelvic Pain Study Group. Randomized controlled trial of depot leuprolide in patients with chronic pelvic pain and clinically suspected endometriosis. *Obstet Gynecol* 1999;93(1):51–58

Owen PR. Prostaglandin synthetase inhibitors in the treatment of primary dysmenorrhea. Outcome trials reviewed. *Am J Obstet Gynecol* 1984;148(1):96–103

Proctor ML, Hing W, Johnson TC, Murphy PA. Spinal manipulation for primary and secondary dysmenorrhea. *Cochrane Database Syst Rev* 2006;3:CD002119

Proctor ML, Latthe PM, Farquhar CM, Khan KS, Johnson NP. Surgical interruption of pelvic nerve pathways for primary and secondary dysmenorrhea. *Cochrane Database Syst Rev* 2005;2:CD001896

Proctor ML, Murphy PA. Herbal and dietary therapies for primary and secondary dysmenorrhea. *Cochrane Database Syst Rev* 2001;00:CD002124

Witt CM, Reinhold T, Brinkhaus B, Roll S, Jena S, Willich SN. Acupuncture in patients with dysmenorrhea: a randomized study on clinical effectiveness and cost-effectiveness in usual care. *Am J Obstet Gynecol* 2008;198(2):166, e1–e8

42 Infertility

Robert L. Barbieri

Definition

Fertility is defined as the capacity to conceive and produce offspring. *Infertility* is the state of a diminished capacity to conceive and bear offspring. In contrast to sterility, infertility is not an irreversible state. The current clinical definition of infertility is the inability to conceive after 12 months of frequent coitus. Infertility prevalence among women aged 15–44 years was 8.5% in 1982 and 7.4% in 2002. Infertility prevalence is greater in older women and possibly in older men. Since the fertility potential of the female partner decreases after 35 years of age, some authorities recommend initiating an infertility evaluation after 6 months of attempting conception in women 35–40 years of age, and immediately in women over 40 years of age.

Causes

In most mammals, including humans, pregnancy requires the effective function of at least five systems or cell types:

1. A competent oocyte
2. A competent sperm
3. A favorable environment in which fertilization can take place
4. A transport system to allow passage of the fertilized oocyte to enter the uterus
5. A prepared endometrium that will accept the implantation of the oocyte and nurture the growing embryo (**Fig. 42.1**).

Abnormalities in any of these five systems can result in infertility.

Based on our current understanding of the causes of infertility, and the most contemporary diagnostic approach to infertility, the most common single causes of infertility are:

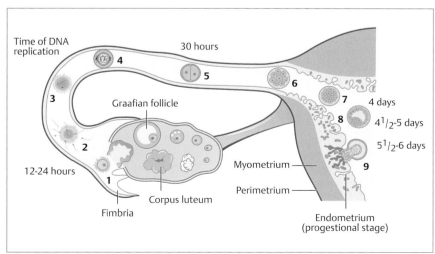

Fig. 42.1 Schematic representation of the transport of the oocyte, sperm and embryo in the female reproductive tract. (1) Ovulation of competent oocyte. (2) Fertilization of oocyte, (3, 4) movement of single cell prezygote through the fallopian tube, (5) multicellular embryo in fallopian tube, (6, 7) arrival of the multicellular embryo into the uterus 4–5 days after ovulation, (8) formation of blastocyst, and (9) implantation into endometrium 5–6 days after ovulation. In an in vitro fertilization cycle, it is common to observe a 2-cell embryo form, about 1 day after fertilization, a 4-cell embryo form about 2 days after fertilization, and a blastocyst about 5 days after fertilization.

1. Male factor: poorly functioning sperm or the absence of sperm (24% of cases)
2. Tubal disease blocking the transport of oocyte, sperm and/or embryo (23% of cases)
3. Anovulatory infertility or poor oocyte function (18% of cases)
4. Unexplained infertility, where no cause of the infertility can be identified (26% of cases)
5. Endometriosis (7% of cases)
6. Other causes, including fibroids and cervical diseases (2% of cases)

Diagnostic Tests

Three diagnostic tests should be performed in almost all couples with infertility:
1. Demonstration of ovulation
2. Semen analysis
3. A hysterosalpingogram to test tubal patency.

In some couples, especially where the female partner is greater than 35 years of age, a test should be performed to assess the size of the remaining ovarian oocyte pool.

Tests of Ovulation

Women who have monthly menses and report moliminal symptoms—such as breast tenderness and dysmenorrhea—are typically ovulatory. In one study, women who reported regular monthly menses were demonstrated to be ovulatory in over 95% of cases. Conversely, women with amenorrhea are likely to be anovulatory (or have uterine adhesions or cervical obstruction preventing menstrual flow). Oligomenorrhea (cycle length >35 days) is typically associated with oligo-ovulation.

The least expensive laboratory method for detecting ovulation is the measurement of the basal body temperature. For most women, the morning basal temperature obtained prior to rising from bed is less than 36.7°C (98°F) before ovulation and more than 36.7°C after ovulation. Progesterone production from the ovary appears to raise the hypothalamic set-point for basal temperature by approximately 0.6°F. The normal luteal phase is typically associated with a temperature rise, above 36.7°C, for at least 10 days in length. Occasionally, basal body temperature recordings may appear monophasic, even in the presence of ovulation. A biphasic pattern is almost always associated with ovulation. If the pattern is biphasic, coitus can be recommended every other day for a period including the five days prior to, and the day of, ovulation.

The main source of progesterone secretion in women is the corpus luteum, which develops from the dominant ovarian follicle after ovulation. Prior to ovulation, the ovary secretes small quantities of progesterone. A serum progesterone level greater than 3 ng/mL is diagnostic of ovulation.. A mid-luteal progesterone concentration less than 10 ng/mL is associated with a lower per-cycle pregnancy rate than progesterone levels above 10 ng/mL. A urine luteinizing hormone (LH) surge is detectable with a home immunoassay kit about 1 day before ovulation. In about 90% of cases, the detection of a urine LH surge is associated with a subsequent ovulation, as demonstrated by an appropriate rise in serum progesterone.

Testing of the Ovarian Oocyte Pool

The oocytes with the best potential for developing into competent embryos appear to be ovulated first. When there are only a small number of oocytes remaining in the ovary, it is likely that these oocytes contain genetic abnormalities that reduce their potential to develop into competent embryos. Detection of women with a low number of ovarian oocytes is predictive of fertility and the effectiveness of fertility treatments.

The best single method for detecting a low number of ovarian oocytes is measurement of serum follicle-stimulating hormone (FSH) during menstrual cycle day 2, 3, or 4 (the second, third or fourth day of menses). This is called the "day 3 FSH" test. During menses, FSH secretion is suppressed by the production of inhibin B from ovarian follicles containing competent oocytes. When the ovarian oocyte pool is small, inhibin B production is low and FSH secretion is increased resulting in serum FSH levels greater than 15 U/L on cycle day 3. Alternatively, serum inhibin B levels can be measured. Low inhibin B levels indicate few remaining ovarian oocytes. However, it is technically challenging to reliably detect low levels of inhibin B. High resolution pelvic sonography can also be used to count the number of follicles (which contain the oocyte) in the ovary. The greater the number of resident follicles detected by ultrasound scanning, the more likely that there is an adequate ovarian oocyte pool.

Semen Analysis

The semen analysis is performed on an ejaculated semen specimen. In some cases, the semen can be obtained by suggesting the couple have sexual intercourse using a condom that contains no spermicide. The semen analysis includes the following measurements: semen volume, sperm concentration, sperm motility, and a microscopic evaluation of sperm morphology. The normal parameters for a semen specimen are listed in **Table 42.1**. In men with one abnormal or borderline semen analysis, it is prudent to repeat the test. If the semen analysis demonstrates a very low sperm concentration (<5 million/mL) a karyotype should be performed to look for defects in the Y chromosome and other problems such as balanced translocations.

Hysterosalpingogram

Obtaining a hysterosalpingogram (HSG) involves the injection of a contrast agent into the cervical os, so that the agent may travel through the uterus and fallopian tubes into the peritoneal cavity. The course of the contrast agent through the reproductive tract is monitored using fluoroscopy. The HSG is very sensitive for detecting tubal disease. It is especially specific for identifying distal tubal occlusion at the fimbriated ends of the tube. In some HSG tests, proximal tubal occlusion at the utero-tubal junction is detected, but follow-up tests such as selective catheterization of the fallopian tubes demonstrates the proximal tube to be patent.

Laparoscopy

In some couples, laparoscopy of the female partner may be of benefit in the diagnosis and treatment of infertility. As noted above, about 7 % of women with infertility have endometriosis, and the only test that can reliably diagnose endometriosis is laparoscopy. If endometriosis is detected at the time of laparoscopy, it can be surgically treated at the same time, which results in an improvement in fertility. Many clinicians reserve laparoscopy for women who have symptoms (severe dysmenorrhea) or physical findings (nodular uterosacral ligaments) suggestive of the disease; and for couples in whom all infertility testing was normal.

Other Tests

Two commonly performed tests, the postcoital test and the endometrial biopsy, are of no value in evaluating most couples with infertility. The postcoital test is performed by getting the couple to have sexual intercourse just prior to ovulation. A speculum exam of the vagina and cervix is performed and a quantity of the cervical mucus is obtained with forceps for examination under the microscope. If motile sperm are present in sufficient quantities the test is normal. If no motile sperm are present, the test is deemed abnormal. In randomized trials of the clinical utility of the postcoital test it was found that it offered no incremental information that was not obtained with the basic three fertility tests; and that it did not influence treatment decisions or fertility outcomes. The test is of no value in evaluating the infertile couple. In the past, the endometrial biopsy was regarded as the "gold standard" for determining whether the endometrium was properly receptive for an incoming embryo. In a well-designed observational study, women with infertility and fertility had similar rates of abnormal, "out of phase" endometrial biopsy results. This indicated that the test cannot discriminate between fertile and infertile women. The endometrial biopsy is of no value in the evaluation of the infertile couple.

Table 42.1 Normal semen parameters

Measurement	Normal range	Comments
Semen volume	2–5 mL	A very low volume may be due to a poorly collected ejaculate or genital tract obstruction.
Sperm concentration	>20 million sperm per mL	Sperm concentration is an important predictor of male fertility. Values less than 10 million sperm per mL are especially indicative of male infertility
Sperm motility	>50 % of sperm should be motile	When sperm concentration is low–normal, good motility may "make up" for the low number of sperm and be associated with good fertility prognosis
Sperm morphology	Evaluation of sperm shape, length, width, volume of acrosome body and assessment of head and tail defects. Using strict criteria, normal morphology is diagnosed when ≥15 % of sperm have normal form. Using lenient criteria, >30 % should have normal form.	Sperm morphology is an important predictor of male fertility.

Treatment

Whenever a clinician approaches the treatment of infertility, alternative choices, such as adoption or remaining childless should be explored with the couple. Treatment of infertility may be stressful for couples and disappointing if it is not successful. In many locales, some aspects of infertility treatment may not be covered by health insurance plans, making treatment an expensive part of a family budget.

Male Factor

Options for the treatment of male factor infertility include: semen donation from a well-screened anonymous donor; intrauterine insemination of the female with the male partner's sperm; and assisted reproductive technology involving in vitro fertilization (IVF) combined with microinjection of a sperm into an oocyte in the laboratory.

Sperm Donation

Donor sperm is typically obtained from men in their 20s who have been thoroughly screened for genetic and sexually transmitted diseases. Donated specimens from these men are cryopreserved in aliquots, which are shipped to the point of clinical care. At the point of care, the sperm specimens are thawed and typically an intrauterine insemination (IUI) is performed to ensure that the maximal number of sperm are delivered high into the reproductive tract. In couples with male factor infertility and a baseline pregnancy rate of 2% per cycle, donor sperm may increase the per cycle pregnancy rate up to 15–25% per cycle. Success of sperm donation is highly dependent on the age of the female partner because, in older women, the ovarian oocyte pool is depleted.

Intrauterine Insemination

In couples where there is a mild male-factor infertility, intrauterine insemination may result in pregnancy. The IUI procedure consists of washing an ejaculated semen specimen to remove prostaglandins, concentrating the sperm in a small volume of culture medium with a high protein concentration which initiates the sperm acrosome reaction, and injecting the sperm suspension directly into the upper uterine cavity using a small catheter threaded through the cervix. IUI deposits a large number of motile sperm high in the female reproductive tract, increasing the number of sperm that reach the ovulated oocyte, and enhancing the pregnancy rate. After coitus, the sperm deposited in the vagina must traverse the cervical mucus, the entire uterus, and the fallopian tube. After IUI, the sperm only need to traverse the fallopian tube. The insemination is timed to take place just prior to ovulation, typically using home urine LH measurement. If the baseline pregnancy rate in an infertile couple is in the range of 2% per cycle, IUI improves the per cycle pregnancy rate to about 4–6% per cycle. A major advantage of the IUI is that it does not require either the male or female partner to take stimulatory hormones.

Intracytoplasmic Sperm Injection

Intracytoplasmic sperm injection (ICSI) is performed by injecting the female partner with FSH and stimulating the development of multiple follicles. The female partner undergoes ultrasound-guided aspiration of the oocytes from the ovary. Once the oocytes are mature, a single sperm is injected into each oocyte using a microscopic injection technique. Remarkably, ICSI can also be used in combination with testicular sperm extraction to produce paternity in men with absolute azoospermia (see Evidence Box 42.1). ICSI has revolutionized the treatment of male factor infertility. In couples with a baseline pregnancy rate in the range of 0–1% per cycle, ICSI may increase the pregnancy rate to 30% per cycle. A major disadvantage of ICSI is that it requires the healthy and normal female partner to take FSH injections to stimulate the development of multiple oocytes. In addition, in some cases of severe male-factor infertility, genetic abnormalities in the Y chromosome can be a cause of the low sperm production. These genetic abnormalities can be passed on to male offspring resulting from ICSI, risking the possibility that those children will be infertile later in their lives.

Tubal Factor

A major cause of tubal obstruction is "subclinical" infection with *Chlamydia trachomatis*. Many women with tubal factor infertility have elevated levels of antibodies to *C. trachomatis*. There is no evidence that treatment with antibiotics will help repair the fallopian tube damage once it has occurred. The options for treatment of tubal factor infertility include surgical repair of the fallopian tube or IVF. Surgical repair of distal fallopian tube occlusion is often successful, but about 30% of pregnancies that occur following surgical repair will be ectopic pregnancies. IVF (see below) is highly effective in treating tubal factor infertility.

Anovulatory Infertility

There are many causes of anovulation (see Chapter 39) and each of these diseases may cause anovulatory infertility. Three of the most common causes of anovulatory infertility are:

1. Hypothalamic hypogonadism due to decreases in gonadotropin-releasing hormone (GnRH), LH, and FSH production
2. Polycystic ovary syndrome (PCOS)
3. Primary ovarian failure

When women present with amenorrhea or oligomenorrhea, signs of anovulation, and oligo-ovulation, serum tests of FSH, prolactin, thyroid-stimulating hormone (TSH) and, if appropriate, testosterone should be obtained. Elevated levels of prolactin and TSH are treated as indicated (see Chapter 39).

Women with primary ovarian failure typically present with amenorrhea or oligomenorrhea, and have persistently elevated serum FSH concentration, indicating a depleted ovarian oocyte pool. The fertility treatment available for these women is donor oocytes from a well-screened donor woman. Women with hypothalamic amenorrhea typically have a history of low body mass index (BMI), or strenuous exercise, or psychosocial stress, or an eating disorder. Therapy focused on resolving the disorder that caused the anovulation is prudent. Alternatively, exogenous injections of FSH and/or LH may be administered to induce ovulation.

PCOS typically presents with the combination of hyperandrogenism, as manifested by hirsutism and an elevated testosterone level, and oligo-ovulation or anovulation. The approach to ovulation induction in PCOS is discussed in detail in Chapter 40. Options available for ovulation induction in infertile women with PCOS include the following:

- weight loss to achieve a BMI below 27 kg/m^2
- treatment with clomiphene citrate pills, typically administered as 50 mg daily for 5 days, which increases pituitary secretion of FSH and LH and results in development of follicle growth and ovulation
- metformin treatment to reverse the insulin resistance present in many women with PCOS
- FSH injections
- ovarian surgery to decrease testosterone production from the many small atretic follicles
- IVF

Unexplained Infertility

Unexplained infertility exists when the three basic tests of infertility are normal. In the female partner ovulation is occurring regularly and the fallopian tubes are normal. In addition the day 3 FSH test should be demonstrated to be normal. In the male partner the semen parameters will have been documented to be normal.

An initial step in the evaluation of the couple with unexplained infertility should be a decision about whether to perform laparoscopy to look for endometriosis and treat it at the time of laparoscopy. Overall about 7% of infertile couples will have endometriosis documented in the female partner. But among couples with normal results from the three basic tests of infertility, about 40% would have endometriosis documented in the female partner, if laparoscopy were performed in all cases. There is evidence from clinical trials that surgical treatment of endometriosis improves fertility (see below). Alternatively, some clinicians prefer not to perform laparoscopy for infertility and proceed directly with the five treatment steps outlined below.

For couples with unexplained infertility, clinical trials have demonstrated that the following stepwise approach to treatment is cost effective:

1. Properly time sexual intercourse using at-home urine LH predictor kits to time ovulation (see Evidence Box 42.2)
2. Improve lifestyle factors that influence fertility (see below)
3. Make use of empiric IUI, which may raise per cycle pregnancy rates from a baseline of 2% to 4–6% per cycle
4. Stimulate double ovulation in the female partner using clomiphene citrate treatment, and use IUI to deliver sperm high into the reproductive tract. This intervention may increase per cycle pregnancy rates from a baseline of 2% to 7–9% per cycle
4. Stimulate triple and quadruple ovulation in the female partner using FSH injections and use IUI to deliver sperm high into the reproductive tract. This intervention may increase per cycle pregnancy rates from a baseline of 2% to 10–15% per cycle. The main disadvantage of this approach is that triplet and quadruplet pregnancy may result. Many clinicians prefer to avoid this step
5. Try IVF. This intervention may increase per cycle pregnancy rates from a baseline of 2% to 30–40% per cycle. The main disadvantage of IVF is that it is resource intensive and may result in a high rate of twin pregnancy.

This stepwise approach to infertility appears to be cost effective (**Table 42.2**).

Table 42.2 Estimated pregnancy rate and cost per treatment cycle in couples with unexplained infertility

Intervention	Per cycle pregnancy rate (%)	Approximate cost per cycle in US dollars 2007
Monitoring urine LH surge using at-home kit	1–3%	50
Intrauterine insemination (IUI)	4–6%	400
Clomiphene citrate (causes double ovulation)	4–6%	100
Clomiphene plus IUI	7–9%	500
Gonadotropin (FSH-only or LH and FSH) injection (causes double and triple ovulation)	4–10%	2000
Gonadotropin injection plus IUI	9–15%	2400
In vitro fertilization	20–40%	17000

FSH, follicle-stimulating hormone; LH, luteinizing hormone.

Endometriosis

Peritoneal and tubal inflammation commonly occur in women with endometriosis and are a potential mechanism linking infertility to the disease. Studies have shown that women with endometriosis have an increased volume of peritoneal fluid, increased peritoneal fluid concentration of activated macrophages, and increased peritoneal fluid concentration of prostaglandins, interleukin-1, tumor necrosis factor, and proteases. These abnormalities in the peritoneal environment may impair gamete, embryo, and fallopian tube function. As an example, peritoneal fluid from women with endometriosis has been reported to inhibit sperm function and ciliary function, thereby possibly reducing fertility.

In women with advanced endometriosis, major pelvic adhesions and scarring contribute to infertility.

As noted above, the "gold standard" for diagnosis of endometriosis is visualization at laparoscopy. Laparoscopic treatment of endometriosis implants by excision or electrosurgical ablation of lesions has been reported to improve fertility. In one trial, 341 women with early stage endometriosis were randomly assigned to a diagnostic laparoscopy combined with surgical resection or ablation of endometriosis lesions or a diagnostic laparoscopy only. During 36 weeks of postoperative follow-up, the per cycle pregnancy rate was significantly higher in the group that underwent surgical resection or ablation

of endometriosis lesions compared with the control group (4.7% vs. 2.4% pregnancy rate per cycle). The cumulative pregnancy rates over the 36 weeks of follow-up in the treatment and control groups were 31% and 18%, respectively. A major advantage of this approach is that the couples did not need to take hormone medications to achieve pregnancy, thereby reducing the risk of multiple gestation pregnancy.

For women with endometriosis who do not become pregnant after laparoscopic surgery, the available treatment options are similar to those for unexplained infertility including: IUI, clomiphene IUI, gonadotropin injections plus IUI, or IVF.

Uterine Factors

Congenital Uterine Anomalies

A definitive cause–effect relationship between uterine anomalies and infertility is not definitively established. However, some uterine abnormalities, such as a septate uterus, appear to be associated with a higher rate of spontaneous abortion than among women with a normal uterus. This may be due to decreased blood flow in the septum, resulting in poor embryo implantation. In infertile women with a septate uterus diagnosed by hysterosalpingography, hysteroscopic resection of the uterine septum is often recommended. Women with a bicornuate uterus may also have a modestly increased risk of spontaneous abortion.

Fibroids

Uterine leiomyomata (fibroids) may be subserosal, intramural, or submucus. Most infertility specialists believe that submucus fibroids may result in infertility. Resection of the submucus fibroid by hysterosocopic resection may result in pregnancy, and will help to improve response to standard fertility treatments, including IVF.

Cervical Factor

Women who have had surgical treatment of cervical dysplasia, such as a cone biopsy, may develop both a mechanical stenosis of the cervical os and a destruction of the glandular elements that produce cervical mucus. Sperm penetration from the vagina through the cervix and into the uterus is facilitated by a patent cervix and adequate cervical mucus. Both cervical stenosis and the absence of cervical mucus can be associated with infertility. Treatment with intrauterine insemination to by-pass the mechanical and mucus-related relative cervical blockade is often effective.

Lifestyle Changes to Improve Fertility and Pregnancy Outcome

Numerous lifestyle choices have been associated with infertility including:

- cigarette smoking by the female and male partners
- obesity in either the female or male partner, or both
- use of caffeine in excess of 500 mg daily (about 4 cups of coffee daily) by the female partner
- consumption of alcoholic beverages, greater than 4 drinks per week by the female partner
- excessive exercise

Since both cigarette smoking and obesity not only impair fertility, but also have major adverse effects on pregnancy, cessation of smoking and normalization of BMI are good goals for infertile couples.

Specific dietary factors may influence the risk of anovulatory infertility. For example, in one prospective study, women who consumed iron supplements were reported to have a 40% lower risk of anovulatory infertility. In another prospective study, dietary patterns characterized by high consumption of mono-unsaturated rather than transfats, vegetable rather than animal protein, low glycemic carbohydrates, high-fat dairy products, and multivitamins were associated with a reduced risk of ovulatory infertility.

Assisted Reproductive Technology

In the United States approximately 4 million live births occur each year. Currently, about 50 000 children are born annually in the United States as the result of IVF treatment. As currently practiced in the United States, the key steps in the IVF treatment process are (**Fig. 42.2**):

1. Stimulate the growth of 10 or more follicles using FSH injections with some adjuvant LH stimulation. Monitor the progress of the follicle growth with serum estradiol measurement and pelvic sonography.
2. Suppress a premature spontaneous endogenous LH surge (which will disrupt the development of the oocytes and trigger a premature ovulation) by administering a GnRH analogue, either a GnRH agonist (using the downregulation phase of the medication) or a GnRH antagonist.
3. Administer an agent to induce the dominant follicles to undergo the final steps of follicle maturation. Most commonly, human chorionic gonadotropin (HCG), which is an LH agonist, is utilized. Alternatively, a bo-

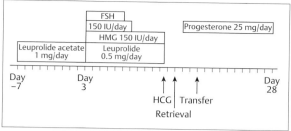

Fig. 42.2 Schematic representation of a typical in vitro fertilization cycle using a gonadotropin-releasing hormone (GnRH) agonist to prevent a premature endogenous luteinizing hormone (LH) surge. The GnRH agonist—in this case, leuprolide acetate—is started prior to the onset of menses in the treatment cycle. On the third day of menses, injections of follicle-stimulating hormone (FSH) and human menopausal gonadotropin (HMG, a mixture of LH and FSH) are initiated and the GnRH agonist dose is decreased. When about 10 follicles have developed, human chorionic gonadotropin (HCG) is administered to initiate the final stages of oocyte maturation. Oocyte aspiration is performed about 36 hours after the HCG injection. Embryos are commonly transferred to the uterus 3 days after oocyte retrieval. Adapted from Davis OK, Rosenwaks Z. In vitro fertilization. In: Keye WR et al. Infertility evaluation and treatment. Philadelphia, PA: WB Saunders, 1995.

lus of GnRH agonist or recombinant LH may be administered.

4. Prior to ovulation of the oocytes, aspirate the oocytes from the follicles using a needle under ultrasonographic guidance. Typically, this occurs about 36 hours after the administration of HCG. On average, about 10 oocytes are obtained at this step, but the range of oocytes harvested is very variable.
5. Incubate the retrieved oocytes with sperm isolated from a semen specimen.
6. On the next day observe the oocytes and determine how many have been fertilized. On average about 60% of the oocytes will fertilize and begin to grow.
7. On the third day after oocyte retrieval, transfer one or two (or more) embryos into the uterus of the female partner using a small plastic catheter. Excess embryos are cryopreserved for use in a future, "natural," non-stimulated cycle.
8. Support the luteal phase of the cycle with exogenous progesterone treatment either as injections or vaginal administration.
9. Check for pregnancy about 2 weeks after embryo transfer. If the pregnancy test is positive, follow the pregnancy ultrasonographically.

In the calendar year 2005 there were over 100 000 assisted reproductive technology cycles including over 80 000 IVF cycles, 16 000 thawed embryo cycles not involving oocyte donation, and 13 000 oocyte donations cycles reported to the Centers for Disease Control and Prevention (**Table 42.3**). About 60% and 4% of the IVF cycles were also combined the ICSI technique and pre-implantation

Table 42.3 Outcomes of in vitro fertilization (IVF) cycles performed in 2005 and reported to the Centers for Disease Control and Prevention and the Society for Assisted Reproductive Technology. Results are stratified by age of the female partner

	Age of the female partner (years)			
	<35	**35–37**	**38–40**	**40–42**
Number of IVF cycles	37 223	20 570	17 805	8337
Percentage of cycles resulting in live births	37%	29%	20%	11%
Average number of embryos transferred	2.4	2.6	3.0	3.3
Percentage of pregnancies with twins	33%	27%	22%	13%
Percentage of pregnancies with triplets or more	4.3%	5.0%	4.4%	2.5%

genetic diagnosis (PGD), respectively. The major fertility indications for IVF were: male factor (17%), tubal factor (10%), decreased ovarian oocyte pool (12%), anovulation (6%), endometriosis (5%), uterine factor (1%), multiple female factors (12%), male and female factors (18%), other and unknown factors (19%). In women under age 35 years, 37% of the IVF cycles initiated resulted in pregnancy with a live birth. Among pregnancies resulting from IVF, 33% were twin gestations and 4.3% were triplets or higher order, multiple gestations. Twin and triplet pregnancy are a major problem associated with IVF because they are associated with increased rates of perinatal mortality, preterm birth, and newborn morbidity (see Chapter 18) In many European fertility centers, embryo transfers are limited to one embryo to reduce the risk of twin and triplet pregnancy. However, single-embryo transfer decreases the pregnancy rate per cycle.

Ovarian Hyperstimulation Syndrome

Gonadotropin injections are commonly used in the treatment of infertility, and are used in especially high doses in IVF. When gonadotropins (FSH and/or LH) are used to stimulate multifollicular development, mild to moderate enlargement of the ovary occurs in as many as 20% of women. Severe enlargement of the ovaries occurs in about 1% of women. Symptoms of ovarian hyperstimulation syndrome (OHSS) include abdominal pain, abdominal distention, nausea, vomiting, diarrhea, and dyspnea. Physical and laboratory findings of OHSS include weight gain, ovarian enlargement, ascites, pleural effusion, hemoconcentration, electrolyte imbalances, renal dysfunction, and thrombosis. Risk factors for OHSS include age under 35 years, low BMI, high doses of FSH, high estradiol con-

centration during the stimulation cycle, increased number and size of follicles, administration of exogenous HCG, a history of PCOS, and cycles in which conception occurs. OHSS is often more severe and has a longer course if a successful pregnancy occurs.

The pathophysiology of OHSS is not completely defined, but during multifollicular development excessive ovarian secretion of vasoactive substances, including vascular endothelial growth factor (VEGF), is believed to trigger the syndrome. VEGF is a potent stimulator of angiogenesis and increases endothelial permeability, possibly by interfering with cellular tight junctions. Other factors that may be involved in the pathogenesis of OHSS include interleukin-6, the renin–angiotensin system and the kinin–kallikrein system. Prevention is best achieved by limiting the dose of gonadotropin administered to young women, and by withholding HCG administration if the serum estradiol level is greater than 1500 pg/mL. Another approach is to change the treatment plan from ovulation induction to an IVF cycle with cryopreservation of all the embryos generated. Treatment includes bed rest, maintenance of intravascular volume, prophylaxis against thrombosis, and surgical correction of ovarian torsion. Physical and laboratory measurements that should be performed daily include measurement of weight and abdominal girth, complete recording of all fluid intake and urine output, measurement of electrolytes, urea nitrogen, albumin, hemoglobin, and coagulation profile.

The initial treatment of OHSS includes preservation of urine output with replacement of fluid volume. Care should be taken not to overhydrate the patient. Early reports suggest that the administration of albumin may help to reduce the risk of OHSS in women with very high estradiol concentrations (over 7000 pg/mL) undergoing IVF. Cabergoline, a dopamine receptor agonist, may block VEGF activation of the endothelial VEGF receptor-2 and be an effective agent to prevent the development of OHSS. In one small clinical trial, women undergoing gonadotropin stimulation for oocyte donation were treated with cabergoline 0.5 mg daily or a placebo for 8 days starting on the day of HCG administration. Compared with placebo, cabergoline was associated with lower hematocrit and less ascites as detected by sonography. The rate of moderate OHSS was 20% in the cabergoline group and 44% in the placebo group. Magnetic resonance imaging studies of endothelial function demonstrated less permeability in the cabergoline group.

Adoption

A difficult decision in fertility treatments is determining when to cease active medical interventions. Throughout the process of fertility treatment, it is prudent to raise the issue of when to cease active intervention and to offer adoption as an alternative method of building a family. It may be useful for couples to simultaneously explore the option of adoption while they are undergoing fertility therapy. If the fertility therapy fails, adoption may help couples cope with the symbolic loss created by their infertility.

Psychosocial Aspects

Many observational studies indicate that stress is associated with infertility; in turn, the treatment of infertility can cause stress. Reducing stress prior to initiating intensive fertility treatments may improve the ability of the couple to successfully complete the treatments recommended. In one small clinical trial, Domar and colleagues reported that treatment of infertile women with a support group or a structured relaxation program was associated with better pregnancy rates with infertility treatment than that observed in a control group.

Inherently, diagnostic and therapeutic procedures offer hope for an imminent successful conception, but each subsequent menstrual cycle rekindles the feeling of loss. Infertility may be perceived by the couple as a loss that is difficult to grieve because the absence of fertility is somewhat intangible. The classic progression of emotions related to a loss is often expressed by the infertile couple. These include the feelings of disbelief and surprise, denial, anger, isolation, guilt, grief, and resolution. Patients wanted their clinicians to recognize their distress and respond in an empathic manner.

Social and Ethical Issues

Worldwide, issues of safe birth and access to contraception take precedence over issues of subfertility. However, in many developed countries, medical resources are sufficient to provide couples who desire to have a family and who have medical diseases that prevent their conception access to high-technology infertility services. Issues related to the fair access to medical resources remains a problem both nationally and worldwide.

IVF and PGD techniques have raised many unique situations that present challenging ethical questions. For example, is it ethical for parents of a child with a life-threatening disease to conceive another child through IVF and PGD who can be a stem cell donor for a hemapoietic transplant for their sick child? A wide range of ethical opinions have been offered in response to this clinical case scenario, ranging from "It should not be allowed" to "It is ethical to proceed with caution after fully consenting all parties." Developing this case further, a couple who were heterogyzgote carriers for an adverse mutation in the *FANCC* gene gave birth to a daughter with Fanconi anemia. The daughter would die unless a hemapoeitic transplant was performed, but a suitable donor was difficult to identify. Using both IVF and PGD, the mother of the child underwent four cycles of IVF that resulted in the creation of 33 embryos, five of which were both an HLA match for her daughter and not homozygous for the deleterious FANCC mutation. In the fourth cycle transfer of one of these embryos resulted in pregnancy. At birth, the umbilical cord blood was collected and used for a hemapoietic transplant in the affected daughter. Both children were reported to be well years after the procedure.

Recently, some couples with a genetic medical issue have asked to have IVF and PGD to ensure that their offspring would have the same genetic issue. For example, couples with a genetic form of deafness have requested IVF and PGD to conceive a child that was also deaf.

The technologies of IVF and PGD create a myriad of opportunities to influence the human genome. In the future the majority of IVF cycles may be performed, not to treat infertility, but to influence the genome of the offspring.

Key Points

- The most common identifiable causes of infertility are: anovulation, poor oocyte quality associated with advancing maternal age, tubal obstruction, poor semen quality including decreased sperm count and/or motility, and endometriosis.
- The three diagnostic tests most clinically useful in the evaluation of an infertile couple are: 1) tests to document ovulation including serum luteal phase progesterone, urine, or serum LH testing or basal body temperature charting, 2) hysterosalpingogram to document tubal patency, and 3) semen analysis. These three tests should be completed early in the evaluation of an infertile couple.

- Lifestyle and mental health improvements that can increase fertility in infertile male and female partners include: timing intercourse to the fertile time of the cycle, stopping smoking, achieving an optimal body mass index, treating anxiety and depression, and reducing stress.
- For the treatment of euestrogenic anovulatory infertility, clomiphene citrate is the most commonly used medication. Clomiphene is a mixed estrogen antagonist-agonist that increases pituitary secretion of follicle-stimulating hormone, thereby stimulating the growth of a competent follicle. About 8% of pregnancies achieved with clomiphene are twin gestations.
- The single most powerful intervention to enhance fertility among infertile couples is *in vitro fertilization* with intracytoplasmic sperm injection, if indicated. However, these procedures are resource intensive.

Evidence Box 42.1

Assisted reproductive technology permits many azoospermic men to father children through the combined procedure of microsurgical sperm extraction followed by intracytoplasmic sperm injection.

Historically, men with azoospermia had a bleak fertility prognosis. Recent advances in assisted reproductive technology permit many azoospermic men to father children through the combined procedure of microsurgical testicular sperm extraction (TESE) followed by intracytoplasmic sperm injection (ICSI). Surprisingly, men with nonobstructed azoospermia have no sperm in their ejaculated semen, but may have a few intratesticular sperm that can be surgically extracted from the testis by identifying seminiferous tubules that appear to be enlarged and removing those tubules for processing in the laboratory. A common cause of absolute azoospermia is Klinefelter syndrome (47,XXY). In a case series of 42 infertile men with Klinefelter syndrome the combined TESE–ICSI procedure resulted in 18 clinical pregnancies with 21 live births.

Schiff JD, Palermo GD, Veeck LL, Goldstein M, Rosenwaks Z, Schlegel PN. Success of testicular sperm injection and intracytoplasmic sperm injection in men with Klinefelter syndrome. J Clin Endocrinol Metab 2005;90:6263–6267.

Evidence Box 42.2

In couples with fertility problems, conception can be enhanced by ensuring that sexual intercourse takes place on the most fruitful days of the menstrual cycle, as determined by monitoring hormones and metabolites in the female partner.

In this study of 221 couples who were planning to become pregnant, the female partner underwent daily monitoring of her urinary estrogen and progesterone metabolites and recorded the timing of sexual intercourse. In 625 menstrual cycles, 192 pregnancies occurred as demonstrated by a positive urine human chorionic gonadotropin level. In this cohort, conception did not occur when sexual intercourse took place 24 hours after ovulation through to the next menses. Pregnancy rates were very low when sexual intercourse occurred more than 5 days before ovulation.

When attempting to enhance fertility, the three best days for recommending sexual intercourse to achieve conception were the day of ovulation and the two days prior to ovulation (see **Table 42.4**).

Wilcox AJ, Weinberg CR, Baird DD. Timing of sexual intercourse in relation to ovulation. N Engl J Med 1995;333:1517–1521.

Table 42.4 Timing of sexual intercourse in relation to ovulation

Day of cycle in relation to day of ovulation	Number of cycles with intercourse only occurring on this one day during the cycle	Pregnancies	Per cycle pregnancy rate for one episode of coitus
−5	12	1	8%
−4	24	4	17%
−3	13	1	8%
−2	28	10	36%
−1	38	13	34%
Ovulation	14	5	36%

Further Reading

Alvarez C, Martí-Bonmatí L, Novella-Maestre E, et al. Dopamine agonist cabergoline reduces hemoconcentration and ascites in hyperstimulated women undergoing assisted reproduction. *J Clin Endocrinol Metab* 2007;92(8):2931–2937

Barbieri RL. The initial fertility consultation: recommendations concerning cigarette smoking, body mass index, and alcohol and caffeine consumption. *Am J Obstet Gynecol* 2001;185(5):1168–1173

Chavarro JE, Rich-Edwards JW, Rosner BA, Willett WC. Diet and lifestyle in the prevention of ovulatory disorder infertility. *Obstet Gynecol* 2007;110(5):1050–1058

Chavarro JE, Rich-Edwards JW, Rosner BA, Willett WC. Iron intake and risk of ovulatory infertility. *Obstet Gynecol* 2006;108(5):1145–1152

Coutifaris C, Myers ER, Guzick DS, et al; NICHD National Cooperative Reproductive Medicine Network. Histological dating of timed endometrial biopsy tissue is not related to fertility status. *Fertil Steril* 2004;82(5):1264–1272

Domar AD, Clapp D, Slawsby EA, Dusek J, Kessel B, Freizinger M. Impact of group psychological interventions on pregnancy rates in infertile women. *Fertil Steril* 2000;73(4):805–811

Guzick DS, Overstreet JW, Factor-Litvak P, et al; National Cooperative Reproductive Medicine Network. Sperm morphology, motility, and concentration in fertile and infertile men. *N Engl J Med* 2001;345(19):1388–1393

Malcolm CE, Cumming DC. Does anovulation exist in eumenorrheic women? *Obstet Gynecol* 2003;102(2):317–318

Marcoux S, Maheux R, Bérubé S; Canadian Collaborative Group on Endometriosis. Laparoscopic surgery in infertile women with minimal or mild endometriosis. *N Engl J Med* 1997;337(4):217–222

Oei SG, Helmerhorst FM, Bloemenkamp KW, Hollants FA, Meerpoel DE, Keirse MJ. Effectiveness of the postcoital test: randomised controlled trial. *BMJ* 1998;317(7157):502–505

Schiff JD, Palermo GD, Veeck LL, Goldstein M, Rosenwaks Z, Schlegel PN. Success of testicular sperm extraction [corrected] and intracytoplasmic sperm injection in men with Klinefelter syndrome. *J Clin Endocrinol Metab* 2005;90(11):6263–6267

Smith S, Pfeifer SM, Collins JA. Diagnosis and management of female infertility. *JAMA* 2003;290(13):1767–1770

Van Voorhis BJ. Clinical practice. In vitro fertilization. *N Engl J Med* 2007;356(4):379–386

Verlinsky Y, Rechitsky S, Schoolcraft W, Strom C, Kuliev A. Preimplantation diagnosis for Fanconi anemia combined with HLA matching. *JAMA* 2001;285(24):3130–3133

Wilcox AJ, Weinberg CR, Baird DD. Timing of sexual intercourse in relation to ovulation. Effects on the probability of conception, survival of the pregnancy, and sex of the baby. *N Engl J Med* 1995;333(23):1517–1521

43 Premenstrual Syndrome

Robert L. Barbieri

Definition

The premenstrual syndrome (PMS) is defined as the presence of both physical and behavioral symptoms that occur repetitively in the luteal phase of the menstrual cycle and functionally interfere with some aspect of the woman's life. Premenstrual dysphoric disorder (PMDD) is a severe form of PMS in which symptoms of irritability, anger, and emotional tension predominate over somatic symptoms such as bloating. The characteristic feature of both PMS and PMDD is the recurrent, cyclic nature of symptoms and a marked on/off nature of the symptoms that begin in the luteal phase of the menstrual cycle and completely remit after the cessation of menses. PMDD is distinguished from PMS by the predominance of mood symptoms, especially anger and irritability.

Diagnosis

PMS and PMDD cannot be diagnosed by histopathologic analysis of a tissue biopsy, nor by measurement of a serum analytes in the laboratory. PMS and PMDD are diagnoses based on the report of symptoms by the patient. There is no universally accepted method for diagnosing PMS and PMDD. Over the past decades, the diagnostic criteria used for these two entities have changed and evolved. It is likely that the diagnostic criteria for PMS and PMDD will continue to change.

A widely used approach for diagnosing PMS is the stepwise algorithm recommended by investigators from the University of California, San Diego.

- **Step 1:** Prospectively document that the symptoms and timing of symptoms are consistent with PMS. The patient must report at least one of the following somatic symptoms for at least 5 days prior to menses in three consecutive menstrual cycles: breast tenderness, abdominal bloating, headache, swollen extremities. In addition, at least one of the following affective symptoms must be present for at least 5 days prior to menses in three consecutive cycles: depression, angry outbursts, irritability, confusion, social withdrawal, fatigue (**Table 43.1**; **Fig. 43.1**).
- **Step 2:** Prospectively document that the bothersome symptoms resolve within 4 days of onset of menses and do not recur until at least cycle day 12.
- **Step 3:** Document that the symptoms are not caused or exacerbated by the use of alcohol or recreational drugs.
- **Step 4:** Document that the symptoms identified in step 1 cause dysfunction in the patient's social or work life as defined by the following criteria: marital or relationship discord confirmed by partner, difficulties in parenting, poor work, or school performance, increased social isolation, legal difficulties, suicidal ideation or somatization with resulting medical interventions.

PMDD is diagnosed based on the criteria in the Diagnostic and Statistical Manual of Mental Disorders, DSM-IV. To

Table 43.1 The diagnosis of premenstrual syndrome is based on self-report of at least one affective and one somatic symptom during the 5 days prior to menses that result in identifiable dysfunction in social or economic performance

Affective symptoms	Somatic symptoms
Depression	Breast tenderness
Angry outbursts	Abdominal bloating
Irritability	Headache
Confusion	Swollen extremities
Social withdrawal	
Fatigue	

Source: From Mortola JF, Girton L, Yen SSC. Am J Obstet Gynecol 1989;161:1682.

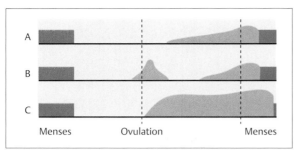

Fig. 43.1 Three patterns of premenstrual symptoms. The red shading represents the timing and severity of the premenstrual symptoms. In all three patterns, the symptoms are most prominent in the luteal phase of the menstrual cycle. Pattern A represents a typical pattern with most symptoms during the second half of the luteal phase and symptom severity peaking late in the luteal phase. In pattern B symptoms are also present around the time of ovulation. Pattern C represents a severe example of premenstrual syndrome with symptoms throughout the luteal phase and extending into the first portion of menses, before subsiding during the following follicular phase.

diagnose PMDD, the clinician needs to prospectively document that characteristic behavioral and physical symptoms are present for 1 week prior to menses and that the symptoms resolve within 5 days of the start of menses. Five symptoms must be present, and at least one symptom must be one of the first four on the list:

- feeling sad or hopeless
- feeling tense, anxious, or on the edge
- marked lability of mood interspersed with frequent tearfulness, and/or
- persistent irritability, anger, and increased interpersonal conflicts
  Other symptoms that qualify include:
- decreased interest in usual activities
- difficulty concentrating
- feeling fatigued
- changes in appetite
- hypersomnia or insomnia
- being overwhelmed or out of control
- other physical symptoms such as breast tenderness or swelling, headaches, joint or muscle pain, bloating, or weight gain

Many women initially thought to have PMS or PMDD have marked symptoms during the follicular phase of the menstrual cycle, well after the cessation of menses. These women most likely have another problem such as an anxiety disorder or depression, rather than PMS or PMDD.

Prevalence and Epidemiology

Using strict definitions of PMDD and PMS, the prevalence of PMDD is reported to be about 4% and the prevalence of PMS has been reported to vary widely among different populations with rates in the range of 5–30%. Multiple studies have reported that premenstrual symptoms have a high degree of heritability. In addition, studies suggest that major depression and PMS are distinct disorders that overlap somewhat, but are not part of single continuum.

Etiology

The etiologies of PMS and PMDD are not well defined. It is highly likely that biological, psychological, and social factors contribute to the development of these two problems. The pathophysiology of PMS and PMDD is thought to involve serotonin deficiency exacerbated by cyclic changes in estradiol and progesterone. Secondary contributions to the pathophysiology of the syndrome likely arise from dysfunction in neuroendocrine systems controlling β-endorphin, γ-aminobutyric acid (GABA) and autonomic nervous system function. Animal experiments have demonstrated that cyclic fluctuations in estradiol and progesterone cause alterations in the serotonin, opioid, and GABA neurotransmitter systems. In women, administration of serotonin agonists ameliorates the symptoms of PMS and PMDD and serotonin antagonists exacerbate the symptoms.

History

The most common somatic symptoms reported by women with PMS are abdominal bloating and fatigue. Breast tenderness and headache are two other frequent symptoms. The most frequent affective symptoms are labile mood and irritability. Other behavioral symptoms include anger, emotional tension, changes in appetite, forgetfulness, and difficulty concentrating.

Most authorities recommend that the symptoms be collected prospectively over two to three menstrual cycles using a standardized menstrual diary (**Table 43.2**). Retrospectively collected data increases the likelihood that a mental health disorder such as anxiety or depression will be inadvertently diagnosed as PMS or PMDD.

Table 43.2 Prospective symptom chart for women with symptoms consistent with premenstrual syndrome

Cycle day	Depression	Angry outbursts	Irritability	Confusion	Social withdrawal	Fatigue	Breast tenderness	Bloating
1								
2								
3								
4								
5								
6								
7								
8								
9								
10								
11								
12								
13								
14								
15								
16								
17								
18								
19								
20								
21								
22								
23								
24								
25								
26								
27								
28								

Source: Adapted from Mortola JF, Girton L, Yen SSC. Am J Obstet Gynecol 1989;161:1682.

Physical Examination and Laboratory Studies

There are no physical examination findings, imaging, or laboratory studies that aid in the diagnosis of PMS or PMDD.

Treatment

Life Style Changes

Life-style interventions proposed as treatments for PMS or PMDD have not been subjected to large scale, rigorous clinical trials. There is some preliminary evidence that aerobic exercise, relaxation training and reflexology may result in modest improvement in symptoms of PMS. As noted below, placebo treatment results in improvement in self-reported symptoms of PMS, making rigorous clinical trials important to understand the relative impact of the "placebo effect" versus active treatment.

Dietary interventions

Calcium supplements, 600 mg of elemental calcium twice daily, have been reported to result in greater symptom improvement than placebo in women with PMS. In one large clinical trial, calcium 600 mg twice daily was superior to placebo in reducing luteal phase symptoms related to negative affect, water retention, food cravings, and lower abdominal pain. Calcium supplements and placebo resulted in similar improvement in reported symptoms during menses. In this study the elemental calcium was administered as two tablets of 750 mg of calcium carbonate in the morning and evening. Each 750 mg calcium carbonate tablet contained 300 mg of elemental calcium.

Pharmacologic Treatment

Serotonin deficiency exacerbated by cyclic changes in estradiol and progesterone are thought to play a primary role in the pathophysiology of PMS and PMDD. Pharmacologic treatment is focused on improving serotonin action or suppressing cyclic changes in estradiol and progesterone.

Selective Serotonin Reuptake Inhibitors

Numerous randomized clinical trials have demonstrated the efficacy of selective serotonin reuptake inhibitors (SSRIs) in the treatment of PMS and PMDD. SSRIs have been demonstrated to improve both somatic and affective symptoms. Agents with proven efficacy include: fluoxetine 20 mg daily (see Evidence Box 43.1), sertraline 50 mg or 100 mg daily, citalopram 10–30 mg daily, and paroxetine 10–30 mg daily.

SSRIs may be given continuously (every day) or intermittently administered only during the luteal phase of the menstrual cycle. Intermittent administration is less costly and has fewer side effects than continuous therapy.

Benzodiazepines

Alprazolam at a dose of 0.25 mg three times daily has been demonstrated in multiple clinical trials to be effective in the treatment of affective symptoms associated with PMS or PMDD. Alprazolam is a second-line treatment for these diseases, because it has more addictive potential than the SSRIs.

Suppressing Cyclic Changes in Estradiol and Progesterone

Gonadotropin-releasing hormone analogues: GnRH agonist analogues cause an initial increase in pituitary secretion of LH and FSH for the first 10 days of administration, but then cause marked suppression of LH and FSH secretion due to both downregulation and desensitization of the pituitary GnRH receptor. The decrease in pituitary secretion of LH and FSH results in suppression of ovarian follicle growth, resulting in a 95% decrease in ovarian estradiol and progesterone production. In turn, serum levels of estradiol and progesterone decrease to the menopausal range and menses cease. Many women treated with GnRH agonist analogues develop hot flushes and accelerated bone loss due to hypoestrogenism.

Numerous small trials have demonstrated that GnRH agonist analogues, such as leuprolide acetate 3.75 mg IM every 4 weeks, are effective for the treatment of PMS and PMDD. GnRH agonists are more effective for the treatment of somatic symptoms and irritability than for depressive symptoms associated with PMS or PMDD.

Bilateral oophorectomy has also been reported to be effective treatment based on case series. Two problems with bilateral oophorectomy as a treatment are that it is irreversible and creates a sudden surgical menopause with a high likelihood of severe menopausal symptoms requiring hormone therapy.

Estrogen–Progestin Contraceptives

In women with PMDD who prefer not to take SSRIs, treatment with an oral contraceptive containing the specialized progestin, drospirenone, results in greater symptom improvement than placebo (see Evidence Box 43.2). Drospirenone is a progestin agonist, mineralocorticoid antagonist, and an anti-androgen. Drospirenone is similar to spironolactone, a mineralocorticoid antagonist and anti-androgen, in its chemical structure.

Treatments not Proven to be Effective

Progesterone

Prescription of progesterone supplements was once a first-line approach to the treatment of PMS. Randomized trials do not support the use of this treatment for PMS.

Dietary Supplements

There is no consistent evidence from controlled trials that dietary supplements such as evening primrose oil (linoleic acid) or ginkgo biloba extract are effective treatment for PMS above their placebo effect.

Bothersome premenstrual symptoms typically consist of a mix of disruptive mood and uncomfortable physical symptoms. The precise pathophysiology of these symptoms is not fully understood, but calcium supplementation, SSRIs, and oral contraceptives are the three interventions that have been demonstrated to have efficacy in treatment of premenstrual symptoms.

Key Points

- Premenstrual syndrome (PMS) is a group of physical and behavioral symptoms that occur in a recurring pattern during the second half of the menstrual cycle. Premenstrual dysphoric disorder (PMDD) is a severe form of PMS with prominent mood changes including irritability and angry outbursts. PMS is common; PMDD occurs infrequently.
- The key to the diagnosis of PMS and PMDD is the collection of a prospective symptom diary over two or more menstrual cycles. Commonly reported somatic symptoms include breast tenderness, abdominal bloating, headache, and swollen extremities. Commonly reported affective symptoms include angry outbursts, irritability, confusion, social withdrawal, and fatigue.
- If symptoms persist during the follicular phase of the menstrual cycle, mental health disorders such as depression or anxiety should be considered.
- Serotonin deficiency exacerbated by cyclic changes in estradiol and progesterone are hypothesized to play a role in the causation of PMDD. Randomized trials have reported that treatment with selective serotonin reuptake inhibitors improve symptoms of PMDD. The magnitude of the improvement compared with placebo is modest.

Evidence Box 43.1

Intermittent dosing with fluoxetine 20 mg daily during the 14 days preceding the onset of menses is an effective treatment for premenstrual dysphoric disorder.

The pathophysiology of premenstrual syndrome (PMS) and premenstrual dysphoric disorder (PMDD) is thought to involve serotonin deficiency exacerbated by cyclic changes in estradiol and progesterone. Pharmacologic treatment is focused on improving serotonin action or suppressing cyclic changes in estradiol and progesterone. Selective serotonin reuptake inhibitors (SSRIs) are first-line therapy for women with PMS or PMDD. Numerous randomized, controlled trials demonstrate the effectiveness of SSRI therapy.

In one trial, 260 women with prospectively documented PMDD were randomized to fluoxetine 10 mg, fluoxetine 20 mg, or placebo dosed daily for 14 days prior to the expected onset of the next menses, for 3 months. The mean age of the patients was 36 years with a mean 10-year history of PMDD. During the first month of treatment, placebo, fluoxetine 10 mg, and fluoxetine 20 mg all resulted in a decrease in symptom severity. Fluoxetine 20 mg produced significantly greater improvement in symptoms than placebo over all 3 months of treatment. Fluoxetine 20 mg was associated with a greater degree of decreased libido than placebo. Placebo treatment was associated with significantly increased self-reported accidental injuries than fluoxetine treatment.

This study, one of the largest clinical trials of treatment of PMDD, indicates that intermittent dosing with fluoxetine 20 mg, for 14 days prior to the expected onset of menses is an effective treatment for PMDD.

Cohen LS, Miner C, Brown E, et al. Premenstrual daily fluoxetine for premenstrual dysphoric disorder: a placebo-controlled, clinical trial using computerized diaries. Obstet Gynecol 2002;100:435–444.

Evidence Box 43.2

Suppression of cyclic changes in ovarian secretion of estradiol and progesterone with an oral contraceptive containing the specialized progestin, drospirenone, is effective treatment for many women with premenstrual dysphoric disorder.

The pathophysiology of premenstrual syndrome and premenstrual dysphoric disorder (PMDD) is thought to involve serotonin deficiency exacerbated by cyclic changes in estradiol and progesterone. Pharmacologic treatment is focused on improving serotonin action or suppressing cyclic changes in estradiol and progesterone. In women with PMDD who prefer not to take selective serotonin reuptake inhibitors, treatment with an oral contraceptive containing the specialized progestin, drospirenone, results in greater symptom improvement than placebo. Drospirenone is a progestin agonist, mineralocorticoid antagonist, and an anti-androgen. Drospirenone is similar to spironolactone, a mineralocorticoid antagonist and anti-androgen, in its chemical structure.

In a large clinical trial, 450 women with prospectively documented PMDD were randomized to treatment with placebo or ethinylestradiol 20 μg plus drospirenone 3 mg daily for 24 days followed by 4 days of placebo pills for 3 months. Many oral contraceptives contain 21 days of hormone pills with 7 days off active treatment. It should be noted that the oral contraceptive used in this study had 24 days of hormone pills and only 4 days off active treatment. The mean age of women in this trial was 32 years Both placebo and the oral contraceptive treatment resulted in an improvement in symptoms of PMDD, but oral contraceptive treatment was superior to placebo across all 3 months of treatment. The oral contraceptive treatment was especially effective in reducing the severity of self-reported depression, hopelessness, guilt, mood swings, and increased appetite/cravings compared with placebo. A positive response, defined as a 50% decrease in symptom score, occurred in 48% of the women taking the oral contraceptive and 36% of the women taking the placebo.

Yonkers KA, Brown C, Pearlstein TB, Foegh M, Sampson-Landers C, Rapkin A. Efficacy of a new low-dose oral contraceptive with drospirenone in premenstrual dysphoric disorder. Obstet Gynecol 2005;106:492–501.

Further Reading

Brown CS, Ling FW, Andersen RN, Farmer RG, Arheart KL. Efficacy of depot leuprolide in premenstrual syndrome: effect of symptom severity and type in a controlled trial. *Obstet Gynecol* 1994;84(5):779–786

Brown J, O'Brien PM, Marjoribanks J, Wyatt K. Selective serotonin reuptake inhibitors for premenstrual syndrome. *Cochrane Database Syst Rev* 2002;00:CD001396

Casper RF, Hearn MT. The effect of hysterectomy and bilateral oophorectomy in women with severe premenstrual syndrome. *Am J Obstet Gynecol* 1990;162(1):105–109

Casson P, Hahn PM, Van Vugt DA, Reid RL. Lasting response to ovariectomy in severe intractable premenstrual syndrome. *Am J Obstet Gynecol* 1990;162(1):99–105

Cohen LS, Miner C, Brown EW, et al. Premenstrual daily fluoxetine for premenstrual dysphoric disorder: a placebo-controlled, clinical trial using computerized diaries. *Obstet Gynecol* 2002;100(3):435–444

Dimmock PW, Wyatt KM, Jones PW, O'Brien PM. Efficacy of selective serotonin-reuptake inhibitors in premenstrual syndrome: a systematic review. *Lancet* 2000;356(9236):1131–1136

Johnson SR. Premenstrual syndrome, premenstrual dysphoric disorder, and beyond: a clinical primer for practitioners. *Obstet Gynecol* 2004;104(4):845–859

Kendler KS, Karkowski LM, Corey LA, Neale MC. Longitudinal population-based twin study of retrospectively reported premenstrual symptoms and lifetime major depression. *Am J Psychiatry* 1998;155(9):1234–1240

Menkes DB, Coates DC, Fawcett JP. Acute tryptophan depletion aggravates premenstrual syndrome. *J Affect Disord* 1994;32(1):37–44

Mortola JF, Girton L, Yen SSC. Depressive episodes in premenstrual syndrome. *Am J Obstet Gynecol* 1989;161(6 Pt 1):1682–1687

Muse KN, Cetel NS, Futterman LA, Yen SC. The premenstrual syndrome. Effects of "medical ovariectomy". *N Engl J Med* 1984;311(21):1345–1349

Pearlstein TB, Bachmann GA, Zacur HA, Yonkers KA. Treatment of premenstrual dysphoric disorder with a new drospirenone-containing oral contraceptive formulation. *Contraception* 2005;72(6):414–421

Rivera-Tovar AD, Frank E. Late luteal phase dysphoric disorder in young women. *Am J Psychiatry* 1990;147(12):1634–1636

Roca CA, Schmidt PJ, Smith MJ, Danaceau MA, Murphy DL, Rubinow DR. Effects of metergoline on symptoms in women with premenstrual dysphoric disorder. *Am J Psychiatry* 2002;159(11):1876–1881

Thys-Jacobs S, Starkey P, Bernstein D, Tian J; Premenstrual Syndrome Study Group. Calcium carbonate and the premenstrual syndrome: effects on premenstrual and menstrual symptoms. *Am J Obstet Gynecol* 1998;179(2):444–452

Yonkers KA, Brown C, Pearlstein TB, Foegh M, Sampson-Landers C, Rapkin A. Efficacy of a new low-dose oral contraceptive with drospirenone in premenstrual dysphoric disorder. *Obstet Gynecol* 2005;106(3):492–501

44 Perimenopause, Menopause, and Postmenopause: Consequences of Ovarian Reproductive Aging

Robert L. Barbieri

In 1900, the life expectancy of US women was 48 years. In 2005, life expectancy for women had increased to 80 years. The median age of menopause has been about 51 years for many centuries. Consequently, the proportion of time women spend in the postmenopausal state has increased dramatically. Determining the impact of ovarian aging and menopause on health is difficult because both aging and menopause affect organ physiology. Detailed scientific information identifying the relative impact on health of aging per se versus menopause is only beginning to become available. It is likely, as our understanding of both aging and menopause improves, that treatment approaches will change significantly.

Definition and Diagnosis

An immutable feature of ovarian biology is the continuous loss of a fixed, nonrenewable pool of oocytes and follicles. The loss of ovarian oocytes begins in utero. At 20 weeks of fetal development, the ovaries contain approximately 7 000 000 oogonia. At birth only 700 000 oocytes remain (**Fig. 44.1**). The loss of oocytes occurs in an exponential manner, meaning that a fixed percentage of oocytes are lost during each given period of time. The rate of loss of oocytes may accelerate after about 37 years of age (**Fig. 44.2**).

Ultimately, the process ends with the loss of all functional oocytes and follicles. This results in: 1) a marked reduction in ovarian estradiol and progesterone production due to the absence of functional follicles, resulting in hot flushes and vaginal symptoms in many women; 2) permanent amenorrhea due to the absence of cyclic ovarian estradiol and progesterone production; and 3) sterility due an absence of functional oocytes.

The continuous loss of ovarian follicles is the key feature of the process of female reproductive aging. The Stages of Reproductive Aging Workshop outlined seven key

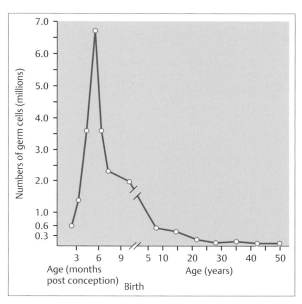

Fig. 44.1 Changes in the total number of oocytes and follicles in human ovaries before and after birth. The number of germ cells in the ovary peaks in utero during the second trimester of gestation. From Baker TG. Radiosensitivity of mammalian oocytes with particular reference to the human female. Reproduced with permission of Elsevier from Am J Obstet Gynecol 1971;110:746–761.

stages in the process of reproductive aging (**Table 44.1**). The staging system is anchored around the final menstrual period (FMP), defined as Stage 0.

Premenopause (reproductive years), is characterized by regular ovulation and cyclic menstrual bleeding, except for intervals of pregnancy and lactation.

The *menopausal transition* occurs beginning about three to five years before the onset of the final menstrual period. It is defined as the onset of variable cycle lengths, usually more than 7 days longer than the normal cycle length, ultimately resulting in multiple skipped cycles and absence of bleeding for more than 60 days. The menopausal transition is caused by increasing inability of the few remaining follicles to grow and ovulate

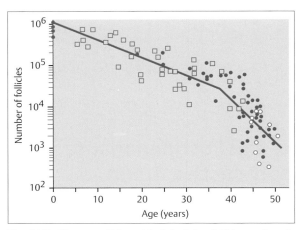

Fig. 44.2 Bi-exponential model of declining follicle numbers in women up to 51 years of age. Accelerated rate of follicle loss appears to occur after age 37 years. From Faddy MI, Gosden R, Gougeon A, et al. Accelerated disappearance of ovarian follicles in mid-life: implications for forecasting menopause. Reproduced with permission of Oxford University Press from Hum Reprod 1992;7:1342-1346.

in monthly cycles, leading to erratic patterns of estradiol and progesterone secretion and corresponding erratic menstrual patterns.

Perimenopause includes both the menopause transition and the 12 months following the final menstrual period. For many authorities the "climacteric" and "perimenopause" are synonyms.

Menopause is the cessation of menstruation, defined as being present after 12 months of amenorrhea following the final menstrual period. The amenorrhea associated with menopause reflects the loss of functional ovarian oocytes and follicles. The median age of onset of menopause is 51 years. In a woman over the age of 45 years, in the absence of other plausible causes, 12 months of amenorrhea is likely to indicate the onset of menopause.

Postmenopause is divided into two phases: the early postmenopause—the first five years following the final menstrual period—and the late postmenopause. During the early postmenopause, ovarian estradiol and progesterone reach nadirs that continue throughout the remainder of life. During early postmenopause, bone loss is accelerated owing to the decrease in ovarian estradiol, progesterone, and androgen production.

Table 44.1 Stages of Reproductive Aging Workshop (STRAW) conceptualization of reproductive aging. An immutable feature of ovarian biology is the continuous loss of ovarian oocytes and follicles, ultimately resulting in loss of all functional oocytes and follicles. The STRAW conceptualization of reproductive aging is anchored around the final menstrual period (FMP)

Stage	Approximate age of onset (years)	Terminology used	Menstrual cycle characteristic	Hormonal patterns
–5	10–16	Menarche (Avg. age 12–13 years)	Irregular and often anovulatory	Normal FSH
–4	16–37	Reproductive life —premenopausal	Regular pattern	Normal FSH, estradiol and progesterone production
–3	37–45	Later reproductive life—premenopausal	Regular pattern	Serum FSH during menses begins to increase
–2	45–50	(Perimenopause) menopausal transition	Cycles of variable length (>7 days different from normal)	Increased serum FSH
–1	45–50	Menopausal transition (Perimenopause)	≥2 Skipped cycles Some cycles >60 days in length	Erratic patterns with some cycles characterized by increased serum FSH, low estradiol, and low progesterone
FMP	**50–51**			
+1	51–56	Early postmenopause	Amenorrhea	High FSH, low estradiol, progesterone and androgen secretion
+2	From 56 to death	Late postmenopause	Amenorrhea	High FSH, very low estradiol, progesterone, and androgen secretion

Source: Modified from Soules MR, Sherman S, Parrott, E, et al. Executive Summary: Stages of Reproductive Aging Workshop (STRAW). Fertil Steril 2001;76:874–878.

Etiology and Epidemiology

The median age of menopause is approximately 51 years of age. About 5 % of women have menopause after 55 years and about 5 % have menopause between 40 and 45 years. About 1 % of women have menopause before age 40 years. Menopause before age 40 years is considered to be clearly abnormal and is diagnosed as premature ovarian failure (see below).

The age of onset of the first menses (menarche) is influenced by body mass, body composition, including body fat, exercise intensity, and general health. Over the centuries there has been a secular trend to an earlier age of menarche, in part, due to an increase in body mass and body fat at earlier ages. However, the age of menopause has not significantly changed for millennia.

Some disease states result in an accelerated loss of ovarian follicles. For example, the genetic disorder 45,X, Turner syndrome, results in the very rapid loss of all ovarian follicles during childhood. At the age of puberty, there are no remaining follicles to secrete the estradiol necessary for breast development and onset of menarche. Consequently women with 45,X are menopausal before they reach menarche. Another genetic disease, galactosemia, results in the accumulation of high concentrations of galactose, an oocyte and follicle toxin, in the blood unless a strict galactose-free diet is consumed. In women with galactosemia who do not follow a galactose-free diet, premature menopause is common. Premature menopause has also been reported in women with myasthenia gravis, probably due to an autoimmune mechanism.

Environmental exposures influence the age of menopause. For example, components of cigarette smoke are thought to be toxic to ovarian oocytes and follicles, resulting in their accelerated loss. The age of onset of menopause is approximately two years earlier in women who smoke. There is a dose-dependent relationship between smoking and early menopause. Alkylating chemotherapy agents, such as cyclophosphamide and radiation, are cytotoxic to both oocytes and follicle cells, and in adequate doses reliably cause premature ovarian failure.

Physiology of Ovarian Aging

Follicle-stimulating hormone (FSH) is the primary hormone controlling the growth of an ovarian follicle. An ovarian follicle must reach a critical size and secrete a critical quantity of estradiol before it can trigger a pituitary luteinizing hormone (LH) surge, which in turn causes the follicle to ovulate. In primates, the feedback control between pituitary FSH and the ovary is set to cause one follicle to grow and ovulate each cycle. From a teleological perspective this tight regulation of FSH decreases the chance of ovulating multiple follicles in one cycle, which reduces the chance of twin and triplet pregnancy. Given the energy intensity of pregnancy, birth, and rearing of offspring among primates, singleton pregnancy is important for the health of the mother and offspring.

Pituitary secretion of FSH is under negative feedback control of hormones secreted by ovarian follicle(s) including estradiol, inhibin A, inhibin B, and progesterone. During premenopause, the functionally "most competent" follicles respond to FSH, grow, secrete estradiol, which suppresses FSH, and ovulate. As women reach approximately 37–41 years of age, the remaining follicles appear to be less responsive to FSH stimulation. This requires the pituitary to secrete increasing quantities of FSH during menses to stimulate the growth of a follicle.

As women enter the perimenopause, some follicles are markedly resistant to FSH stimulation. In a perimenopausal woman, when an available follicle is intensely resistant to FSH, the pituitary secretes massive amounts of FSH in an attempt to cause the follicle to grow and secrete estradiol. If the follicle does not respond, the cycle is characterized by high levels of FSH, low levels of estradiol and light menstrual bleeding. These cycles are often anovulatory. In a subsequent cycle, if the next available follicle(s) is somewhat more responsive to FSH, the massive quantities of FSH released throughout the previous cycle may carry over into the following cycle, causing the follicle to grow quickly and secrete excessive amounts of estradiol. The excessive estradiol secretion, in turn, exerts negative feedback on FSH, causing FSH levels to fall to levels observed in young premenopausal women. Therefore, this cycle is characterized by low levels of FSH during most of the cycle, abnormally high levels of estradiol, and heavy menses. The oscillation between cycles with poor follicle responsiveness (high FSH, low estradiol, light menses) and an overstimulated follicle (low FSH, high estradiol, heavy menses) is a major feature of the perimenopause interval.

The oscillation between light and heavy menses is often troubling to perimenopausal women. To prevent the FSH-follicle oscillation, pituitary secretion of FSH must be definitively suppressed. Suppression of pituitary FSH cannot be accomplished with doses of estrogen–progestin typically used to treat hot flushes and vaginal symptoms (**Tables 44.2, 44.3**). Suppression of pituitary FSH secretion during the perimenopausal stage requires the doses of estrogen–progestin used in standard hormonal contraceptives, which are in general about five to eight times higher than doses used in hormone therapy for postmenopausal women.

When all functional ovarian follicles are depleted, there is no hormonal negative feedback control of FSH secretion. Circulating FSH is markedly increased in postmenopausal women. Circulating estradiol, progesterone, inhibin A, and inhibin B are markedly decreased in postmenopausal women.

Table 44.2 Standard and low dose treatments for hot flushes in postmenopausal women. A major guideline for hormone treatment is to prescribe the lowest dose for the shortest period of time that will achieve the therapeutic goal *

Preparation	Generic	Brand name	Low dose	Standard dose
Estrogens				
Oral	Conjugated equine estrogen (CEE)	Premarin	0.3 mg, 0.45 mg	0.625 mg
	Estradiol	Estrace	0.25 mg, 0.5 mg	1.0 mg
Transdermal	Estradiol	Menostar, Alora, Climara, Vivelle	0.014 mg, 0.025 mg, 0.0375 mg	0.05 mg, 0.1 mg
Progestins				
Oral	Medroxyprogesterone acetate (MPA)	Provera	1.5 mg, 2.5 mg	5 mg, 10 mg
	Progesterone	Prometrium	100 mg	200 mg
Vaginal	Progesterone tablet	Endometrin	100 mg	
	Progesterone gel	Crinone	45 mg (4% gel) or 90 mg (8% gel)	
Combination Estrogens–Progestins				
Oral continuous	CEE plus MPA	Prempro	0.3 mg CEE plus 1.5 mg MPA	0.625 mg CEE plus 2.5 mg MPA
Transdermal continuous	Estradiol plus norethindrone acetate	Activella		1 mg estradiol plus 0.5 mg norethindrone

* For women with a uterus, administer an estrogen–progestin regimen, either cyclically or continuously. For estrogen–progestin cyclic regimens, select both an estrogen and progestin. Administer the estrogen continuously and administer the progestin either 14 days every month (calendar days 1–13), or 14 days every 3 months. For estrogen–progestin continuous regimens, administer both an estrogen and progestin daily. For women without a uterus, administer only an estrogen as a continuous regimen.

Table 44.3 Standard treatments for vaginal symptoms, such as dryness, in postmenopausal women. Nonhormonal preparations include Replens, a polycarbophil-based vaginal moisturizer

Preparation	Generic	Brand	Low dose	Standard dose
Vaginal rings	Estradiol acetate	Femring vaginal ring		0.05 mg daily, 0.1 mg daily
	Estradiol	Estring	0.0075 mg daily	
Vaginal tablets	Estradiol	Vagifem	0.025 mg daily	
Vaginal cream	Conjugated equine estrogen (CEE)	Premarin vaginal cream	0.3 mg CEE weekly (0.5 g of cream weekly)	0.3–1.0 mg CEE daily (0.5–2.0 g of cream daily)
	Estradiol (0.01%)	Estrace	0.2 mg weekly (2 g of cream weekly)	0.2–0.4 mg daily (2–4 g of cream daily)

Clinical Presentation

History

Many symptoms have been reported to be associated with perimenopause and postmenopause, but symptoms caused by aging may confound these associations. After carefully controlling for aging, the perimenopause and postmenopause are thought to be reliably associated with four symptoms:

1. Menstrual irregularity leading to amenorrhea
2. Hot flushes
3. Vaginal dryness
4. Sleep disturbance, caused in part by the hot flushes

Menstrual Cycle Irregularity

As defined in the STRAW staging system, the onset of perimenopause is first characterized by irregular menstrual cycle length, with a pattern more than 7 days different from the patient's typical menstrual cycle length. In some women, the onset of menstrual cycle irregularity results in more frequent menses with cycle lengths less than 24 days. Almost all menstrual cycles less than 24 days in length are anovulatory cycles. In other women, the onset of menstrual cycle irregularity results in less frequent menses with cycle lengths greater than 35 days. As the patient approaches the final menstrual period, they may experience cycles more than 60 days in length. From a simple viewpoint, this represents a "skipped period."

Hot Flushes

The perimenopause and postmenopause are often characterized by the onset of hot flushes, which occur in most women. Both rapidly changing serum concentrations of estradiol (perimenopause) and very low concentrations of estradiol (postmenopause) are thought to destabilize hypothalamic regulatory centers, resulting in the phenomenon of hot flushes. Hot flushes occur most frequently in the perimenopausal transition. Hot flushes are less commonly reported by Chinese and Japanese women. Hot flushes typically begin as the sudden onset of the sensation of warmth or heat on the face, neck, and chest, which may spread throughout the body. The sensation can be intense and associated with sweating followed by chills and shivering. Hot flushes are especially common at night and may wake the patient from sleep. Severe hot flushes can prevent women from entering stages of deep sleep associated with dreaming, and may contribute to insomnia and irritability.

Hot-flush–like symptoms may also be caused by hyperthyroidism, carcinoid, and pheochromocytoma. Medications that may cause hot flushes include anti-estrogens such as tamoxifen, aromatase inhibitors such as letrozole or anastrozole, and GnRH analogues such as leuprolide, niacin, and nitrates.

For most women, hot flushes will improve in about 30% of women in a few months and in 90% of women within 5 years. About 10% of women will experience hot flushes, often without improvement, for many years.

Vaginal Symptoms

The prevalence of vaginal symptoms, including dryness, discomfort, itching and dyspareunia, increases from about 10% in the perimenopause to over 50% in the late postmenopause. Vaginal symptoms are probably due to low levels of estradiol and androgens, and aging. Postmenopausal women have decreased vaginal blood flow and decreased vaginal secretion; and increased fragmentation of vaginal elastin.

As noted above, after carefully controlling for aging, the perimenopause and postmenopause are thought to be reliably associated with four symptoms:

1. Menstrual irregularity leading to amenorrhea
2. Hot flushes
3. Vaginal dryness
4. Sleep disturbance, caused in part by hot flushes.

However, many perimenopausal and postmenopausal women report symptoms of sexual dysfunction, mood and cognitive changes, and urinary incontinence. These symptoms are sometimes attributed to the process of ovarian aging, but little evidence supports a direct causative relationship.

Sexual Dysfunction

Many factors may cause perimenopausal and postmenopausal women to report decreased sexual desire. These factors include:

- decreases in ovarian and adrenal production of estradiol and androgens
- vaginal dryness
- psychosocial stress including simultaneously caring for children, parents, home-life, and being employed full-time
- a waning feeling of intimacy, support, and closeness with their partner

If a hormone plays a role in the development of postmenopausal hypoactive sexual desire disorder, clinical trial evidence indicates that testosterone plays a greater role than estradiol. In one clinical trial of naturally menopausal women with hypoactive sexual desire disorder, 549 women were randomized to treatment with a testosterone-releasing transdermal patch (300 µg/day) or a placebo. Treatment with a testosterone patch significantly increased the frequency of satisfying sexual activity and sexual desire.

Mood Changes

Mood changes, including symptoms consistent with depression and anxiety disorders, are best understood using a biopsychosocial model that emphasizes the multifactorial nature of depression and anxiety. Mood changes, depression, and anxiety are influenced by genetic, biological, psychological, and social factors. Ovarian aging may influence mood and symptoms of depression and anxiety by causing hot flushes, which interfere with the quality of sleep. For women with both postmenopausal symptoms and depression, treatment with selective serotonin reuptake inhibitors may be more effective than treatment with estrogen–progestin hormone therapy. In one clinical trial, 40 women with postmenopausal symptoms and clinical depression were randomized to treatment with escitalopram (Lexapro) 10–20 mg daily, or to estrogen–progestin hormone treatment, ethinyl estradiol 5 mg plus norethindrone acetate 1 mg daily (FemHRT). After 8 weeks of treatment, symptoms of depression improved in 75% of women treated with escitalopram and 25% of women treated with estrogen–progestin ($P = 0.01$). Menopausal symptoms improved in 56% of women treated with escitalopram and 31% of women treated with estrogen–progestin ($P = 0.03$).

Cognition

Many women report that they experienced a change in cognitive function during the transition from the premenopausal to postmenopausal stage. However, prospective studies indicate that neither ovarian aging nor estrogen or progestin therapy has a major impact on cognition or reported quality of life.

Urinary Incontinence

Reported symptoms of incontinence increase with aging, but there is no strong evidence that estradiol or progesterone influences the rate of increase of symptoms of incontinence observed with aging. In postmenopausal women, estrogen–progestin therapy was associated with a significant increase in reported symptoms of incontinence within 4 months of initiating treatment.

Physical Examination

There are few physical findings associated with ovarian aging. In the perimenopausal and postmenopausal stages, the vaginal skin becomes thinner with areas that are pale and lack rugae. The thin vaginal mucosa is associated with visible blood vessels and areas of petechial hemorrhage. Erythema of the vagina and peri-urethra are also common. The vaginal pH increases to a range of 6 to 7, much higher than the 4.5 observed in premenopausal women. In postmenopausal women vaginal pH cannot be used to aid in the diagnosis bacterial vaginosis or trichomoniasis.

Laboratory Testing

Menopause is diagnosed clinically based on menstrual cycle history (12 months of amenorrhea), age of the woman (over 45 years), and associated symptoms such as hot flushes. If laboratory confirmation is necessary or desired, serum FSH should be measured. In a young woman who has developed prolonged amenorrhea, FSH (along with prolactin, TSH, and a pregnancy test) should be measured to determine whether premature ovarian failure has occurred.

Premature (Primary) Ovarian Failure

Premature ovarian failure (POF) occurs when all ovarian follicles and oocytes have been depleted before 40 years of age. Presenting symptoms are similar to those observed in naturally occurring menopause. POF may be due to autoimmune oophoritis. Women with POF should be evaluated for other autoimmune diseases such as systemic lupus erythematosus, polyglandular failure, Addison disease, and myasthenia gravis. About 3% of women with POF will develop Addison disease. POF may be associated with genetic disorders such as the fragile X syndrome (premutations in the *FMR1* gene). In general, women are treated with contraceptive doses of estrogen–progestin to help prevent bone loss and the development of osteoporosis. Women with POF may become pregnant through oocyte donation.

Surgical Menopause

The surgical removal of all ovarian tissue in a premenopausal woman, abruptly causes a dramatic decrease in circulating estradiol and progesterone. Women undergoing surgical menopause may have more pronounced and severe symptoms than women with natural menopause. These women are typically treated with either contraceptive doses of estrogen–progestin, or postmenopausal hormone therapy (five to eight times lower doses than in contraceptive formulations).

Treatment

Menopausal Hot Flushes

A major challenge in identifying effective treatments for hot flushes is the observation that hot flushes will resolve in the majority of women, with time, without treatment. Given this fundamental observation, placebo-controlled trials are mandatory before efficacy can be established. A corollary is that if hot flushes often resolve with observation, "placebos" will appear to be effective in the treatment of hot flushes.

There is no consistent evidence from high quality clinical trials for the effectiveness of the following in the treatment of hot flushes:
- acupuncture
- yoga
- dong quai
- evening primrose oil
- ginseng
- kava
- red clover extract
- black cohosh
- soy products
- vitamin E

Estrogen Treatment

Multiple randomized, placebo-controlled trials have reported that estrogen reduces the frequency of hot flushes by about 80% or more. Relief is typically clearly noted within 4 weeks of initiating therapy. An evolving research goal is to identify the lowest dose of estrogen replacement that will reliably improve hot flushes. It appears that very low doses of estrogen are often effective in treating hot flushes.

In postmenopausal women with a uterus, treatment with estrogen will cause endometrial hyperplasia and cancer. Consequently, when treating these women with estrogen, a progestin must be added to the regimen to prevent hyperplasia and cancer. Progestins are typically administered continuously with the estrogen, or cyclically. In postmenopausal women without a uterus, estrogen may be administered without progesterone.

In postmenopausal women, estrogen and estrogen–progestin treatment may be associated with adverse effects including deep venous thrombosis and stroke (See Evidence Box 44.1). These adverse effects have influenced the recommendation that when treating hot flushes with hormone therapy, the lowest dose, for the shortest interval consistent with efficacy should be administered.

Continuous therapy, cyclic therapy—monthly cycles, and cyclic therapy—seasonal cycles: Estrogen-only hormone therapy is typically given continuously, without interruption. Estrogen–progestin hormone therapy may be given in many different temporal sequences. The main objectives are to reduce the menopausal symptoms with estrogen and prevent endometrial hyperplasia with the progestin. Estrogen–progestin therapy may be given continuously without interruption. This regimen has the greatest likelihood of producing the fewest days of uterine withdrawal bleeding. Some women on continuous estrogen-progestin therapy will develop light bleeding that occurs at irregular intervals with varying days of bleeding, and is difficult to predict (breakthrough bleeding). With cyclic monthly regimens, estrogen is given continuously, and progestin is given for 12–14 days (calendar days 1–13) each month. With cyclic seasonal regimens, estrogen is given continuously and progestin is given for 14 days every 3 months. Cyclic seasonal regimens are associated with fewer days of uterine withdrawal bleeding than cyclic monthly regimens. Cyclic monthly regimens are likely to be associated with the greatest number of days of bleeding, but the fewest unexpected days of bleeding of the three regimens.

Nonestrogen Treatment

Doses of progestins in the upper range of the those ordinarily administered, such as medroxyprogesterone acetate 20 mg daily, reduce the frequency of hot flushes. The serotonin–norephinephrine reuptake inhibitor, venlafaxine, and its active metabolite, desvenlafaxine, are both effective in reducing the frequency of hot flushes and are an alternative to estrogen or progestin treatment of hot flushes.

Cessation of Hormone Therapy

If hormone therapy is abruptly discontinued, the return of hot flushes may be pronounced. When discontinuing therapy it is wise to taper hormone therapy over an extended period.

Vaginal Symptoms

In postmenopausal women, vaginal symptoms may be effectively treated with vaginal moisturizers or estrogen. A polycarbophil-based vaginal moisturizer (Replens) available without a prescription provides symptom improvement similar to that observed with estrogen. Vaginal estrogen provides symptom improvement in the majority of postmenopausal women with vaginal symptoms, such as dryness. Vaginal estrogen therapy is available in creams, tablets, or hormone-releasing vaginal rings. Given the potential adverse effects associated with oral estrogen and oral estrogen–progestin treatment, when hormones are used to treat vaginal symptoms they should ordinarily be administered vaginally.

Osteoporosis

Osteoporosis is a disease of the bone caused both by low bone mass and by disordered bone microarchitecture, which manifests as low-trauma fractures. About 50% of postmenopausal women will experience a clinically significant osteoporotic fracture of the spine or hip. Among postmenopausal women with a hip fracture, 50% will be unable to walk independently after the fracture heals, causing a great deal of morbidity.

Osteoporosis is currently diagnosed by the measurement of bone mineral density (BMD), and is present when the BMD is below –2.5 standard deviations of the mean BMD of a normal young person of the same sex (T-score). A T-score of –2.5 is associated with more than fourfold increased risk of fracture compared with a T-score of zero. A previous history of low-trauma fracture markedly increases the risk of future fractures, regardless of the BMD measurement.

Most experts recommend that all women over 65 years of age be offered a BMD test, typically using dual x-ray absorptiometry (DXA) testing. In addition, all postmenopausal women with a risk factor for low-trauma fracture, such as a premenopausal amenorrhea, very low body mass, or current cigarette smoking may also be offered a BMD test.

The prevention and treatment of osteoporosis begins with adequate weight-bearing exercise, vitamin D supplements at doses in the range of 800 IU daily, and adequate calcium intake, typically 1000–1500 mg daily. It is important to note that the standard recommended supplement dose of vitamin D, 400 IU, is not adequate to prevent osteoporosis and low-trauma fractures. Eight hours of walking per week is associated with a 50% decrease in the risk of hip fracture.

Bisphosphonates, including alendronate (70 mg orally weekly), risedronate (70 mg orally twice-monthly), ibandronate (150 mg orally monthly or 3 mg by intravenous bolus every 3 months), and zoledronic acid (5 mg by intravenous infusion annually) are the primary treatments for osteoporosis. These agents reduce the risk of fracture by about 45% in postmenopausal women with osteoporosis. At the doses used for the treatment of osteoporosis these agents have few side effects. At higher doses, such as those used to treat patients with cancer metastasis to bone, these agents can be associated with osteonecrosis of the jaw. To minimize the risk of osteonecrosis of the jaw, some authorities recommend that postmenopausal women discontinue bisphosphonates for 3 months prior to major dental surgery, such as a tooth implant.

Estrogen and estrogen–progestin treatment are also effective in the treatment of postmenopausal osteoporosis, reducing the risk of future fractures by about 35%. For women with both hot flushes and osteoporosis, estrogen, or estrogen–progestin treatment is a logical approach to treating both conditions simultaneously. In women with only osteoporosis, bisphosphonates are usually recommended, because they are unlikely to be associated with deep venous thrombosis or stroke, two adverse effects that may be caused by hormone therapy.

Raloxifene, a selective estrogen receptor modulator (SERM) that has both estrogen agonist activity on bone and estrogen antagonist activity on the uterus, is approved for the treatment of osteoporosis. Calcitonin nasal spray (200 IU daily) is also approved for the treatment of osteoporosis. Neither agent is widely used for the treatment of osteoporosis.

Since raloxifene is approved to reduce the risk of breast cancer in women at high risk for the disease, if a woman at high risk of breast cancer has osteoporosis, raloxifene might be the logical agent to use in this situation. Calcitonin appears to reduce pain associated with an osteoporotic fracture. For a patient with an osteoporotic fracture and significant pain that is not responsive to standard treatments, calcitonin may be of value both to prevent future fractures and to reduce the pain symptoms.

Recombinant parathyroid hormone (PTH), administered as a daily subcutaneous injection is approved for the treatment of osteoporosis. Unlike the bisphosphonates and estrogen, which improve bone density by reducing bone resorption, PTH increases bone formation and is the only anabolic bone medicine currently approved for use.

Cardiovascular Disease

Estrogen has both beneficial and adverse effects on the vascular system. Estrogen and estrogen–progestin clearly induce alterations in the vascular and coagulation system, which increases the risk of both deep venous thrombosis and stroke. Estrogen–progestin, when administered to women in the late postmenopause, also increases the risk of cardiovascular events such as myocardial infarction. However, estrogen and estrogen–progestin may decrease the risk of cardiovascular events such as myocardial infarction when administered to women in the early postmenopause. The discordant effect of hormone therapy in the early and late postmenopause is termed the "timing hypothesis." The basis of the timing hypothesis may be that during the early stages of arterial plaque formation, estrogen stabilizes the plaque and prevents the accumulation of lipid and calcium in the plaque. In the later stages of arterial plaque formation, estrogen may have reduced beneficial effect, permitting the thrombotic tendency of estrogen to allow further evolution of the plaque and its clinical consequences.

Breast Cancer

Breast cancer is known to be a hormonally sensitive tumor. In postmenopausal women at high-risk for developing breast cancer, anti-estrogens, such as raloxifene or tamoxifen, reduce the risk of developing breast cancer. In women with estrogen-receptor positive invasive breast cancer, anti-estrogens such as raloxifene or tamoxifen and aromatase inhibitors such as letrozole decrease the rate of recurrence of the disease. In one clinical trial, 434 women with breast cancer were randomly assigned to receive two years of hormone therapy (estrogen-alone in women with a hysterectomy, and estrogen–progestin in women with an intact uterus) versus nonhormonal treatment. After a median follow-up of 2 years, 26 women in the hormone therapy group and 7 in the nonhormone therapy group had a breast cancer recurrence yielding a relative risk of 3.5 (95% CI, 1.5 to 8.1) in the hormone-treated women. The study was stopped because of the statistically significant increased risk of recurrent breast cancer. Most oncologists prefer that women with breast cancer do not receive hormone therapy

The Future of Hormone Therapy

A contemporary goal of hormone therapy is to use the lowest effective doses of native estradiol and progesterone that achieve the clinical goal. Very low doses of oral or transdermal estradiol may be effective in the treatment of vasomotor symptoms in many postmenopausal women. For example, transdermal estradiol 14 µg or 25 µg daily, administered using a transdermal patch, is effective for the treatment of vasomotor symptoms in many women. In the recent past, transdermal estradiol doses in the range of 50–100 µg daily were commonly used for hormone treatment. In addition, more clinicians are using native ("natural) micronized progesterone in hormone therapy regimens for postmenopausal women with an intact uterus, rather than "synthetic" progestins such as medroxyprogesterone acetate.

The result of the Women's Health Initiative has taken postmenopausal hormone therapy in the direction of using the lowest doses of hormones for the shortest period of time that achieves treatment efficacy. In addition, the Women's Health Initiative has clearly demonstrated that hormone therapy should only be used for the treatment of clinical symptoms, such as hot flushes, that are caused by the menopause.

Key Points

- In developed countries, women live about 30 years of their lives in the postmenopause period.
- Perimenopausal and postmenopausal women may be affected by symptoms associated with hypoestrogenism, including vasomotor symptoms and vaginal dryness. Hypoestrogenism is also the most common cause of osteoporosis resulting in vertebral and hip fractures.
- In most women, hot flushes will resolve without treatment. For women with symptomatic hot flushes who desire treatment, transdermal or oral estrogen is very effective medication. For women with a uterus, a progestin such as oral micronized progesterone, must be given to prevent estrogen-induced endometrial hyperplasia.
- For women with vaginal dryness, direct application of estrogen to the vaginal epithelium is optimal because it minimizes systemic dosing. Vaginal estrogen treatment is available in creams, tablets, and vaginal rings.
- Osteoporosis is best treated with an oral bisphosphonate.

Evidence Box 44.1

Hormone therapy has both significant beneficial and adverse effects in postmenopausal women.

The Women's Health Initiative (WHI) is one of the largest trials executed by the National Institutes of Health. This trial demonstrated both beneficial and adverse effects of estrogen and estrogen–progestin hormone therapy. One demonstrated beneficial effect was a reduction in osteoporotic fractures of the spine and hip. Demonstrated adverse effects included an increased risk of deep venous thrombosis and stroke. The publication of the results of the WHI resulted in a marked decrease in the use of hormone therapy by postmenopausal women. Currently, the main indication for hormone therapy in the postmenopause is to treat hot flushes and vaginal symptoms. Hormone therapy should be used at the lowest dose, for the shortest period of time compatible with achieving the therapeutic goal.

The Women's Health Initiative (WHI) was a randomized trial of estrogen and estrogen–progestin in healthy, mostly late postmenopausal women, with an average age of 63 years. The objective of the study was to determine the impact of hormone therapy on cardiovascular, breast, and bone disease in healthy postmenopausal women. For both estrogen and estrogen–progestin treatment, hormone therapy was associated with an increased risk of deep venous thrombosis and stroke compared with placebo. For both estrogen and estrogen–progestin treatment, hormone therapy was associated with a decreased risk of hip and vertebral fracture compared with placebo. Estrogen–progestin treatment was associated with an increased risk of cardiovascular events and incidence breast cancer compared with placebo. In contrast, estrogen-only treatment was not associated with these adverse effects. This study resulted in the conclusion, that hormone therapy should only be used to treat hot flushes or vaginal symptoms at the lowest dose for the shortest period of time consistent with effective treatment. Hazard ratios (95 % CI) of various events during treatment with hormone therapy or placebo are given in **Table 44.4**.

Rossouw JE, Anderson GL, Prentice RL, et al. Risks and benefits of estrogen plus progestin in healthy postmenopausal women: principal results from the Women's Health Initiative randomized controlled trial. JAMA 2002;288:321–323.

Anderson GL, Limacher M, Assaf AR, et al. Effects of conjugated equine estrogen in postmenopausal women with hysterectomy: the Women's Health Initiative randomized controlled trial. JAMA 2004;291:1701–1712.

Evidence Box 44.2

Conjugated equine estrogen (Premarin) has both estrogen agonist and antagonist properties.

Conjugated equine estrogen (Premarin) is one of the most widely used estrogens for hormone replacement. Originally, conjugated equine estrogen was obtained by extracting sulfated estrogens (conjugates) from pregnant mare's urine, hence "Premarin" (PREgnant MARe's urINe). Currently, as noted in the Food and Drug Administration's description of the drug, Premarin is a mixture of conjugated estrogens obtained from natural sources occurring as estrogen sulfates blended to represent the average composition of material derived from pregnant mare's urine. The dominant estrogen in conjugated equine estrogen (CEE) is estrone sulfate, a major circulating estrogen metabolite and precursor in humans (and horses). Estrone sulfate is well absorbed into the circulation and has a prolonged half-life compared with native estradiol. Estrone sulfate can be converted to estrone and then to estradiol, the biologically active estrogen, in most tissues. Other components of CEE include 17α-dihydroequilin, 17α-estradiol, and 17β-dihydroequilin. There is laboratory evidence that both 17α-dihydroequilin and 17α-estradiol may be partial estradiol antagonists, while estrone sulfate and 17β-dihydroequilin are estrogen agonists. Consequently, the mixture in conjugated equine estrogen may result in a compound that has both estrogen agonist and antagonist properties, similar to what might be expected from a selective estrogen receptor modulator (SERM). The partial estrogen antagonist properties of conjugated equine estrogen may account for the paradoxical observation that Premarin, when used alone for hormone therapy in postmenopausal women, is not associated with an increased risk of breast cancer. For example, in the Women's Health Initiative, after a mean follow-up of 7.1 years, the risk of invasive breast cancer in women treated with daily conjugated equine estrogen versus placebo was 0.80 (95 % CI, 0.62 to 1.04; $P = 0.09$). When the data were analyzed based on the subject's adherence to the assigned regimen, a significant reduction in invasive breast cancer risk was observed in the women who reliably took their conjugated equine estrogen compared with placebo, hazard ratio 0.67 (95 % CI 0.47 to 0.97; $P = 0.03$). In contrast, the pure estrogen agonist, estradiol, does appear to increase the risk of breast cancer in postmenopausal women.

Anderson GL, Limacher M, Assaf AR, et al. Effects of conjugated equine estrogen in postmenopausal women with hysterectomy: the Women's Health Initiative randomized controlled trial. JAMA 2004;291:1701–1712.

Dey M, Lyttle CR, Pickar JH. Recent insights into the varying activity of estrogens. Maturitas 2000;34(Suppl 2):S25–S33.

Table 44.4 Comparison of estrogen and estrogen–progestin interventions

Intervention	Conjugated equine estrogen 0.625 mg daily or placebo	Conjugated equine estrogen 0.625 mg plus medroxyprogesterone acetate 2.5 mg daily or placebo
Sample size	9739	16 608
Mean age of subjects (years)	63	63
Mean duration of hormone use (years)	6.8	5.2
Coronary heart disease	0.91 (0.75 to 1.12)	**1.29 (1.02 to 1.63)**
Breast Cancer	0.77 (0.59 to 1.01)	**1.26 (1.00 to 1.59)**
Stroke	**1.39 (1.10 to 1.77)**	**1.41 (1.07 to 1.85)**
Thromboembolism	1.34 (0.87 to 2.06)	**2.13 (1.39 to 3.25)**
Osteoporotic hip fracture	**0.61 (0.41 to 0.91)**	**0.67 (0.47 to 0.96)**
Osteoporotic vertebral fracture	**0.62 (0.42 to 0.93)**	**0.65 (0.46 to 0.92)**

Further Reading

Anderson GL, Limacher M, Assaf AR, et al; Women's Health Initiative Steering Committee. Effects of conjugated equine estrogen in postmenopausal women with hysterectomy: the Women's Health Initiative randomized controlled trial. *JAMA* 2004;291(14):1701–1712

Bakalov VK, Vanderhoof VH, Bondy CA, Nelson LM. Adrenal antibodies detect asymptomatic auto-immune adrenal insufficiency in young women with spontaneous premature ovarian failure. *Hum Reprod* 2002;17(8):2096–2100

Clarkson TB. Can women be identified that will derive considerable cardiovascular benefits from postmenopausal estrogen therapy? *J Clin Endocrinol Metab* 2008;93(1):37–39

Cramer DW, Harlow BL, Xu H, Fraer C, Barbieri R. Cross-sectional and case-controlled analyses of the association between smoking and early menopause. *Maturitas* 1995;22(2):79–87

Cramer DW, Barbieri RL, Fraer AR, Harlow BL. Determinants of early follicular phase gonadotrophin and estradiol concentrations in women of late reproductive age. *Hum Reprod* 2002;17(1):221–227

Dey M, Lyttle CR, Pickar JH. Recent insights into the varying activity of estrogens. *Maturitas* 2000;34(Suppl 2):S25–S33

Grady D. Clinical practice. Management of menopausal symptoms. *N Engl J Med* 2006;355(22):2338–2347

Hays J, Ockene JK, Brunner RL, et al; Women's Health Initiative Investigators. Effects of estrogen plus progestin on health-related quality of life. *N Engl J Med* 2003;348(19):1839–1854

Holmberg L, Anderson H; HABITS steering and data monitoring committees. HABITS (hormonal replacement therapy after breast cancer—is it safe?), a randomised comparison: trial stopped. *Lancet* 2004;363(9407):453–455

Rossouw JE, Anderson GL, Prentice RL, et al; Writing Group for the Women's Health Initiative Investigators. Risks and benefits of estrogen plus progestin in healthy postmenopausal women: principal results From the Women's Health Initiative randomized controlled trial. *JAMA* 2002;288(3):321–333

Shifren JL, Davis SR, Moreau M, et al. Testosterone patch for the treatment of hypoactive sexual desire disorder in naturally menopausal women: results from the INTIMATE NM1 Study. *Menopause* 2006;13(5):770–779

Soares CN, Arsenio H, Joffe H, et al. Escitalopram versus ethinyl estradiol and norethindrone acetate for symptomatic peri- and postmenopausal women: impact on depression, vasomotor symptoms, sleep, and quality of life. *Menopause* 2006;13(5):780–786

Soules MR, Sherman S, Parrott E, et al. Executive summary: Stages of Reproductive Aging Workshop (STRAW). *Fertil Steril* 2001;76(5):874–878

Steinauer JE, Waetjen LE, Vittinghoff E, et al. Postmenopausal hormone therapy: does it cause incontinence? *Obstet Gynecol* 2005;106(5 Pt 1):940–945

Woods NF, Smith-Dijulio K, Percival DB, Tao EY, Taylor HJ, Mitchell ES. Symptoms during the menopausal transition and early postmenopause and their relation to endocrine levels over time: observations from the Seattle Midlife Women's Health Study. *J Womens Health (Larchmt)* 2007;16(5):667–677

45 The Biology of Cancer

Robert L. Barbieri

Two characteristic features of cancer cells are unrestrained proliferation and invasion into adjacent structures (**Fig. 45.1**). The mechanisms by which normal adult cells develop the capacity for both unrestrained proliferation and invasiveness are not full characterized, but altered function of genomic DNA is critical to the phenotype. Genomic DNA can be permanently altered by many mechanisms. Relevant to gynecological disease, the biological mechanisms that can alter the function of genomic DNA include viral infection (cervical cancer), excess hormonal stimulation (endometrial cancer), and various mutations that reduce the cell's capacity for DNA repair or that disrupt cell cycle control checkpoints(endometrial and ovarian cancer). These mechanisms are explored in this chapter, using examples from gynecologic cancer.

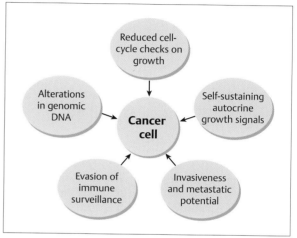

Fig. 45.1 Characteristics and behavior of cancer cells.

Cervical Cancer is Caused by the Human Papilloma Virus

In 1983, zur Hausen reported the presence of human papilloma virus (HPV) types 16 and 18 in cervical cancer biopsies. Subsequent research led to an understanding of the molecular mechanisms by which infection with HPV-16 and HPV-18, if left untreated, cause cervical cancer. HPV type 16 and 18 infections have also been shown to cause cancer of the vulva, vagina, penis, anus, and mouth. The circle of medical science, from molecular discovery to effective patient and population treatment, was closed in 2005 when a vaccine for HPV-16 and HPV-18 to combat cancer became widely available. In 2008, zur Hausen received the Nobel Prize in Medicine for this important discovery. Zur Hausen has gone on to discover that polyomaviruses can cause skin cancer. The role of viruses in the etiology of cancer continues to evolve.

HPV infection is endemic among sexually active men and women. There are over 115 types of HPV infection and over 40 types are specific for the anogenital epithelium. In most cases, infection with HPV results in latent infection without symptoms, physical findings, or cellular changes in the cervix. In some cases, HPV infection results in active infection 2–8 months after initial exposure, which results in cellular changes in the cervix including nuclear enlargement, multinucleation, and perinuclear cytoplasmic clearing. These cellular findings are often diagnosed on cervical cytology as low-grade squamous intra-epithelial neoplasia. Immunological response to the infection may result in resolution or chronic infection. If the HPV integrates into the cell genome, high-grade squamous intra-epithelial lesions and cancer may result. The HPV types that are most likely to result in genomic integration and cancer are 16, 18, 45, 59, and 35. Integration of HPV into the genome results in overexpression of E6 and E7, two HPV proteins that release the cell from cell cycle checkpoints.

The viral E6 protein binds to the tumor suppressor gene p53 (which blocks the progression of cells through the late G_1 phase), reducing its activity and increasing its degradation. This reduction in expression of p53 releases the cell from the G_1 cell-cycle checkpoint, and permits the cell to replicate more rapidly. In addition, normal levels of p53 activity prevent cells with DNA damage from proliferating. Reduction in p53 activity is associated with chromosome instability, increasing the likelihood that additional detrimental mutations will accrue.

The viral E7 protein binds to the retinoblastoma protein (Rb) which causes the release and activation of transcription factor E2F, which promotes cell proliferation. In addition, when E7 is released by infected cells it causes an increase in the production of interleukins 6 and 8, which in turn increases the rate of cell proliferation. The ability of certain HPV types to integrate into the genome, overexpress E6 and E7, and thereby decrease the function of two important tumor suppressor proteins, p53 and Rb, is central to the oncogenic potential of these types. It is likely that the double-hit on two important tumor suppressor networks, p53 and Rb, is critical to evading normal cell mechanisms for restraining growth.

Endometrial Cancer is Caused by Unopposed Estrogen Stimulation

Estradiol stimulates endometrial cell proliferation. Progesterone blocks estradiol stimulation of endometrial cells. In the high concentrations observed in pregnancy, progesterone can cause terminal differentiation of endometrial cells to form decidua. These cells have markedly reduced capacity for further proliferation. The essence of the estradiol-induced proliferation of the endometrium and the progesterone-induced secretory differentiation and block of further proliferation represents the ebb–flow of the endometrium during the menstrual cycle. Estradiol causes the endometrium to grow, progesterone stops the growth and prepares (by differentiation) the endometrium for implantation. At menses, withdrawal of both the estradiol and progesterone disrupts the integrity of the endometrium and results in menstrual bleeding. With the next cycle, increase in ovarian production of estradiol causes the endometrium to stabilize, start growing, and stop bleeding.

Constant estradiol stimulation of the endometrium results in the development of type I, endometrioid, endometrial cancer. These lesions have characteristic mutations in the PTEN, k-ras and beta-catenin genes and demonstrate DNA microsatellite instability. The PTEN (phosphatase and tensin homologue) gene is a suppressor of estrogen-stimulated endometrial cell growth. Mutations in the *PTEN* gene that result in loss of function cause greater endometrial cell growth in response to a given concentration (dose) of estradiol. In addition, endometrial cancer cells appear to sometimes amplify the estrogen receptor gene, resulting in overexpression of active estrogen receptor, further sensitizing the cell to the growth-promoting effects of estradiol stimulation.

Endometrial and Ovarian Cancers are Caused by Germ-Line Mutations in DNA Mismatch Repair Genes

Lynch syndrome is an autosomal dominant disease caused by a germ-line mutation in one of several DNA mismatch repair (MMR) genes. It is responsible for about 2% of all endometrial cancers and 10% of endometrial cancers occurring in women of less than 50 years of age. The job of the DNA MMR proteins is to correct DNA base mismatches, and to repair short insertion or deletion mismatches. These errors occur at a low frequency (1 time in a million) during the base pairing process of DNA replication. At least six related genes produce proteins that work together to repair DNA mismatches. These six genes are hMSH2, hMLH1, hPMS1, hPMS2, hMSH6, and hMLH3. Recognition of mismatches is done by heterodimeric combinations of MSH2/MSH6 and MSH2/MSH3. Repair of mismatches is done by heterodimeric combinations of MLH1/PMS2, MLH1/PMS1, and MLH1/MLH3.

Inactivation of both alleles of one of the six *MMR* genes can lead to defective MMR, the accumulation of DNA errors, and eventually a series of critical mutations that result in cell proliferation and invasiveness. In most cases, patients with Lynch syndrome have a germ line mutation in one allele of a *MMR* gene. The second allele is inactivated by a mutation (2nd hit), loss of heterozygosity, or epigenetic silencing by hypermethylation. Loss of both alleles of either MSH2 or MLH1 cause over 90% of cases of Lynch syndrome.

There are specific genotype–phenotype relationships in the Lynch syndrome. The colon cancer risk is 50–70% in women with either the MSH2 or MLH1 mutations. However, the risk of endometrial cancer is greater in women with MSH2 mutations (40%) than in women with MLH1 mutations (27%). Women with MSH6 mutations have the greatest rate of endometrial cancer (70%).

When parents with the Lynch syndrome marry they run the risk of having children with bi-allelic MMR loss in the germ-line. This condition is rare, but typically results in the childhood onset of hematological and brain cancer.

Breast and Ovarian Cancers can be Caused by Mutations in BRCA1 and BRCA2

The *BRCA1* gene codes for a 220 kDa multifunctional protein that participates in regulations of transcription, repair of damaged DNA, control of cell-cycle, and ubiquitination of proteins. BRCA1 likely participates in multiple cell system functions by binding to a large number of diverse partner proteins. Over 600 unique deleterious mutations in BRCA1 have been reported. Most of these mutations cause the production of a truncated protein that has lost various degrees of function. A deleterious mutation in BRCA1 is present in approximately 0.2% of the general population and 2% of the Ashkenazi Jewish population.

Inactivation of both alleles of the *BRCA1* gene can lead to increased cell proliferation and the accumulation of additional DNA errors, resulting in the accumulation of a series of critical mutations that cause increased cell proliferation and invasiveness. Women with a germ-line mutation in one allele of the *BRCA1* gene may have the second allele inactivated by mutation or loss of heterozygosity. The inheritance pattern is autosomal dominant with high penetrance. This results in an increased lifetime risk of breast cancer (60%) and ovarian cancer (40%). Interestingly, in women with BRCA1 mutations, the ovarian cancer appears to begin in the epithelium of the fallopian tube and then metastasizes to the ovary (Evidence Box 45.1).

BRCA2 is a DNA repair gene. A germ-line mutation resulting in loss of function of BRCA2, followed by mutations in a somatic cell, can result in loss of BRCA2 expression and the development of both breast and ovarian cancer. In women with germ-line mutations of *BRCA2*, the lifetime risk of breast cancer is about 60% and the lifetime risk of ovarian cancer is about 20%. *BRCA2* mutations increase the risk for male breast cancer.

Women who discover that they are carriers of BRCA mutations often experience significant psychological distress as they attempt to navigate a personal pathway through multiple treatment options including risk- reducing bilateral mastectomy and bilateral salpingoophorectomy.

Evolving Issues in Cancer Biology

Multistep Process of Carcinogenesis

During the lifetime of somatic cells, mutations can accumulate in the parent cell and its descendent cells through many mechanisms, including chemical and radiation induced mutagenesis. Some mutations give the affected cell a growth advantage over neighboring cells and result in the progeny of the mutated cells outnumbering the wild-type cells. From within this clonal population, a cell(s) can accumulate additional mutations providing additional growth advantage that permits accelerating clonal expansion. Eventually the cell may be released from cell-cycle checkpoints, increase proliferation, and acquire invasive properties.

The multistep process of carcinogenesis is well studied in colon cancer, where initial mutations result in the development of clonal adenomas and later mutations within the adenoma can lead to colon cancer. Mutations in the adenomatous polyposis gene occur early in the multistep process, and mutations in p53 tend to occur late in the process. In addition to point mutations, additional mechanisms that can cause accelerating cell proliferation and acquisition of invasiveness include: DNA methylations, gene rearrangements, gene amplification, and deletions.

Oncogenes

Many genes participate in cell growth pathways. When these genes become mutated they may become more active, resulting in enhanced cell proliferation. *K-ras* is a cellular oncogene that participates in increasing cell proliferation in many tumors. The ras oncogene products are G-like proteins that transmit a growth signal from the cell membrane to the nucleus. Mutations that create resistance to GTP hydrolysis by GTPase leaves the ras proteins in an active form that drives cell proliferation.

Angiogenesis

Growing tumor cells must be able to create a rich blood supply to support their growing metabolic needs. Most tumor cells produce vascular endothelial growth factor (VEGF), which binds to VEGF-2 receptors on endothelial cells and stimulates angiogenesis. Hypoxia is common in solid tumors. Hypoxia stimulates VEGF production. In addition to tumor production of VEGF, host platelets and tumor-associated stromal cells also produce VEGF. A humanized monoclonal antibody against

VEGF (bevacizumab) has been demonstrated to improve survival in patients with advanced colon cancer or non–small-cell lung carcinoma. Other small molecule inhibitors of VEGF receptors and platelet-derived growth factor receptors have also been approved for the treatment of cancer (sorafenib, sunitinib).

Immunology

Many tumor cells express novel proteins due to multiple mutations or viral infection that conferred proliferative advantages. The immune system can respond to these unique antigens and modulate the growth of tumor cells. Tumor antigens can serve as a target for treatment. The administration of monoclonal antibodies against the tumor antigen HER2 (trastunzumab) is clinically effective in breast cancer. Many laboratories are trying to develop vaccines to unique tumor cell antigens.

Tumors can fight back against the host immune system by producing immunosuppressive molecules such as transforming growth factor beta and soluble Fas ligand. In addition, the tumor can attract regulatory T cells that suppress antitumor effector T cells.

Cancer Stem Cells

Stem cells that reside in tumors appear to be key to the early proliferation and later maintenance of cancer. In human breast cancer, a low prevalence cell that is CD44-positive and CD24-negative is the cell with the greatest ability to propagate the tumor in immunosuppressed mice. These stem cells can differentiate into all the cellular elements of a mammary gland when given a favorable environment. Cancer treatment that kills the prevalent, non–stem-cell tumor cells may not be especially effective, because stem cells can proliferate and regenerate the tumor.

Epigenetics

Epigenetics is the study of changes in gene expression and phenotype that are caused by chemical changes which do not alter the DNA sequence. Methylation of DNA is the best-studied epigenetic mechanism. Methylation of DNA tends to suppress expression of the methylated gene. In many human tumors there is global hypomethylation causing expression of many genes that should not be expressed in adult cells. Paradoxically, hypermethylation of tumor suppressor genes, including tumor suppressor micro-RNA genes, may help release tumor cells from

controlled growth. Chemical modifications of histone proteins, such as lysine acetylation, arginine methylation and serine phosphorylation, can also cause epigenetic changes that influence phenotype.

Key Points

- All cancer is caused by changes in genomic DNA that permit dysregulated cell growth.
- Changes in genomic DNA that may permit excessive cell growth include mutations that cause: 1) the loss of activity of tumor suppressor genes; 2) the activation of tumor inducing genes; 3) gene rearrangements that result in novel oncogenic proteins; and 4) the insertion of viral oncogenes.
- Cervical cancer can be caused by integration into genomic DNA of the viral oncogenes E6 and E7 found in HPV-16. E6 reduces the activity of the tumor suppressor gene p53 and E7 reduces the activity of retinoblastoma (Rb) protein, thereby increasing the proliferative activity of the cell.
- Endometrial cancer can be caused by continuous exposure to critical levels of estradiol. Estradiol stimulates continuous proliferation of endometrial gland cells, increasing the rate of mutation, ultimately resulting in neoplasia.

Evidence Box 45.1

In women with BRCA1 mutations, ovarian cancer may actually begin in the distal portion of the fallopian tube, so risk-reducing surgery requires both removal of the ovary and the fallopian tube.

Women with BRCA1 mutations are at increased risk for breast and ovarian cancer. Several studies of BRCA1-positive women have demonstrated that the fallopian tube may have a central role in the development of ovarian cancer. In a study of 94 healthy women who were BRCA1 carriers and opted for risk-reducing salpingo-oophorectomy six cancers were detected.[*] Of the six cancers, two were in the fallopian tube only, three were present simultaneously in both the tube and ovary, and one was present in only the ovary.

In another series of BRCA1-positive women undergoing risk-receding salpingo-oophorectomy five cancers or pre-invasive lesions were detected.[**] All five tumors were in the fallopian tube. In pathological analysis of fallopian tube lesions in women with BRCA1, mutations in p53 were commonly observed.[***] Mutations in the p53 tumor suppressor gene that result in loss of function are causally linked with many types of cancers. In BRCA1 women, the inciting pelvic cancer lesion may start in the distal fallopian tube and then spread to the ovary.

[*] **Finch A, Shaw P, Rosen B, Murphy J, Narod SA, Colgan TJ. Clinical and pathologic findings of prophylactic salpingo-oophorectomies in 159 BRCA1 and BRCA2 carriers. Gynecol Oncol 2006;100:58–64.**

[**] **Medeiros F, Muto MG, Lee Y, et al. The tubal fimbria is a preferred site for early adenocarcinoma in women with familial ovarian cancer syndrome. Am J Surg Pathol 2006;30:230–236.**

[***] **Lee Y, Miron A, Drapkin R, et al. A candidate precursor to serous carcinoma that originates in the distal fallopian tube. J Pathol 2007;211:26–35.**

Further Reading

Cid-Arregui A, Juárez V, zur Hausen H. A synthetic E7 gene of human papillomavirus type 16 that yields enhanced expression of the protein in mammalian cells and is useful for DNA immunization studies. *J Virol* 2003;77(8):4928–4937

Esteller M. Epigenetics in cancer. *N Engl J Med* 2008;358(11):1148–1159

Fearon ER, Vogelstein B. A genetic model for colorectal tumorigenesis. *Cell* 1990;61(5):759–767

Finch A, Shaw P, Rosen B, Murphy J, Narod SA, Colgan TJ. Clinical and pathologic findings of prophylactic salpingo-oophorectomies in 159 BRCA1 and BRCA2 carriers. *Gynecol Oncol* 2006;100(1):58–64

Kennedy RD, Quinn JE, Johnston PG, Harkin DP. BRCA1: mechanisms of inactivation and implications for management of patients. *Lancet* 2002;360(9338):1007–1014

Kerbel RS. Tumor angiogenesis. *N Engl J Med* 2008;358(19):2039–2049

Lebeau A, Grob T, Holst F, et al. Oestrogen receptor gene (ESR1) amplification is frequent in endometrial carcinoma and its precursor lesions. *J Pathol* 2008;216(2):151–157

Lee Y, Miron A, Drapkin R, et al. A candidate precursor to serous carcinoma that originates in the distal fallopian tube. *J Pathol* 2007;211(1):26–35

Llobet D, Pallares J, Yeramian A, et al. Molecular pathology of endometrial carcinoma: practical aspects from the diagnostic and therapeutic viewpoints. J Clin Pathol 2008, e-pub

Medeiros F, Muto MG, Lee Y, et al. The tubal fimbria is a preferred site for early adenocarcinoma in women with familial ovarian cancer syndrome. *Am J Surg Pathol* 2006;30(2):230–236

Münger K, Phelps WC, Bubb V, Howley PM, Schlegel R. The E6 and E7 genes of the human papillomavirus type 16 together are necessary and sufficient for transformation of primary human keratinocytes. *J Virol* 1989;63(10):4417–4421

Pett M, Coleman N. Integration of high-risk human papillomavirus: a key event in cervical carcinogenesis? *J Pathol* 2007;212(4):356–367

zur Hausen H. Novel human polyomaviruses—re-emergence of a well known virus family as possible human carcinogens. *Int J Cancer* 2008;123(2):247–250

46 Gestational Trophoblastic Disease: Molar Pregnancy

Robert L. Barbieri

Definition

Gestational trophoblastic diseases (GTDs) are a group of five interrelated disorders of trophoblast epithelium of the placenta, which lead to placental tumors. Of the five forms of GTD, two forms, complete hydatidiform mole (**Fig. 46.1**) and partial hydatidiform mole, tend to have a benign course and are cured in the majority of cases by evacuating the uterus with a suction dilation and curettage. Three forms of GTD are malignant: invasive mole, choriocarcinoma, and placenta site trophoblastic tumor. Malignant forms of GTD are referred to as gestational trophoblastic neoplasia (GTN) and are typically treated with chemotherapy and hysterectomy if appropriate. Malignant forms of GTD most commonly arise from the malignant transformation of a complete hydatidiform mole, but they may occur following any type of gestation including term pregnancy, ectopic pregnancy, or spontaneous abortion. Malignant GTD is curable in most cases.

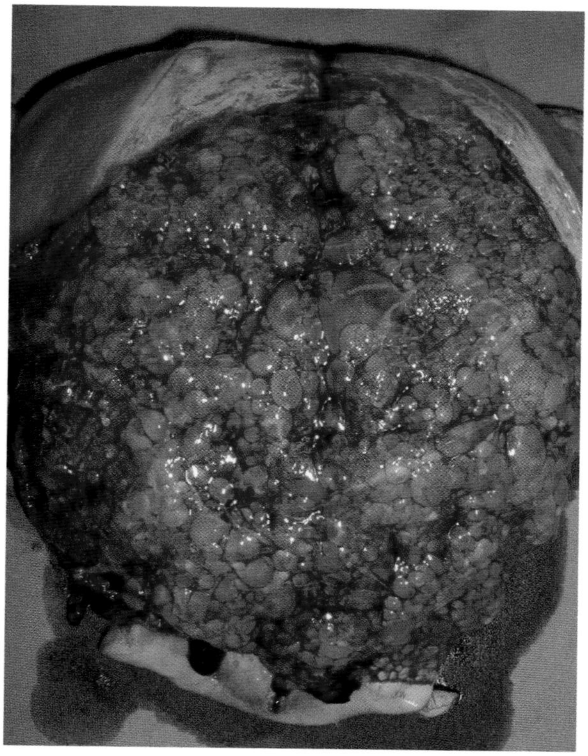

Hydatidiform mole, which may be complete or partial, is the most common type of GTD and represents over 80% of all cases. This chapter will focus on these two presentations of the disease. Malignant GTD will be reviewed briefly at the end of the chapter.

Fig. 46.1 Gross pathology of a complete hydatidiform mole in a hysterectomy specimen. From Sidney Southwest Arpa Health Service. New South Wales, Australia.

Hydatidiform Mole

Etiology

All hydatidiform moles have abnormal DNA complements, which are the result of abnormal fertilization of an oocyte (**Table 46.1**). In the case of complete hydatidiform mole, an empty oocyte is fertilized by a sperm that duplicates its chromosome material, or, less commonly, an empty oocyte is fertilized of by two sperm. A partial mole arises from the fertilization of an oocyte by two sperm resulting in triploidy.

Table 46.1 Characteristic features of complete and partial hydatidiform molar pregnancy

	Complete hydatidiform mole	Partial hydatidiform mole
Karyotype	90% of cases 46,XX; 10% of cases 46,XY	90% of cases triploid—69,XXX or 69,XXY
Source of sex chromosomes	All sex chromosomes are of *paternal* origin	One set of chromosomes are of maternal origin, and two sets of paternal origin
Villi swelling	Diffuse swelling of all villi	Focal swelling, scalloped villi
Trophoblast hyperplasia	Marked, circumferential around villi	Minimal, focal
Fetal tissue	None	Present
Immunocytochemistry	Intense staining for human chorionic gonadotropin	Intense staining for placental alkaline phosphatase
Malignant sequelae	About 20% of cases	2% of cases

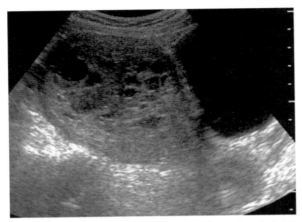

Fig. 46.2 Ultrasonographic presentation of complete hydatidiform mole.

Diagnosis and Initial Monitoring of Disease Activity

In countries where diagnostic ultrasonography is widely available, most hydatidiform moles are diagnosed by this technique in the first trimester of pregnancy. Almost all women with hydatidiform mole present with first trimester uterine bleeding. Due to the bleeding, pelvic ultrasound examination is routinely obtained to assess the status of the pregnancy. Complete hydatidiform mole is diagnosed when the ultrasound scan demonstrates the characteristic "snow storm" of multiple small cystic structures, which is the ultrasonographic presentation of multiple swollen villi (**Fig. 46.2**). Partial hydatidiform mole typically are thought to be missed abortions on ultrasonography, but when the uterus is evacuated, full pathological analysis demonstrates the presence of a mole. Women with suspected molar pregnancy should have a suction dilation and curettage to obtain placental tissue for final pathological diagnosis. In 80% of cases of complete hydatidiform mole, suction dilation and curettage cures the disease. In

20% of cases the disease persists requiring later chemotherapy. In 98% of cases of partial hydatidiform mole, suction dilation and curettage cures the disease.

After dilation and curettage, serum human chorionic gonadotropin (HCG) levels are followed weekly. An HCG level that reaches less than 5 mIU/mL indicates that the disease is cured. Following evacuation of a complete or partial hydatidiform mole, on average it takes 100 days or 60 days, respectively, for the HCG to reach less than 5 mIU/mL. (After a normal pregnancy, HCG levels return to normal after 4 weeks.) An HCG level that does not decrease (plateau of HCG for 3 weeks), or increases by 10%, or remains at greater than 5 mIU/mL after 26 weeks of measurement indicates the presence of persistent hydatidiform mole. In this situation, 75% of the cases represent an invasive mole and 25% represent choriocarcinoma.

Pathology

Complete hydatidiform moles are characterized by diffuse and marked swelling of the villi. Partial hydatidiform moles are characterized by focal swelling of the villi and the presence of embryonic tissue (**Table 46.1**).

Prevalence and Epidemiology

About 1 in 1000 pregnancies are complicated by hydatidiform mole. In Asia and Latin America, higher rates of mole have been reported. The two main risk factors are a history of a previous GTD pregnancy (1% risk of recurrence) and maternal age younger than 20 years or older than 35 years. Other minor risk factors are cigarette smoking, nulliparity, and history of infertility.

History, Physical Examination, and Laboratory Studies

Most women with complete hydatidiform mole present with vaginal bleeding in the first trimester of pregnancy. Diagnostic ultrasonography is ordered to evaluate the source of bleeding and the diagnosis is made. The increasing availability of high-quality ultrasound imaging and the widespread use of this technology in pregnancy has resulted in a marked change in the initial presentation of the disease.

Prior to the availability of ultrasonography, the diagnosis of GTD was typically made at 16 weeks' gestation, early in the second trimester. In the past, an enlarged uterus (50% of cases), theca lutein cysts, anemia (50% of cases), hyperthyroidism (7% of cases), and preeclampsia (27% of cases) were common findings in women with GTD. In the modern era, with wide availability of high-quality sonography, the diagnosis of GTD is typically made at about 10 weeks gestation. With early diagnosis, the only symptom may be first trimester vaginal bleeding. In the modern era it is unusual to see a patient with GTD present with hyperthyroidism or preeclampsia (<1% of cases). Early in the first trimester it is more difficult to identify cases of GTD by ultrasonography. This means that highly experienced sonologists who focus on obstetric and gynecologic imaging are more likely to make an early diagnosis. Partial hydatidiform moles typically present as missed abortions. Evacuation of the uterus results in pathological identification of the partial mole.

Treatment

As noted above, the treatment of both complete and partial hydatidiform moles is evacuation of the uterus with suction dilation and curettage. Following suction dilation and curettage, serum HCG is measured weekly. In 80% of cases of complete hydatidiform mole, this results in cure of the disease as represented by an HCG level of less than 5 mIU/mL. Once the HCG level reaches less than 5 mIU/mL, it is uncommon for that value to be exceeded. In 20% of cases, HCG levels do not decrease to this level.

Following dilation and curettage, 98% of cases of partial hydatidiform mole are cured. Prior to suction dilation and curettage, a complete blood count, renal, liver, and thyroid function tests are obtained to assess for systemic manifestation of the disease. A type and screen is obtained to facilitate the availability of red blood cells if needed for transfusion. Routine imaging of the liver, chest, and brain is not necessary. In order to prevent another pregnancy during the initial interval of weekly HCG measurements, highly effective contraception should be recommended, such as prescrition of an oral contraceptive.

In 20% of cases, HCG levels do not decrease to less than 5 mIU/mL and chemotherapy is given to eradicate the persistent disease. In general, women with persistent disease should be referred to a trophoblast disease center. Women with persistent disease should have a thorough evaluation for the presence of detectable metastatic disease, including pelvic ultrasound exam and computed tomography of the thorax. If either of these studies demonstrate metastatic or persistent tumor, imaging of the brain and liver is indicated. In most cases if pelvic sonography and computed tomography of the thorax are negative for metastases, then brain and liver imaging will also be negative. In women with known choriocarcinoma, complete imaging of the pelvis, thorax, liver, and brain should be obtained before treatment. In women who have completed their family, hysterectomy may be a useful adjuvant to single agent chemotherapy in order to reduce the bulk of residual and invasive disease.

Staging

Staging of GTN is based on the International Federation of Gynecologists and Obstetrician's system:

- Stage I: persistently elevated hCG levels and tumor confined to the uterus
- Stage II: tumor outside of the uterus, but limited to vagina or pelvic
- Stage III: pulmonary metastases
- Stage IV: metastatic disease at nonpulmonary sites such as brain, liver, and kidneys

For women with stage I disease who are at low risk, single-agent chemotherapy with methotrexate or dactinomycin is used to treat persistent disease. Risk can be assessed using a complex scoring system which assesses points for the following factors: patient age, type of antecedent pregnancy, interval between pregnancy and start of chemotherapy, pretreatment HCG level, size of largest tumor, site of metastases, number of metastases, and history of prior chemotherapy.

Methotrexate is commonly administered as an intramuscular injection once weekly with or without leucovorin rescue. Normal cells can be rescued from the toxic effects of methotrexate on folate metabolism by leucovorin (folinic acid). In contrast gestational trophoblast tumor cells accumulate large quantities of methotrexate metabolites and cannot be easily rescued by leucovorin from the toxic effects of methotrexate. Dactinomycin is as effective as methotrexate, but is associated with more side effects such as nausea and vomiting.

After chemotherapy, HCG levels are monitored weekly and should decrease rapidly. Multiple courses of single-agent therapy may be given to achieve an HCG level of less than 5 mIU/mL. Over 80% of women with persistent disease will be cured by a single-agent regimen. In cases where multiple courses of single-agent chemotherapy do not result in normalization of the HCG, multiagent chemotherapy is administered (see section below on Gestational Trophoblastic Neoplasia).

False-Positive Serum HCG Measurements

The treatment regimen recommended above is highly dependent on the monitoring of serum HCG to determine whether persistent disease is present. In rare circumstances, laboratories will report a serum HCG value greater than 5 mIU/mL, but further testing will demonstrates that there is no HCG in the serum. These false-positive laboratory results are thought to be due to antibodies in the patient's serum that interfere with the HCG assay. Interfering antibodies are present in low concentration in the urine. If a false-positive result is suspected, a simultaneous urine assay for HCG should be performed. A positive serum HCG and a negative urine HCG should prompt additional testing with highly reliable and specific HCG assays. In normal sera that does not contain interfering antibodies, sequential dilution of the sera should result in an appropriate sequential decrease in the measured HCG values. For example, diluting the serum 1 : 1 with control sera should result in a 50% decrease in measured HCG; diluting the serum 1 : 3 should result in a 75% decrease in measured HCG. In sera that contain interfering antibodies, sequential dilution does not result in the expected decrease in measured HCG.

Malignant Disease: Gestational Trophoblastic Neoplasia

Three forms of GTD are malignant: invasive mole, choriocarcinoma, and placenta site trophoblastic tumor (PSTT). These malignant forms of GTD are referred to as gestational trophoblastic neoplasia (GTN). As indicated by the terminology, invasive mole is characterized by invasion of trophoblastic tissue into the myometrium of the uterus. Choriocarcinoma is characterized by sheets of anaplastic cytotrophoblasts and syncytiotrophoblasts without chorionic villi.

GTN occurs following about 20% of the cases of complete hydatidiform mole and less than 5% of cases of partial hydatidiform mole. If histological samples are available, persistent disease following a complete hydatidiform mole demonstrates invasive mole in 75% of cases and choriocarcinoma in 25% of cases. Persistent trophoblastic disease following a spontaneous abortion, ectopic pregnancy or term pregnancy is always caused by choriocarcinoma or PSTT. Choriocarcinoma occurs in approximately 1 in 30000 pregnancies. PSTT is very rare and is managed by hysterectomy with chemotherapy if indicated. All women with malignant GTD should be referred to a center specializing in this disease.

Treatment

Persistent GTD that is resistant to single agent chemotherapy and high-risk malignant GTN are typically treated with multiagent chemotherapy. A commonly used multiagent regimen includes etoposide, methotrexate with leucovorin rescue, and dactinomycin on days 1 and 2 followed by cyclophosphamide and vincristine on day 8 (EMA/CO therapy). Therapy is repeated every 2 weeks until HCG is less than 5 mIU/mL and all radiographic evidence of active malignant disease has resolved. Therapy is then continued for another three cycles to consolidate the cure. Using this regimen the overall 5-year survival rate is about 90%.

Molar pregnancy was reported by ancient Greek physicians based on the visual identification of the grossly swollen placental villi ("cluster of grapes"). In the modern era, molar pregnancy is diagnosed based on ultrasonographic findings. The first trimester diagnosis of molar pregnancy has dramatically altered the presentation of the disease, with most patients presenting with no systemic symptoms. In most cases, the disease resolves following evacuation of the uterus.

Key Points

- Most women with complete molar pregnancy present with vaginal bleeding in the first trimester of pregnancy. In developed countries, the diagnosis is typically suspected based on a ultrasonographic examination during the first trimester to evaluate the cause of vaginal bleeding.
- The treatment of molar pregnancy is evacuation of the uterus followed by sequential measurement of serum human chorionic gonadotropin (HCG). Suction curettage is the preferred method of evacuation of the uterus. Following evacuation, if the HCG level quickly falls to undetectable levels, the tumor is cured. If the HCG level rises or does not fall, postevacuation chemotherapy may be necessary to cure the tumor.
- Single agent intravenous methotrexate with leucovorin rescue is the most commonly used chemotherapy for a stage I, persistent gestational trophoblastic neoplasm.

Evidence Box 46.1

Women treated for complete hydatidiform mole are considered to be in complete remission once their serum level of human chorionic gonado tropin has fallen to 5 mIU/mL or less.

For women with complete hydatidiform mole diagnosed by ultrasonography, standard treatment is uterine evacuation with suction dilation and curettage. Following uterine evacuation, serum HCG is measured sequentially. Women are diagnosed as having complete remission of their trophoblast tumor when their HCG level becomes undetectable (<5 mIU/mL). Historically, women were required to demonstrate an

HCG level of less than 5 mIU/mL for 6 months in order to be diagnosed as in complete remission. However, data from one center indicates that once a woman achieves a single HCG level of less than 5 mIU/mL it is highly likely that she has entered a complete remission. In this study, the course of 1029 women with complete hydatidiform mole was analyzed. 15% of the patients developed persistent gestational trophoblastic neoplasia. Of the 85% of patients who entered remission, 99.8% were demonstrated to have entered a complete remission once their HCG level became undetectable. A sensitive HCG assay with a lower limit of sensitivity of 5 mIU/mL had better performance characteristics for determining complete remission than an HCG assay with a lower limit of sensitivity of 10 mIU/mL.

Wolfberg AJ, Feltmate C, Goldstein DP, et al. Low risk of relapse after achieving undetectable hCG levels in women with complete molar pregnancy. Obstet Gynecol 2004;104:551–554.

Further Reading

Berkowitz RS, Goldstein DP. Chorionic tumors. *N Engl J Med* 1996;335(23):1740–1748

Bower M, Newlands ES, Holden L, et al. EMA/CO for high-risk gestational trophoblastic tumors: results from a cohort of 272 patients. *J Clin Oncol* 1997;15(7):2636–2643

Cole LA. Phantom hCG and phantom choriocarcinoma. *Gynecol Oncol* 1998;71(2):325–329

Curry SL, Schlaerth JB, Kohorn EI, et al. Hormonal contraception and trophoblastic sequelae after hydatidiform mole (a Gynecologic Oncology Group Study). *Am J Obstet Gynecol* 1989;160(4):805–809, discussion 809–811

Hammond CB, Weed JC Jr, Currie JL. The role of operation in the current therapy of gestational trophoblastic disease. *Am J Obstet Gynecol* 1980;136(7):844–858

Hassadia A, Gillespie A, Tidy J, et al. Placental site trophoblastic tumour: clinical features and management. *Gynecol Oncol* 2005;99(3):603–607

Kohorn EI. The new FIGO 2000 staging and risk factor scoring system for gestational trophoblastic disease: description and critical assessment. *Int J Gynecol Cancer* 2001;11(1):73–77

Rotmensch S, Cole LA. False diagnosis and needless therapy of presumed malignant disease in women with false-positive human chorionic gonadotropin concentrations. *Lancet* 2000;355(9205):712–715

Soto-Wright V, Bernstein M, Goldstein DP, Berkowitz RS. The changing clinical presentation of complete molar pregnancy. *Obstet Gynecol* 1995;86(5):775–779

Wells M. The pathology of gestational trophoblastic disease: recent advances. *Pathology* 2007;39(1):88–96

Wolfberg AJ, Feltmate C, Goldstein DP, Berkowitz RS, Lieberman E. Low risk of relapse after achieving undetectable HCG levels in women with complete molar pregnancy. *Obstet Gynecol* 2004;104(3):551–554

47 Vulvar and Vaginal Lesions

Robert L. Barbieri

Types of Lesion

Palpable Lesions

Common, palpable, nonpigmented lesions of the vulva-vagina include Bartholin Cyst, condylomata acuminata, skin tags (achrochordons), and vaginal wall cysts.

Bartholin Cyst and Abscess

The Bartholin glands are located at the 4-o'clock and 8-o'clock positions at the vulvovaginal junction. Normal Bartholin glands are about 0.5 cm in diameter with a duct that is about 2 cm in length. They secrete fluid and provide moisture to the vagina. When the Bartholin duct is blocked fluid may accumulate in the cyst causing a large swelling of the labia. If the fluid in the blocked gland becomes infected the cyst becomes an abscess and can be exceedingly painful and erythematosus. About 10% of

Bartholin abscesses are associated with *Neisseria gonorrhoea* or *Chlamydia trachomatis* infections.

The lifetime risk of developing a Bartholin cyst is about 1%. Asymptomatic Bartholin cysts do not need therapy. If a Bartholin cyst produces symptoms such as vulvar discomfort it may be treated by marsupialization (**Fig. 47.1**) or by placement of a balloon catheter into the cyst (Word catheter). The balloon catheter simultaneously drains the cyst and helps to create a new duct to prevent recurrence of the cyst. If an abscess is present, a typical antibiotic regimen includes ceftriaxone 250 mg intramuscular injection in a single dose (to cover for *Escherichia coli* and *N. gonorrhoea*) plus metronidazole 500 mg orally twice daily for 7 days. If *C. trachomatis* is present, azithromycin 1 g orally as a single dose is recommended.

Very rarely the Bartholin gland may be the site of origin for an adenocarcinoma or squamous cell carcinoma. Bartholin cysts and abscesses are typically fluid-filled. A solid tumor of the Bartholin glands should raise suspicion of a cancer. Women over the age of 40 years with a Bartholin cyst, abscess, or solid tumor should undergo resec-

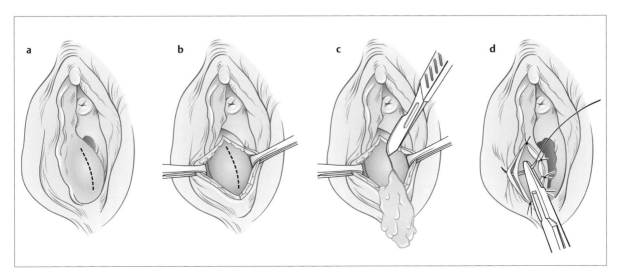

Fig. 47.1 Surgical approach to the marsupialization of a Bartholin cyst.

tion of the gland to allow for definitive histological diagnosis to ensure that cancer is not present.

Condylomata Acuminata

Anogenital warts are caused by infection with human papilloma virus, most commonly subtypes HPV-6 and HPV-11. Endogenous immune surveillance helps to prevent condylomata from growing to a large size in immune competent women. Immunosuppressed women, such as those with HIV disease or organ transplant recipients, are at increased risk of developing large condylomata. For example, in a study of over 700 women, condylomata were present in 7 % of women with HIV and 1 % of women who were HIV-negative. When condylomata grow into large exophytic masses they can interfere with vaginal intercourse and vaginal delivery. Condylomata lata, a dermatological manifestation of secondary syphilis, are flatter than condylomata acuminata.

Skin Tag

A skin tag or achrochordons is a flesh-colored, pedunculated outgrowth of normal skin on a stalk or wide base. Skin tags usually occur in sites of friction such as the inguinal area, axilla, or neck. They are associated with insulin resistance, which occurs in obesity, polycystic ovary syndrome, and diabetes.

Vaginal Wall Cysts

Vaginal wall cysts, which are typically located in the lateral or posterior walls of the vagina, may be caused by embryonic remnants of the müllerian or wolffian ducts (Gartner duct cyst) or from epidermal inclusion cysts. Endometriosis cysts occasionally involve the vaginal wall. Imaging studies such as magnetic resonance imaging may be helpful in identifying whether the cysts are simple fluid-filled structures or contain solid components. Imaging is also helpful in detecting additional small cysts that could not be detected by physical examination. Asymptomatic vaginal wall simple cysts do not need to be drained or excised. If symptoms are presents, such as pressure or pain symptoms, urinary incontinence, or pain with intercourse, the cysts can be excised or marsupialized, or drained. Anterior vaginal wall cysts near the introitus may be urethral diverticulum.

Molluscum Contagiosum

Molluscum is caused by a poxvirus and results in raised, dome-shaped skin lesions with an umbilicated center. Crural folds are a common site for molluscum lesions along with the axilla, and antecubital and popliteal fossae. Molluscum is spread by skin-to-skin contact. Molluscum occurs commonly in children. Molluscum is uncommon in adults unless they are immunosuppressed due to HIV infection, chemotherapy, or chronic glucocorticoid treatment. Genital lesions should be treated to prevent spread by genital contact. Standard treatment involves removal of the lesions with cryotherapy, electrosurgery, or laser. Small studies have reported that topical application of cantharidin or concentrated potassium hydroxide may be successful in eradicating the lesions.

Pigmented lesions

Acanthosis Nigricans

Acanthosis nigricans (AN) is a velvety, mossy, verrucuous hyperpigmented skin change which usually presents in the nape of the neck, in the axillae, beneath the breasts, and on the inner thighs. The salient histological features are papillomatosis, hyperkeratosis, and hyperpigmentation. Achrochordons are often present in association with AN. The majority of cases of AN are caused by insulin resistance and friction in the intertrigonous areas. Occasionally, AN is a manifestation of an occult adenocarcinoma of the gastrointestinal tract or lung. In women, AN is often associated with polycystic ovary syndrome and diabetes, and it may be present in women with endometrial hyperplasia or endometrial cancer.

Melanocytic Nevi

Melanocytic nevi are a benign proliferation of a type of melanocyte, the nevus cell. Women with lightly pigmented skin and women with intense sun exposure are more likely to develop melanocytic nevi.

Atypical Nevi and Melanoma

Atypical nevi are benign proliferations of nevus cells that share some of the features of melanoma. Women with multiple atypical nevi are at increased risk for melanoma. Melanoma is the sixth most common cancer in young women. Less than 1 % of melanomas arise on the vulva or vagina. In contrast to common melanomas in sun-exposed areas that occur in young women, most vulvar melanomas occur in women of 50–70 years of age. However, melanoma is a cause of up 10 % of malignant tumors involving the vulva. Vaginal melanoma is extremely rare. Common clinical features of melanoma may be recalled using the mnemonic A, B, C, D, E: **A**symmetry, irregular **B**orders, **C**olor variability, **D**iameter greater than 6 mm, and **E**nlargement or **E**volution of the color, size, or borders of the lesion. If clinical examination raises the possibility of atypical nevi or melanoma, a skin biopsy is recommended.

White Plaques or Patches

Lesions due to lichen sclerosus, lichen planus, and lichen simplex chronicus are discussed in Chapter 30.

Pustules and Vesicles

Skin Abscess

Skin abscesses are collections of pus within the dermis and deeper tissues. A furuncle ("boil") is an abscess of a hair follicle that extends into the subcutaneous tissue underlying the dermis. A carbuncle is a coalescence of multiple abscesses of hair follicles with multiple sites of drainage. Up to 50% of cases of skin abscesses are caused by *Staphylococcus aureus* infection (either methicillin-sensitive or methicillin-resistant). For small furuncles, treatment with warm compresses may be effective. For larger abscesses, incision and drainage is a preferred approach.

Hidradenitis Suppurativa

Hidradenitis suppurativa is a chronic disease characterized by multiple occluded abscesses of follicles that involve the intertrigonous areas of the axillae, groin, and intramammary folds. The occluded abscesses cause painful nodules which may resolve or open to the surface, releasing purulent drainage. Early stage lesions are managed with diet, including low glycemic index and non-dairy diets, and topical antibiotics, including clindamycin 1% lotion twice daily. Lesions may also be injected with glucocorticoids such as triamcinolone 10 mg/mL, with injection of 0.1 to 0.5 mL into each lesion. More advanced lesions are managed with local or wide excision of the affected areas.

Herpes Simplex Virus

This disease is discussed in Chapter 31.

Scabies

Scabies is caused by infection with the mite, *Sarcoptes scabiei*. It is transmitted by direct contact with an infected person. The infection is typically manifested by intense pruritis, especially at night, and small erythematosus papules. Secondary staphylococcal infections may complicate the process. Treatment of scabies is with topical permethrin (5%) or oral ivermectin, 200 µg/kg.

Ulcers and Fissures

Aphthous Ulcers

In adolescents, painful aphthous ulcers may occur during or after a viral illness such as influenza A. Girls may present with severe genital pain a chief complaint. Sexually transmitted diseases such as herpes simplex virus and fungal disease should be excluded.

Behçet Disease

Behçet disease is a systemic vasculitis that causes chronic and relapsing mucocutaneous aphthous ulcers and additional systemic disease, including genital ulcers and uveitis. There are no definitive laboratory tests for establishing the diagnosis, which is made based on clinical criteria. Consensus criteria for the diagnosis include recurrent oral aphthous ulcers at least three times per year plus two additional findings from the following: 1) genital ulcers, 2) uveitis, or 3) skin lesions such as erythema nodosum. There are few large clinical trials to guide the treatment of Behçet disease. The most commonly used medications are colchicine and glucocorticoids.

Crohn Disease

Crohn disease is a bowel inflammatory process that often results in the development of fistula between the bowel mucosa and other epithelial surfaces including the perianal, vaginal, and perineal skin. Approximately 30% of patients with Crohn disease have perianal involvement. Fistulas to the perianal, vaginal, and perineal skin are often first diagnosed by the passage of flatus or stool through the fistula. Primary treatment of the fistulas may include anti-inflammatory agents such as infliximab plus antibiotics such as metronidazole.

Syphilis Chancre, Chancroid, Lymphogranuloma Venereum, Granuloma Inguinale

These lesions are discussed in Chapter 31.

Vulvar Intra-epithelial Neoplasia

Vulvar intra-epithelial neoplasia (VIN) is a premalignant lesion that may progress to vulvar cancer if untreated. The most common symptom is vulvar pruritis. The lesions are usually raised, multifocal, in non–hair-bearing locations and can be of any color: white, red, pink, gray, or brown.

The usual type of VIN, representing 95% of cases, occurs mostly in premenopausal women and is related to exposure or infection with HPV. Multifocal VIN, usual type, is associated with infection with HPV subtypes 16,

18, and 31 and should be regarded as premalignant lesions. The differentiated type of VIN represents 5% of cases, usually occurs in postmenopausal women, is unifocal, and may be associated with lichen sclerosus (see Chapter 30). VIN, differentiated type, may be found near a lesion of squamous cell carcinoma.

If VIN is suspected, colposcopy and multiple biopsies are warranted. Treatment of VIN will help to prevent invasive vulvar cancer. Wide local excision is often recommended. Alternative treatments include laser ablation of the lesions or treatment with topical imiquimod. If the lesions are in a periclitoral, perianal, and periurethral location, topical treatment or laser ablation may help to minimize deformity and loss of function. Widespread use of HPV vaccination could prevent the majority of cases of VIN.

Vulvar Cancer

Vulvar cancer is the fourth most common gynecologic cancer, following uterine, ovary, and cervical cancer. Most vulvar cancers are diagnosed in postmenopausal women. The most common symptom is pruritis. Other symptoms include vulvar bleeding or an enlarged groin lymph node. Vulvar cancers most often present with a single plaque, ulcer, or raised mass lesion. In 5% of cases the lesions are multifocal. The definitive diagnosis requires biopsy of the suspicious lesion(s).

Two pathways to the development of vulvar cancer are HPV infection with oncogenic subtypes and chronic dermatological inflammation such as occurs with the diseases lichen sclerosus and lichen planus (Evidence Box 47.1). HPV infection with the oncogenic subtypes 16 and 33 cause approximately 50% of vulvar cancers. Women with previously treated cervical cancer are at increased risk for developing vulvar and vaginal cancer. Most vulvar cancers are squamous cell carcinomas, but other histological types include melanoma, basal cell carcinoma, extramammary Paget disease, Bartholin gland adenocarcinoma, and soft tissue sarcoma.

Vulvar cancers spread by direct extension to adjacent tissues, by lymphatic spread to regional lymph nodes, including superficial and deep inguinal and femoral lymph nodes, and less commonly by blood-borne dissemination.

Vulvar cancers are staged using a surgical-pathological system involving tumor diameter, depth of stromal invasion, status of regional lymph nodes, and evidence of distant metastasis (**Table 47.1**). Inguinal and femoral lymph node status and age of the patient are the most important predictors of disease progression and survival . Consequently, staging must involve sampling of these lymph nodes, except for women with stage IA disease.

Table 47.1 Surgical–pathological staging and survival in vulvar cancer

Stage		5-year survival rate
I	Tumor confined vulva or perineum, Lesion ≤2 cm in diameter.	77%
IA	Stromal invasion ≤1 mm.	
IB	Stromal invasion >1 mm.	
II	Tumor confined vulva or perineum, Lesion >2 cm in diameter. Negative lymph nodes	55%
III	Tumor of any size with spread to lower urethra or anus and/or unilateral regional lymph node involvement	31%
IV		<10%
IVA	Tumor invades upper urethra or bladder or rectal mucosa or pelvic bones or bilateral regional lymph node involvement.	
IVB	Any distant metastasis	

Historically, vulvar cancers were treated with radical vulvectomy including removal of the entire vulva to the deep fascia of the thigh, the pubic periosteum, and inferior fascia of the urogenital floor. Radical vulvectomy may result in significant loss of function and morbidity. Alternative surgical approaches that achieve a tumor-free surgical margin of more than 1 cm wide may cause less loss of function and morbidity. One such approach is a three-incision technique (**Fig. 47.2**). Another approach is local excision of the vulvar tumor with unilateral inguinal and femoral lymph node dissection. Altered body image following radical surgery for vulvar cancer may be improved by vulvovaginal reconstruction. Women with multiple positive lymph nodes may be treated with adjuvant radiotherapy to the groin. Women with advanced stage cancer may be treated with postoperative radiotherapy to the vulva. Recurrences and metastasis may be treated with surgery, radiotherapy, and/or chemotherapy.

Vaginal Intra-epithelial Neoplasia

Vaginal intra-epithelial neoplasia (VAIN) is far less common than cervical or vulvar intra-epithelial neoplasia. Most women with VAIN have no symptoms, but some present with vaginal discharge or postcoital bleeding. Bimanual examination may detect raised lesions in the vagina. Cytology, HPV DNA testing, colposcopy, and vaginal biopsy are important studies in the diagnosis of VAIN. In

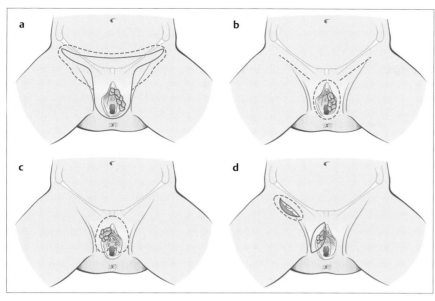

Fig. 47.2a–d Approaches to resection of vulvar cancer.
a Modified butterfly incision.
b Triple incision method preserving skin along the inner thighs.
c Anterior horseshoe incision.
d Unilateral incision in the groin and elliptical excision of the primary vulvar lesion. Reproduced with permission from Elkas JC, Berek, JS. Vulvar cancer: staging, treatment and prognosis. In: UpToDate, Basow DS (Ed), UpToDate, Waltham, MA, 2009 (www.uptodate.com).

a woman who has had a total hysterectomy, vaginal cytology (Pap smear) that demonstrates atypical or dysplastic cells should be followed by a colposcopy with biopsy to look for VAIN.

VAIN is classified into three categories, depending on the depth of epithelial involvement with the lesions as assessed with biopsy and histological analysis. In VAIN 1 the lesion involves the upper third of the epithelium. In VAIN 2 the lesion involves two-thirds of the epithelium. VAIN 3 involves more than two-thirds of the epithelium. Most women with VAIN are diagnosed between 40 and 60 years of age and most have concurrent epithelial neoplasia of the cervix and/or vulva. HPV infection is a likely cause of many cases of VAIN. The mature differentiated squamous epithelium of the vagina is less likely to be infected with HPV than the cervical transformation zone.

Surgical excision is the most commonly used treatment for VAIN. Surgical excision also permits a complete histological analysis of the lesion(s). Alternative treatments include laser ablation of the lesions or topical application of 5-fluorouracil.

Vaginal Cancer

Vaginal cancer is an uncommon malignancy representing less than 1% of gynecologic tumors. Most women present with vaginal bleeding or a watery, pinkish discharge. Vaginal cancers may be small and difficult to detect. Some are first diagnosed during the work-up of an abnormal cervical–vaginal cytology screening. Most vaginal cancer lesions are squamous cell carcinomas (>80%), but melanoma, sarcoma, and adenocarcinoma may also primarily involve the vagina. In most cases of vaginal squamous cell cancer, infection with HPV subtypes 16 and 18 are the likely etiological cause. Vaginal cancer is staged surgically (**Table 47.2**). Surgery and radiotherapy are the main approaches to treatment of vaginal cancer.

Table 47.2 Surgical staging and survival in vaginal cancer

Stage		5-year survival rate
I	Tumor confined to vaginal mucosa	67%
II	Tumor involves submucosal extension	39%
IIA	Submucosal extension but no involvement of parametrium.	
IIB	Involvement of parametrium, but no extension to pelvic side wall.	
III	Tumor extends to pelvic side wall	33%
IV		
IVA	Tumor involves mucosa of bladder or rectum or extends outside pelvis	19%
IVB	Distant metastasis	<10%

Key Points

- Vulvar cancer is the fourth most common gynecologic cancer after uterine, ovary, and cervical cancer.
- Women with vulvar cancer typically present with vulvar itching or vulvar bleeding. The definitive diagnosis is made by vulvar biopsy.
- Vulvar cancer can be caused by infection with human papilloma virus subtypes HPV-16 or HPV-33, or chronic dermatological inflammation such as occurs with lichen sclerosus.
- Vulvar cancer is treated surgically with excision of the primary lesion and sampling of local and regional lymph nodes.

Evidence Box 47.1

Vulvar squamous cell carcinoma is probably caused by two different etiologies: HPV infection, and chronic dermatological inflammation due to lichen sclerosus.

The vulvectomy specimens of 78 women with squamous cell cancer of the vulva were studied by histological and human papilloma virus (HPV) DNA detection techniques. Fifty-one women had a keratinizing squamous cancer and 27 had nonkeratinizing (warty or basaloid) squamous cancer. Of the 51 women with a keratinizing squamous cancer, 71% had an associated histological diagnosis of lichen sclerosus. (Lichen sclerosus is chronic inflammatory dermatological condition of the vulva. Most women with lichen sclerosis have itching. Histological characteristics of lichen sclerosus included marked inflammation and epithelial thinning.) None of the 27 women with nonkeratinizing tumors had a coexisting histological diagnosis of lichen sclerosus. Of the 27 women with nonkeratinizing cancers, 81% were positive for HPV DNA. The most frequently detected HPV subtypes were HPV-16 and HPV-33. Of the 51 women with keratinzing tumors only 4% had HPV DNA detected. The mean age of the women in the two groups was 73 years for the keratinzing tumors and 57 years for the nonkeratinizing tumors. This observational study suggests that there are two pathways to the developement of vulvar squamous cell carcinoma.

Hording U, Junge J, Daugaard S, Lundvall F, Poulsen H, Bock JE. Vulvar squamous cell carcinoma and papillomaviruses: indications for two different etiologies. Gynecol Oncol 1994;52:241–246.

Further Reading

Balamurugan A, Ahmed F, Saraiya M, et al. Potential role of human papillomavirus in the development of subsequent primary in situ and invasive cancers among cervical cancer survivors. *Cancer* 2008; 113(10, Suppl)2919–2925

Blecharz P, Karolewski K, Bieda T, et al. Prognostic factors in patients with carcinoma of the vulva—our own experience and literature review. *Eur J Gynaecol Oncol* 2008;29(3):260–263

Castle PE, Schiffman M, Bratti MC, et al. A population-based study of vaginal human papillomavirus infection in hysterectomized women. *J Infect Dis* 2004;190(3):458–467

Conley LJ, Ellerbrock TV, Bush TJ, Chiasson MA, Sawo D, Wright TC. HIV-1 infection and risk of vulvovaginal and perianal condylomata acuminata and intraepithelial neoplasia: a prospective cohort study. *Lancet* 2002;359(9301):108–113

Ferreira M, Crespo M, Martins L, Félix A. HPV DNA detection and genotyping in 21 cases of primary invasive squamous cell carcinoma of the vagina. *Mod Pathol* 2008;21(8):968–972

Höckel M, Dornhöfer N. Vulvovaginal reconstruction for neoplastic disease. *Lancet Oncol* 2008;9(6):559–568

Hørding U, Junge J, Daugaard S, Lundvall F, Poulsen H, Bock JE. Vulvar squamous cell carcinoma and papillomaviruses: indications for two different etiologies. *Gynecol Oncol* 1994;52(2):241–246

International Study Group for Behçet's Disease. Criteria for diagnosis of Behçet's disease. *Lancet* 1990;335(8697):1078–1080

Pradhan S, Tobon H. Vaginal cysts: a clinicopathological study of 41 cases. *Int J Gynecol Pathol* 1986;5(1):35–46

Stehman FB, Look KY. Carcinoma of the vulva. *Obstet Gynecol* 2006;107(3):719–733

48 Cervical Neoplasia and Cancer

Robert L. Barbieri

Cervical Neoplasia

Definition

Cervical neoplasia represents a disease continuum from low-grade cervical neoplastic lesions to invasive and metastatic cancer (**Fig. 48.1**). Most cases of cervical neoplasia are caused by infection with human papilloma virus (HPV). For women infected with oncogenic HPV sub-types, it may take 5 to 10 years or more for the disease to progress from low-grade cervical neoplasia to invasive cancer. This relatively long disease progression interval makes cervical neoplasia an optimal target for population screening.

Unique nomenclature is used to describe cervical neoplasia based on cytology assessment (Papanicolaou [Pap] smear test) and histological assessment (cervical tissue biopsy) (**Table 48.1**). Cervical cancer is staged using clinical examination (**Table 48.2**). Unlike ovarian and endometrial cancer, cervical cancer is not surgically staged.

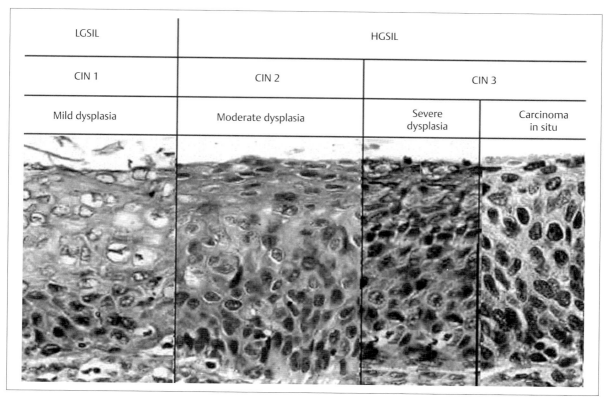

LGSIL	HGSIL		
CIN 1	CIN 2	CIN 3	
Mild dysplasia	Moderate dysplasia	Severe dysplasia	Carcinoma in situ

Fig. 48.1 Histology of cervical intra-epithelial lesions. For nomenclature key, see **Table 48.1**. Modified with permission from Holschneider, CH. Cervical intraepithelial neoplasia: Definition, incidence and pathogenesis. In: UpToDate, Basow DS (Ed), UpToDate, Waltham, MA, 2009 (www.uptodate.com).

Table 48.1 Unique nomenclature is used to describe cervical neoplasia based on cytology or histological changes

Cytology assessment—Pap smear	
Negative for intra-epithelial lesion or malignancy	
Atypical squamous cells (ASC) of undetermined significance (ASC-US)	
Low-grade squamous intra-epithelial lesion (LSIL)	
High-grade squamous intra-epithelial lesion (HSIL)	
Squamous cell carcinoma	
Histological assessment—cervical tissue biopsy	
Normal	
Cervical intra-epithelial neoplasia 1 (CIN 1)	Dysplastic cellular changes are confined to the basal third of the epithelium
Cervical intra-epithelial neoplasia 2 (CIN 2)	Dysplastic cellular changes are confined to the basal two-thirds of the epithelium
Cervical intra-epithelial neoplasia 3 (CIN 3)	Dysplastic cellular changes are greater than two-thirds of the epithelial thickness
Cancer	

Table 48.2 FIGO* staging of cervical cancer

FIGO stage	Characteristics
0	**Carcinoma in situ**
I	**Cervical carcinoma confined to the cervix/uterus**
IA	*Invasive carcinoma diagnosed by microscopy*
IA1	Stromal invasion less than 3 mm in depth and 7 mm in lateral spread
IA2	Stromal invasion between 3 mm and 5 mm in depth
IB	**Clinically visible lesion confined to the cervix**
IB1	Clinically visible lesion 4 cm or less in greatest dimension
IB2	Clinically visible lesion greater than 4 cm in greatest dimension
II	**Cervical cancer invades beyond the cervix/uterus but not to pelvic side-wall or to the lower third of the vagina**
IIA	No parametrial invasion
IIB	Parametrial invasion
III	**Cervical cancer extends to the pelvic side-wall and/or involves the lower third of the vagina and/or causes hydronephrosis**
IIIA	Tumor involves lower third of vagina, no extension to pelvic side-wall
IIIB	Tumor extends to pelvic side-wall or causes hydronephrosis
IV	**Cervical cancer extends beyond the pelvis and/or involves the bladder or rectal epithelium**
IVA	Spread to adjacent organs such as the bladder and/or rectum
IVB	Distant metastases

* International Federation of Gynecology and Obstetrics.

Prevalence and Epidemiology

HPV infection is endemic, and the majority of sexually active men and women will have had an HPV infection by the time they are 50 years of age. In a recent survey of almost 2000 females, the prevalence of HPV infection—as detected by a polymerase chain reaction technique performed on cellular material obtained from a vaginal swab—was about 27%. Most HPV infections are cleared within 18 months of infection. There are over 100 different subtypes of HPV, each with a unique biology and oncogenic potential, of which 40 subtypes are specific for the anogenital epithelium. HPV-6 and HPV-11 cause about 90% of condylomatous genital warts. These subtypes are unlikely to cause cervical cancer, because they do not integrate into the genome and disrupt cell turnover. HPV subtypes 6 and 11 may cause low-grade cervical lesions such as LSIL or CIN 1. HPV subtypes 16 and 18 cause about 75% of all cervical cancers. These two high-risk subtypes persist in cells and may integrate into the genome, increasing cell mitosis. HPV-16 and HPV-18 cause both low-grade and high-grade lesions. The other HPV subtypes that may cause cervical cancer are 31, 33, 35, 39, 45, 51, 52, 56, 58, 59, 68, 69, and 82.

Etiology

HPV infection of a cervical or vaginal cell causes cellular changes including nuclear enlargement, multinucleation, hyperchromasia, and perinuclear cytoplasmic halos that can be detected by cytological or histological assessment. The HPV infection may be reversed by the recruitment of macrophages and lymphocytes and the production of anti-HPV antibodies. Immunosuppression increases the risk of an HPV infection progressing to high-grade lesions. Alternatively, certain HPV subtypes may integrate into the genome causing high-grade lesions and eventually cervical cancer. HPV infection also causes many cases of vaginal, vulvar (see Chapter 47), anal, and penile cancer. Integration of the HPV virus into the genome results in the overexpression of two viral genes, E6 and E7. HPV E6 increases the degradation of p53 and E7 inactivates the retinoblastoma protein (Rb), which are the products of two important tumor suppressor genes. Reduced expression of these two tumor suppressor genes results in increased mitotic activity of the infected cell with the potential for additional mutations leading to cancer.

Prevention

L1 and L2 are the encapsulating proteins for HPV. L1 molecules, which are specific for each HPV subtype, self-assemble into hollow viruslike particles with high immunogenicity. Two HPV vaccines are currently available: a bivalent vaccine for HPV subtypes 16 and 18; and a quadrivalent vaccine for HPV subtypes 6, 11, 16, and 18. The quadrivalent vaccine is parenterally administered in three doses at 0, 2, and 6 months. In one trial of the quadrivalent vaccine, 552 women with a mean age of 20 years were randomized to vaccination with the active vaccine or a placebo with 3 years of follow-up. Protection against cervical intra-epithelial neoplasia (CIN) caused by HPV subtypes 6, 11, 16, and 18 occurred in 100% of the women in the study. In the women treated with placebo injections, 7 cases of CIN infection caused by these four subtypes were detected. No genital warts due to HPV-6 or HPV-11 occurred in the treated group. In the women in the placebo group 4 cases of genital warts occurred. This trial stimulated the completion of very large-scale clinical trials, which have confirmed the protective effect of HPV vaccination (Evidence Box 48.1).

Data from multiple clinical trials indicate that HPV vaccination does not significantly alter the course of HPV infection in those women already infected prior to vaccination. However, if a woman is infected with one specific HPV subtype, for example HPV-11, at the time of vaccination, the vaccine is protective against the other subtypes, for example, 6, 16, and 18, to which the patient has not yet been infected. Consequently, HPV vaccination is most cost-effective when administered prior to exposure to the virus, which typically occurs after sexual debut. The current quadrivalent vaccine is recommended for females from 9 to 26 years of age. It is likely that studies will demonstrate that it is also effective for older women who have not yet been exposed to all four subtypes contained in the vaccine. Vaccination of males would reduce the prevalence of HPV infection, but in some economic models vaccination of males is less cost-effective than vaccination of females. Males in high-risk groups may be candidates for vaccination. In resource-limited settings, it may be very difficult to provide the vaccine to either females or males because of the expense.

Screening

The primary method of screening for cervical neoplasia caused by HPV infection is cervical cytology (Pap smear). Molecular testing for HPV nucleotides may be performed in conjunction with cervical cytology, or as a follow-up test for certain cervical cytology results. Screening for cervical neoplasia should begin about 3 years after the onset of sexual activity and no later than 21 years of age. From 21 to 30 years of age screening using cervical cytology should be performed every year. After 30 years of age, if recent screening has been normal, cervical cytology can be performed every 2–3 years.

Cervical–Vaginal Cytology

Cells from the cervix and vagina are sampled by using a brush or spatula on the exocervix, and using a brush or cotton swab on the endocervix. In the standard Papanicolaou (Pap) test the cells are transferred to a glass slide and chemically fixed before the sample dries. In the liquid-based approach, the cells are transferred to a liquid transport medium. The cells of interest are separated from the liquid medium by filtration and then transferred to a glass slide for cytological analysis. Women preparing for a Pap smear should avoid scheduling the test during menses and avoid douching, sexual intercourse, or the use of tampons for 48 hours before the scheduled test to avoid reducing the number of available cervical cells for interpretation. The sensitivity and specificity of cervical cytology for the detection of cervical neoplasia CIN 2, or worse, is approximately 80% and 95% respectively. The sensitivity of Pap smears for detecting adenocarcinoma of the cervix is lower than for detecting squamous carcinoma.

Human Papilloma Virus (HPV) Testing

DNA testing for HPV may be performed by signal amplification using an in situ hybridization technique or polymerase chain reaction amplification. In one signal amplification assay, the liquid used to collect the cervical specimen is treated with a base to release viral DNA. The DNA is hybridized with specific RNA probes that target high-risk HPV subtypes. The RNA–DNA hybrids are captured onto a solid surface using antibodies. The captured RNA-DNA hybrids are detected with antibodies linked to an alkaline phosphatase signaling system that emits chemiluminescence, which can be measured photometrically. The test is "positive" if high-risk subtype specific DNA sequences are detected. If no high-risk subtypes are detected the test is reported as "negative". Negative tests would be reported in the setting of no HPV infection or infection with low-risk HPV subtypes. Primary screening using only HPV testing is highly sensitive (90%) but has relatively low specificity (85–90%). This would result in a large number of women being referred for colposcopy. HPV infections are often transient and the majority of women with HPV infections never develop a neoplastic lesion.

Utilizing Both Cervical Cytology and HPV Testing

One approach to screening is to use primarily cervical cytology testing (every 1–3 years) and only use HPV testing to stratify women with atypical squamous cells of uncertain significance (ASC-US) into a low-risk group that can return to normal screening intervals or into a high-risk group that should followed up with colposcopy. A second approach is to simultaneously use both cervical cytology and HPV testing for primary screening of women over the age of 30 years. If both tests are negative, the patient has an extremely low chance of having significant cervical neoplasia and may wait 3–5 years before being re-screened (**Table 48.3**). The sensitivity and specificity of the combined test for the detection of cervical neoplasia CIN 2, or worse, is approximately 98% and 93%, respectively. HPV testing has less of a role in women 20–30 years of age because many of them have transient infection with a high-risk HPV subtype.

As technology develops, direct testing to identify the presence or absence of the most oncogenic HPV subtypes, 16, 18, and 45, may help to guide clinical decision making. Women with these oncogenic HPV subtypes are at the greatest risk of progressing to advanced cervical neoplastic lesions.

Cervicoscopy, Cervicography, and Speculoscopy

Direct visual inspection of the cervix using an acetic acid or iodine wash and magnification has been proposed as a screening method in low-resource environments. These techniques all have low specificity and are not recommended for use in countries with access to cytology or HPV DNA testing.

Diagnosis

Condylomata acuminata: These lesions typically present as single or multiple papules on the posterior introitus, labia majora and/or labia minora. Most condylomata are caused by infection with HPV-6 or HPV-11. The definitive diagnosis is made by skin biopsy. Cervical and vaginal cytology and colposcopy are warranted to evaluate the extent of the HPV disease.

Cervical neoplasia: If neoplasia is suspected based on positive cervical cytology and/or HPV DNA testing, colposcopy with directed biopsies should be performed. If the patient has a history of anal receptive intercourse, anoscopy should be performed. To begin the colposcopy, 3% to 5% acetic acid is swabbed on the cervix and vagina because areas of epithelial dysplasia contain dense nuclei that cause the tissue to turn white after acetic acid treatment. The cervical epithelium is then visualized with a colposcope which is a microscope with 2× to 25× magnification settings and a 30-cm focal length. Areas of white epithelium and abnormal vascularization are identified and a few biopsies are obtained for histological confirmation. For women with advanced lesions, an endocervical curettage is obtained to assess involvement of the junction of the squamous epithelial (outer cervix) and columnar (endocervical canal) cells, the so-called transformation zone.

Table 48.3 Approach to women undergoing cervical neoplasia screening with both cervical cytology and human papilloma virus (HPV) DNA testing

Cervical cytology result	HPV DNA testing result	Recommended testing
Negative for intra-epithelial lesion or malignancy	Negative	Repeat screening in 3–5 years
Negative for intra-epithelial lesion or malignancy	Positive for high-risk HPV subtypes	Repeat combined test in one year.
Atypical squamous cells (ASC) of undetermined significance (ASC-US)	Negative	Repeat cervical cytology alone in 1 year
ASC-US	Positive for high-risk HPV subtypes	Colposcopy
Low-grade or high-grade squamous intra-epithelial lesion (LSIL) (HSIL)	Either negative or positive	Refer for immediate colposcopy

Treatment

Following diagnosis with colposcopy directed biopsy, advanced cervical intra-epithelial neoplasias are typically treated by ablative or excisional therapy to destroy the neoplastic cells. Ablative therapy options include cryotherapy or laser therapy. Excisional therapies included surgical conization with a scalpel ("cold-knife" conization), electrosurgical excision with a loop, or laser conization.

If the colposcopy directed biopsies demonstrate a histological CIN 1 lesion and the initial cytology indicated a low-grade lesion, a reasonable option is to follow the patient expectantly. In many cases, the patient's immune system will eventually clear the HPV infection, and both the cervical cytology and the colposcopy will return to normal. In one trial only 10–15 % of women with CIN 1 progressed to an advanced lesion with 2 years of follow-up. These women can be managed with follow-up cervical cytology at 6 and 12 months, or HPV testing at 12 months.

If the colposcopy directed biopsies demonstrate a histological CIN 1 lesion and the initial cytology indicated a *high*-grade lesion there is a persistent concern that a high-grade lesion was not detected at the time of colposcopy. These women can be offered expectant management as above, or they may warrant excisional therapy that is both diagnostic and therapeutic. If managed expectantly, these women should have both cytology and colposcopy performed at 6 and 12 months.

CIN 2 and 3 lesions are routinely treated with ablative or excisional therapy, unless the patient is an adolescent or pregnant. Expectant management of CIN 2 is not a good option, because progression to CIN 3 or invasive cancer will occur in 25 % and 5 % of cases, respectively. If micro-invasive disease is suspected, a surgical conization with a scalpel is often performed to provide the best assessment of the depth of the neoplastic lesion.

Adolescents have a very high rate of regression of CIN 2 and CIN 3 lesions. For adolescents with CIN 2, expectant management with follow-up colposcopy is recommended. For adolescents with CIN 3, ablation or excisional therapy is recommended. Pregnant women are at risk for spontaneous abortion if aggressively treated for CIN. In addition, expectant management of pregnant women with CIN 2 and 3 lesions is associated with a high rate of regression following completion of the pregnancy. Consequently, CIN 2 and 3 are typically managed expectantly in pregnant women.

Treatment of CIN is associated with long-term adverse outcomes. For example, surgical conization with a scalpel and electrosurgical excision with a loop are associated with an increased risk of preterm delivery in future pregnancies. An excisional procedure with a depth greater than 1 cm appears to increase the risk of preterm delivery and preterm premature rupture of the membranes.

Given these concerns, the minimal amount of cervical tissue necessary to treat the lesion should be excised. Cervical stenosis is a long-term complication of treatment that may be associated with hematocolpos and pelvic pain.

Cervical Cancer

Staging

If histology demonstrates invasive cervical cancer, the patient undergoes staging to plan therapy. The FIGO (International Federation of Gynecology and Obstetrics) system is the most commonly used staging system for cervical cancer (**Table 48.2**; **Fig. 48.2**). The majority of women with advanced stage cervical cancer will die of their disease within 5 years (**Table 48.4**). The FIGO system is a clinical staging system and permits the following diagnostic studies in determining the stage: physical examination of the pelvis and assessment of groin and supraclavicular adenopathy; colposcopy, endocervical curettage, conization, hysteroscopy, cystoscopy and proctoscopy, intravenous pyelogram; and plain radiographic examination of the lungs and skeleton. Results from positron emission tomography, magnetic resonance imaging, or computed tomography cannot be utilized to assign a FIGO stage, but they may be of clinical use in planning treatment.

Treatment

Patients with minimal cervical cancer lesions (stage IA, IB1, small IIA lesions) can be treated with radical hysterectomy or radiotherapy. Radical hysterectomy is a procedure where the entire uterus and cervix is removed en-bloc along with the adjacent parametrial tissue and the upper one-third of the vagina. The parmetrium includes the round, broad, cardinal, and uterosacral ligaments. Radical hysterectomy is routinely combined with pelvic and para-aortic lymphadenectomy to assess the spread of disease. If the surgical specimen reveals positive resection margins, positive lymph nodes, or metastases into the parametrium, the patient is at high risk of recurrence and chemoradiotherapy or radiotherapy should be recommended. Chemoradiotherapy is more effective than radiotherapy alone. In chemoradiotherapy, the patient gets standard radiotherapy, 50 Gy in about 30 fractions to the pelvic field, plus four cycles of cisplatin plus 5-fluorouracil. Compared with radiotherapy alone, chemoradiotherapy is associated with 31 % reduction in the risk of death, and a decrease in the rate of local and distant metastases.

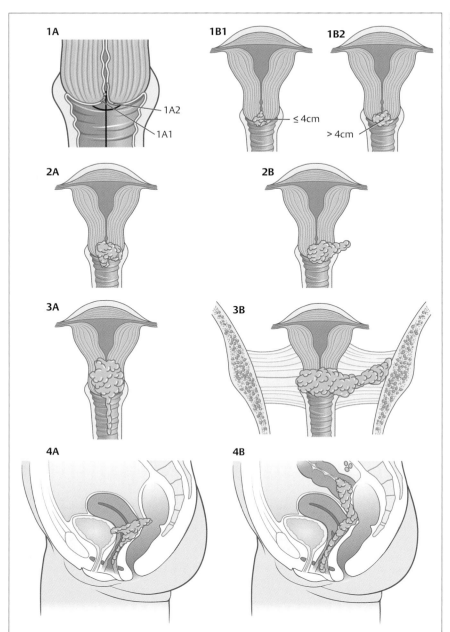

Fig. 48.2 Schematic examples of the FIGO (International Federation of Gynecology and Obstetrics) staging system for cervical cancer. For nomenclature key, see **Table 48.2**.

Radiotherapy is an accepted primary treatment modality for stage IA, IB, and IIA cervical cancer. In one randomized trial of radiotherapy versus radical hysterectomy plus adjuvant radiotherapy, 5-year disease-free rates were similar in both groups, 73% and 84% respectively. The two main techniques for radiotherapy of cervical cancer are external photon beam radiotherapy or brachytherapy. Brachytherapy is commonly performed using a technique that involves using an applicator to place a 137-Cs or 192-Ir source in close proximity to the cervical tumor. Both ra-

diotherapy and radical hysterectomy may lead to vaginal shortening and scarring, which adversely impacts sexual function. For women with advanced stage (stages IIB, III, IVA) cervical cancer, combination chemotherapy and radiotherapy are often recommended.

Table 48.4 Survival for patients with cervical cancer by FIGO *
stage

FIGO stage		5-year survival rate
I		Cervical carcinoma confined to the cervix/uterus
	IA1	99%
	IA2	96%
	IB1	88%
	IB2	79%
II		Cervical cancer invades beyond the cervix/uterus but not to pelvic side-wall or to the lower third of the vagina
	IIA	69%
	IIB	65%
III		Cervical cancer extends to the pelvic side-wall and/or involves the lower third of the vagina and/or causes hydronephrosis
	IIIA	40%
	IIIB	43%
IV		Cervical cancer extends beyond the pelvis and/or involves the bladder or rectal epithelium.
	IVA	20%
	IVB	15%

* International Federation of Gynecology and Obstetrics.
Source: Adapted from Benedet JL, Odicino F, Maisonneuve P, et al. Carcinoma of the cervix uteri. Int J Gynecol Obstet 2003;83(Suppl 1):41–78.

Global Burden of Cervical Cancer

In many developing countries cervical cancer is the most common cancer and the most common cause of cancer death among women. Nearly 80% of cervical cancer cases in the world occur in developing countries. Lack of access to screening and treatment makes cervical cancer a major health burden in these countries. Given the lack of access to screening resources, authorities have explored the effectiveness of alternative screening algorithms. In one proposed algorithm all woman would be screened once in their life at age 35 years. This approach is estimated to reduce the risk of cancer by 30% and to be a relatively low-cost intervention. Screening techniques that have been explored in resource-constrained regions include standard cervical cytology, DNA testing for HPV infection, and direct visual inspection of the cervix after application of acetic acid or iodine. If the cost of HPV vaccination could be reduced, widespread vaccination of women in developing countries would be an important

intervention. The high incidence of cervical cancer in developing countries is a global health problem that could potentially be solved by the application of standard medical interventions which are widely available in developed countries.

Key Points

- Cervical cancer is the third most common gynecologic malignancy, after endometrial and ovarian cancer.
- Most cases of cervical cancer are caused by oncogenic human papilloma viruses, including HPV-16 andHPV-18. The viral genes, E6 and E7 can integrate into genomic DNA and inactivate two tumor suppressor genes, p53 and Rb.
- Vaccination for HPV-16 and HPV-18 reduces the risk of both cervical intra-epithelial neoplasia and cancer.
- Cervical cancer is preceded by an orderly transition from normal cervical epithelium through multiple stages of worsening intra-epithelial neoplasia to invasive cancer. This progression takes many years, making this an optimal tumor for screening, which is done by cervical cytology (Pap smear). An alternative to screening with cytological techniques is to directly test for the oncogenic HPV viruses, including HPV-16 and HPV-18.
- The treatment of cervical cancer usually involves surgical treatment including hysterectomy, removal of adjacent parametrial tissue and the upper third of the vagina, and pelvic and para-aortic lymphadenectomy.

Evidence Box 48.1

Human papilloma virus (HPV) vaccine prevents cervical neoplasia and anogenital lesions in HPV-naive women. To be maximally effective, the HPV vaccine must be administered before the sexual debut of the patient.

Study 1: In the Future II study, 12 167 women, aged from 15 to 26 years were randomized to placebo injections or quadrivalent HPV-6, -11, -16, -18 vaccine (three doses: 0, 2, and 6 months). One month after completion of vaccine, those women who were not infected with HPV-16 or HPV-18 were then followed for 3 years. In this group of HPV-naive women, among the vaccinated group (N = 5305) one woman developed a CIN 3 lesion due to HPV-16 and no women developed a CIN 2 lesion. Among the HPV-naive women in the placebo group (N = 5260), 28 developed CIN 2 and 29 developed CIN 3. HPV-16 accounted for 35 of the lesions and HPV-18 for 11 of the lesions. This represents a vaccine efficacy of 98% (95% CI, 86% to 100%).

Study 2: In a companion study to assess the effects of the quadrivalent vaccine on anogenital lesions, 5455 women, aged 16 to 24 years were randomized to placebo injections or quadrivalent HPV-6, -11, -16, -18 vaccine (three doses: 0, 2, and 6 months). One month after completion of vaccine, those women who were not infected with HPV-6, -11, -16, or -18 were then followed up for 3 years. The primary endpoints were the incidence of genital warts, vulvar or vaginal intra-epithelial neoplasia or cervical cancer. In this group of HPV-naive women, among the vaccinated group (N = 2261) no woman developed any HPV-related lesion. Among the HPV-naive women in the placebo group (N = 2279) the following lesions were detected: vulvar condyloma (47 women), vaginal condyloma (6 women), vulvar intra-epithelial neoplasia (18 women), CIN 1 (49 women), CIN 2 (21 women), CIN 3 (17 women), and adenocarcinoma in situ (6 women). This represents a vaccine efficacy of 100%.

The Future II Study Group. Quadrivalent vaccine against human papillomavirus to prevent high-grade cervical lesions. N Engl J Med 2007;356:1915–1927.

Garland SM, Hernandez-Avila M, Wheeler CM, et al. Quadrivalent vaccine against human papillomavirus to prevent anogenital diseases. N Engl J Med 2007;356:1928–1943.

Further Reading

Benedet JL, Odicino F, Maisonneuve P, et al. Carcinoma of the cervix uteri. *Int J Gynaecol Obstet* 2003;83(Suppl 1):41–78

Bulkmans NW, Berkhof J, Rozendaal L, et al. Human papillomavirus DNA testing for the detection of cervical intraepithelial neoplasia grade 3 and cancer: 5-year follow-up of a randomised controlled implementation trial. *Lancet* 2007;370(9601):1764–1772

Cox JT, Schiffman M, Solomon D; ASCUS-LSIL Triage Study (ALTS) Group. Prospective follow-up suggests similar risk of subsequent cervical intraepithelial neoplasia grade 2 or 3 among women with cervical intraepithelial neoplasia grade 1 or negative colposcopy and directed biopsy. *Am J Obstet Gynecol* 2003;188(6):1406–1412

Cox T, Cuzick J. HPV DNA testing in cervical cancer screening: from evidence to policies. *Gynecol Oncol* 2006;103(1):8–11

Cuzick J, Clavel C, Petry KU, et al. Overview of the European and North American studies on HPV testing in primary cervical cancer screening. *Int J Cancer* 2006;119(5):1095–1101

Dunne EF, Unger ER, Sternberg M, et al. Prevalence of HPV infection among females in the United States. *JAMA* 2007;297(8):813–819

Garland SM, Hernandez-Avila M, Wheeler CM, et al; Females United to Unilaterally Reduce Endo/Ectocervical Disease (FUTURE) I Investigators. Quadrivalent vaccine against human papillomavirus to prevent anogenital diseases. *N Engl J Med* 2007;356(19):1928–1943

Goldie SJ, Gaffikin L, Goldhaber-Fiebert JD, et al; Alliance for Cervical Cancer Prevention Cost Working Group. Cost-effectiveness of cervical-cancer screening in five developing countries. *N Engl J Med* 2005;353(20):2158–2168

Kyrgiou M, Koliopoulos G, Martin-Hirsch P, Arbyn M, Prendiville W, Paraskevaidis E. Obstetric outcomes after conservative treatment for intraepithelial or early invasive cervical lesions: systematic review and meta-analysis. *Lancet* 2006;367(9509):489–498

Landoni F, Maneo A, Colombo A, et al. Randomised study of radical surgery versus radiotherapy for stage Ib–IIa cervical cancer. *Lancet* 1997;350(9077):535–540

FUTURE II Study Group. Quadrivalent vaccine against human papillomavirus to prevent high-grade cervical lesions. *N Engl J Med* 2007;356(19):1915–1927

Villa LL, Costa RL, Petta CA, et al. Prophylactic quadrivalent human papillomavirus (types 6, 11, 16, and 18) L1 virus-like particle vaccine in young women: a randomised double-blind placebo-controlled multicentre phase II efficacy trial. *Lancet Oncol* 2005;6(5):271–278

49 Uterine Leiomyomas

Jon Ivar Einarsson

Etiology

Uterine leiomyomas, more commonly referred to as uterine fibroids, are benign tumors that arise from the myometrium of the uterus. The uterus is mostly composed of smooth muscle cells, designed to expand with the growing pregnancy and to help with vaginal delivery by contracting forcefully at the end of gestatation. Uterine fibroids can form underneath the endometrium (submucosal), in the myometrium (intramural), or underneath the uterine serosa (subserosal) (**Fig. 49.1**). Why fibroids are formed is not well understood. There are some genetic abnormalities in the smooth muscle cells that increase the risk for developing fibroids, and they seem to be under hormonal control, although the precise mechanism of this is not fully understood either.

Epidemiology

Uterine fibroids are very common and are found in 40–60% of reproductive age women. When examining surgically removed uteri from women of all ages, up to 80% of them are found to have some fibroids present. Some of the factors that influence the development of uterine fibroids are listed in **Table 49.1**. African-American women have higher risk for developing uterine fibroids than Caucasian women. Other risk factors for developing uterine fibroids include nulliparity (never carried a pregnancy beyond 20 weeks' gestation), obesity, alcohol consumption, and genetic predisposition. It has also been proposed that high consumption of red meat and ham could increase the risk of fibroids, while consumption of fruit and vegetables could decrease the risk for fibroids; however, this has not been conclusively proven. Consistent use of birth control pills may lower the risk for developing uterine fibroids, although some studies show contrary findings.

Table 49.1 Factors that influence the development of uterine fibroids

Increased risk
40 years or older
African-American race
Family history of uterine fibroid tumors
Nulliparity
Obesity
Decreased risk
More than five pregnancies
Postmenopausal status
Prolonged use of oral contraceptives
Smoking
Use of depot medroxyprogesterone acetate (Depo-Provera)

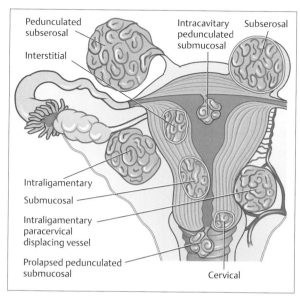

Fig. 49.1 Various subtypes of uterine fibroids based on location. Reproduced courtesy of Dr. William J. Mann.

Symptoms

Uterine fibroids can cause abnormal uterine bleeding, pelvic pressure, and can have a negative effect on fertility. In general, fibroids that press on and distort the endometrium can cause abnormal bleeding. This includes submucosal fibroids and large intramural fibroids. When the fibroids grow larger, the uterus expands and puts pressure on adjacent organs, such as the rectum and the urinary bladder. This can lead to a feeling of fullness, constipation, and frequent urination. In extreme cases the uterus can be the size of a full-term pregnancy, reaching all the way up to the liver and diaphragm. Fibroids usually do not cause extreme pain; however, sometimes a fibroid might lose its blood supply due to rapid growth. This causes the fibroid to die (degenerate), which can cause severe pain. The pain will usually get better over a period of few days, but sometimes requires a surgical intervention. Fibroids that press on the endometrium probably decrease fertility, since this can interfere with the implantation of the embryo. Currently, no well-designed randomized clinical trials evaluating the effects of fibroids on fertility have been published. However, based on the best available evidence, it seems that removing uterine fibroids that distort the uterine cavity improves fertility in such women.

Diagnosis

Large fibroids can usually be identified during a regular abdominal exam or a pelvic exam. Ultrasonography can identify most fibroids and is easily performed in a doctor's office. The addition of saline infusion sonohysterography can help to identify fibroids that are inside the uterine cavity. Office hysteroscopy is also an excellent tool to detect uterine fibroids inside the uterine cavity. Magnetic resonance imaging (MRI) gives very accurate information about the exact location and size of the fibroids. It is a useful tool to determine appropriate treatment options, such as removal of the uterine fibroids (myomectomy), embolization or focused ultrasound (see below), or a hysterectomy. MRI can also be helpful in determining if there is something else in the uterus that is causing the symptoms, such as adenomyosis or a leiomyosarcoma (cancer of the uterine muscle). It is, however, the most expensive diagnostic option and should be used selectively.

Treatment for Uterine Fibroids

It is important to note that since fibroids are not cancerous, no treatment at all is probably the best option for women who are asymptomatic. The traditional treatment for uterine fibroids involves either removing the fibroids or the uterus via a laparotomy incision. Hysterectomy has usually been recommended for women who are not planning to have any more children, since there is a 15–20% risk that the symptoms will not improve following a myomectomy, thereby requiring additional surgery. However, some women may want to conserve their uterus even though they are not planning a future pregnancy. It is important to respect their wishes as long as they fully understand the risks and benefits associated with their decision. In addition to performing a hysterectomy or a myomectomy via a laparotomy incision, there are a number of minimally invasive and noninvasive options currently available, or in development, for this condition. Some of these surgical and nonsurgical options are discussed below (**Table 49.2**).

Medical Treatment

Gonadotropin-Releasing Hormone Agonists

The growth of uterine fibroids seems to be influenced by estrogen and progesterone. By modulating the effects of these hormones it is possible to significantly decrease the size of the fibroids. Gonadotropin-releasing hormone (GnRH) is normally produced in the hypothalamus and controls the ovarian production of estrogen and progesterone by influencing pituitary production of luteinizing hormone and follicle-stimulating hormone.

When a synthetic version of GnRH (GnRH agonist) is administered to a woman, there is an inital 2-week period of stimulation of hormone production, but then the system becomes oversaturated and the production of estrogen and progesterone shuts down temporarily. GnRH agonists are usually injected into muscle in long-acting formulations that have an effect for 1 or 3 months. They can also be administered daily using a nasal spray. In 3 months, GnRH agonists can shrink uterine size by one-third and the fibroid size by half. In addition, vaginal bleeding usually stops completely. Symptom relief from pressure or bleeding is therefore common. Unfortunately, GnRH agonists have significant side effects associated with hypoestrogenism, such as night sweats, hot flushes, irritability, vaginal dryness, and difficulty sleeping. In addition, long-term use is associated with significant bone loss (estrogen stimulates bone formation). Because of this, use GnRH agonists for longer than 6 months is not recommended. It is possible to reduce the side effects of

Table 49.2 Treatment options for uterine fibroids

Option	Advantages	Disadvantages	Good option for
Medical treatment	Noninvasive	No currently available long-term option	Poor surgical candidates
		Needs to be used until menopause	Patients reluctant to have surgery
Myomectomy	Effective	Recurrence rate requiring surgery	Women who want to become pregnant
	Often possible to perform laparoscopically	Adhesion formation	
		Risk of uterine rupture	
Hysterectomy	Permanent solution to the problem	Relatively invasive procedure	Women who are not considering further childbearing
		Precludes childbearing	
Uterine fibroid embolization	Minimally invasive	Not suitable for all candidates	Poor surgical candidates
		Complications most common following hospital discharge	Patients reluctant to have surgery
MRI-guided focused ultrasound	Noninvasive	Not suitable for all candidates	Poor surgical candidates
		Not as effective as other treatment options	Patients reluctant to have surgery

the GnRH therapy by using a very low dose of estrogen or progesterone (add-back therapy). It is generally recommended to wait at least 4 weeks before starting the add-back therapy, in order to get a maximum effects on the fibroids.

Because GnRH agonist therapy can only be used for a short period and because the effects are quickly reversed, GnRH agonist therapy is mostly used to reduce the size of uterine fibroids before surgery. This facilitates the removal of the uterus or fibroids at the time of surgery. The maximal effect on uterine size is reached at 3 months, and therefore it is not necessary to treat women longer preoperatively.

Selective Progesterone Receptor Modulators

An intense search is in progress for a suitable long-term medical treatment for fibroids. One promising option seems to be medications called selective progesterone receptor modulators (SPRMs). These medications interact with cell receptors that respond to progesterone and change the effect that progesterone has on cells. One of these, called Mifepristone, has been found to be effective in reducing the size and symptoms of fibroids. However, the effects of long-term use are unknown and Mifepristone has been associated with an increased risk for endometrial hyperplasia. Another SPRM that shows promise is Asoprisnil. Early studies indicate that this medication is effective in decreasing symptoms and uterine size with no effect on endometrial function (Evidence Box 49.1). Time will tell whether this type of medication may be generally adopted, but early results are encouraging.

Birth Control Pills

Birth control pills do not seem to be very helpful to treat symptoms associated with uterine fibroids; however, they are effective in treating abnormal bleeding due to problems with ovulation and may decrease the growth rate of uterine fibroids. Possibly, the abnormal bleeding experienced might not be due to the fibroids, and therefore a 3 month trial of birth control pills is appropriate in selected cases.

Hormonal Intrauterine Device

The progesterone intrauterine device (IUD) marketed as Mirena might be effective in reducing abnormal uterine bleeding associated with fibroids; however, the size and growth of the uterine fibroids are probably not affected.

Surgical Treatment

Myomectomy should be the surgical option of choice in women who want retain their fertility. Other options such as uterine artery embolization, uterine artery occlusion, cryomyolysis, and focused ultrasound are usually not recommended for women who want to have more children. There are nevertheless some women who have become pregnant after these procedures and successfully carried their babies to term without complications. Most of these women became pregnant following uterine artery embolization. The number of complications associated with such pregnancies was significantly greater than in women who did not have these procedures. This may in part be explained by other, underlying health problems which might have increased the risk for pregnancy complications in these women. Nevertheless, women who want to become pregnant in the future should choose to have either an abdominal or a laparoscopic myomectomy.

Myomectomy

Myomectomy, or removal of uterine fibroids, is commonly performed in women who want to retain their fertility. It depends largely on the surgeon's skill and experience as to which cases can be performed laparoscopically rather than via laparotomy. In general, cases where intramural fibroids larger than 10 cm across and more than three fibroids are removed at the time of surgery are associated with a higher complication rate. Fibroids that are located in the broad ligament or in the cervix can also be challenging to remove laparoscopically.

A major limiting factor is laparoscopic suturing. Suturing laparoscopically is a very advanced skill and most gynecologists do not have the capability to do this properly. It is critical to close the uterine incision adequately, since this most likely impacts the risk for uterine rupture during a subsequent pregnancy. Remember that most women who have a myomectomy are hoping to carry a pregnancy to term after the procedure. If the hysterotomy scar

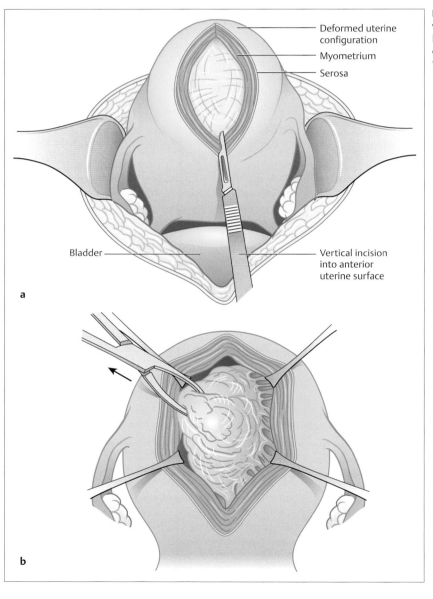

Fig. 49.2a–d Myomectomy. **a** Initial vertical incision into the anterior uterine surface. **b** Fibroid removal: a towel clamp is placed on the myoma for traction to aid in dissection.

Deformed uterine configuration

Myometrium

Serosa

Bladder

Vertical incision into anterior uterine surface

a

b

Fig. 49.2c, d ▶

is weak, the uterus can rupture as the uterus expands and the uterine wall becomes thinner. This can be very dangerous for mother and child, in some cases leading to neonatal death and a peripartum hysterectomy.

Surgical principles: The basic surgical principles are the same whether a myomectomy is performed laparoscopically or via a laparotomy (**Fig. 49.2**). An incision is made into the uterine serosa and carried down all the way to the fibroid. The fibroid is then gently freed from the uterus by pulling on it and cutting away its attachments. Once the fibroid is removed the uterine incision needs to be closed properly, since this helps to prevent uterine rup-

ture in a future pregnancy. This is the most challenging part when performing the procedure laparoscopically, because it involves a lot of suturing. The uterine incision is closed in layers, usually three to four, depending on the depth of the uterine incision. The fibroid itself is removed via the abdominal incision, or with a morcellator in the case of laparoscopy.

A laparoscopic morcellator is a long, hollow cylinder with a sharp circular blade on one end. A grasper is inserted through the morcellator and the tissue is pulled toward the circular blade. The blade is activated by pressing a button or a pedal, resulting in rapid circular blade motion. By pulling the tissue into the blade, the fibroid

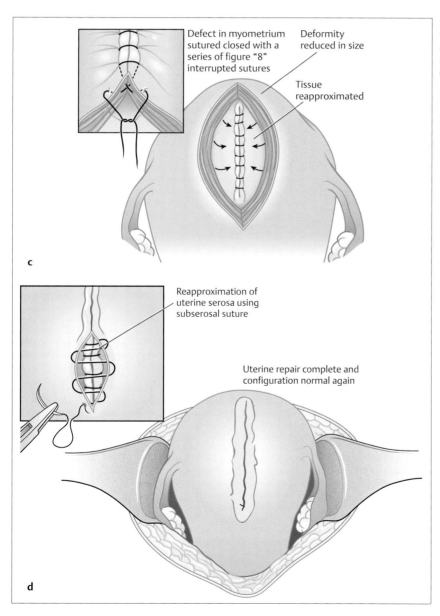

Defect in myometrium sutured closed with a series of figure "8" interrupted sutures

Deformity reduced in size

Tissue reapproximated

c

Reapproximation of uterine serosa using subserosal suture

Uterine repair complete and configuration normal again

d

Fig. 49.2c, d Myomectomy. **c** The defect in the myometrium is closed with a series of "figure-of-eight" interrupted sutures. **d** End result [to come]. Reproduced courtesy of Dr. William J. Mann.

can be removed from the abdomen in long strips of tissue, similar to apple cores. Using this techniqe, large amounts of tissue can be removed through an opening measuring 1.2–1.5 cm wide.

Due to the challenge of laparoscopic suturing, a hybrid procedure called laparoscopically assisted myomectomy (LAM) has been developed. By means of this technique, the fibroid is released laparoscopically as previously described and then a small laparotomy incision (4–5 cm wide) is made above the pubic hairline. The fibroid is removed through this incision and the uterus is sutured through it as well. This technique is well suited when dealing with a large number of fibroids, or when the physician is not proficient in laparoscopic suturing. It is not well suited to fibroids that are located on the back of the uterus, since it is difficult to reach this area through a small incision.

A recently available alternative is the da Vinci robot for the myomectomy. The da Vinci robot consists of three or four mechanical arms that are controlled by the surgeon from a separate control unit (console). The arms of the robot can carry various instruments and the instruments can move freely at the tip, allowing freedom of movement similar to that which the human wrist offers during open surgery. In addition, the surgeon has a three-dimensional vision of his environment through the control unit. This makes suturing easier for the less experienced laparoscopic surgeon. The robot has some disadvantages, including lack of tactile sensation, that is, the surgeon is not able to feel how hard or soft an organ is or how tightly a knot is being tied and has to rely completely on visual cues. The robot is also bulky and set up times are longer due to the amount of time it takes to drape and connect the robotic arms prior to starting the surgery. The robot is also expensive and the current version uses slightly larger trocars than the trocars used in standard laparoscopy cases, resulting in slighly larger abdominal scars.

Uterine Artery Embolization

In appropriately selected patients, uterine artery embolization (UAE) can be an effective treatment option, especially for women who, for a variety of reasons, are not favorable surgical candidates. UAE is performed by an interventional radiologist. A small catheter is placed into a blood vessel in the groin and threaded up to the uterine artery under radiographic guidance. Once the catheter is in the right place, small particles are released into the blood stream that subsequently become stuck in the blood vessels supplying the fibroids. This reduces or stops blood flow to the fibroids, which in turn causes them to die and shrink. This technique is also sometimes called uterine fibroid embolization (UFE), since it can sometimes be performed more selectively by targeting individual fibroids rather than the main blood supply of the uterus. The UFE procedure itself usually takes about an hour to complete.

UFE is very effective in properly selected patients, with over 85 % of patients reporting significant improvement in symptoms, even on long-term follow-up. Patients with multiple fibroids or large fibroids have slightly less favorable outcomes. In addition, patients with submucosal fibroids are traditionally considered to be unsuitable candidates for this procedure, since treatment failure is high and there is some risk of abscess formation. Finally, patients with pedunculated fibroids on a stalk that is narrower than 2 cm are not good candidates for UFE due to the risk of developing fibroid necrosis and subsequent infection.

Following the procedure, patients commonly suffer some pain and discomfort due to fibroid necrosis, which causes inflammation and swelling of the uterus. Patients are usually admitted for one or two days following UFE for pain control. Fever is common (due to the inflammation) and some patients experience nausea. These symptoms gradually improve over time and most patients are back to normal in about 10–14 days. When compared with abdominal myomectomy, the two treatments were equally effective, but patients who had UFE had a shorter hospital stay (1 vs. 2.5 days) and were able to return to normal activities quicker (15 vs. 44 days). A recent study comparing laparoscopic myomectomy and UFE found that return to normal activities was similar in both groups, but complications were more common in the UFE group (Evidence Box 49.2).

Laparoscopic Uterine Artery Occlusion

Laparoscopic Uterine Artery Occlusion (LUAO) is an alternative to UFE, where the uterine artery is located and permanently clamped using laparoscopy. The uterus regains its blood supply through collateral routes within 6 hours; however, the fibroids are not able to do this and die off. A recent comparative study between UFE and LUAO found the two procedures to be equally effective in reducing bleeding when measured with pictorial charts. However, more women in the LUAO group complained of excessive bleeding 6 months after the procedure than women in the UFE group. There was significantly less pain associated with the LUAO than UFE. LUAO is a promising alternative to UFE, especially when there are large fibroids or pedunculated fibroids present. This allows the physician to remove the large fibroids during the LUAO procedure, which might help to relieve pressure symptoms better than uterine fibroid embolization.

Vaginal Uterine Artery Occlusion

This is an experimental technique by which the uterine arteries are located vaginally with the help of ultrasound imaging and temporarily clamped for 6–8 hours. As mentioned above, when the uterine artery is clamped, the uterus regains its blood supply within 6 hours, but the fibroids are not able to do this and die off. The patients are usually offered an epidural or spinal analgesia and are temporarily admitted to hospital while the clamp is on the uterine arteries. Once the clamp is removed, patients are able to go home the same day. The preliminary results are promising, but more studies are needed before this technique becomes available as a treatment option for the general public.

Laparoscopic Myolysis

This technique involves localizing the uterine fibroids laparoscopically and destroying them with either extreme heat or cold. Usually, a needle is inserted into the fibroid and the tip of the needle is heated or cooled to destroy the fibroid. Preliminary studies indicate significant reduction in fibroid volume and also significant improvement in symptoms.

The ideal candidate should have no more than four fibroids and no fibroid larger than 10 cm. The advantage over myomectomy is that here no suturing is required. However, the destruction of the fibroid can result in the formation of extensive scar tissue and possibly a weak uterine wall. Myolysis is therefore not recommended for women planning to have more children and is considered experimental at present.

Magnetic Resonance-Guided Focused Ultrasound

This is an outpatient procedure, where MRI is used to locate the fibroids and multiple ultrasound beams are focused on a small part of the fibroid at a time. The focused ultrasound waves create a lot of heat which destroys the uterine fibroid. The procedure takes place in a radiology suite with the patient lying prone on an MRI table. The procedure time is two to three hours.

Early studies are promising for this technique; however, because of lack of long-term safety data it is not a good option for women who wish to retain their fertility. Other patients who are not well suited for this procedure are patients with submucous fibroids, multiple fibroids, fibroids near the bowel or bladder, or fibroids where abdominal scars are in the path of the ultrasound beams. Magnetic resonance-guided focused ultrasound is also relatively expensive and should be used only on selected patients until better long-term follow-up results are available.

Uterine Sarcomas

Arising from the uterine myometrium, these tumors are rare with an incidence of only approximately 17 per million women annually. The incidence seems to be higher in African-American women, long-term users of tamoxifen, and in women with a history of pelvic radiation. Uterine sarcomas are divided into five subgroups according to their histological origin, with the two most common types being carcinosarcoma and leiomyosarcoma. These tumors typically present with abnormal uterine bleeding, but other presenting symptoms include pain, foul-smelling vaginal discharge, and pelvic pressure. Traditionally, a rapidly growing uterus has been considered a risk factor for developing a uterine sarcoma; however, this has not been confirmed in the literature.

Uterine sarcomas are aggressive tumors and difficult to distinguish from uterine fibroids on imaging studies. Patients diagnosed with a uterine sarcoma have a poor prognosis with a recurrence rate of 53–71 % in early stage tumors treated with a hysterectomy. Hysterectomy with removal of both adnexa is the standard therapy, but adjuvant therapy with radiation and chemotherapy is commonly used, although the efficacy of this treatment is controversial.

Key Points

- Uterine leiomyomas are the most common benign tumors in women.
- Uterine leiomyomas that cause no symptoms usually do not need treatment and may be followed over time by physical examination and imaging studies.
- Uterine leiomyomas that cause menorrhagia can be treated with hormones, uterine artery embolization, or surgical removal of the tumors.
- Submucus leiomyomas may be associated with infertility and in those cases surgical removal is warranted.
- Hysterectomy is one of the most commonly performed surgical procedures. The most common indication for hysterectomy is uterine leiomyomas causing menorrhagia.

Evidence Box 49.1

Asoprisnil is a selective progesterone receptor modulator that shows promise in the treatment of uterine fibroids.

Asoprisnil is a selective progesterone receptor modulator that suppresses endometrial and myometrial growth with apparently minimal side effects. In a recent randomized clinical trial, 129 women with leiomyomas were randomized to take Asoprisnil (5, 10, or 25 mg) or placebo orally daily for 12 weeks. Asoprisnil suppressed uterine bleeding in 28%, 64%, and 83% of subjects at doses of 5, 10, and 25 mg, respectively, and reduced leiomyoma and uterine volumes. Leiomyoma volume was reduced by 36% after 12 weeks in the 25-mg group. Asoprisnil was associated with follicular-phase estrogen concentration and minimal hypoestrogenic symptoms.

According to this first randomized trial, Asoprisnil seems to be well tolerated and effective in controlling uterine bleeding and reducing leiomyoma volume. Further studies with larger patient cohorts and long-term follow-up need to be conducted before Asoprisnil can be recommended for general use, however the results of this initial study are encouraging.

Chwalisz K, Larsen L, Mattia-Goldberg C, Edmonds A, Elger W, Winkel CA. A randomized, controlled trial of asoprisnil, a novel selective progesterone receptor modulator, in women with uterine leiomyomata. Fertil Steril 2007 Jun;87(6):1399–1412.

Evidence Box 49.2

A randomized trial comparing uterine artery embolization with surgery showed mixed results, with no clear advantage overall for either approach.

Hysterectomy and myomectomy have been the standard of care for treatment of uterine fibroids. A recent randomized trial compared these traditional treatments with uterine artery embolization to evaluate and compare efficacy and safety of these two treatment modalities. For the comparison 106 patients were randomized to embolization, while 51 underwent surgery (43 hysterectomies and 8 myomectomies). The primary outcome was quality of life at 1 year of follow-up, as measured by the Medical Outcomes Study 36-Item Short-Form General Health Survey (SF-36). There were no 1 year. The embolization group had a shorter median duration of hospitalization than the surgical group (1 day vs. 5 days) and a shorter time before returning to work. At 1 year, symptom scores were better in the surgical group. Twelve percent of patients in the embolization group experienced adverse events in the first year while there were adverse events in 20% of patients in the surgery groups. This difference was not statistically significant. The majority of adverse events in the surgery group occurred during the initial hospitalization, while most complications in the embolization group occurred after hospital discharge. Nine percent of patients in the embolization group required repeated embolization or hysterectomy for inadequate symptom control.

While embolization was associated with faster recovery and shorter hospital stay in this study, there were significant number of late complications requiring re-admission and in some cases repeat surgery. Designing a randomized trial comparing embolization with vaginal or laparoscopic hysterectomy may be an appropriate next step, since these minimally invasive surgical techniques are gradually becoming the standard of care for most cases of hysterectomy.

Edwards RD, Moss JG, Lumsden MA, et al. Committee of the Randomized Trial of Embolization versus Surgical Treatment for Fibroids. Uterine-artery embolization versus surgery for symptomatic uterine fibroids. N Engl J Med 2007 Jan 25;356(4):360–370.

Further Reading

Advincula AP, Song A. The role of robotic surgery in gynecology. *Curr Opin Obstet Gynecol* 2007;19(4):331–336

Borgfeldt C, Andolf E. Transvaginal ultrasonographic findings in the uterus and the endometrium: low prevalence of leiomyoma in a random sample of women age 25-40 years. *Acta Obstet Gynecol Scand* 2000;79(3):202–207

Brooks SE, Zhan M, Cote T, Baquet CR. Surveillance, epidemiology, and end results analysis of 2677 cases of uterine sarcoma 1989-1999. *Gynecol Oncol* 2004;93(1):204–208

Cantuaria GH, Angioli R, Frost L, Duncan R, Penalver MA. Comparison of bimanual examination with ultrasound examination before hysterectomy for uterine leiomyoma. *Obstet Gynecol* 1998;92(1):109–112

Chiaffarino F, Parazzini F, La Vecchia C, Chatenoud L, Di Cintio E, Marsico S. Diet and uterine myomas. *Obstet Gynecol* 1999;94(3):395–398

Chwalisz K, Larsen L, Mattia-Goldberg C, Edmonds A, Elger W, Winkel CA. A randomized, controlled trial of asoprisnil, a novel selective progesterone receptor modulator, in women with uterine leiomyomata. *Fertil Steril* 2007;87(6):1399–1412

Cook JD, Walker CL. Treatment strategies for uterine leiomyoma: the role of hormonal modulation. *Semin Reprod Med* 2004;22(2):105–111

Cramer SF, Patel A. The frequency of uterine leiomyomas. *Am J Clin Pathol* 1990;94(4):435–438

Day Baird D, Dunson DB, Hill MC, Cousins D, Schectman JM. High cumulative incidence of uterine leiomyoma in black and white women: ultrasound evidence. *Am J Obstet Gynecol* 2003;188(1):100–107

Dueholm M, Lundorf E, Hansen ES, Ledertoug S, Olesen F. Evaluation of the uterine cavity with magnetic resonance imaging, transvaginal sonography, hysterosonographic examination, and diagnostic hysteroscopy. *Fertil Steril* 2001;76(2):350–357

Dueholm M, Lundorf E, Hansen ES, Ledertoug S, Olesen F. Accuracy of magnetic resonance imaging and transvaginal ultrasonography in the diagnosis, mapping, and measurement of uterine myomas. *Am J Obstet Gynecol* 2002;186(3):409–415

Dueholm M, Lundorf E, Olesen F. Imaging techniques for evaluation of the uterine cavity and endometrium in premenopausal patients before minimally invasive surgery. *Obstet Gynecol Surv* 2002;57(6):388–403

Edwards RD, Moss JG, Lumsden MA, et al; Committee of the Randomized Trial of Embolization versus Surgical Treatment for Fibroids. Uterine-artery embolization versus surgery for symptomatic uterine fibroids. *N Engl J Med* 2007;356(4):360–370

Eisinger SH, Bonfiglio T, Fiscella K, Meldrum S, Guzick DS. Twelve-month safety and efficacy of low-dose mifepristone for uterine myomas. *J Minim Invasive Gynecol* 2005;12(3):227–233

Fennessy FM, Tempany CM, McDannold NJ, et al. Uterine leiomyomas: MR imaging-guided focused ultrasound surgery—results of different treatment protocols. *Radiology* 2007;243(3):885–893

Fennessy FM, Tempany CM. MRI-guided focused ultrasound surgery of uterine leiomyomas. *Acad Radiol* 2005;12(9):1158–1166

Ferenczy A, Richart RM, Okagaki T. A comparative ultrastructural study of leiomyosarcoma, cellular leiomyoma, and leiomyoma of the uterus. *Cancer* 1971;28(4):1004–1018

Fiscella K, Eisinger SH, Meldrum S, Feng C, Fisher SG, Guzick DS. Effect of mifepristone for symptomatic leiomyomata on quality of life and uterine size: a randomized controlled trial. *Obstet Gynecol* 2006;108(6):1381–1387

Flake GP, Andersen J, Dixon D. Etiology and pathogenesis of uterine leiomyomas: a review. *Environ Health Perspect* 2003;111(8):1037–1054

Goldberg J, Pereira L, Berghella V, et al. Pregnancy outcomes after treatment for fibromyomata: uterine artery embolization versus laparoscopic myomectomy. *Am J Obstet Gynecol* 2004;191(1):18–21

Goodwin SC, Bradley LD, Lipman JC, et al; UAE versus Myomectomy Study Group. Uterine artery embolization versus myomectomy: a multicenter comparative study. *Fertil Steril* 2006;85(1):14–21

Goodwin SC, Spies JB, Worthington-Kirsch R, et al; Fibroid Registry for Outcomes Data (FIBROID) Registry Steering Committee and Core Site Investigators. Uterine artery embolization for treatment of leiomyomata: long-term outcomes from the FIBROID Registry. *Obstet Gynecol* 2008;111(1):22–33

Hald K, Kløw NE, Qvigstad E, Istre O. Laparoscopic occlusion compared with embolization of uterine vessels: a randomized controlled trial. *Obstet Gynecol* 2007;109(1):20–27

Kaunitz AM. Progestin-releasing intrauterine systems and leiomyoma. *Contraception* 2007; 75(6, Suppl)S130–S133

Landon MB, Hauth JC, Leveno KJ, et al; National Institute of Child Health and Human Development Maternal-Fetal Medicine Units Network. Maternal and perinatal outcomes associated with a trial of labor after prior cesarean delivery. *N Engl J Med* 2004;351(25):2581–2589

Lethaby A, Vollenhoven B, Sowter M. Pre-operative GnRH analogue therapy before hysterectomy or myomectomy for uterine fibroids. *Cochrane Database Syst Rev* 2001;2(2):CD000547

Lichtinger M, Herbert S, Memmolo A. Temporary, transvaginal occlusion of the uterine arteries: a feasibility and safety study. *J Minim Invasive Gynecol* 2005;12(1):40–42

Major FJ, Blessing JA, Silverberg SG, et al. Prognostic factors in early-stage uterine sarcoma. A Gynecologic Oncology Group study. *Cancer* 1993; 71(4, Suppl)1702–1709

Marshall LM, Spiegelman D, Barbieri RL, et al. Variation in the incidence of uterine leiomyoma among premenopausal women by age and race. *Obstet Gynecol* 1997;90(6):967–973

Meredith RF, Eisert DR, Kaka Z, Hodgson SE, Johnston GA Jr, Boutselis JG. An excess of uterine sarcomas after pelvic irradiation. *Cancer* 1986;58(9):2003–2007

Odunsi K, Moneke V, Tammela J, et al. Efficacy of adjuvant CYVADIC chemotherapy in early-stage uterine sarcomas: results of long-term follow-up. *Int J Gynecol Cancer* 2004;14(4):659–664

Ohgi S, Nakagawa K, Inoue H, Yasuda M, Saito H. Uterine artery embolization should not be recommended without careful consideration in the treatment of symptomatic uterine fibroids. *J Obstet Gynaecol Res* 2007;33(4):506–511

Parazzini F, Negri E, La Vecchia C, Fedele L, Rabaiotti M, Luchini L. Oral contraceptive use and risk of uterine fibroids. *Obstet Gynecol* 1992;79(3):430–433

Parker WH, Fu YS, Berek JS. Uterine sarcoma in patients operated on for presumed leiomyoma and rapidly growing leiomyoma. *Obstet Gynecol* 1994;83(3):414–418

Platz CE, Benda JA. Female genital tract cancer. *Cancer* 1995; 75(1, Suppl)270–294

Ratner H. Risk factors for uterine fibroids: reduced risk associated with oral contraceptives. *Br Med J (Clin Res Ed)* 1986;293(6553):1027

Reed SD, Newton KM, Thompson LB, McCrummen BA, Warolin AK. The incidence of repeat uterine surgery following myomectomy. *J Womens Health (Larchmt)* 2006;15(9):1046–1052

Rha SE, Byun JY, Jung SE, et al. CT and MRI of uterine sarcomas and their mimickers. *AJR Am J Roentgenol* 2003;181(5):1369–1374

Ross RK, Pike MC, Vessey MP, Bull D, Yeates D, Casagrande JT. Risk factors for uterine fibroids: reduced risk associated with oral contraceptives. *Br Med J (Clin Res Ed)* 1986;293(6543):359–362

Schwartz SM, Marshall LM, Baird DD. Epidemiologic contributions to understanding the etiology of uterine leiomyomata. *Environ Health Perspect* 2000;108(Suppl 5):821–827

Sizzi O, Rossetti A, Malzoni M, et al. Italian multicenter study on complications of laparoscopic myomectomy. *J Minim Invasive Gynecol* 2007;14(4):453–462

Somigliana E, Vercellini P, Daguati R, Pasin R, De Giorgi O, Crosignani PG. Fibroids and female reproduction: a critical analysis of the evidence. *Hum Reprod Update* 2007;13(5):465–476

Stewart EA. Uterine fibroids. *Lancet* 2001;357(9252):293–298

Taniguchi F, Harada T, Iwabe T, Yoshida S, Mitsunari M, Terakawa N. Use of the LAP DISK (abdominal wall sealing device) in laparoscopically assisted myomectomy. *Fertil Steril* 2004;81(4):1120–1124

Wegienka G, Baird DD, Hertz-Picciotto I, et al. Self-reported heavy bleeding associated with uterine leiomyomata. *Obstet Gynecol* 2003;101(3):431–437

Zupi E, Sbracia M, Marconi D, Munro MG. Myolysis of uterine fibroids: is there a role? *Clin Obstet Gynecol* 2006;49(4):821–833

50 Endometrial Cancer

Robert L. Barbieri

Endometrial cancer is the most common gynecologic malignancy (**Fig. 50.1**). After breast, lung, and colon cancer, it is the fourth most common cancer in women living in developed countries. Of all cancers in women, about 6% are due to endometrial cancer.

Definition

Endometrial cancer is a pathological diagnosis, which is made when histological study indicates disruption of the normal endometrial epithelial cell and glandular growth and architecture with *invasion of neoplastic epithelium into the underlying stroma*. The abnormal pattern of growth and architecture is most often caused by somatic mutations that reduce the normal mechanisms which constrain uncontrolled cell growth.

A precursor to endometrial cancer is endometrial hyperplasia. Simple endometrial hyperplasia has a low rate of progression to endometrial cancer. Complex endometrial hyperplasia, including cellular atypia, has a higher rate of progression to endometrial cancer.

Endometrial cancer is often characterized as type I (primarily induced by hormone imbalance: too much estrogen and too little progesterone) and type II (not primarily related to hormone imbalance). Type I endometrial cancer typically presents histologically as a low-grade tumor with endometrioid features. Type I endometrial cancer is primarily induced by extended endometrial stimulation by estrogen without exposure to progesterone. Common clinical conditions where there is chronic exposure to estrogen without exposure to progesterone include: 1) anovulatory states such as the polycystic ovary syndrome; 2) exogenous estrogen therapy without progestin treatment; 3) obesity; and 4) estrogen-secreting granulosa cell tumors. Obesity and insulin resistance can cause anovulation resulting in the common triad of endometrial cancer, diabetes, and hypertension. Type II

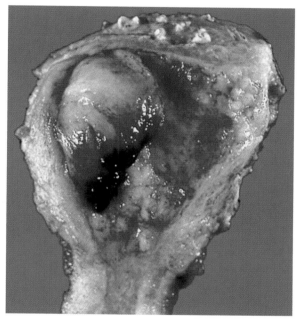

Fig. 50.1 Endometrial cancer in a hysterectomy specimen. The uterus has been cut open to assess the extent of the cancer. From: Silverberg, SG, Kurman, RJ. Tumors of the Uterine Corpus and Gestational Trophoblastic Disease. AFIP Atlas of Tumor Pathology, version 2.0, American Registry of Pathology, Washington DC 1995.

endometrial cancer is unrelated to estrogen stimulation and commonly presents histologically as a high-grade tumor with papillary serous or clear cell features. Women with type II endometrial cancer tend to be older with a history of more pregnancies than those with type I disease. Of all cases of endometrial cancer about 75% are type I and 25% are type II.

Etiology

Type I endometrioid endometrial cancers have characteristic mutations in the PTEN, k-ras and beta-catenin genes and demonstrate DNA microsatellite instability. The PTEN (phosphatase and tensin homologue) gene is a suppressor of estrogen-stimulated endometrial cell growth. Mutations in the *PTEN* gene that result in loss of function cause greater endometrial cell growth in response to a given concentration (dose) of estradiol. Type II serous endometrial cancers often have mutations in p53, which is a tumor suppressor gene that blocks the progression of cells through the late G_1 phase. Loss of function mutations in *p53* releases somatic cells from the G_1 cell cycle checkpoint and permits the cells to replicate more rapidly. In addition, normally expressed wild-type p53 prevents cells with DNA damage from proliferating. Loss of function mutations in p53 is associated with chromosome instability increasing the likelihood that additional detrimental mutations will accrue. In the Lynch syndrome (also called the hereditary nonpolyposis colorectal cancer syndrome), autosomal dominant *germ-line* mutations in the DNA mismatch repair genes, *MLH1*, *MSH2*, *MSH6*, or *PMS2*, cause a multiorgan cancer syndrome associated with colon, ovary, and endometrial cancer. Among women less than 50 years of age with endometrial cancer, about 10% have the germline mutations characteristic of the Lynch syndrome.

Epidemiology

The median age of diagnosis is 61 years with most women diagnosed between 50 and 70 years of age. A number of exposures reduce the risk of developing endometrial cancer, including multiparity, estrogen–progestin contraceptive use, chronic progestin therapy, and cigarette smoking. Exposures that increase the risk of developing endometrial cancer include advancing age, obesity, chronic estrogen treatment without concomitant progestin treatment, tamoxifen therapy, and nulliparity.

Prevention

Exposure to estrogen, unopposed by progestin, is a major risk factor for endometrial cancer. In obese women, fat cells containing aromatase produce excess extra-ovarian estrogen. In addition, obesity is often associated with anovulation, reducing progesterone secretion. Any intervention that reduces the prevalence of obesity will likely reduce the risk of endometrial cancer. Increasing exercise and reducing glycemic load are two interventions that likely reduce the risk of endometrial cancer. Unlike tamoxifen, which acts as an estrogen agonist in the endometrium and increases the risk of endometrial cancer, a related compound, raloxifene, is an anti-estrogen in the endometrium. Raloxifene use reduces the risk of endometrial cancer by about 50% in postmenopausal women.

History

Abnormal patterns of uterine bleeding, especially in postmenopausal women, may be caused by endometrial lesions such as endometrial hyperplasia, endometrial cancer, polyps, or submucus fibroids. Women with a uterus who take estrogen, but no progestin, are at high risk of developing endometrial hyperplasia and cancer. Tamoxifen, a mixed estrogen agonist–antagonist, which acts as an estrogen agonist in the endometrium, is associated with an increased risk of endometrial cancer. A history of diabetes, hypertension, and/or obesity should increase the clinical suspicion that endometrial cancer may be present.

Physical Examination

Obesity and hypertension are common physical findings in women with endometrial cancer. Acanthosis nigricans, a dermatological finding observed in women with insulin resistance, may be present in some women with endometrial hyperplasia or cancer. Most cases of endometrial cancer are stage I. Other than bleeding from the uterus, there may be no additional abnormal findings on physical examination.

Diagnosis

All postmenopausal women with abnormal bleeding should have an endometrial biopsy, which has more than 95% sensitivity for detecting endometrial cancer. To fully evaluate the uterine cavity and endometrium, a hysteroscopy is often combined with an endometrial biopsy, especially if a recent endometrial biopsy did not reveal

Table 50.1 Common pathological findings on endometrial biopsy in postmenopausal women with uterine bleeding. In this study 1168 postmenopausal women with uterine bleeding underwent an endometrial biopsy

Endometrial lesion: final diagnosis	Prevalence
Endometrial or vaginal atrophy	59%
Endometrial polyp	12%
Endometrial cancer	10%
Endometrial hyperplasia (may be a precursor to endometrial cancer)	10%
Hormone effect	7%
Hematometra	2%
Cervical neoplasia	<1%

Source: Karlson B, Granberg S, Wikland M, et al. Transvaginal ultrasonography of the endometrium in women with postmenopausal bleeding. A Nordic multicenter study. Am J Obstet Gynecol 1995;172:1488–1494.

the cause of the bleeding. In postmenopausal women with uterine bleeding who completed a thorough evaluation, the causes of the bleeding are listed in **Table 50.1**. If an endometrial biopsy cannot be accomplished, or is refused by the patient, a transvaginal sonogram that demonstrates an endometrial thickness ≤4 mm is associated with a very low rate of endometrial cancer. In women with endometrial cancer, a cervical cytology specimen will demonstrate endometrial cancer cells in about 40% of cases.

Screening

General population screening for endometrial cancer is not recommended. Women with average or moderately increased risk of developing endometrial cancer should be taught the risks of the disease and its typical symptoms, including postmenopausal bleeding. They should be encouraged to seek health care at the first sign of postmenopausal bleeding. This group includes women with obesity, diabetes, insulin resistance, or women taking tamoxifen. Women with a uterus taking estrogen but no progestin should have an endometrial biopsy at least yearly. Women with Lynch syndrome have a 50% chance of developing endometrial cancer and a 10% chance of developing ovarian cancer. They should be offered hysterectomy and bilateral salpingo-oophorectomy after they complete their family. Until they have a hysterectomy, they should have an annual endometrial biopsy.

Staging and Surgical Treatment

Endometrial cancer is staged surgically. Surgical staging is both diagnostic and therapeutic. The surgical staging procedure should include total hysterectomy, bilateral salpingo-oophorectomy, cytological assessment of peritoneal washings, biopsy of suspicious lesions and, if warranted, retroperitoneal lymph node sampling. The FIGO (International Federation of Gynecology and Obstetrics) staging system is presented in **Table 50.2**. In addition to staging, the tumor is histologically graded with regard to the extent of differentiation of the adenocarcinoma, with grade 1 representing tumors with less than 5% solid, nonsquamous or morular components. Grade 3 represents tumors with more than 50% solid, nonsquamous or morular components. Surgical staging for endometrial cancer results in a diagnosis of synchronous ovarian cancer in 5% of women.

In young women wishing to preserve ovarian function, oophorectomy may be deferred, but the patient

Table 50.2 The FIGO* staging system for endometrial cancer

FIGO stage			5-year survival rate
I	Tumor limited to the uterine corpus		
	A	Tumor limited to endometrium	91%
	B	Tumor invades up to 50% of width of myometrium	90%
	C	Tumor invades more than 50% of the width of myometrium	81%
II	Tumor extends into cervix, but does not extend outside uterus		
	A	Tumor limited to endocervical glands	78%
	B	Tumor invades stoma of the cervix	71%
III	Local and regional spread		
	A	Tumor involves uterine serosa and/or adnexae or cancer cells in peritoneal fluid	60%
	B	Tumor extends into vagina	30%
	C	Tumor metastases in pelvic or para-aortic lymph nodes	52%
IV	Tumor invades nonreproductive organs		
	A	Tumor invades bladder or bowel	15%
	B	Distant metastases	17%

*International Federation of Gynecology and Obstetrics.

should understand the risk of synchronous ovarian cancer with microscopic disease foci. Pelvic and para-aortic lymph nodes should be assessed by inspection and palpation. Suspicious lymph nodes should be removed for histological study. Many oncology surgeons prefer to routinely perform a complete pelvic lymphadenectomy and para-aortic lymphadenectomy to maximize the number of nodes sampled to assess nodal disease. Since the uterine fundus drains to the para-aortic nodes and the lower uterine segment drains to the iliac lymph nodes, both pelvic and para-aortic lymphadenectomy are necessary for full nodal sampling. An alternative approach is to avoid lymph node dissection in women at the lowest risk of metastasis and recurrence, and those with endometrioid tumors grade 1 or 2 with less than 50% invasion of the myometrium.

The surgical procedure can be accomplished with a standard abdominal laparotomy incision, or by laparoscopy with or without the assistance of a surgical robot. In a systematic review of randomized trials of surgical treatment of endometrial cancer, laparoscopic surgery was associated with decreased surgical complications, less blood loss, shorter hospital stay, and more rapid return to work compared with laparotomy surgery. Cancer-free survival is similar in women who have either laparotomy or laparoscopic surgery.

Adjuvant Treatment

The most significant prognostic factors are surgical stage, histological grade, and depth of myometrial invasion. Women with endometrial cancer can be assigned to three risk groups: low, intermediate, or high. Adjuvant therapy is tailored for each risk group.

Low risk: Women with grade 1 or 2 histology and invasion limited to less than 50% of the myometrium (stage IA or IB) are at low risk for disease recurrence. Total abdominal hysterectomy–bilateral salpingo-oophorectomy (TAH-BSO) is the definitive therapy for these women and they do not need to be offered adjuvant therapy.

Intermediate risk: Women with stage IC tumors or IA/IB, grade 3 tumors are at intermediate risk for recurrence of disease and may be offered adjuvant radiotherapy. In these women radiotherapy does not improve survival but reduces the risk of local disease recurrence.

High risk: Women with stage IC/grade 3 tumors and women with stage IIA or greater disease are at high risk of cancer recurrence. These women should have undergone maximal cytoreductive surgery with their TAH-BSO. All high-risk women should be offered adjuvant therapy. For women with high-risk cancer and organ-confined extra-uterine disease, radiotherapy is often recommended. For women with stage III or stage IV disease, adjuvant chemotherapy with doxorubicin and cisplatin results in better survival compared with whole abdominal radiotherapy (see Evidence Box 50.1). For women with gross residual disease or who have not received radiotherapy, the addition of paclitaxel to doxorubicin and cisplatin may improve response.

Post-treatment Follow-up

Most recurrences occur within 3 years of initial treatment. Approximately half of recurrences occur in the vagina or pelvis, and the remainder occur in the upper abdomen or lung. Most recurrences are associated with symptoms such as vaginal bleeding, abdominal or pelvic pain, cough, or unintended weight loss. The standard recommended follow-up includes physical exam and cervical cytology every 6 months for 2 years and then annually.

Treatment of Recurrent Disease

Radiotherapy, chemotherapy, and surgery are all utilized in the treatment of recurrent disease. Surgery and/or radiotherapy may be appropriate for site specific lesions, such as those in the vaginal vault. For widely metastatic recurrent disease, chemotherapy with doxorubicin, cisplatin, and paclitaxel may provide short-term benefit.

Uterine Sarcoma

Uterine sarcomas are uncommon tumors, representing less than 5% of all uterine cancers. They arise either from the connective tissue elements of the endometrium or the myometrium. Most sarcomas present as postmenopausal uterine bleeding with an enlarged uterus. The three common types of uterine sarcomas in adults are endometrial stromal sarcoma, leiomyomsarcoma, and undifferentiated endometrial sarcoma. Endometrial stromal sarcomas arise from the stromal elements of the endometrium and are typically well-differentiated tumors that are indolent in their clinical behavior. Leiomyosarcomas arise from myometrial cells. Histology demonstrates more than 10 mitoses per high power field, prominent cellular atypia, and areas of tumor necrosis.

Key Points

- Endometrial cancer is the most common gynecologic malignancy.
- There are two types of endometrial cancer. Type I is primarily induced by a hormone imbalance characterized by too much estrogen stimulation and too little progesterone to block estrogen-induced endometrial proliferation. A type I tumor typically presents as a low-grade tumor with endometrioid features. A type II tumor is not caused by estrogen stimulation and often presents as a high-grade tumor with papillary-serous or clear cell features.
- Women with endometrial cancer typically present with abnormal uterine bleeding. The cancer is diagnosed by endometrial biopsy. All postmenopausal women with uterine bleeding must have an endometrial sampling.
- The treatment of endometrial cancer is surgical and usually includes hysterectomy, bilateral salpingo-oophorectomy and staging of the tumor.

Evidence Box 50.1

Chemotherapy is more effective than whole-abdominal irradiation for the treatment of stage III or IV endometrial cancer.

Historically surgery and radiotherapy were the main treatments for advanced endometrial cancer. This clinical trial demonstrated that surgery plus chemotherapy is more effective than surgery plus radiotherapy for the treatment of advanced endometrial cancer.

In this trial, 396 women with stage III or IV endometrial cancer who had surgical staging (total hysterectomy, bilateral salpingo-oophorectomy, pelvic washings for cytology, lymph node dissection) were randomized to receive whole-abdominal irradiation (30 Gy in 20 fractions with a 15-Gy boost) or chemotherapy with seven cycles of doxorubicin 60 mg/m^2 plus cisplatin 50 mg/m^2. Following the surgical treatment, more than 85% of the subjects had only microscopic cancer at entry into the study. The median follow-up was 74 months. At 60 months, adjusting for stage, 55% of the chemotherapy and 42% of the irradiation patients were alive (death hazard ratio 0.68 favoring chemotherapy, P <0.01). At 60 months, 50% of the chemotherapy patients and 38% of the irradiation patients were disease-free. Greater acute toxicity including gastrointestinal toxicity, thrombocytopenia, neutropenia and infection was observed in the women treated with chemotherapy. Treatment contributed to the deaths of 4% of the chemotherapy patients and 2% of the irradiation patients.

Randall ME, Filiaci VL, Muss H, et al. Randomized phase III trial of whole-abdominal irradiation versus doxorubicin and cisplatin chemotherapy in advanced endometrial carcinoma: a Gynecologic Oncology Group Study. J Clin Oncol 2006;24:36–44.

Further Reading

de la Orden SG, Reza MM, Blasco JA, Andradas E, Callejo D, Pérez T. Laparoscopic hysterectomy in the treatment of endometrial cancer: a systematic review. *J Minim Invasive Gynecol* 2008;15(4):395–401

DeMichele A, Troxel AB, Berlin JA, et al. Impact of raloxifene or tamoxifen use on endometrial cancer risk: a population-based case-control study. *J Clin Oncol* 2008;26(25):4151–4159

Karlsson B, Granberg S, Wikland M, et al. Transvaginal ultrasonography of the endometrium in women with postmenopausal bleeding—a Nordic multicenter study. *Am J Obstet Gynecol* 1995;172(5):1488–1494

Lu KH, Schorge JO, Rodabaugh KJ, et al. Prospective determination of prevalence of lynch syndrome in young women with endometrial cancer. *J Clin Oncol* 2007;25(33):5158–5164

Malzoni M, Tinelli R, Cosentino F, et al. Total laparoscopic hysterectomy versus abdominal hysterectomy with lymphadenectomy for early-stage endometrial cancer: a prospective randomized study. Gynecol Oncol 2008

Patel AV, Feigelson HS, Talbot JT, et al. The role of body weight in the relationship between physical activity and endometrial cancer: results from a large cohort of US women. *Int J Cancer* 2008;123(8):1877–1882

Randall ME, Filiaci VL, Muss H, et al; Gynecologic Oncology Group Study. Randomized phase III trial of whole-abdominal irradiation versus doxorubicin and cisplatin chemotherapy in advanced endometrial carcinoma: a Gynecologic Oncology Group Study. *J Clin Oncol* 2006;24(1):36–44

51 Ovarian and Fallopian Tube Cysts and Tumors

Robert L. Barbieri

Ovarian Tumors

Evaluation of the Adnexal or Ovarian Mass

One of the common problems in gynecology is determining the optimal approach to the management of an adnexal or ovarian cyst or tumor. The term "adnexal" refers to both the fallopian tube and ovary and the connective structures immediately adjacent, including the upper portion of the broad ligament and mesosalpinx. It is often difficult to definitively determine if an adnexal lesion arises in the fallopian tube or ovary until surgical exploration. Consequently, "adnexal" is ordinarily used to indicate ambiguity about the structure causing the cyst or tumor.

The point prevalence of an ovarian cyst or tumor is about 8 % in premenopausal women and 2 % in postmenopausal women. Surgical exploration and cyst or tumor removal are required if there is a suspicion of malignancy. Central to the problem is using available data to make an estimate of the likelihood that a tumor is benign or malignant. In general, three factors guide the management of an adnexal or ovarian mass: the menopausal status of the patient; the appearance of the ovarian cyst or tumor on ultrasound imaging; and a serum CA-125 measurement.

Many different ovarian structures can give rise to cysts and tumors (**Fig. 51.1**). The approach to an ovarian cyst or tumor varies for premenopausal and postmenopausal women. In premenopausal women the differential diagnosis is very broad (**Table 51.1**) and ultrasonography plays the key role in determining whether the tumor is benign or malignant, and whether the tumor requires surgery. Ultrasonographic findings which suggest that a malignant tumor is present include: a solid tumor with irregular borders; ascites; four or more papillary structures in the cyst or tumor; diameter greater than 10 cm; and Doppler demonstration of significant blood flow into the cyst or tumor. Ultrasonographic findings which suggest that an ovarian cyst is benign include: a unilocular cyst; no solid component greater than 0.7 cm in diameter; smooth cyst or tumor surfaces; and Doppler demonstration of no significant blood flow into the cyst or tumor.

In premenopausal women the most commonly detected adnexal cyst is a functional ovarian cyst, which arises from the normal process of ovarian follicular growth, ovulation, and corpus luteum formation. The epithelium lining of an ovarian follicular cyst has basal tight junctions that permit the epithelium to secrete fluid into the closed space, permitting the cyst to grow. Most follicular cysts resolve over one or two months and can be followed to resolution using pelvic ultrasound examination.

In postmenopausal women, ultrasonography plus measurement of serum CA-125 play the key role in assessing whether the tumor is malignant. In postmenopausal women with an ovarian cyst or tumor, a CA-125 level equal to or greater than 35 IU/L suggests the presence of an ovarian or fallopian tube malignancy. In premenopausal women the CA-125 level is often elevated due to benign pelvic diseases such as endometriosis or

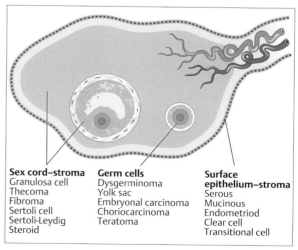

Sex cord–stroma	Germ cells	Surface epithelium–stroma
Granulosa cell	Dysgerminoma	Serous
Thecoma	Yolk sac	Mucinous
Fibroma	Embryonal carcinoma	Endometriod
Sertoli cell	Choriocarcinoma	Clear cell
Sertoli-Leydig	Teratoma	Transitional cell
Steroid		

Fig. 51.1 The myriad of ovarian tumor histological subtypes are derived from the surface epithelium–stroma, germ cells, or sex cord–stromal elements. Adapted from UpToDate – Origins of ovarian tumors.

Table 51.1 Differential diagnosis of ovarian and adnexal cysts and tumors in premenopausal women

Processes arising from the ovary
Simple follicular cysts
Corpus luteum cysts
Hemorrhagic cysts
Polycystic ovary syndrome
Theca lutein cysts
Endometrioma
Sex cord stromal tumors
Germ cell tumors • Mature teratoma (dermoid) • Immature (malignant) teratoma

Ovarian epithelial tumors
• Benign ovarian epithelial tumors
  – Serous cystadenoma
  – Mucinous cystadenoma
• Malignant ovarian epithelial tumors
  – Serous ovarian cancer
  – Mucinous ovarian cancer
  – Endometrioid ovarian cancer
  – Clear cell ovarian cancer

Processes arising from outside the ovary
Hydrosalpinx
Paraovarian cyst
Peritoneal inclusion cyst
Ectopic pregnancy
Pedunculated fibroid
Diverticular abscess
Colon cancer
Fallopian tube cancer
Inflammatory bowel disease
Pancreatic pseudocyst
Pelvic kidney

fibroid tumors. Consequently, in premenopausal women the CA-125 measurement is not specific for the diagnosis of ovarian malignancy. CA-125 is much more sensitive and specific for the diagnosis of ovarian malignancy in postmenopausal women, in whom a CA-125 level greater than 100 IU/L strongly suggests the presence of an ovarian malignancy. Many authorities recommend that a postmenopausal woman with an ovarian cyst or tumor and a CA-125 level greater than 100 IU/L should be immediately referred to a gynecologic oncologist, so that cy-

toreductive surgery can be accomplished, if necessary, at the initial surgery.

Ovarian Torsion

Ovarian torsion involves the twisting of the ovary around its pedicle causing a reduction or cessation in blood flow to the ovary, which incites severe lower abdominal pain, nausea, and pelvic tenderness. Ovarian torsion is a common gynecologic emergency. The presentation is non-pecific with both severe abdominal/pelvic pain and an adnexal mass being present in over 85 % of women with torsion. Laparoscopy is required to definitively diagnose or exclude ovarian torsion. When the diagnosis of ovarian torsion is raised in a woman with lower abdominal/pelvic pain and an ovarian or fallopian tube cyst, laparoscopy is required to confirm that the diagnosis is correct. If blood flow to the ovary has ceased, all ovarian tissue on the affected side may die within 12 hours unless the ovary and vascular pedicle are untwisted at surgery.

Epithelial Ovarian Tumors

Ovarian Tumors of Low Malignant Potential

Ovarian tumors of low malignant potential (also known as borderline tumors) have two common histological patterns: serous (histology similar to the fallopian tube), or mucinous (histology similar to the cervix glands). Ovarian tumors of low malignant potential are often unilateral and stage I or II at the time of diagnosis and surgical treatment. Conservative surgical approaches with preservation of fertility can be achieved by performing a unilateral salpingo-oophorectomy and staging, thereby conserving the contralateral ovary and uterus. Chemotherapy does not play a significant role in the treatment of these tumors.

Ovarian Epithelial Cancer

Ovarian cancer is the most common gynecologic malignancy that causes death. Following breast, lung, and colon cancer, it is the fourth most common cause of cancer death in women living in developed countries. Of all cancer deaths in women, about 6 % are due to ovarian cancer. Ninety percent of ovarian tumors are epithelial, consisting of five histological subtypes: serous, mucinous, endometrioid, clear cell, or transitional cell. These histological types recapitulate the development of the müllerian tract:
- The serous histology best resembles the epithelium of the fallopian tube.
- The mucinous histology best resembles the epithelium of the cervix.

- The endometrioid histology resembles the endometrium.
- The clear cell histology resembles the pelvic peritoneum.

Most cases of ovarian epithelial cancer (OEC) are diagnosed in women between 40 and 65 years of age.

Epidemiology: The lifetime risk of developing OEC is 1.5%. Most women with OEC will die of the disease. Repetitive ovulation and stimulation by gonadotropins are two proposed mechanisms which link various reproductive exposures and the risk of ovarian cancer. Exposures that reduce the risk of developing OEC include:
- prolonged use of estrogen–progestin contraceptives
- multiparity
- tubal ligation
- prolonged intervals of breast-feeding

Exposures and diseases that increase the risk of OEC include:
- infertility and nulliparity
- early menarche or late menopause
- endometriosis
- exposure to talc

Germ-line mutations in *BRCA1*, *BRCA2* and the DNA repair genes (*MSH2*, *MLH1*, *PMS1*) are associated with an increased risk of ovarian cancer. Interestingly recent pathological studies suggest that in women with BRCA1 mutations, ovarian cancer lesions actually begin in the distal fallopian tube and then spread to the ovary and other peritoneal surfaces (see Chapter 45).

History and physical examination: OEC is a "silent" killer. It is often very difficult to diagnose OEC prior to its reaching an advanced stage (stage III or IV). Most medical organizations recommend against screening in the general population. But recent recommendations are to be vigilant about early symptoms of ovarian cancer to pursue early detection. The six symptoms that are most highly and reliably associated with a diagnosis of ovarian cancer are pelvic pain, abdominal pain, increased abdominal circumference, abdominal bloating, early satiety, and difficulty eating. Up to 70% of women with ovarian cancer report these symptoms for up to a year before their cancer diagnosis. If these symptoms occur at least 12 days a month, investigations including physical examination, CA-125 testing, and pelvic sonography may be warranted.

Physical examination using bimanual pelvic examination to detect an ovarian tumor has low sensitivity and specificity. In overweight and obese women it is unusual to palpate an adnexal mass on bimanual examination, even if a large cystic structure is demonstrated on ultrasound imaging (low sensitivity). In thin, premenopausal women, it is usual to palpate an ovary, but unless the ovary is significantly enlarged (>5 cm) it is unlikely to represent an ovarian tumor. In postmenopausal women, all palpated adnexal masses should be evaluated with a pelvic ultrasound exam and CA-125 measurement. For premenopausal women with an adnexal mass palpated on bimanual pelvic examination, pelvic ultrasonography is usually warranted.

Pelvic ultrasonography and CA-125 measurement: Ultrasonographic findings which suggest that a malignant tumor is present include: a solid tumor with irregular borders; ascites; four or more papillary structures in the cyst or tumor; diameter greater than 10 cm; and Doppler demonstration of significant blood flow into the cyst or tumor. Ultrasound findings which suggest that an ovarian cyst or tumor is benign include: a unilocular cyst; no solid component greater than 0.7 cm; smooth cyst or tumor surfaces; Doppler demonstration of no significant blood flow into the cyst or tumor.

Postmenopausal women with a simple ovarian cyst of less than 5 cm in diameter and a normal CA-125 level (<35 IU/L) can typically be followed-up with serial physical examination and pelvic ultrasound exam.

In postmenopausal women with a serum CA-125 level equal to or greater than 35 IU/L, ovarian cancer is often present. In premenopausal women, elevated serum CA-125 levels may be due to cancer or other benign gynecologic lesions such as endometrioma cysts of the ovary. More than 80% of women with OEC have an elevated serum concentration of CA-125 (≥35 IU/L). OEC with a serous histology is more likely to show an elevated CA-125 level than OEC with a mucinous histology.

Prior to surgical resection of a suspicious ovarian mass, women should be screened for colon cancer, have a recent mammogram, and undergo cervical cytology.

Surgical–pathological diagnosis: Surgical removal of a concerning adnexal cyst is the only method for definitively identifying the histology of the cyst and is simultaneously the first step in staging and treatment of ovarian tumors. Gynecologic oncologists are more likely to thoroughly complete a full surgical staging than general gynecologists and therefore, when available, they should lead the surgical diagnosis and treatment of these lesions. The FIGO (International Federation of Gynecology and Obstetrics) staging system is presented in **Table 51.2**. Sixty percent of women with OEC present at stage III or IV disease, which is associated with a less than 30% 5-year survival rate. The late stage of diagnosis and the high mortality rate makes OEC a fearsome cancer.

The steps in the surgical staging procedure include:
1. Collection of peritoneal fluid and peritoneal washings for cytology
2. Removal of affected adnexa and examination of a frozen section to confirm the diagnosis

Table 51.2 Ovarian cancer 5-year survival rate by FIGO* stage

Stage		Description	5-year survival rate
I		Tumor limited to the ovaries	
	A	Growth limited to one ovary, capsule intact	89%
	B	Growth limited to two ovaries, no malignant peritoneal cells	65%
	C	Tumor on surface of ovary or peritoneal fluid has cancer cells	78%
II		Tumor extends beyond ovary to the pelvic organs	
	A	Metastases to the uterus or fallopian tubes.	79%
	B	Metastases to other pelvic tissues.	64%
	C	Stage IIA or IIB tumor with ruptured ovarian capsule, or peritoneal fluid has cancer cells.	68%
III		Tumor extends to peritoneal implants outside the pelvis or positive lymph nodes	
	A	On visual surgical inspection, tumor limited to the pelvis, but microscopic analysis demonstrates tumor seeding on peritoneal surfaces outside the pelvis	49%
	B	Tumor implants present on peritoneal surfaces, <2 cm in diameter.	41%
	C	Peritoneal implants >2 cm and/or tumor positive retroperitoneal or inguinal lymph nodes.	29%
IV		Tumor has distant metastasis. Cancer cells in a pleural effusion or liver parenchymal tumor is stage IV.	13%

* International Federation of Gynecology and Obstetrics.

3. Biopsies of peritoneal surfaces, including the cul-de-sac, bladder peritoneum, paracolic gutters, and bowel mesentery
4. Total omentectomy
5. Pelvic and para-aortic node sampling
6. Appendectomy
7. Completion of hysterectomy and bilateral salpingo-oophorectomy
8. Cytoreduction of all visible lesions

For optimal cytoreduction, bowel resection, stripping of disease from the diaphragm, and splenectomy may be necessary. Radical debulking may include distal pancre-atectomy, liver resection, and dissection of tumor from the porta hepatis. Optimal cytoreduction involves leaving no cancer lesion more than 1 cm in diameter. At the end of the procedure a peritoneal port may be placed to allow for intraperitoneal chemotherapy. This extensive pelvic–abdominal surgery carries a high postoperative morbidity, including an increased risk for thromboembolic events, massive shifts in fluids, hemorrhage, and infection.

Treatment: *Platinum plus paclitaxel are standard agents for the treatment of advanced ovarian cancer.* Approximately 60% of women with ovarian cancer present with stage III or IV disease. The standard approach to their treatment is optimal cytoreductive surgery (which also achieves accurate surgical staging) followed by platinum-based chemotherapy. Clinical trials comparing tumor response to dual-agent treatment with cyclophosphamide and doxorubicin versus doxorubicin and platinum demonstrated that complete response rate was 51% with platinum-based regimen compared with a 26% response with the doxorubicin regimen. Carboplatin and cisplatin are equally efficacious in the treatment of ovarian epithelial cancer. Beginning in 1990s, paclitaxel plus platinum began to replace doxorubicin plus platinum for chemotreatment of ovarian cancer.

The biology of ovarian cancer is characterized by spread of metastases along peritoneal surfaces. The "pumping" action of the diaphragm with each breath may contribute to the circulation of tumor cells throughout the abdomen along peritoneal surfaces. Intraperitoneal (IP) chemotherapy with paclitaxel permits achieving peritoneal concentrations up to 1000 times greater than those achieved by intravenous (IV) treatment. Randomized clinical trials have demonstrated that IV paclitaxel plus IP cisplatin and paclitaxel resulted in superior survival than treatment with IV paclitaxel plus cisplatin alone, that is 66 months versus 50 months, respectively (Evidence Box 51.1). A common approach is to place an IP catheter at the conclusion of cytoreductive surgery in order to facilitate IP chemotherapy, if surgical staging demonstrates that postoperative chemotherapy is warranted.

Ovarian Cancer in Pregnant Women

The five most common cancers diagnosed during pregnancy are breast, thyroid, cervix, lymphoma, and ovary. About 2% of pregnant women have a clinically significant ovarian cyst or tumor and of these lesions about 1% are malignant OECs and 1% are ovarian tumors of low malignant potential. Among pregnant women with an ovarian tumor or cyst, only surgical resection can achieve a definitive diagnosis. Ultrasonography is often used to estimate the risk of malignancy and to determine whether surgery should occur during the pregnancy or await delivery. For a woman with ovarian cancer diagnosed during pregnancy, chemotherapy treatment is guided by the trimester of pregnancy. If a woman is within 3 weeks of delivery, chemotherapy is usually delayed until delivery. If a woman is in the third trimester but delivery is not imminent, treatment with carboplatin or cisplatin is often recommended.

Cancer Metastatis to the Ovary

Extra-ovarian cancers metastatic to the ovary represent about 5% of ovarian tumors. Bowel and breast cancers are the most likely to metastasize to the ovary. These tumors metastatic to the ovary are often called Krukenberg tumors. The histology of these tumors typically demonstrates mucinous carcinomas with Signet-ring patterns. In addition, lymphomas, bladder, and head and neck tumors may metastasize to the ovary.

Risk-Reducing Bilateral Salpingo-Oophorectomy in Women at High Risk for Ovarian Cancer

Women with germ-line mutations in BRCA1, BRCA2 or DNA repair genes are at increased risk for ovarian and breast cancer. These women may opt for risk-reducing bilateral salpingo-oophorectomy when they have completed their family. This surgery reduces the risk of ovarian, fallopian tube, or primary peritoneal cancer by about 90%. At the time of risk-reducing surgery, about 5% of women are diagnosed as having an occult ovarian or fallopian tube cancer. Risk-reducing surgery must include a salpingectomy because many ovarian cancers begin in the distal portion of the fallopian tube in these women.

Germ Cell Tumors

Consistent with their name, germ cell tumors arise from primordial germ cells of the ovary and include the following tumor types: teratoma (mature, immature and monodermal), dysgerminoma, yolk sac tumors, embryonal carcinoma, and choriocarcinoma. They represent about 20% of all ovarian tumors and most commonly occur in women 10–30 years of age. The most common germ cell tumor is the mature teratoma, also commonly referred to as a "dermoid" cyst. Women with germ cell tumors often present with pelvic or lower abdominal pain. The tumor is typically identified on pelvic sonography obtained in response to the symptom of pelvic pain. These tumors are

Table 51.3 Ovarian germ cell serum tumor markers

Tumor	Serum HCG	Serum AFP	Serum LDH
Immature teratoma	No	No	No
Choriocarcinoma	Yes	No	Sometimes
Embryonal carcinoma	Yes	Yes (70% of cases)	Sometimes
Dysgerminoma	Not usually (10% are positive for HCG)	No	Yes
Endodermal sinus tumor	No	Yes	No

HCG, human chorionic gonadotropin; AFP, α-fetoprotein; LDH, lactate dehydrogenase.

most often unilateral. Unlike malignant OECs which are typically stage III, most germ cell tumors are stage I. Most germ cell tumors secrete tumor markers which can used to follow the success of surgical therapy (**Table 51.3**).

Teratomas

Mature teratomas, the "dermoid" cysts, are the most common of all germ cell tumors. They are benign, usually cystic lesions, containing tissue from all embryonic layers including ectodermal (accounting for the hair, sebaceous material, and skin seen in these tumors), mesodermal, and endodermal components. About 10% of these tumors are bilateral. The Rokitansky tubercle is a solid nodule located at the junction between the teratoma and the ovary. This area has the greatest cellular variety making it a focus for pathological analysis. Cystectomy is definitive therapy. If inspection of the contralateral ovary is normal, it need not be biopsied. During surgery the sebaceous contents may spill, which can cause peritonitis if left in the abdomen.

Monodermal teratomas are specialized tumors that contain a predominant histological cell type such as thyroid tissue (struma ovarii) or a carcinoid tumor.

Immature teratomas are rare teratomas that contain immature cells differentiating toward nerve, bone, muscle, and glands. The tumors are graded histologically based on the amount of immature neural elements. Tumor grade is a predictor of extra-ovarian spread of disease.

Dysgerminomas

All dysgerminomas are malignant. Dysgerminomas are the female manifestation of a tumor similar to the male testicular seminoma. Dysgerminomas account for only 2% of all germ cell tumors, but 50% of all malignant germ cell tumors. They typically occur in young women. Phenotypic females with a Y chromosome are at increased risk of developing a gonadoblastoma, which then can evolve to contain a dysgerminoma. In these women both gonads need to be surgically removed. If the dysgerminoma is limited within the capsule of the ovary, salpingo-oophorectomy is curative in almost all cases. Chemotherapy may be recommended when the tumor has extended beyond the ovary.

Endodermal Sinus Tumor

Endodermal sinus tumor has histological features similar to the endodermal sinuses of the rodent yolk sac and is derived from the primitive yolk sac. These tumors occur in girls, teenagers, and young women. The tumors are usually treated with both surgery and bleomycin, etoposide, and cisplatin.

Embryonal Carcinoma

Embryonal carcinoma is a rare germ cell tumor that resembles the embryonal carcinoma of the testis and occurs in teenagers. It is very aggressive and is usually treated with both surgery and bleomycin, etoposide, and cisplatin.

Choriocarcinoma

This tumor is discussed in Chapter 46.

Sex Cord–Stromal Tumors

Sex cord-stromal tumors arise from granulosa, thecal, and stromal cells of the ovary. These cells are neither germ cells nor epithelial cells. These tumors account for about 5% of all ovarian tumors. Thecal cells are the ovarian homologue of testicular Leydig cells, and granulosa cells are the ovarian homologue of Sertoli cells. Consequently, some tumors of the granulosa and thecal cells can take on histological features of Leydig or Sertoli cells. Most ovarian sex cord-stromal tumors secrete steroid hormones. In the normal ovary the granulosa cell secretes estradiol, and the thecal and stromal cells secreteandrogens. When a girl has a sex cord-stromal tumor (granulosa cell) secreting estrogen, she may present with precocious puberty or, if secreting androgen (thecal cell), she may present with virilization.

Fibromas

Fibromas are the most common sex cord–stromal tumors. They are benign solid tumors that most commonly occur in postmenopausal women and do not secrete estrogen or androgen. The presence of an ovarian fibroma plus ascites or pleural effusion is the "Meigs syndrome" and is likely caused by the secretion of vasoactive peptides, such as vascular endothelial growth factor, from the tumor. Unilateral salpingo-oophorectomy is the definitive treatment for a fibroma.

Granulosa–Stromal Cell Tumors

These represent about 70% of all sex cord–stromal tumors and occur in females of all ages. In the adult subtype of granulosa cell tumors, the cells arrange themselves in clusters around a central cavity, the so-called "Call–Exner body." Since the tumors can secrete estrogen, abnormal uterine bleeding is a common symptom and endometrial hyperplasia is often diagnosed on endometrial biopsy. Left untreated, granulosa cell tumors can cause endometrial cancer. The average diameter of a granulosa cell tumor at the time of diagnosis is about 10 cm. These masses are sufficiently large that they can often be detected on bimanual pelvic examination. Granulosa cells and granulosa cell tumors (and some mucinous epithelial ovarian tumors) produce inhibin A, inhibin B, and anti-müllerian hormone (AMH) in large quantities. Measurement of inhibin B, inhibin A, or AMH can be used as a tumor marker.

Complete surgical resection is the first-line treatment of granulosa cell tumors. In postmenopausal and perimenopausal women, and women with advanced disease, the surgical procedure of choice is a total hysterectomy plus bilateral salpingo-oophorectomy with pelvic and para-aortic lymph node dissection. In young women with stage I disease, a unilateral salpingo-oophorectomy along with peritoneal cell cytology and multiple biopsies is appropriate treatment if preservation of reproductive potential is desired. In all women with a granulosa cell tumor, endometrial biopsy to rule out cancer is necessary. For women with stage IA disease, surgery is definitive therapy and no adjuvant treatment is needed. Recurrence can be assessed by sequential measurement of inhibin B.

In women with advanced disease, chemotherapy with bleomycin, etoposide, and cisplatin is the preferred regimen.

Thecomas

Thecomas are benign, large, solid, unilateral ovarian tumors that arise from the theca cells of the ovary and typically occur in postmenopausal women. Thecomas typical consist of mixes of thecal and granulosa cells, and secrete estrogen. Abnormal uterine bleeding due to unopposed estrogen stimulation of the endometrium is a common presenting symptom. Since thecomas typically occur in postmenopausal women, the recommended therapy is total hysterectomy plus bilateral salpingo-oophorectomy.

Sertoli–Leydig Cell Tumors

These tumors resemble the histology of the testis, with hollow or solid tubules surrounded by cells with a Sertoli appearance and Leydig-like cells in the stroma. Most of these tumors are large and unilateral. They produce androgens resulting in a clinical picture ranging from hirsutism to full virilization (balding, clitoromegaly, deep voice, upper body muscle prominence). For women who have completed childbearing, total hysterectomy plus bilateral salpingo-oophorectomy is recommended. Unilateral salpingo-oophorectomy is appropriate for women desiring to preserve fertility. Metastatic disease or recurrence, which occurs in about 20% of cases, is most often treated with bleomycin, etoposide, and cisplatin.

Fallopian Tube and Mesosalpingeal Cysts

Vestigial structures derived from the wolffian duct, tubal epithelium, or peritoneum can develop into simple cysts in the mesosalpinx. Cystic structures can form from the serosa at the distal end of the fallopian tube producing the hydatid cysts of Morgagni.

Fallopian Tube Cancer

Adenocarcinoma of the fallopian tube is an uncommon tumor and represents less than 1% of gynecologic malignancy. Many women with fallopian tube malignancy are diagnosed between age 50 and 60 years. Women with fallopian tube malignancy often present with a watery vaginal discharge (due to fluid secretion into the tubal lumen) or bleeding, an adnexal cyst, and lower abdominal pain. The CA-125 level is typically elevated in women with fallopian tube cancer. These tumors are surgically staged using a FIGO system similar to that used for ovarian cancer (see **Table 51.2**).

Key Points

- Ovarian cancer is the second most common gynecologic malignancy, after endometrial cancer. Ovarian cancer is commonly diagnosed at an advanced stage of the disease, stage III or stage IV. Consequently, it is the most common cause of death from gynecologic malignancy.
- Ultrasonography is commonly used to help differentiate a benign ovarian cyst from a cyst with the potential to be malignant. Ultrasonographic findings which suggest an ovarian

cyst is benign include: a unilocular cyst; no solid component; smooth cyst or tumor surfaces; no blood flow into the cyst on Doppler imaging; and a cyst <5 cm in diameter.
- The serum tumor marker CA-125 is useful in identifying postmenopausal women with an ovarian cyst who may be at increased risk for ovarian cancer.
- Women who are suspected of having ovarian cancer should be referred to specialists for initial treatment.
- The initial step in the treatment of ovarian cancer is complete surgical staging and maximal resection of disease, also known as cytoreductive surgery.
- Following surgery, chemotherapy for ovarian cancer often includes platinum and paclitaxel. The biology of ovarian cancer is characterized by the spread of metastases along peritoneal surfaces. Intraperitoneal chemotherapy should be considered in women with advanced ovarian cancer.

Evidence Box 51.1

The combination of optimal cytoreductive surgery plus both intravenous and intraperitoneal chemotherapy significantly improves the survival of women with stage III ovarian cancer.

In this trial 415 women with stage III ovarian cancer who had undergone optimal cytoreductive surgery (defined as residual tumor nodules <1 cm in diameter) were randomized to receive six treatment cycles of either standard intravenous chemotherapy with paclitaxel plus cisplatin, or experimental chemotherapy with intravenous paclitaxel plus intraperitoneal cisplatin plus paclitaxel. The median survival was 50 months in the standard intravenous chemotherapy group and 66 months in the experimental intravenous plus intraperitoneal therapy group (P <0.03). In the subgroup of women from this trial who underwent a "second look" surgical staging and treatment operation, 41% of the women in the standard intravenous chemotherapy group and 57% of the women in the experimental group had a complete pathological response with no residual tumor.

Although the experimental therapy was associated with the longest median survival ever reported in a large trial for stage III ovarian cancer, significant side effects were experienced by these women. Women treated with combined intravenous plus intraperitoneal chemotherapy had significantly more leukopenia, thrombocytopenia, abdominal pain, and gastrointestinal and neurologic symptoms than women receiving standard intravenous chemotherapy. The combined intravenous plus intraperitoneal chemotherapy was so toxic that only 42% of the women in this group were able to complete the full 6 cycles of the protocol. In contrast, 83% of the women in the standard intravenous therapy group completed 6 cycles of chemotherapy.

Optimal outcome with combined intravenous and intraperitoneal chemotherapy requires successful cytoreductive surgery and the placement of an intraperitoneal catheter. To minimize surgery it is often best to place an intraperitoneal catheter at the end of the cytoreductive surgery, so that it can be used postoperatively without requiring another operation.

Armstrong DK, Bundy B, Wenzel L, et al. Intraperitoneal cisplatin and paclitaxel in ovarian cancer. N Engl J Med 2006;354:34–43.

Further Reading

Armstrong DK, Bundy B, Wenzel L, et al; Gynecologic Oncology Group. Intraperitoneal cisplatin and paclitaxel in ovarian cancer. *N Engl J Med* 2006;354(1):34–43

Goff BA, Mandel LS, Drescher CW, et al. Development of an ovarian cancer symptom index: possibilities for earlier detection. *Cancer* 2007;109(2):221–227

Omura GA, Bundy BN, Berek JS, Curry S, Delgado G, Mortel R. Randomized trial of cyclophosphamide plus cisplatin with or without doxorubicin in ovarian carcinoma: a Gynecologic Oncology Group Study. *J Clin Oncol* 1989;7(4):457–465

Pectasides D, Pectasides E, Psyrri A. Granulosa cell tumor of the ovary. *Cancer Treat Rev* 2008;34(1):1–12

Timmerman D, Testa AC, Bourne T, et al. Simple ultrasound-based rules for the diagnosis of ovarian cancer. *Ultrasound Obstet Gynecol* 2008;31(6):681–690

Part VI Human Sexuality

52 Sexuality

Robert L. Barbieri

Sexuality is a central part of human experience (**Fig. 52.1**). Sexual dysfunction is the inability to participate as desired in a sexual relationship. The causes of sexual dysfunction are complex. Problems of sexual function are best approached with a biopsychosocial model that recognizes the important contribution of biological, psychological, and social–cultural factors in sexual health.

Sexual Identity

Across mammalian species, haploid gametes can be reliably assigned to two categories: sperm (male), and oocytes (female). In contrast, it is not possible to assign all people to parallel, rigid, sexual identities such as male and female. Sexual identity is more plastic than biological or anatomical sex. Many people have blended sexual identities that combine features of male and female sexuality. In addition, about 1 in 10000 people who are genetically and anatomically male, strongly prefer a female sexual identity, and vice versa. Trans-sexuals are estranged from their own sex organs and seek a gender identity of the opposite sex. Transgendered individuals are estranged from their own sex organs but do not desire to seek full reassignment to the opposite sex, and seek an in-between sexual status.

Among many mammalian species, during embryonic development and fetal life, the brain is programmed toward a male or female pattern of sexuality. The programming is manifested in morphologic differences in brain nuclei and is associated with sex-specific behaviors such as copulatory positions. The programming occurs in fetal life and the dimorphic patterns of behavior become observable after being activated by the hormones of puberty. Fetal androgens appear to play a major role in causing differentiation of the brain nuclei to a male pattern. In humans, fetal programming is influenced by events in childhood and adolescence.

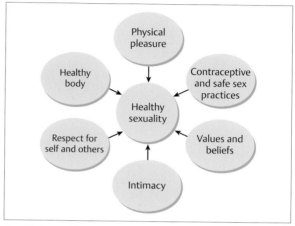

Fig. 52.1 Health sexuality is the product of multiple dimensions.

Sexual Response in Men and Women

Masters and Johnson posited that in men and women there are four stages of sexual response: excitement, plateau, orgasm, and resolution. Building on this linear model of sexual response, later investigators replaced excitement with two phases: desire, and arousal. This culminated in a five-stage linear model of sexual response:

1. Desire
2. Arousal
3. Plateau
4. Orgasm
5. Resolution

Recent models of sexual response have emphasized that a circular model, where sequential responses overlap and build on previous stimuli, may be more accurate. Recent models also emphasize the importance of emotional intimacy and the quality of the relationship between the two partners in the achievement of sexual health.

Sensory input and psychological fantasy stimulate the arousal response. In men, sexual arousal is anatomically evident by the development of penile tumescence or erection. In women arousal may result in vasocongestion of the clitoris, vagina, vulva, breasts and areola, transudation of vaginal fluid, and nipple erection. In men orgasm is manifested by contractions of the vas deferens, seminal vesicles, and prostate followed by contractions of the urethra and penile base muscles, which accompanies ejaculation. In women orgasm most often occurs separately from sexual intercourse, with manual or oral stimulation of the clitoris. In women, during orgasm the upper one-third of the vagina tents and becomes enlarged, while the lower one-third of the vagina narrows from muscular contractions involving the perineal, bulbocavernosus, and pubococcygeal muscles.

Table 52.2 Prevalence in men of lack of interest in sex, climax too early, and unable to maintain an erection stratified across four age groups (N = 1249)

Age group (years)	Lack of interest in sex (%)	Climax too early (%)	Unable to maintain an erection (%)
18–29	14%	30%	7%
30–39	13%	32%	9%
40–49	15%	28%	11%
50–59	17%	31%	18%

Source: Adopted from Laumann EO, Paik A, Rosen RC. Sexual dysfunction in the United States: prevalence and predictors. JAMA 1999;281:537–544.

Sexual Dysfunction in the General Population

Sexual dysfunction is the presence of disturbances in sexual desire and/or in the psychophysiological changes associated with the sexual response cycle. Approximately 40% of women and 30% of men report sexual dysfunction. Common problems reported by heterosexual women are: 1) a lack of interest in sex; 2) an inability to achieve orgasm; 3) pain caused by sexual intercourse; 4) lack of pleasure with sex; and 5) trouble lubricating (**Table 52.1**). Common problems reported by heterosexual men are: 1) lack of interest in sex; 2) orgasm occurs too early; 3) trouble maintaining an erection; 4) inability to achieve orgasm; and 5) anxiety about sexual performance (**Table 52.2**). In both men and women, poor overall health, mental health problems, poverty, and a history of sexual abuse increase the risk of sexual dysfunction.

Table 52.1 Prevalence in women of lack of interest in sex, inability to achieve an orgasm, and pain caused by sexual intercourse stratified across four age groups (N = 1486)

Age group (years)	Lack of interest in sex (%)	Unable to achieve orgasm (%)	Pain during sexual intercourse (%)
18–29	32%	26%	21%
30–39	32%	28%	15%
40–49	30%	22%	13%
50–59	27%	23%	8%

Source: Adopted from Laumann EO, Paik A, Rosen RC. Sexual dysfunction in the United States: prevalence and predictors. JAMA 1999;281:537–544.

The Sexual History

The majority of women and men will not volunteer to their clinician that they are having sexual problems. In one study only 3% of patients volunteered that they had a sexual problem, but when the same group of patients was directly asked by their clinician about sexual issues, 20% reported a sexual problem. It is important for clinicians to provide a supportive environment to discuss sexual problems, and to actively inquire about their presence. If a sexual disorder is identified, it may be helpful for the clinician to explicitly comment that these disorders are common in their practice and that it can be difficult for patients to openly discuss intimate sexual issues, but that by discussing these issues improvement will likely occur.

The sexual history may be initiated by asking, "Do you have any concerns about your sex life?" Additional open-ended questions that may be helpful include: Are you having sexual relations currently? With men or women or both? If you are not having sex, when did you last have intercourse? Are you satisfied with the frequency and quality of your sexual experiences? How many sexual partners do you have? What is the emotional quality and intimacy of your relationship with your sex partner(s)? A more thorough approach to the sexual history is presented in **Table 52.3**.

If a sexual concern is identified, the patient should describe her problem in detail, in her own words. Many women will report that they have decreased "libido," but on further questioning an orgasm or pain disorder is identified. Asking the patient to describe in detail a typical sexual interaction with her partner can be helpful too: Who initiates sexual play? What is the frequency of sexual relations? Are you feeling receptive when your partner initiates sexual play?

Table 52.3 The thorough sexual history uses a multifaceted approach to explore the factors influencing sexual health

Approach to the patient
Sexual function is influenced by many factors including biological, psychological, and social factors. Most sexual problems are best approached using a biopsychosocial model.

Chief Complaint and creation of a supportive environment
Elicit, in her own words, the concern the patient has with sex and sexual function. What problems are present in most situations? Have you had a change in your interest in sex? Do you have trouble becoming aroused or sufficiently lubricated? Are you able to have an orgasm by self-stimulation or with your partner? Do you have pain with sex?
Use open-ended questions. Explicitly acknowledge the potential embarrassment of the topic. Reassure the patient that sex problems are common. Counsel the patient that it is good to address these issues

Biological factors
• Evaluate the presence of chronic disease such as diabetes, cardiovascular, neurologic, or mental health diseases • Evaluate the impact of current medications on sexual function • Consider previous surgery, including pelvic surgeries, and obstetric history • Inquire about menstrual history and ovulatory status

Psychological factors
• Evaluate evidence for depression, anxiety, or premenstrual dysphoric disorder • Assess use of alcohol, recreational drugs, and tobacco • Inquire whether the patient has a history of sexual abuse or domestic violence. As a child, did the patient experience sexual touching? Assess relationships and sexual experiences during childhood and adolescence • Assess emotional intimacy of the couple • Inquire about sexual thoughts and fantasies

Social factors
• Evaluate family problems that might create stress, including problems with children and aging parents • Evaluate satisfaction with work and concerns about finances

Table 52.4 Approach to completing a gynecologic examination in women with sexual dysfunction.

Nongenital	Evidence for vascular disease: hypertension, decreased distal pulses.
	Evidence for musculoskeletal disease.
	Evidence of neurological disease.
External genitalia	Sparse pubic pilosebaceous units suggest low androgen levels.
	Assess for lichen sclerosis or lichen planus.
	Assess for fungal or viral diseases.
	Assess for dermatitis.
	Assess for atrophy.
	Assess clitoris for phimosis, adhesions
Introitus and vagina	Assess for evidence of inflammation or point tenderness.
	Assess for abnormalities of hymen.
	Assess for adequacy of estrogen stimulation of epithelium and the degree of lubrication.
Cervix, pelvic ligaments, pelvic muscles, adnexa	Assess for trigger points.
	Assess uterosacral ligaments for nodularity, thickening or tenderness.
	Assess adnexa for masses or tenderness.
	Assess uterus for size and tenderness.
Rectal	Assess for the presence of an anal wink

Source: Adopted from Basson R. Sexual desire and arousal disorders in women. N Engl J Med 2006;354:1497–1506.

The patient's medical history should also be assessed, because many chronic illnesses (diabetes, hypertension, cardiovascular diseases, cancer, neurologic disease), mental health issues (depression, anxiety), pain syndromes, or previous pelvic surgery (cystocele, rectocele repair) may influence sexual function. Many cardiovascular and mental health medications can contribute to sexual dysfunction.

A paper-based sexual function questionnaire, the Female Sexual Function Index, is available at the Web site: http://www.fsfi-questionnaire.com/, along with a scoring system. The 19 question instrument permits the differentiation of disorders of desire, arousal, lubrication, orgasm, satisfaction, and pain.

The physical examination can be tailored to the specific problem elicited on history. A general approach to the physical exam is presented in **Table 52.4**.

Common Sexual Problems in Women

Desire Disorders

There are two well-described sexual desire disorders:
1. Hypoactive sexual desire disorder (HSDD), which is the persistent or recurrent deficiency or absence of

sexual fantasies and/or sexual receptivity that causes personal distress

2. Sexual aversion disorder (SAD), which is defined as the persistent or recurrent extreme aversion to all, or almost all, sexual contact with a partner that causes personal distress. SAD is an extreme aversion to sexual contact and is similar to a phobia.

Arousal Disorders

There are two sexual arousal disorders:

1. Female sexual arousal disorder (FSAD) is the inability to attain or maintain sufficient sexual excitement due to either a lack of psychological excitement or a lack of physical manifestations of excitement such as absence of vaginal secretions. For example, a woman who is not lubricating and distressed by this fact may have FSAD.

2. Persistent genital arousal disorder (PGAD) is the persistent intrusive feeling of sexual arousal, such as vaginal congestion, in the absence of any sexual desire or interest that causes personal distress. An example of FSAD is a woman with an engorged clitoris and vaginal fullness, who is at work and has no conscious sexual fantasies or thoughts of sexual excitement. Some experts liken this condition to priapism in men.

Orgasm Disorders

Female orgasm disorder (FOD) is the persistent difficulty or delay in achieving an orgasm following sufficient sexual stimulation or arousal that causes personal distress. It can be primary, as in the case of a woman who has never experienced an orgasm, or secondary, as in the case of a woman who is unable to achieve orgasm owing to medication, aging, or medical problems.

Pain Disorders

There are four female sexual pain disorders: dyspareunia, vulvodynia, vaginismus, and noncoital nonsexual pain disorder.

Dysparuenia

Dyspareunia is the persistent or recurrent presence of genital pain associated with sexual intercourse that causes distress or interpersonal difficulty. Dyspareunia is commonly reported to occur at the entrance to the vagina, or deep in the pelvis, especially with penile thrusting, or both. Women with vulvovaginal disease are at increased risk for dyspareunia.

Vulvodynia

Vulvodynia is a common cause of sexual pain. It is a disorder of the vulva characterized by burning, stinging, rawness, and irritation. In vulvodynia there are not visible infectious, inflammatory, or neoplastic lesions. Vulvodynia may be provoked by sexual or nonsexual contact or unprovoked. Vestibulodynia refers to a subgroup of women with vulvodynia, where pain is localized to the vestibule and can be provoked by light contact.

Vaginismus

Vaginismus is the recurrent or persistent involuntary spasm of the musculature of the outer third of the vagina, which interferes with vaginal penetration and causes personal distress. In many women vaginismus is related to musculoskeletal problems that cause muscle spasm of the pelvic floor. Some women who have been sexually abused may develop vaginismus.

Noncoital Nonsexual Pain Disorder

Noncoital nonsexual pain disorder is the presence of genital pain during sexual stimulation that does not involve intercourse. The most common manifestation of this problem is clitorodynia which is the presence of pain or hypersensitivity with clitoral stimulation.

Treatment of Female Sexual Dysfunction

Most authorities recommend that the treatment of female sexual dysfunction include multiple modalities that reflect the complex biopsychosocial factors that cause the problem. For example, a treatment plan might include cognitive behavioral therapy, sex therapy, and appropriate medicines. The combination of cognitive behavioral therapy and sex therapy has been demonstrated to be superior to no treatment in one clinical trial.

Cognitive Behavioral Therapy

Cognitive behavioral therapy (CBT) focuses on modifying thoughts and emotions that are not constructive to a satisfying sexual life. Issues that may be explored include:
- self concepts about body image and body function
- developing constructive patterns of communication
- enhancing erotic stimulation and nongenital contact
- exploring approaches to building a more intimate and loving relationship, reducing disrespectful treatment of the partner

Sex Therapy

Sex therapy includes sensate focus experiences and bibliotherapy. The goal of sensate focus exercises is to increase the couple's emotional closeness and mastery of erotic stimulation. In an example of a sensate focus exercise, the couple is instructed to lie together in a warm, safe, cozy, and romantic setting. The couple is instructed to avoid genital intercourse and to begin by touching hands, face, and nongenital body parts. The couple gradually increases their touching in more intimate areas. In succeeding sensate focus sessions the couple gets undressed and begins to touch genital areas and touch breasts. The couple is encouraged to communicate their sensations and desires. Ultimately, penetrative sexual intercourse is recommended. Bibliotherapy, the reading of erotic material with or without self-stimulation or partner-stimulation, is another approach to developing more responsive sexual function.

Moisturizers and Lubricants

For women with a dry vagina or who have difficulty lubricating before sexual intercourse, the use of a moisturizing agent on a regular basis and a lubricant during intercourse may be helpful. One long-acting vaginal moisturizer is a polycarbophil biopolymer (Replens) that sticks to the vaginal epithelium and slowly releases water to produce a moist coating over the vaginal epithelium. A water-soluble lubricant such as Astroglide or K-Y Personal lubricant can be used with sexual intercourse. Some authorities recommend the use of vegetable oils, such as Crisco or olive oil as oil-based lubricants.

Physical Therapy and Mechanical Stimulators

The Eros therapy device is a handheld vacuum device that is applied in the area of the clitoris and is thought to increase blood flow to the genital area by creating a light suction effect. It is used three to four times per week either before sexual relations, or independent of sex.

Hormonal Medications

Estrogen

Women with a dry vagina who do not respond sufficiently to treatment with a moisturizer and lubricant can be offered low-dose vaginal estradiol treatment. In hypoestrogenic women, vaginal estradiol can acidify vaginal pH, increase the growth of the vaginal epithelium, and increase vaginal and cervical secretions. Many authorities believe that vaginal estradiol is the most effective treatment for women with severe vaginal dryness. Vaginal estradiol can be effective when it is administered in very low doses, such as 10–25 µg of estradiol daily. (Preovulatory ovarian estradiol production is in the range of 300 µg daily). Vaginal tablets of estradiol are available in doses of 10 µg and 25 µg. A vaginal estradiol ring, Estring, releases 6–9 µg of estradiol daily. Another vaginal estradiol ring, Femring, releases 50–100 µg of estradiol daily. Vaginal estradiol creams are available formulated as native estradiol, estrone sulfate, or conjugated equine estrogens.

Estrogens clearly improve vaginal dryness in postmenopausal women, and may improve sexual function in these women. However, in women whose main complaint is decreased desire or arousal, estrogen has not been definitively demonstrated to improve sexual function.

Androgens

With aging and the menopause transition, serum levels of androgens decrease, including dehydroepiandrosterone, androstenedione, and testosterone. In women with adrenal insufficiency, replacement of androgens has been reported to improve sexual function, including improvements in desire, arousal, and frequency of satisfying sexual relations. In women who undergo bilateral oophorectomy, circulating testosterone and androstenedione decrease to a greater degree than the decrease observed with menopause or aging alone. In these women, testosterone treatment has been reported to increase the frequency of satisfying sexual relations, but the clinical impact is modest, averaging about one more satisfying sexual experience per month (see Evidence Box 52.1). Androgen treatment is clearly not a panacea for postmenopausal women with sexual dysfunction.

Nonhormonal Medications

Zestra is an over-the-counter topical treatment that has been reported to improve sexual function in women with female sexual arousal disorder. Zestra is an oil-based blend of borage seed oil, primrose oil, *Angelica* root extract, *Coleus forskohli* extract, ascorbyl palmitate, dl-α-tocopherol, and fragrances. It is applied to the vulva a few times per week. It should not be used on the introitus because this increases the risk of causing a sensation of burning. In one pilot study, Zestra increased sexual arousal compared with placebo.

ArginMax is an over-the-counter oral nutritional supplement that contains l-arginine, ginseng, ginkgo biloba, damiana leaf, multiple vitamins, and minerals. It is thought to increase blood flow to the genital organs and facilitates arousal. In one clinical trial women treated with ArginMax reported increased desire and sexual intercourse compared with women treated with placebo.

Adolescent Sexuality

Approximately 50% of high school students have had sexual intercourse. The prevalence of sexual intercourse increases from about 25% at age 15 years to about 60% at age 18 years. Among many adolescents, contraceptives and safe-sex practices are not consistently used and many unintended pregnancies and sexually transmitted diseases (STDs) occur in this age group. Parents may be reluctant to discuss contraceptive and STD issues with adolescents, and health care providers play a lead role in providing this counseling to adolescents. Clinicians should

ensure that these discussions occur in private and away from parents or peers. Clinicians can reduce the discomfort of adolescents to discuss issues of sexual health by being comfortable asking about sexual orientation and contraceptive practices.

Postpartum Sexual Dysfunction

Most women resume sexual intercourse within 6 weeks following delivery. The majority of postpartum women report decreased sexual desire. Women who are breast-feeding are more likely to report decreased desire and dry vagina than women who are not. Breast-feeding is associated with less ovarian estradiol production and a greater risk of vaginal dryness. In postpartum women with vaginal dryness, a moisturizer and lubricant, or vaginal estradiol may be help improve vaginal lubrication.

Sexuality in Chronic Illness

There is a high prevalence of sexual dysfunction in people with chronic diseases and in the final years of life. Among patients receiving some care at hospices about two-thirds reported problems with sexual interest or activity. Interestingly, less than 10% of patients in palliative care programs reported being asked about their sexual function. In the evaluation of sexual problems of patients near the end of life there is a high prevalence of fatigue, dyspnea, depression, and altered body image, and these factors should be evaluated. Counseling and treatment should focus on giving patients permission to express their sexuality, providing medical information as needed to address specific problems, and giving suggestions to enhance sexual function (moisturizers and lubricants).

Sexuality in Older Adults

With aging, men and women report decreases in sexual activity. At 65–74 years and 75–85 years of age, 40% and 17% of women, resectively, report sexual activity with a partner in the past 12 months. Among the same two age groups, 22% and 16% reported masturbating within the past 12 months. Women in poor health reported less sexual activity and less satisfying sexual activity. Women were less likely than men to discuss their sex problem with a physician. Counseling and treatment may focus on giving permission to express their sexuality and suggestions to enhance sexual function.

Sexual activity is an important contributor to perceived quality of life for most people. Surveys indicate that most clinicians are not routinely exploring the issue of sexuality with their patients.

Key Points

- The linear model of sexual response: 1) desire, 2) arousal, 3) plateau, 4) orgasm, and 5) resolution has evolved into a more circular model, where sequential responses overlap and build on previous stages.
- The majority of men and women will not volunteer to their clinicians that they are having sexual problems. Screening for sexual problems requires establishing an empathic and supportive environment and directly asking questions such as: Do you have any concerns about your sex life? Are you having sexual relations currently? Are you satisfied with the frequency and quality of your sexual experiences? What is the emotional quality and intimacy of your relationship with our sex partner(s)?
- There are two recognized disorders of sexual desire: hypoactive sexual desire disorder, and sexual aversion disorder.
- There are two recognized disorders of sexual arousal: female sexual arousal disorder, and persistent genital arousal disorder.
- There are four female sexual pain disorders: dyspareunia, vulvodynia, vaginismus, and noncoital nonsexual pain disorder.
- Sexual disorders are best approached using a biopsychosocial model and are best treated with multimodal interventions that include cognitive behavioral therapy, sex therapy, and appropriate medical interventions and medications.

Evidence Box 52.1

Following oophorectomy, testosterone replacement modestly increases sexual desire and frequency of satisfying sexual activity.

After bilateral oophorectomy, estradiol production is reduced by 95% and testosterone production decreases by 50% and such women are often treated with estrogen replacement but seldom receive testosterone replacement. Testosterone may influence sexual function in women. The purpose of this clinical trial was to test whether testosterone influences sexual function in women after bilateral oophorectomy.

Women between 24 and 70 years of age (mean age 50 years) who reported decreased sexual desire after bilateral salpingo-oophorectomy, and were already receiving estrogen replacement therapy, were randomized to receive placebo (*N* = 119) or one of 3 doses of transdermal testosterone: 150 µg/day (*N* = 107), 300 µg/day (*N* = 111), or 450 µg/day (*N* = 111) for 24 weeks. Sexual desire and frequency of satisfying sexual activity were assessed throughout the trial. Of the volunteers, 71% completed the 24-week trial. Transdermal testosterone had a dose-dependent effect on sexual desire and activity. Testosterone at a dose of 150 µg/day did not significantly improve sexual function compared with placebo. Testosterone at doses of 300 µg/day and

450 µg/day increased self-reported sexual desire and the frequency of satisfying sexual relations compared with placebo. Testosterone at a dose of 300 µg/day significantly increased the frequency of satisfying sexual activity by an average of 1 episode per month, a modest clinical effect. Testosterone replacement did not significantly increase the frequency of orgasm compared with placebo. Eleven percent of the volunteers withdrew from the study because of side effects. The long-term safety of testosterone replacement has not been established and the treatment is not approved by the Food and Drug Administration.

This trial indicates that testosterone replacement has a modest, positive clinical effect on sexual function in women with low sexual desire following oophorectomy. Clearly, testosterone replacement is not a "wonder drug" for the treatment of sexual dysfunction.

Braunstein GD, Sundwall DA, Katz M, et al. Safety and efficacy of a testosterone patch for the treatment of hypoactive sexual desire disorder in surgically menopausal women. Arch Int Med 2005;165:1582–1589.

Further Reading

Arlt W, Callies F, van Vlijmen JC, et al. Dehydroepiandrosterone replacement in women with adrenal insufficiency. *N Engl J Med* 1999;341(14):1013–1020

Basson R. Clinical practice. Sexual desire and arousal disorders in women. *N Engl J Med* 2006;354(14):1497–1506

Braunstein GD, Sundwall DA, Katz M, et al. Safety and efficacy of a testosterone patch for the treatment of hypoactive sexual desire disorder in surgically menopausal women: a randomized, placebo-controlled trial. *Arch Intern Med* 2005;165(14):1582–1589

Ferguson DM, Steidle CP, Singh GS, Alexander JS, Weihmiller MK, Crosby MG. Randomized, placebo-controlled, double blind, crossover design trial of the efficacy and safety of Zestra for Women in women with and without female sexual arousal disorder. *J Sex Marital Ther* 2003;29(Suppl 1):33–44

Glazener CM. Sexual function after childbirth: women's experiences, persistent morbidity and lack of professional recognition. *Br J Obstet Gynaecol* 1997;104(3):330–335

Ito TY, Polan ML, Whipple B, Trant AS. The enhancement of female sexual function with ArginMax, a nutritional supplement, among women differing in menopausal status. *J Sex Marital Ther* 2006;32(5):369–378

Laumann EO, Paik A, Rosen RC. Sexual dysfunction in the United States: prevalence and predictors. *JAMA* 1999;281(6):537–544

Lindau ST, Schumm LP, Laumann EO, Levinson W, O'Muircheartaigh CA, Waite LJ. A study of sexuality and health among older adults in the United States. *N Engl J Med* 2007;357(8):762–774

Segraves RT, Balon R. Sexual Pharmacology: Fast Facts. New York: WW Norton, 2003:420

Swaab DF, Chung WC, Kruijver FP, Hofman MA, Ishunina TA. Sexual differentiation of the human hypothalamus. *Adv Exp Med Biol* 2002;511:75–100, discussion 100–105

Trudel G, Marchand A, Ravart M, Aubin S, Turgeon L, Fortier P. The effect of a cognitive-behavioral group treatment program on hypoactive sexual desire in women. *Sex Relat Ther* 2001;16:145–164

Tylee A, Haller DM, Graham T, Churchill R, Sanci LA. Youth-friendly primary-care services: how are we doing and what more needs to be done? *Lancet* 2007;369(9572):1565–1573

53 Domestic Violence and Sexual Assault

Robert L. Barbieri

Domestic Violence

Definition

Domestic violence is defined as controlling or violent behavior by a person against an intimate partner. It necessarily involves at least two people: a perpetrator, and a victim. In some relationships a recurrent cycle of violence and reconciliation is observed (**Fig. 53.1**). Domestic violence is a breach of the human rights of the victim and destroys trust in the relationship. Domestic violence may include physical abuse, sexual assault, emotional abuse, social isolation, economic control, and even murder. Indirectly, children, adolescents, and other adults may be psychologically harmed by witnessing domestic violence in their home. Domestic violence represents a major health burden. It is difficult to detect without routine screening of at-risk populations.

Detection

Routine screening is required to detect most cases of domestic violence. A single question has been demonstrated to increase the rate of detection: "At any time, has a partner hit, kicked, or otherwise hurt or threatened you?" A set of three questions that helps to detect domestic violence in pregnant women is:

1. "Within the last year, have you been hit, slapped, kicked, or otherwise physically hurt by someone?"
2. "Since you have been pregnant, have you been hit, slapped, kicked, or otherwise physically hurt by someone?"
3. "Within the last year has anyone forced you to have sexual activities?"

The screening for domestic violence must be performed in a private setting without the presence of anyone but

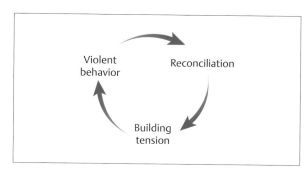

Fig. 53.1   Three stages in a recurring cycle of domestic violence.

the patient and clinician. A minority of patients initially object to being screened for domestic violence, but empathic support usually overcomes initial resistance to answer the question(s). Prefacing the direct question with a preamble, such as: "Violence is so common in our society, I ask all my patients about their exposure to violence" may help to overcome the resistance of some patients to responding to the question. An alternative to routine screening of all patients is to screen for domestic violence in patients known to be at increased risk: female emergency room patients and trauma victims, pregnant women, women with sexually transmitted diseases and women with chronic pain symptoms such as abdominal or pelvic pain, or headaches. Pediatricians have reported that detection and treatment of domestic violence may be the most effective means of preventing child abuse.

Prevalence and Epidemiology

Domestic violence is a worldwide problem. In large population surveys, about 5 % of women reported at least one episode of domestic violence within the past year and about 25 % reported a lifetime history of domestic violence. The Centers for Disease Control and Prevention (CDC) reports that domestic violence in the United States causes approximately 1200 deaths and 2 million injuries to women each year. Victims of domestic violence are more likely to smoke cigarettes, report risky sexual behaviors, and be disabled. They are also at increased risk for heart disease, stroke, asthma, and arthritis. The majority of women murdered by an intimate partner have had multiple contacts with the health care system in the year before their death.

Approximately 10% of pregnant women are victims of domestic violence. Domestic violence may begin during a pregnancy or pregnancy may accelerate its intensity and frequency. Homicide is an important cause of death of pregnant women. Domestic violence during pregnancy may be associated with adverse pregnancy outcomes, including an increased risk of delivering a low birth weight infant.

Factors that increase the risk of being a victim of domestic violence include poverty, low education level, unemployment, being unmarried, and having young children. Being a victim of domestic violence increases the risk of an affective disorder such as depression, and increases the risk of reporting symptoms including abdominal and pelvic pain.

Domestic violence is common in heterosexual, gay, and lesbian relationships. In heterosexual relationships 95% of the victims are women. Children who experience domestic violence have an increased risk of affective disorders, aggression, and impulsivity. Children with a parent who is a victim of domestic violence may be at increased risk for obesity and diabetes when they become adults. Children can be protected against the adverse effects of domestic violence by experiencing supportive relationships inside and outside the home.

Etiology

Anger is a common human emotion. Many people are unable to manage their anger in socially acceptable forms, and when angry they behave violently against inanimate objects, animals, pets, and other people. Targeting an intimate partner is a complex expression of anger that often triggers a cycle of violence, followed by apologies and an interval of increased intimacy, followed by another episode of violence. Murder is an extreme manifestation of anger and violence in an intimate relationship. Women are more likely to be murdered by an intimate partner than all other types of assailants.

Treatment

Most physicians are not experts in the treatment of domestic violence. Physicians who diagnose domestic violence should refer the patient to specialized resources that typically include specialized social workers and

domestic violence experts. Social workers will typically spend considerable time with the patient exploring important aspects of domestic violence, such as what to do in a crisis, identification of safe houses and methods of transport to the safe house, and ways to find money and obtain the legal documents needed to escape the abusive relationship.

RADAR

A simple mnemonic to guide the clinical approach to domestic violence is "RADAR." This mnemonic represents a five-step detection and treatment process:
1. R—Routinely screen patients for domestic violence
2. A—Ask a direct question such as: "At any time, has a partner hit, kicked or otherwise hurt or threatened you?"
3. D—Document your findings in the medical record
4. A—Assess patient safety, including issues such as "Are there guns in the home?", "Have there been threats of suicide/homicide?", "Has there been violence toward the children?"
5. R—Refer to a specialist in domestic violence, often a highly trained and experienced social worker

Sexual Assault

Definition

Sexual assault is a sexual act performed by one person on another without consent. Sexual assault is an act of control and aggression. Victims do not cause the sexual assault.

Prevalence and Epidemiology

Women make up 90% of the victims of sexual assault. It is difficult to make a precise estimate of the prevalence of sexual assault because most incidents are never reported. For women, the lifetime risk of experiencing a sexual assault is estimated to be between 20% and 35%. According to national data sources, in the United States since 1994 the rate of forcible rape has been decreasing. Many victims of sexual assault are adolescents and children. In one survey, about 50% of females who reported being sexually assaulted were less than 18 years of age. Most women know their attacker.

Comprehensive Care of the Sexual Assault Victim

The hospital-based emergency department is the primary point of care for the majority of rape victims. Specialized nurses who are part of the Sexual Assault Nurse Evaluation (SANE) program often provide, supervise, or coordinate the care of victims of sexual assault. Areas of focus for the treatment of victims of sexual assault include: rapid access to treatment by a specialized team of clinicians; assessment and treatment of bodily injuries with a focus on genital trauma; psychological assessment and support; pregnancy assessment and prevention; preventive treatment of sexually transmitted diseases; and collection of forensic data including toxicology testing for the presence of date-rape drugs.

History

Important historical items include details of the assault including time, location, weapons, force, threats; history of loss of consciousness, physical description of the assailant, specifics of the sexual contact, areas of trauma, bleeding and exposure to blood from the assailant, hygiene activities following the assault, and history of recent consensual sexual activity.

Physical Examination and Laboratory Studies

The victim needs to completely undress and should disrobe on a surface, such as a sheet, that can be used to capture any evidence that falls from her clothes. Bodily trauma should be assessed and documented in detail with support from photographs. Many providers in the SANE program will perform colposcopic examination to increase the detection of minor trauma. An ultraviolet light source can help identify proteins, such as present in semen, and foreign debris on the skin.

The following items need to be collected to complete the forensic examination: all the victim's clothing, swabs of the mouth, vagina and rectum, combed scalp and pubic hair specimens, control samples of the victim's scalp and pubic hair, fingernail scrapings and clippings, a tube of blood, and saliva. The forensic material must be sealed and stored to maintain a valid "chain of evidence."

To assist in the medical care of the victim, testing for chorionic gonadotropin (HCG), syphilis, and hepatitis B should be performed. Sites of sexual contact can be sampled for gonorrhea and Chlamydia. If the victim plans to take antibiotic therapy as a preventive step, these cultures can be deferred. If loss of consciousness was reported, toxicology testing for flunitrazepam (Rohypnol) can be performed.

Treatment

The CDC recommends prophylactic treatment for Chlamydia and gonorrhea for victims of sexual assault. Empiric therapy includes: 1) ceftriaxone 125 mg intramuscularly to prevent gonorrhea, 2) azithromycin 1 g orally as a single dose or doxycycline 100 mg twice daily for 7 days to prevent Chlamydia, and 3) metronidazole 2 g orally as a single dose to prevent trichomoniasis. The CDC also recommends hepatitis B vaccination for those patients who were not previously vaccinated. The CDC recommends against the use of hepatitis B immune globulin because of cost–benefit considerations. Prophylactic treatment with antiviral drugs to prevent human immunodeficiency virus (HIV) following sexual assault is controversial. The CDC recommends giving patients postexposure prophylaxis for HIV for 3–7 days, with a follow up visit to consider the pros and cons of ongoing prophylaxis. The risk of HIV infection is low after a single sexual assault.

Postcoital contraception should be offered to all women who are raped. A preferred regimen is levonorgestrel 1.5 mg orally, as a single dose. Given the number of medications offered to the patient, an antiemetic should be offered or prescribed.

Psychological support is an important part of the treatment and healing of rape victims. All rape victims should be offered a referral to a mental health specialist. Immediately following a sexual assault, the victim may experience anger, anxiety, shame, guilt, obsessive and intrusive thoughts, and insomnia. In a later phase vivid dreams and nightmares; musculoskeletal, abdominal and pelvic pain symptoms; and phobias may occur. Following a sexual assault, post-traumatic stress disorder (PTSD), depression, and chronic anxiety may develop. Up to 50% of women who have experienced a sexual assault develop PTSD. Selective serotonin reuptake inhibitors improve the symptoms of PTSD in victims of sexual assault (see Evidence Box 53.1)

Approximately 2 weeks after the sexual assault the patient should be seen for follow-up pregnancy testing and assessment of mental health needs. Follow-up testing for sexually transmitted diseases is performed if the patient has relevant symptoms, or did not take the preventive antibiotic therapy. Follow-up HIV and syphilis testing may be performed 12 and 24 weeks after the assault.

Key Points

- Domestic violence is common and under-reported. In population-based surveys about 5% of women report at least one episode of domestic violence within the past year. About 25% of women report at least one episode of domestic violence during their lifetime.
- Routine, confidential screening is required to detect most cases of domestic violence. An empathic supportive perspective is important in eliciting open answers to questions concerning domestic violence. A preamble such as "Violence is so common in our society, I ask all my patients about their exposure to violence" followed by direct questions such as: "During the past year have you been hit, slapped, kicked or otherwise physically hurt by someone?" may help to elicit open responses.
- Social workers and experts in domestic violence help to guide the treatment of the victim.
- Sexual assault is common. For women, the lifetime risk of sexual assault is about 20–35%. Women under 18 years of age are at greatest risk of sexual assault.
- Evaluation and treatment of sexual assault is best provided in a comprehensive setting by health care providers with specialized training. Victims of sexual assault should receive prophylactic treatment for Chlamydia and gonorrhea, hepatitis B vaccination, if not previously received, and counseling about prophylactic treatment with antiviral drugs to prevent human immunodeficiency virus. Postcoital contraception should be offered to all women who are raped. Up to 50% of women develop post-traumatic symptoms following a sexual assault. Extended mental health care should be offered to victims.

Further Reading

Stein DJ, Ipser JC, Seedat S. Pharmacotherapy for post-traumatic stress disorder (PTSD). *Cochrane Database Syst Rev* 2006;25:CD002795

Brady K, Pearlstein T, Asnis GM, et al. Efficacy and safety of sertraline treatment of posttraumatic stress disorder: a randomized controlled trial. *JAMA* 2000;283(14):1837–1844

Centers for Disease Control and Prevention (CDC). Adverse health conditions and health risk behaviors associated with intimate partner violence—United States, 2005. *MMWR Morb Mortal Wkly Rep* 2008; 57(5, 5)113–117

Centers for Disease Control and Prevention. Sexually transmitted diseases treatment guidelines 2006. *MMWR Morb Mortal Wkly Rep* 2006;55(RR11):1–100

Kessler RC, Sonnega A, Bromet E, Hughes M, Nelson CB. Post-traumatic stress disorder in the National Comorbidity Survey. *Arch Gen Psychiatry* 1995;52(12):1048–1060

Nerøien AI, Schei B. Partner violence and health: results from the first national study on violence against women in Norway. *Scand J Public Health* 2008;36(2):161–168

Thomas C, Hyppönen E, Power C. Obesity and type 2 diabetes risk in midadult life: the role of childhood adversity. *Pediatrics* 2008;121(5):e1240–e1249

Evidence Box 53.1

Selective serotonin reuptake inhibitors improve the symptoms of post-traumatic stress disorder in victims of sexual assault.

Following sexual assault, post-traumatic stress disorder (PTSD) may occur in up to 50% of victims. In a systematic review of 35 randomized trials using selective serotonin reuptake inhibitors to treat PTSD, these antidepressants were demonstrated to reduce flashbacks, arousal, and avoidance.[*] In one clinical trial, 187 outpatients with PTSD were randomized to treatment with sertraline (25 mg daily for 1 week, followed by upward dose titration to a mean dose of about 150 mg daily) or placebo. 62% of the subjects in the study had experienced a sexual or physical assault prior to developing PTSD.[**] For the subjects treated with sertraline and placebo, the overall improvement rate was 53% and 32%, respectively. The subjects treated with sertraline reported significantly less avoidance, numbing, and arousal. Sertraline treatment was associated with a significant improvement in self-reported quality of life scores. Insomnia was the side effect reported significantly more often with sertraline than with placebo treatment (16% vs. 4%).

[*]**Stein DJ, Ipser JC, Seedat S. Pharmacotherapy for post-traumatic stress disorder. Cochrane Database Syst Rev 2006;00:CD002795.**

[**]**Brady K, Pearlstein T, Asnis GM, et al. Efficacy and safety of sertraline treatment of posttraumatic stress disorder. JAMA 2000;283:1837–1844.**

Part VII Professional Behavior, Ethics, and Legalitis

54 Medical Economics and Social Issues

Robert L. Barbieri

Population Health Promotes Economic Growth and Stability

There is a strong relationship between population health and economic growth and stability. In general, countries with strong, growing, and stable economies have better overall population health than do poor countries. In general within a country, wealthy individuals and families have better health and more access to high quality health care than do poor individuals and families. The strong relationship between health and economic prosperity both at the global and individual levels is a major challenge to clinicians. As part of their professional commitment, clinicians need to be engaged in trying to provide equitable access to health care for all members of their community.

Two key links between health and economic growth are longevity and small family size. As the health of a population improves longevity increases. As longevity increases the educational and skill level of members of the society increases, in turn increasing their economic productivity. OB/GYN practitioners help to ensure the birth of healthy children, thereby initiating the path to a long and healthy life. In general, as family size decreases, investment in each child increases, resulting in better educated and more economically productive adults. According to one report, as the growth rate of the population of a country increases by 1%, the rate of growth of domestic product decreases by 0.4% (Bloom DE, Williamson J. Demographic transitions and economic miracles in emerging Asia. World Bank Econ Rev 1998;12:419–455). OB/GYN practitioners play a key role in helping families achieve their optimal size.

Health Economics Issues in Developed Countries

In many developed countries, controlling the rate of growth of health care costs and ensuring high quality are critical health economics issues. As a thought experiment, it is not sustainable for the health care costs to grow at a rate of 10% per year and gross domestic product (GDP) to grow at a rate of 4% per year. Eventually the entire GDP would be spent on health care.

The amount of gross domestic product (GDP) spent on health care varies substantially among developed countries (**Fig. 54.1**). Most developed countries are taking multiple steps to attempt to control the rate of rise of health care costs including:
- reducing health care waste
- increasing the use of low-cost generic medications
- requiring extensive evidence-based review of all new technologies and medications before they become available for use
- implementing an interoperable, nationwide system of electronic health records
- improving long-term management of chronic conditions
- reducing the use of expensive interventions in the last few weeks of life
- reducing administrative costs of managing health insurance plans
- increasing primary prevention activities
- replacing per-case payments with capitation for a population or case-rates
- directly or indirectly rationing health care

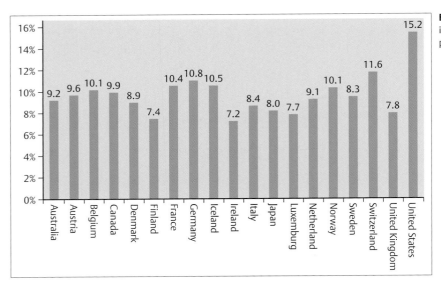

Fig. 54.1 Total health care spending as a percentage of gross domestic product in 2003.

Reducing Waste: Lean Engineering

Reducing health care waste can take many forms, including avoiding unnecessary tests and procedures. Toyota engineers developed the concept of "lean production systems," which is the never-ending pursuit of perfection by eliminating unnecessary steps and waste in the production process. In health care, common causes of waste include:
- waiting (patients waiting in the emergency department for admission and treatment, physicians waiting for a test result)
- queuing of work (delaying performing a lab test until there are a 100 samples ready for testing)
- production defects (failed venipuncture, medication errors)
- unnecessary steps in production process (forcing providers to complete duplicate paperwork, moving patients from unit to unit)
- inefficient transportation systems
- overproduction (preparing medications just in case they need to be used)
- unnecessary movement and searching (looking for a missing chart or missing piece of equipment)

Using the lean production method, Toyota engineers have achieved high levels of reliability, quality, and cost-control. Health systems are in the process of systematically redesigning work using these proven methods.

Generic Medications

In the United States a 90-day supply of a generic osteoporosis medication, alendronate, costs $10. A 90-day supply of the same brand-name product costs in the range of $200. The widespread use of generic medications has the potential to reduce overall health care costs. A modest concern is that the use of generics will reduce the money available to pharmaceutical firms for research and development of new drugs.

Effectiveness Review of All New Drugs and Technology

Many new drugs and technologies are expensive but offer only a modest improvement in health outcomes. Most health insurers have evidence-based processes for trying to limit the introduction of new technologies and procedures that are supported by limited evidence. For example, some insurers require the publication of three high-quality clinical trials that demonstrate the clinical utility of a new technology or procedure before they will reimburse for the innovative technology or new procedure. A modest disadvantage of this approach is that it can delay the access of patients to promising, but as yet unproven, treatments.

Interoperable National Health Record

An electronic health record opens opportunities for health savings through the use of decision-support software to encourage the use of generic medications, reduce the use of unnecessary imaging studies, avoid duplication of testing, and ensure timely provision of preventive care services such as vaccinations. Key concerns with an electronic health record include the protection of the patient's privacy and provisions to "hide" especially sensitive medical information.

Long-Term Management of Chronic Health Conditions

It is estimated that 10% of patients create 70% of all health care costs. Many of these patients have chronic conditions such as diabetes, emphysema, and heart failure, which may be best managed in an outpatient setting by midlevel providers such as nurse practitioners and physician assistants. By proactively ensuring patients are incorporating healthy behaviors (such as taking their medicines) in their daily activities, expensive hospitalizations can be reduced.

Reducing the Use of Expensive Interventions in the Last Weeks of Life

A substantial percentage of all health care expenditure occurs in the last year of life. Wide geographic variation exists in the total value of health care interventions provided in the last year of life. This suggests that regional culture and practice patterns influence the intensity of health care provided in this period. Reducing the variation in health care expenditures in the last year of life will likely reduce the rate of growth of health care costs.

Reducing Administrative Costs of Managing Health Insurance

Most economists believe that when analyzed in a narrow context, the best approach to reducing administrative costs in the health care system is to move to a single-payor system such as the Medicare system for all citizens. A major concern with this cost-saving intervention is that it is likely that the range of choices for clinicians and patients will be reduced and innovation might be slowed. Government control of all health care choices is likely to result in some limitations of benefits, reduction in service quality for some citizens, and potential delays in care.

Increasing Primary Prevention Activities

Prevention activities such as vaccinations improve population health but may not dramatically reduce health care costs in most developed countries that are already reaping the benefits of prevention activities. Primary prevention activities that focus on healthy life styles, such as maintaining an optimal body mass index, have not received sufficient attention and are likely to reduce the costs of major diseases such as diabetes and heart disease. Many preventive services that have been documented to have

Table 54.1 Preventive health services that provide the greatest improvement in health and have a positive economic impact

Highly effective preventive services that are routinely provided to most people	Highly effective preventive services that are often not routinely provided
Vaccinate children	Screen for tobacco use and provide tobacco cessation counseling
Screen for cervical cancer	Screen for vision impairment in adults >65 years of age
Screen newborns for hemoglobinopathies, phenylketonuria, and congenital hypothyroidism	Assess adolescents and adults for alcohol and drug use and counsel on both
Screen for hypertension	Screen for colorectal cancer among all adults >50 years of age
Vaccinate adults >65 years of age for influenza	Screen for Chlamydia among women aged 15–24 years
Screen for hyperlipidemia	Vaccinate adults >65 years of age against pneumococcal disease
Screen for breast cancer among women 50–69 years of age	

Source: Adopted from Coffield AB, Maciosek MV, McGinnis JM, et al. Priorities among recommended clinical preventive services. Am J Prev Med 2001;21:1–9.

a positive health and economic impact are not routinely provided by clinicians (**Table 54.1**).

Ceasing Per-Case Payments

Many clinicians are compensated based on per-case payments for each interaction with a patient. The per-case payment system does not systematically create incentives for integrating care and reducing the overall costs of treating a disease, nor does it focus on the quality of care across all clinical events. Per-case payment systems are most useful for encouraging clinicians to provide care in acute settings, but are less effective at enhancing the integration of care for chronically ill people. Per-case payment systems may also stimulate over-utilization of services.

However, all options to replace per-case payments have both strengths and weaknesses. For example, in some countries total health care spending has a fixed budget ceiling. A strength of this system is that all parties can anticipate the total economic impact of all health care costs in a given year, which is helpful in budget and workforce planning. A weakness of the approach is that if all health care dollars are spent after 10 months of the budget year, the providers will not be reimbursed for the care they provide in the last 2 months of the year, thereby reducing the providers' willingness to provide care toward the end of each budget cycle.

Professional Liability Reform

Professional liability concerns cause clinicians to practice defensive medicine. This results in the overuse of the most expensive technology and interventions in order to avoid the rare possibility of "missing a diagnosis." Defensive medical practices are a major driver of health care costs in countries with substantial medical tort litigation activity.

Rationing Health Care

In many cultures, the idea of rationing health care is not warmly embraced. In countries with government-controlled health care systems, rationing of care typically causes the rise of a parallel health system for those individuals wealthy enough to pay directly for their services. In the end this can result in a "two tier" health care system based on economic factors.

Many governments have attempted to create "soft" rationing systems that do not impact the majority of citizens but prevent access to some costly services that only a small number of citizens would use. This approach reduces the adverse political impact that would occur if rationing were experienced by a large number citizens. An example of "soft" rationing is the Oregon Health Plan's prioritized list of health services. To reduce the rate of growth of health care costs, leaders in Oregon rank-ordered 700 diagnoses and treatments based on their potential health impact for the entire population. The top 80% of the 700 items were approved for funding and the remaining 20% of treatments were denied coverage. For example, surgical procedures for terminally ill patients were determined to be not reimbursable. Important health services, such as dental services, were placed near the top of the list and were reimbursed for the first time, thereby increasing population health. Basically the plan implements the idea that expensive medical interventions that might have marginal benefits for a single patient will not be funded if it means that funds will be diverted from medical interventions that clearly help large numbers of people.

Improving Quality

The value of a service or product is defined by both its cost and quality. As developed countries struggle to control the rate of rise in health care costs, they also are systematically dealing with the issue of quality of services. Managers of health systems recognize that if services are going to be costly, they had better be able to demonstrate that the services are of a high quality. Health system managers are making ever-increasing efforts to improve quality through a number of interventions:

- using evidence-based approaches to plan medical care, thereby reducing unnecessary interventions of marginal benefit
- reducing medication errors by using computerized physician order entry combined with computerized systems for medication administration
- reducing surgical errors, such as wrong-site surgery, by implementing surgical checklists (**Table 54.2**)
- planning for an optimal response to infrequent high-acuity emergency medical events by team training, simulations, and credentialing of clinicians
- increasing transparency by publishing hospital-specific complication rates, adverse events, and patient-satisfaction scores on public Web sites

Table 54.2 World Health Organization Surgical Checklist. The purpose of the surgical checklist is to improve the quality of surgical care

Preoperative checklist
Confirm patient identity, surgical site, planned procedure, and completion of consent form.
Mark surgical site if applicable to reduce the risk of wrong-site surgery
Anesthesia team completes safety checklist
Pulse oximeter is placed on patient and is functioning
Review patient's allergies
Identify if patient has a difficult airway or is at risk for aspiration
Identify if patient is at risk for more than 500 cc blood loss given the planned procedure
Surgical team checklist immediately prior to starting surgery
All surgical team members introduce themselves and identify their roles
Surgeon, anesthesiologist and surgical nurse confirm correct patient, surgical site, and planned procedure
Surgeon alerts team to potential unexpected or critical steps and planned duration of operation

Table 54.2 Continued

Surgical nurse confirms sterility and adequacy of equipment
Surgical team confirms that antibiotic prophylaxis has been begun prior to incision, if appropriate
All essential imaging studies are available in operating room
Postoperative checklist
Surgical nurse and team agree that the instruments, needles and sponges are all accounted for at the end of the operation
The surgical nurse verbally confirms that the surgical specimen is labeled correctly
Equipment problems are identified for repair
Surgical team reviews the procedure and identifies any concerns for the recovery of patient

Source: Haynes AB, Weiser TG, Berry WR, et al. A surgical safety checklist to reduce morbidity and mortality in a global population. *N Engl J Med* 2009;360:491–9.

Health Disparities

Health and economic status are highly correlated. People who are wealthy tend to have better health than people who are poor. The poverty–disease cycle creates serious issues of disparities in health care, especially as the range of wealth varies greatly in a single population or country. In one analysis of longevity in the United States, low-income and residence in counties with high homicide rates among adult men (>1%) was associated with a marked decrease in life expectancy.

Health Economics Issues in Countries with Rapidly Growing Economies

The GDP of most developed countries is growing at a rate of 3–5% per year. In China, India and Brazil, the gross domestic product is growing at a rate of 7–10% per year. As these populous countries rapidly expand their economies, unique challenges are occurring in their health care systems. A major feature of the economic growth in these countries is the rapid rise of both a middle class and a class of millionaires. These newly minted, economically privileged individuals are demanding access to a wider range of health care services. In response, parallel systems of health care, including a state-sponsored system and a private-pay system, are developing in parallel. There is a great need to build more infrastructure, such as

high technology hospitals and surgical units and a need for more clinicians in high technology specialties.

Health Economics Issues in Developing and Poor Countries

Many poor countries struggle to provide basic medical services such as obstetric and pediatric care for their citizens. In the 1600s in Plymouth Massachusetts, about 1% of pregnant women died in childbirth and 20% of children died at birth or in the first year of life. In many poor countries of the world, these very high maternal and neonatal mortality rates are still prevalent in the 21st century. Contrast this with the figures in the developed world of 0.01% of pregnant women dying in childbirth and 0.5% of children dying in childbirth or in the first year of life. Access to basic maternity services, such as the availability of operative delivery, blood replacement, uterotonics and antibiotics would significantly improve population health in poor countries.

Life expectancy is dramatically different in poor countries compared to wealthy countries. In many wealthy countries life expectancy is in the range of 80 years, while in poor countries life-expectancy is in the range of 50 years. Many poor countries need to develop basic infrastructure in order to improve population health. These basic needs include access to clean water, clean air, sanitation, control of infectious agents and a stable cadre of nurses and doctors. Infectious diseases are major contributors to illness in poor countries. For example, in some countries, 10% or more of the population is infected with human immunodeficiency virus. These infections create great suffering and reduce economic productivity. A new challenge in poor countries is the flight of indigenous, highly trained health care workers from poor countries to wealthy countries to pursue their professional careers. This immigration pattern reduces the ability of poor countries to manage their public health interventions, further contributing to the cycle of poverty and disease.

Key Points

- Adequate health care enhances the economic productivity and competitiveness of a society by ensuring a productive and long-living work force. Paradoxically in highly developed, economically advantaged countries, governments are actively trying to reduce the rate of growth of health care costs. Continuous increases in health care costs greater than the overall growth of an economy result in reduced resources available for other social programs such as education and anti-poverty interventions.
- In developed countries it is difficult to control the rate of growth in health care costs because of an aging population and the availability of new expensive treatment options that flow from medical innovation.

- Options to control the rate of growth of health care costs include: reduction of waste in the medical system; use of generic medications; review of all new drugs and technologies for cost-effectiveness; creation of a national electronic health record; use of active medical management for costly chronic health conditions; reduction of the use of expensive interventions in the last month of life; reduction of administrative costs of managing the health care system; increasing primary prevention activities; and transition from per-case payments to capitation and rationing of health care.

Evidence Box 54.1

Regional variations in health care costs offer an opportunity to optimize health care and reduce expenses by studying best practices from geographic areas with good outcomes and low costs.

Based on data from 2006, there are marked regional variations in health care costs across geographic regions in the United States.[*] For example, in Manhattan, New York average 2006 Medicare spending was $12114 per year per enrolled person. In contrast, in Minneapolis, Minnesota, average 2006 Medicare spending was $6705 per year per person. Arguably health care in Minneapolis is on par with the care provided in Manhattan. In fact, some data suggests that health outcomes in Minneapolis are superior to those in Manhattan. What accounts for the wide difference in cost between Minneapolis and Manhattan?

The cost difference is unlikely to be due to "technology" per se, because physicians and patients in both Manhattan and Minneapolis have access to similar medical technology. It is also unlikely that physicians in Minneapolis are inappropriately rationing care to the citizens of that city. Data suggests that physicians in Manhattan and Minneapolis have adopted different processes for utilizing health care resources.

In one research study, common clinical scenarios, such as stable angina or typical gastroesophageal reflux, were presented to physicians from low-cost and high-cost regions.[**] Physicians from high-cost regions were more likely to refer these patients to subspecialists than those from low-cost regions. Subspecialists are more likely to intensively use technology, such as advanced imaging procedures, which increases the cost of care for the condition. In the same study, when presented with a case of an 85-year-old man with an exacerbation of end-stage congestive heart failure, the physicians form high-cost regions were more likely to admit the patient to a hospital intensive care unit, while physicians from low-cost regions were more likely to keep the patient

home and not admit the patient to the hospital. If the clinical practices of physicians from low-cost regions could be transferred to high-cost regions it is likely that the rate of rise of health care costs could be reduced.

Substantial research indicates that physicians are the most responsible decision makers in the amount of care received by their patients. If physicians adopt clinical processes that are strongly supported by evidence and guidelines, and avoid clinical recommendations that are discretionary or not supported by the evidence, it is likely that health care costs could be substantially reduced.

[*]**Fischer ES, Bynum JP, Skinner JS. Slowing the growth of health care costs—lessons from regional variation. N Engl J Med 2009;36:849–852.**

[**]**Sirovich B, Gallagher PM, Wennberg DE, Fisher ES. Discretionary decision making by primary care physicians and the cost of US health care. Health Affairs 2008;27:813–823.**

Further Reading

Bodenheimer T. The Oregon Health Plan—lessons for the nation. First of two parts. *N Engl J Med* 1997;337(9):651–655

Coffield AB, Maciosek MV, McGinnis JM, et al. Priorities among recommended clinical preventive services. *Am J Prev Med* 2001;21(1):1–9

Denny CC, Emanuel EJ, Pearson SD. Why well-insured patients should demand value-based insurance benefits. *JAMA* 2007;297(22):2515–2518

Emanuel EJ, Fuchs VR. The perfect storm of overutilization. *JAMA* 2008;299(23):2789–2791

Mirvis DM, Bloom DE. Population health and economic development in the United States. *JAMA* 2008;300(1):93–95

Mongan JJ, Ferris TG, Lee TH. Options for slowing the growth of health care costs. *N Engl J Med* 2008;358(14):1509–1514

Murray CJ, Kulkarni SC, Michaud C, et al. Eight Americas: investigating mortality disparities across races, counties, and race-counties in the United States. *PLoS Med* 2006;3(9):e260–e271

Pham HH, Ginsburg PB, McKenzie K, Milstein A. Redesigning care delivery in response to a high-performance network: the Virginia Mason Medical Center. *Health Aff (Millwood)* 2007;26(4):w532–w544

Rubin RJ, Mendelson DN. How much does defensive medicine cost? *J Am Health Policy* 1994;4(4):7–15

Woolhandler S, Campbell T, Himmelstein DU. Costs of health care administration in the United States and Canada. *N Engl J Med* 2003;349(8):768–775

55 Provider–Patient Communications and Interactions

Hugh E. Mighty

The provider–patient relationship is a complex and dynamic one with several characteristics that differentiate it from other human relationships. It is a relationship in which the physician historically has been assumed to possess most of the expertise and authority. Until the last couple of decades, it was expected that the provider would use this expertise and authority to make decisions for the patient, and patients were expected to follow medical recommendations.

With the advent of the Internet and other readily available sources of medical information and advice, as well as the increased focus on patient-centered care, the provider–patient relationship has shifted away from this paternalistic model. Rather, it has become an increasingly consumer-driven model of care, in which patients are also viewed as having expertise and authority, many of whom expect to be actively involved in most decisions regarding their care. This new model presents both opportunities and challenges to interactions between health care providers and their patients.

This chapter reviews the core values and principles that should guide provider–patient interactions, and discusses the critical role of effective communication in prompting positive provider–patient interactions. It also explores some common challenges to effective interactions between health care providers and their patients.

Core Values

Pellegrino identifies six virtues that are "indispensable for attainment of the ends of medicine":
1. Fidelity to trust
2. Benevolence
3. Intellectual honesty
4. Courage
5. Compassion
6. Truthfulness

We have modified this list slightly and added respect and collegiality, because of the increasingly multicultural environment in which physicians must work. **Table 55.1** gives a brief explanation of these seven key virtues.

Table 55.1 Key virtues of the physician

Fidelity to trust	Patients, upon seeking the help of a physician, entrust the physician with their wellbeing. The doctor has an obligation to be true to that trust
Benevolence	The provider should act in a manner that promotes the welfare and best interest of the patient and avoids harming the patient
Intellectual honesty	The physician must know the bounds of his or her knowledge and be willing to admit when this is the case and seek assistance from others. The physician should present information to the patient in a balanced, unbiased, and truthful manner. The physician should avoid misrepresenting the value of certain treatment options over others, especially if personal financial gain is to be had from these options
Courage	Providers sometimes have to put themselves in harm's way or into uncomfortable situations to care for or defend the rights of their patients. The physician needs physical, emotional, and intellectual courage
Compassion	The physician should interact with the patient with empathy and understanding- in a way that reflects how they want to be treated themselves or how they would want a loved one treated
Respect	The physician should be courteous and show tolerance for others. He or she should take into account the feelings, needs, beliefs, thoughts, and wishes of the patient
Collegiality	The provider must show respect for other providers and staff members and work with them in a way that promotes the best interests of the patients they care for

Adapted with permission from Pellegrino ED. Professionalism, profession and the virtues of the good physician. Mt Sinai J Med 2002; 69(6):378–384.

Provider–Patient Communications

Effective communication is the foundation upon which the provider–patient relationship must be built. Providers must learn how to both elicit from their patients key information that helps guide diagnosis and communicate back to patients information on their diagnosis and treatment options in a way which can be comprehended and trusted. Providers who can master the skills of effective communication with their patients are more likely to have patients who are satisfied with the care they receive, who are more compliant with treatment recommendations, and who are less likely to sue for an unanticipated outcome.

Results of numerous research studies suggest that patients who have a positive relationship with their health care provider are more likely to have improved health outcomes. The recognition of the importance of both communication and interpersonal skills, and of the fact that these skills can be taught, has led accrediting and licensing entities, including the Accreditation Council for Graduate Medical Education (ACGME), to include these skills as a core competency.

Eliciting All Pertinent Information From a Patient at Interview

Gathering information from the patient is a critical component of each provider–patient encounter. The patient can provide key data regarding symptoms that can help guide diagnosis, information about individual circumstances that can affect disease progression and likelihood of treatment success, and information regarding side effects and symptom improvement, worsening, or resolution that may help the provider monitor the success of the treatment and/or management plan.

The process of information sharing by the patient is facilitated if the encounter is patient-centered rather than clinician centered. Unfortunately, too many clinical encounters are guided by, and focus on, the provider. One study found three common features of such provider-focused care: 1) Clinicians do a majority of the talking even when they are obtaining a history; 2) They ask nearly six closed-ended questions for every one open-ended question; 3) They often interrupt the patient when he or she is trying to provide information or ask a question.

Not giving patients adequate time to be heard or not letting them provide other pertinent information can be particularly dangerous, since the patient often has information that is critical to a timely diagnosis. In addition to knowing how to listen and what questions to ask and when, the clinician must know how to ask questions in a way that will maximize the chances that the patient will share complete and accurate information.

The provider must be especially sensitive to the choice of words as well as any body language that may interfere with the patient's willingness to share information. This is especially important in the field of obstetrics and gynecology in which providers often need to ask about sensitive topics such as reproductive choices and sexual activity—topics about which most patients will be hesitant and cautious to share information.

The patient may not fully understand why the provider needs this very private information. Therefore, when discussing such sensitive issues, it may be helpful to share with the patient the reason for the question, and help her to understand its relevance to her health.

For example, when asking whether a patient whether she has sex with men, women, or both, the provider can explain that certain conditions such as cervical cancer are most common among women who have sex with men. Or, when asking about a history of sexually transmitted infections, the provider can explain that Chlamydia or gonorrhea can cause a condition that can lead to infertility, or that a herpes outbreak during labor and birth can cause a dangerous infection in the newborn.

The provider should reassure the patient that the information gathered will be used to improve the care provided to her and will be kept confidential. Another helpful strategy to relieve patient anxiety regarding questions about sensitive topics, when relevant, is to "normalize" the question. In other words, the provider can let the patient know that the question is routinely asked of all patients.

The provider can even show the patient that these questions are written into the preprinted prenatal record. For example, questions eliciting a thorough history of gynecologic infections, including sexually transmitted infections, are a part of every routine first obstetric visit.

Although checklists and medical forms can help expedite health care encounters and ease documentation, they can also lead patients to omit information that may be important for the provider to know. The same situation can occur when providers ask questions that the patient can answer with a simple "yes" or "no" or other one-worded answers. These are called closed-ended questions. Such questions are sometimes necessary.

However, it is also necessary at times for the provider to elicit additional relevant information. Asking open-ended questions is a useful way to elicit such information. Some examples of valuable open-ended questions are as follows:

- Tell me about how you first noticed something was wrong.
- Tell me about other things that you feel are important for me to know about you or your medical history.
- What things do you feel may be obstacles to your taking your medication as directed?

- Tell me what you know about the IUD [intrauterine device] and why you think it is a good option for you.

When the patient has provided any information, the physician can ensure that he or she has heard and interpreted this information correctly by asking additional questions for clarification and by stating back to the patient what was said. The following is an example of how this works: "Ms. Jones, if I understand you correctly, you feel that the IUD would be a good form of birth control for you, because you are pretty sure that you do not want any more children, but are not ready for a permanent form of birth control such as a tubal ligation. Is this correct?" "Furthermore, I hear you saying that you are worried about the cancer risks associated with hormonal methods of birth control. Is this correct?" "Are there any other concerns that might affect your choice of birth control method?"

The provider should make sure to ask such questions in a nonjudgmental tone of voice, using words that are easy to understand and avoiding medical jargon. When the patient is answering a question, the provider should refrain from interrupting her or from completing her sentences. Studies have shown that physicians interrupt patients in their opening statement in the vast majority of visits, when the patient has barely had time to talk about her health issues.

When providers interrupt in this manner, they run the dual risks of having the patient shut down and not share vital information and of "nontracking" the conversation, that is, shifting the focus of the visit to what the physician, rather than the patient, perceives to be relevant. As has been mentioned earlier, this can lead to delays in diagnosis or, even worse, to a misdiagnosis.

The physician's body language during the encounter and his or her listening skills are equally as important as determining what questions to ask and how to ask them. Listening is an active form of communication. As Freeman summarizes:

> "Listening is not simply hearing words. It involves a concerted effort to listen to the way the words are said, to recognize the feelings underlying the spoken word and to be aware of what the patient has left out of their narrative. This last aspect of listening has been called 'listening with the third ear.'"

Thus, the provider needs to be aware not only of what is being said, but of both his or her own body language and that of the patient's. The provider should make ample eye contact with the patient—which is easier if the patient and the provider are at the same eye level (both sitting down, for example). Furthermore, although it is often necessary to take notes on the medical chart as the patient provides information, if the provider looks only at the chart and not the patient, he or she may miss some important nonverbal cues from the patient. It is also important to take a

break from charting, if the patient is disclosing sensitive information or is upset or otherwise emotional.

In addition to putting down the chart and looking at the patient, leaning forward and nodding are other examples of body language that encourages the patient to share information. Physicians should avoid body language that gives the patient the message that they are in a rush or that the information being conveyed is not important. This negative body language includes standing up while the patient is talking, looking at a watch or clock, turning one's back on the patient to chart, or standing next to the door.

Griffith et al. (see Further Reading) utilized a scoring system of seven nonverbal cues in their study of the effect of the provider's nonverbal communication skills on patient satisfaction:
1. Facial expressivity
2. Frequency of smiling
3. Frequency of nodding
4. Frequency of eye contact
5. Body lean (forward vs. backward)
6. Body posture (closed vs. open)
7. Tone of voice.

Finally, in addition to the factors described above, the provider should try to create a physical environment in which the patient is comfortable and more likely to be able to participate in a healthy exchange of information with the provider. The temperature in the examination room should be comfortable and the room should be set up in a manner that protects the patient's privacy. This includes privacy curtains or screens and exam tables that are positioned, if possible, parallel to the door so that if someone were to walk in during a pelvic exam, the patient's genital area would not be exposed.

If the provider needs to elicit an extensive history (i.e., more than a couple of questions), the patient should be allowed to stay dressed and then given some time in private to change into an exam gown. The patient should be provided with gowns of appropriate size. If a pelvic exam is to be conducted, sheets should be provided, so that the patient can drape her legs and keep her buttocks and genital area covered until just before the pelvic exam, and re-cover herself immediately afterward. If the patient has brought a support person(s) or children with her, she should be allowed to determine whether she wants them to remain in the room for the exam and, if she does, where they should sit or stand during the exam.

Summary

In summary, the following tips will facilitate a patient's sharing of complete and accurate information during the provider–patient encounter:
- Introduce yourself to the patient and shake her hand.
- Allow the patient to answer in her own words.

- Do not interrupt the patient or put words in her mouth.
- Ask open-ended questions that will elicit information form patient in her own words.
- Maximize eye contact.
- Lean forward, nod, and give other active nonverbal cues to the patient that you are listening, including when you are charting.
- Let the patient know why you are asking questions of a sensitive nature.
- Normalize the questions for the patient.
- Stop charting if the patient is having a hard time with a question or becomes emotional.
- Repeat what the patient says, so that you can be sure that you fully understood the patient.
- Assure the patient of the confidential nature of the information she is sharing.
- Avoid body language that indicates that you are in a hurry.
- Make the physical environment as comfortable as possible.
- Protect the patient's privacy.

Delivering Information to a Patient

Many of the same guidelines of effective communication discussed above apply as well to clinical encounters in which a provider needs to convey, rather than elicit, information. In these circumstances, however, the provider has the additional challenges of providing information in a clear manner, and then of ensuring that the patient has indeed understood the information being conveyed.

Ensuring the information being relayed to a patient is being assimilated is particularly important when a patient needs to make a decision regarding treatment, and when a provider is giving a patient instructions on patient-administered medications and/or treatments. The process of providing information to the patient, allowing the patient to ask questions, answering the questions, ensuring patient comprehension, and obtaining and documenting a patient's agreement to a particular management plan and/or treatment, is known as *informed consent.*

The process of obtaining informed consent prior to a medical intervention became standard practice following a series of legal cases in the 1950s and 1960s, where patients successfully sued for injury sustained during treatments or surgeries which the patients claimed they would not have undergone had they fully known and understood the risks involved. Whereas it may be difficult to obtain and document informed consent in a manner that will stand up to any and all legal claims, the process of giving patients complete, accurate, and truthful information regarding their disease/condition prognosis and treatment options is not only a legal but also a professional expectation. **Table 55.2** summarizes the process and key components of informed consent.

In general, when conveying information to a patient, a provider needs to be honest and truthful. He or she needs to use language that the patient can understand. Educational handouts can be very helpful in this respect. Such handouts are available for many medical conditions and are often also available in multiple languages. Providers may also want to create their own handouts on topics about which they commonly have to educate patients. The patient can keep the handout to read at her own pace later, which is particularly helpful when dealing with a new di-

Table 55.2 The process of informed consent*

Outcome	Purpose	Legal issues/caveats
Assess the patient's ability to provide informed consent	Is the patient a minor?	Depending on State laws and the condition/procedure you are obtaining consent for, minors may not be able to provide consent. Many, but not all, States allow minors to consent to treatment related to reproductive health
	Is the patient temporarily or permanently incompetent?	Patients who are mentally incapacitated (e. g., mentally retarded, intoxicated, altered psychological state) may not be able to provide informed consent. Depending on the circumstance, the provider may need to obtain consent from a legally appointed decision-maker, wait until the patient regains competence, or may need to seek a court order. In cases of emergency, the provider may need to forgo the process of inform consent (see below)
	Can the patient understand the information being presented?	If the patient does not speak fluent English, an interpreter should be brought in to assist in the process. The provider should avoid medical jargon and speak in terms that the patient can understand. The provider may want to use appropriate printed handouts
	Is the patient an autonomous decision-maker?	The provider should try to make a determination regarding the autonomy of the patient in making treatment decisions, and take steps to ensure that the patient is free from coercion
	Is this an emergency situation?	In cases of an emergency when the patient is unconscious or otherwise incapable of providing consent, and when the patient's life or health is in danger without prompt attention, the law permits treatment without a patient's explicit consent

Table 55.2 Continued

Outcome	Purpose	Legal issues/caveats
Provide information regarding treatment/procedure	Diagnosis/condition that is being treated	This should include some information on how provider has arrived at diagnosis, an assessment of how confident the provider is regarding the diagnosis, the expected course of the condition or disease, and a prognosis for the patient without treatment
	Recommended treatment/procedure and reason for recommendation	The recommended treatment should be the one that is most likely to benefit the patient regardless of the cost and whether or not the patient has insurance that covers this treatment or procedure. It should also be a recommendation that is based on accepted standard of care. If the recommended treatment is not considered standard of care (or if it is experimental) the patient should be informed of this fact and why this is nonetheless the recommended treatment. Off-label use of devices and medications should be explained to the patient
	Potential risks and benefits of treatment or procedure	This should be based on current data
	Estimation of probability of success of treatment or procedure	This should also be based on current data. Never guarantee an outcome. The patient should be told that estimations of probability of success are usually based on grouped data and that it is impossible to know how specific patients will respond and whether or not there will be complications
	Alternatives to the recommended treatment and their risks and benefits and probability of success	These should include all alternatives regardless of cost or patient's insurance coverage and should also including the alternative of nontreatment
	Risks of nontreatment	
Allow time for questions, discussion, and clarification		Make sure that the patient has some time to process the information (in nonurgent cases, it may be prudent to allow patient a day or two to consider treatment options). Answer questions truthfully and let the patient know if there is something you do not know or are unsure about
Assess understanding		Ask the patient to put into her own words her understanding of her diagnosis and/or treatment options and the risks of treatment and nontreatment
Document consent or informed refusal		It is a MUST to document the consent process. Requirements for preprinted and signed consent forms vary by State and by type of treatment and procedure, so the provider should be familiar with State and institutional laws, regulations, and guidelines. The physician should always write a note in the medical record about the informed consent process, but a note in the medical record will not suffice if there is a requirement for a written and signed consent form. If the patient refuses treatment, this must be carefully documented as well

*These are general guidelines: the amount and type of information that a provider must disclose to a patient in the course of informed consent depends on State law, case law, statutes and regulations. Providers need to be aware of these and institutional requirements.

agnosis and feeling overloaded with information. Written instructions on treatment plans, how to take medication, and when and who to contact to report problems can also facilitate a healthy provider–physician relationship. However, studies have shown that the average person reads at an eighth-grade level, and many adults have either basic or below-basic literacy. Thus, patients may have limited literacy and the content of both spoken and written information may need to be adapted. The use of pictures, diagrams, and videos may help convey educational messages in an effective manner to individuals with limited literacy.

Giving Bad or Difficult News to Patients

Providers in the field of obstetrics and gynecology often have to give patients bad or difficult news. However, they often are woefully unprepared for how to break bad or difficult news in a manner that minimizes trauma to the patient, the family, and even for themselves. Such news may including letting someone know that they have tested positive for Chlamydia or HIV, or telling a pregnant woman that her child has a birth defect.

Girgis and Sanson-Fisher (see Further Reading) reported the results of a multidisciplinary consensus group convened in order to create guidelines on how to break bad news to patients (**Table 55.3**). An interesting finding in the literature search conducted by this consensus group is that although providers tended to view professional detachment as a desirable quality in the delivery of bad news to a patient, patients found such professional detachment upsetting and even traumatizing. Recurrent themes from the providers' point of view include feelings of being unprepared to break bad news to patients and dealing with the emotional aftermath of such disclosures.

Some providers said they didn't believe that psychosocial support should be part of their job description.

This physician attitude contrasts with patients' often-expressed desires for their provider to give them complete and honest information in a caring and compassionate manner, and to be empathetic and serve as a source of support.

Balancing the need for clinical objectivity with the need for compassionate bedside manner can be a gargantuan task. During the difficult exchanges that follow the disclosure of bad news, providers and patients alike must remember that medicine, as much as it is a science, is also an art practiced by humans on humans. Therefore, empathy from both parties toward the other will help to make it more likely for these difficult encounters to be therapeutic rather than traumatic.

Table 55.3 Giving bad news

Key ingredients	Further instructions
Choose one person to give the news	The provider giving the news should be someone who the patient knows and trusts and has been involved in her care. If this person is not readily identifiable, try to choose someone who is skilled at delivering bad news. The physician who has been guiding the care/diagnosis should be present, if at all possible, even if he or she is not the one who will be breaking the news.
Allot enough time	Make sure that there is ample uninterrupted time both to both give the news and to spend time with the patient after the news has been delivered. The end of an office session or a time when a provider does not have other commitments are good options. The provider(s) should avoid responding to nonemergency phone calls or pagers during that time
Prepare	Preparations should include practicing what will be said as well as assembling resources that may be helpful. The provider should try to anticipate the patient's questions and informational needs and have the necessary resources (including written materials or even additional providers) available
Ensure that the place where the news will be given is comfortable and private	The room where the news will be disclosed should be private. If possible there should be a phone in the room in case the patient needs to call family or loved ones. Make water and tissues available
Facilitate the presence of family members/support	The patient should be encouraged to bring or call in family or other support people
Be straightforward and honest but avoid being blunt, cold, or detached	Patients want and deserve full and honest information. They also want and deserve this information in a compassionate and empathetic manner. Acknowledge the difficulty of situation and your own shortcomings/discomfort but avoid using detachment as a coping mechanism. If you cannot do this for a patient, you should find a provider who can, and be present to support that provider and answer questions. Do not avoid the patient, this will engender feelings of abandonment and mistrust
Encourage and allow the patient to express emotions	Make sure that the patient knows that she can cry and voice her emotions. Acknowledge that she may need some time before she can talk further. Give her the option to have you leave the room. Do not rush her.
Assess the patient's understanding and emotional status and her immediate information and support needs	Ensure that she has understood the diagnosis and prognosis. Assess whether she needs some educational materials and help her obtain them. Make sure that she is not in danger of hurting herself including an assessment of her ability to drive herself home
Arrange for follow up visit	Make plans to have her return (within 24 hours if possible) to discuss the management plan and next steps, including support services and assistance with disclosure to others. Ensure that she knows how to reach you or other appropriate support in the intervening time

Reproduced with permission from Girgis A, Sanson-Fisher RW. Breaking bad news: consensus guidelines for medical practitioners. J Clin Oncol 1995; 13(9):2449–2456

Disclosing Medical Errors to Patients

Although disclosing bad news is a daunting task, disclosing a medical error can be terrifying. Studies reveal that a majority of patients want to be told about medical errors. Furthermore, there is mounting pressure from patient safety movements for mandated error disclosure. However, the fear of a punitive patient response keeps most providers from letting their patients know when they have made an error. Currently, there is only a 30% error disclosure rate.

Although most physicians agree with the ethics of disclosing medical errors, and an increasing number of institutions have policies in place to promote disclosure of medical errors, these policies are often not accompanied by guidelines on how to disclose an error, nor are they embedded in a broader system to protect the provider or hospital from the medical liability such disclosure may create. It must be emphasized that most medical errors are not due to the medical negligence of individual providers, but rather are systems-related.

Most patients, however, view medical error as failure by an individual provider. Until providers have some protection from the risk of rising malpractice premiums, loss of liability, and multimillion dollar jury awards, it is unlikely that medical error disclosure rates will increase significantly. It is worth noting that there are numerous efforts to bring about the changes necessary that allow for medical error disclosure in a way that protects both physicians and patients.

Special Challenges in the Provider–Patient Relationship

There are particular circumstances and patient characteristics and patient populations that can create challenges to effective provider–patient interaction and/or communication. These include cultural differences, language barriers, limited literacy, status differences between provider and patient, and personality issues.

Cross-Cultural Interactions

As the population in a country grows more diverse, healthcare providers must become competent in providing care to patients who come from different ethnic and cultural backgrounds from themselves. The impact of these cultural and language differences on the provider–patient relationship has not been studied extensively. However, concerns regarding the possibility that these differences may contribute to the disparities in health outcomes among racial and ethnic minorities has prompted an increased focus on promoting cultural competence in the training of physicians and other healthcare providers.

Although a comprehensive discussion of cultural competency in health care is outside the scope of this chapter, the following offers some basic pointers to what can be helpful. Knowing key phrases in a patient's language can be helpful, for example. However, the provider must keep in mind that even if he or she is fluent in the patient's language, there is more to cultural competency than language.

Likewise, although becoming familiar with some of the customs and beliefs of particular ethnic groups that a provider may frequently encounter may be helpful, customs and beliefs can vary greatly, even within individual countries or ethnic groups, depending on geographic location, socioeconomic status, and other similar factors.

Simply learning about specific beliefs and behaviors common to a certain group can lead to errors of oversimplification of a patient's experience or of stereotyping. It may be more useful to think of cultural competency as human relationship building rather than memorizing a "laundry list" of customs and beliefs associated with a particular group of people.

In developing cultural competency skills there are some essential points that providers should keep in mind:

- There are cultural norms regarding how individuals communicate and interact with those of different genders, socioeconomic groups, and perceived status or authority. These may significantly impact the clinical encounter.
- There are cultural beliefs regarding disease causation and treatment. These can include beliefs regarding foods, temperature, and specific activities.
- Similarly, the provider needs to be aware of the possibility that the patient also may be seeking simultaneous care from a traditional healer or using traditional remedies. The provider must avoid dismissing these beliefs and alternative approaches and work instead to understand how they shape the individual's response to illness and approach to treatment. There are differences as to what things are valued—for example, old age, independence, etc.
- There are cultural differences in how decisions are made and who makes a final decision.
- A key component of cultural competency is recognizing one's own biases as well as recognizing the fact that there are customs, beliefs, and norms that guide physician behavior just as there are for patient behavior.

The patient explanatory model has been described as a way for healthcare providers to gain an understanding of how these factors affect the clinical encounter. This patient explanatory "is the patient's understanding of the cause, severity, and prognosis of an illness; the expected treatment; and how illness affects his or her life. In essence, it is the meaning of the illness for the patient."

This model is often referred to in the context of dealing with patients of different cultures. However, since every individual patient has specific beliefs and values that vary from the provider's, this model can be helpful in all clinical encounters.

The following set of questions, which derived from the classic work of Kleinman et al. (see Further Reading), can guide providers in finding out from a patient how their beliefs and norms affect their understanding and experience of illness and disease.

- What do you think caused the problem?
- Why do you think it started when it did?
- What do you think your illness does to you?
- How does the illness work?
- How severe is your illness? How long do you think will it last?
- How do you think it should be treated?
- Who gives you advice about this illness?
- Who can help you treat it?
- Have you seen a healer or other doctor for this illness?
- What are you afraid of with this illness?
- What are your goals or results you want from treatment?

From this information the provider can understand the patient's model for the illness, and then can compare the patient model to his or her own medical/physician model of the illness. Kleinman et al. recommend discussing openly with the patient how these two models are similar or different, and work with the patient to negotiate a management plan. It is especially important to work with the patient to identify parts of the patient's model that may interfere with appropriate care (or that may be dangerous) and collaborate with the patient to create a shared model that meets the therapeutic goal.

Communicating With Patients of Limited Language Skills

As previously indicated, a growing number of patients do not speak the dominant language of their country as their primary language. Depending on the language proficiency of the patient, it may be necessary to obtain an interpreter. In the United States, for example, organizations receiving federal funds are obligated by law to provide free of charge appropriate interpretation services, either by bilingual staff or by proficient interpreters. Even when not required by law, however, the use of interpreters is highly recommended. Patients who need an interpreter but for whom one is not obtained have the lowest satisfaction of all patient groups with the interpersonal aspects of their clinical encounter.

Failure to obtain appropriate translation can result in harmful, if not deadly, consequences. In a much publicized case in the United States, the failure to obtain adequate translator services was cited as the main contributor to a Spanish-speaking 18-year-old in Florida being incorrectly diagnosed as being a drug abuser when, in reality, he had a brain aneurysm. The patient ended up with quadriplegia and his family successfully sued and was awarded $71 million. **Table 55.4** includes some guidelines on the effective use of interpreters in medical encounters.

Table 55.4 Model guidelines for the use of interpreters

Talk to the interpreter prior to starting the exchange with the patient. Let the interpreter know the relevant background, so that he or she can familiarize before entering the patient's room
Review with the interpreter the goal of the exchange (e. g., to let the patient know that you are recommending that her baby be delivered via cesarean section)
Review with the interpreter your expectation that the interpretation be without omissions, editing, or editorializing
Ask the interpreter to let you know if there is something he or she does not understand or needs repeated, or if there is something the patient does not understand and needs to be repeated
Have the interpreter introduce himself or herself and then have the interpreter introduce you
Position yourselves so that everyone can have eye contact (i.e., the patient can see both the interpreter and the provider; the provider can see the patient and the interpreter, and the interpreter can see both the patient and the provider)
Talk to the patient not to the interpreter
Speak slowly, clearly, and pause to let the translator speak
If there is a confusing response to a question or the patient asks something that does not make sense, ask for clarification
Ask for a verbatim translation if confusion persists
After the encounter, meet with the interpreter to assess normality of exchange and to ask whether the interpreter feels that there was any confusion or any additional information or cultural clarification (keep in mind, however, that language proficiency does not equal cultural proficiency, and that an interpreter may not be able to evaluate the encounter for cultural misunderstandings)
If a professional interpreter is not available and you need to use an ad hoc translator:
Assess level of proficiency
Never use a minor unless it is an emergency and nobody else is available
Make sure that the patient agrees to having the ad hoc translator
Keep in mind the limitations of the ad hoc translator, including potential conflict of interest and lack of expertise in medical translation

Adapted from: Guidelines for Use of Medical Interpreter Services. Washington, DC: Association of American Medical Colleges, 2009

Interactions with Patients Who Are Research Subjects

Due to a history of gross violations of human rights conducted in the name of medical research—most notably the Tuskegee Syphilis Study and the experiments conducted by the Nazis in World War II—the National Research Act was signed into US law in 1974, creating the National Commission for the Protection of Human Subjects of Biomedical and Behavioral Research. This commission was asked to identify the ethical principles and guidelines for research involving human subjects. The Belmont Report (see Further Reading) summarizes the work of the Commission and is required reading for any investigator hoping to conduct research involving human subjects. Many of the issues such as autonomy and informed consent that are addressed in the Belmont Report and other documents guiding the treatment of human research subjects are addressed in Chapter 56 on ethics, and in the section above on informed consent.

Key points to remember are that patients cannot be the subjects of research studies unless they have voluntarily gone through an informed consent process within the context of an approved protocol that has gone through review by an institutional review board (IRB), or unless such an entity has determined that the research activity (such as retrospective chart review) is exempt from the requirement of informed consent.

Similarly, providers must remember that those activities that are part of an IRB-approved research study are subject to specific review and reporting requirements as outlined by the IRB, whether or not these activities are part of the routine care provided to a patient. Under the US federal law outlining the protection of human subjects in research conducted or supported by any federal department or federal agency, pregnant women and fetuses in utero are both considered "vulnerable" populations and that there are specific restraints on the use of either group as research subjects.

Dealing With Difficult Patients

Despite every effort to create a positive relationship with a patient, there are times that a patient may exhibit a pattern of annoying, disruptive, disrespectful, or even threatening behavior. If a patient threatens or assaults a provider or staff member, law enforcement should be contacted. In other cases of abusive or noncompliant behavior, however, providers should draw boundaries but also try to re-engage the patient in a positive relationship. This may require that someone sit down with the patient not only to explain why the behavior is not acceptable, but also to hear from the patient the reasons for her behavior.

Terminating the Provider–Patient Relationship

There are times when patients have valid grievances with their medical care. Once this grievance is acknowledged and/or addressed, there may be a resolution to the behavior. There are times, however, when the behavior may persist and it may become necessary for the provider to terminate the provider–patient relationship.

Although a provider has the right to terminate care of a patient who has become disruptive, noncompliant, or abusive, certain steps must be taken to help ensure that a claim of abandonment will not be filed against the provider. These steps include the following:

- Contact the patient's insurer to find out their policy regarding termination—put a copy of this termination policy in the chart.
- Send a certified letter stating that you are terminating your interaction with the patient, but that you will continue the relationship for 30 days for emergent issues (or whatever is required by the insurer). Put a copy of the letter in the patient's chart.
- Consider contacting a risk management professional and/or a lawyer.
- If desired or required by the patient's insurance company, assist the patient in finding another provider. Keep in mind that if a patient is pregnant and in her third trimester, she may not be able to find another provider during the pregnancy.
- Assist the patient in transferring her medical record and in any other documentation needs she may have in order to transfer her care to another provider. Patients with government insurance may be harder to terminate and may require the involvement of mediation services or a second chance for the patient with another provider within same practice/group.
- If the patient becomes violent, or threatens violence at any time, law enforcement should be contacted.

Physician–Physician Interactions

Although this chapter is about patient–physician communication and interactions, the manner in which providers relate to each other can have a significant impact on the provider–patient relationship and is, therefore, mentioned here briefly. Adversarial, disrespectful, or confrontational relationships between providers can lead to poor patient satisfaction with their care, and even to medical error.

In the United Sates, the Joint Commission recently released a Sentinel Even Alert on behaviors that undermine a culture of safety. In its review of hospitals for accreditation, it now requires that hospitals "create and implement a process for managing disruptive and inappropriate behaviors." Such behaviors include not only aggressive outbursts such as yelling, intimidation, use of insults and threats, but also passive disruptive behaviors such as refusal to answer questions, failure to answer pagers or phone calls, or refusal/failure to share with another provider important patient information.

Key Points

- Interpersonal and communications skills are now clearly recognized as core competencies for physicians in training.
- Research has demonstrated that these skills can be taught and that providers who have undergone training in communication perform better in Objective Structured Clinical Examinations and have higher satisfaction scores from standardized patients.
- No longer can these skills be viewed as personality characteristics that a provider either has or lacks, but rather they must be viewed in the same way as the other core skills that a student must acquire in his or her medical training.
- Like many of these other skills, communication and interpersonal skills must be continuously reviewed, evaluated, practiced, and refined.

Further Reading

The Belmont Report: Ethical Principles and Guidelines for the Protection of Human Subjects of Research. 1978; DHEW Publications No. (05)78-0012

Berry DL, Wilkie DJ, Thomas CR Jr, Fortner P. Clinicians communicating with patients experiencing cancer pain. *Cancer Invest* 2003;21(3):374–381

Carrillo JE, Green AR, Betancourt JR. Cross-cultural primary care: a patient-based approach. *Ann Intern Med* 1999;130(10):829–834

Commission TJ. Behaviors that undermine a culture of safety. *Sentinel Event Alert* 2008;(40):1–3

Freeman R. The psychology of dental patient care. 9. Communicating effectively: some practical suggestions. *Br Dent J* 1999;187(5):240–244

Girgis A, Sanson-Fisher RW. Breaking bad news: consensus guidelines for medical practitioners. *J Clin Oncol* 1995;13(9):2449–2456

Griffith CH III, Wilson JF, Langer S, Haist SA. House staff nonverbal communication skills and standardized patient satisfaction. *J Gen Intern Med* 2003;18(3):170–174

Kleinman A, Eisenberg L, Good B. Culture, illness, and care: clinical lessons from anthropologic and cross-cultural research. *Ann Intern Med* 1978;88(2):251–258

Morales LS, Cunningham WE, Brown JA, Liu H, Hays RD. Are Latinos less satisfied with communication by health care providers? *J Gen Intern Med* 1999;14(7):409–417

Pellegrino ED. Professionalism, profession and the virtues of the good physician. *Mt Sinai J Med* 2002;69(6):378–384

56 Clinical Ethics in Obstetrics and Gynecology

Hugh E. Mighty and Jenifer Fahey

There are times when physicians are called upon by their patients or colleagues to help make difficult medical decisions. There also are times when physicians may disagree with decisions that their patients or colleagues have made. In either case, the physician must be able to analyze the situation in a systematic fashion in order to provide advice in a way that promotes the patient's best interest. Preparing medical students to take on this professional responsibility should be an essential goal in medical education.

This chapter provides a brief overview of clinical ethics, including a review of core principles of medical ethics followed by a section on common ethical dilemmas that are specific to the field of obstetrics and gynecology. It also includes representative case studies to highlight relevant points and provides students with some general guidelines for ethical decision-making.

Medical Ethics

Background

Ethics is the branch of philosophy concerned with the study or evaluation of human behavior/conduct to identify the norms, rules, values, and principles that guide our moral life. Medical ethics is an example of "applied ethics," in which these values, norms, or principles are used to guide decision-making in actual cases where the best course of action is not clearly evident. Because medical knowledge often is not enough to guide medical decision-making, it is important for health practitioners to have an understanding of key concepts in the field of ethics, and learn how to conduct a careful and disciplined analysis of ethical dilemmas that may confront them in the clinical arena.

Western medical ethics traces its roots to antiquity and the beginning of the Hippocratic tradition, which emphasizes the concept of duty to patient and provides guidelines for physician behavior when interacting with patients. Many of the same core concepts of medical ethics found in the earliest writings on the subject can be found in the Code of Ethics of the American Medical Association (AMA), first adopted in 1847. In the 1970s, Beauchamp and Childress published their seminal modern text on medical ethics, *The Principles of Biomedical Ethics,* in which they identify beneficence, nonmaleficence, autonomy, and justice as the four, core moral principles of biomedical ethics. Since then, a principle-based approach (also known as "principalism") has come to dominate the medical ethics arena.

A common criticism of this principle-based approach, however, is that although it provides a helpful way to study an ethical problem, it is of limited use in guiding decision-making in clinical practice. This is due, in large part, to the fact that in many clinical cases these principles are actually in conflict with one another, and there is no clear hierarchy among them to help resolve such ethical dilemmas. Furthermore, the principle-based approach relies heavily on moral rules and theories but underemphasizes contextual issues, such as gender relations, standards of practice, economics, cultural considerations, and legal issues, which affect both patient and provider decision-making.

In such situations, the clinician may have to draw on other resources or theoretical frameworks to help guide decision-making. A summary of some of the moral theories that guide medical ethics is included in **Table 56.1**.

Principles of Medical Ethics

Regardless of the criticisms of a principle-based approach, beneficence, nonmaleficence, autonomy, and justice are still widely accepted as core principles in medical ethics. A brief definition of these four principles can be found in **Table 56.2** and below in more detail.

Table 56.1 Examples of moral theories

Virtue ethics	Moral conduct should be guided by virtues such as kindness, compassion, respect for others, etc.
Professional ethics	Moral conduct should be guided by the standards that are outlined by accredited/well-trained group of professionals
Utilitarian ethics	Moral conduct should be guided by the balance of the total good or total bad consequences of actions in a way that maximizes good/value
Kantian ethics	Moral conduct should be guided by the acceptability of an action if this action were generalized to all similar situations
Feminist ethics	Moral conduct should take into account gender considerations to ensure that there is not harmful gender bias in one's actions
Rights-based ethics	Moral conduct should ensure that basic individual rights (autonomy, privacy, confidentiality) are upheld
Communitarian ethics	Moral conduct should ensure that communal values are upheld

Table 56.2 Core principles of medical ethics as they pertain to the physician's actions

Autonomy	The physician should respect the right of the patient to make decisions regarding their care
Beneficence	The physician should act in a way that promotes the patient's best interests and promotes patient wellbeing
Nonmaleficence	The physician should avoid harming the patient
Justice	The physician should give the patient what is his or her due and should treat similar patients equally

Autonomy

Autonomy, or self-rule, in the context of ethics is the quality of moral independence. In the realm of medical ethics, it is manifested as the right to make one's own decisions. To be an autonomous entity the individual must be: (1) free from coercion or other controlling influence or influences, and (2) possess the capacity for "intentional action." Respect for autonomy in medical decision-making is understood to mean that if these two standards for autonomy are reasonably met, the individual has the right to make decisions regarding their medical care, even if

the decision conflicts with what the provider believes is in their best interest.

The term "reasonably" is used because humans are rarely fully free of controlling influence. So, although a provider may not always be able to determine whether a patient is truly an autonomous entity, he or she should make a reasonable effort to determine whether there are controlling influences that significantly compromise the patient's autonomy. It is also understood that a physician should not take actions that exert a controlling influence on the patient.

There are many times when treatments and procedures will compromise the capacity for intentional action. Self-administration of narcotics or other psychotropic medications are good examples. Thus, the patient should not be asked to make medical decisions in this compromised state. Furthermore, it is clearly unethical to purposely compromise a patient's capacity for intentional action with this compromised capacity being the end goal. It is the principle of autonomy, and the obligation to try to ensure that the patient is an autonomous entity, which underlies the concept of informed consent. Informed consent is a central concept to ethical decision-making, which is discussed in detail in Chapter 55 and 57.

Beneficence and Nonmaleficence

The obligation to do good (beneficence), along with the obligation not to inflict harm on others (nonmaleficence), are closely related principles that are central to medical ethics. Their importance to medical ethics dates back to antiquity, when it is believed that Hippocrates (or one of his students) included them in the oath taken by new physicians, now commonly known as the Hippocratic Oath. Included in the same statement within the oath is the principle of justice: "I will apply dietetic measures for the benefit of the sick according to my ability and judgment; I will keep them from harm and injustice."

If medicine is the science and art of promoting health and wellbeing by treating, alleviating, and curing disease, it can then be argued that beneficence is the driving ethical principle of medicine. However, all ethical principles, including beneficence and the obligations derived from these principles, are bounded and sometimes even overridden by other principles and obligations. Quite often, for example, the obligation to "do good" for a patient, which is derived from the principle of beneficence, comes into conflict with an obligation derived from another key ethical principle—the obligation to respect patient autonomy.

Justice

Justice is the concept of giving to each person what is his or her due. In the realm of medical ethics it includes the obligations to provide to each patient that to which he or she is entitled, to allocate resources fairly, and to treat all patients equally. It is a complex principle prone to the effects of context and individual bias, including the physician's background and experience.

What is perceived as just by an individual or group of individuals can vary greatly from what others may believe to be just. Furthermore, in a system of unequal distribution of resources, the physician is handicapped in his or her ability to be truly just. For example, regardless of severity of disease, patients with health insurance will often have access to care more readily than those who do not.

In nonemergency situations, the physician has an obligation to promote the wellbeing of each individual patient, and is not expected to take into consideration these system-wide dilemmas of distributive justice during individual clinical encounters. However, advocating for a just allocation of health care resources and not taking actions that compound inequalities in our health care system are ethical obligations of the physician. In emergency or mass casualty situations, however, physicians *will* have to take into consideration the limited availability of resources and make decisions as to whom to treat and in what order.

In addition to the principles outlined above, there are values or "moral rules" that also are an important part of ethical decision-making and behavior in the medical arena. These include, but are not limited to, veracity (telling the truth); respect for patient's privacy, confidentiality, and dignity as well as professionalism, compassion, and collegiality. Some of these concepts are also discussed in more detail in Chapter 55 on communication and provider–patient interactions.

A number of professional medical organizations and associations have created documents that translate these principles and moral rules into prescriptive statements on physician conduct, ethical medical decision-making, and provider–patient relationships. The AMA's Code of Ethics included in **Table 56.3** is an example of such a document. The American College of Obstetricians and Gynecologists (ACOG) also has a Code of Ethics, which is very similar to that of the AMA.

Table 56.3 The American Medical Association's Code of Ethics

I	A physician shall be dedicated to providing competent medical care, with compassion and respect for human dignity and rights
II	A physician shall uphold the standards of professionalism, be honest in all professional interactions, and strive to report physicians deficient in character or competence, or engaging in fraud or deception, to appropriate entities
III	A physician shall respect the law and also recognize a responsibility to seek changes in those requirements which are contrary to the best interests of the patient
IV	A physician shall respect the rights of patients, colleagues, and other health professionals, and shall safeguard patient confidences and privacy within the constraints of the law
V	A physician shall continue to study, apply, and advance scientific knowledge, maintain a commitment to medical education, make relevant information available to patients, colleagues, and the public, obtain consultation, and use the talents of other health professionals when indicated
VI	A physician shall, in the provision of appropriate patient care, except in emergencies, be free to choose whom to serve, with whom to associate, and the environment in which to provide medical care
VII	A physician shall recognize a responsibility to participate in activities contributing to the improvement of the community and the betterment of public health
VIII	A physician shall, while caring for a patient, regard responsibility to the patient as paramount
IX	A physician shall support access to medical care for all people

Reproduced with permission from American Medical Association. Code of Medical Ethics. Chicago, Ill: American Medical Association, 2008.

Ethical Dilemmas in Obstetrics: the Fetus as Patient

Maternal Autonomy vs. Fetal Beneficence

Ethical decision-making in obstetrics and gynecology is complicated by several factors that are peculiar to the field. The most significant of these in the practice of obstetrics is that the provider is simultaneously caring for two patients—the mother and the fetus—both of whose interests the provider owes a duty to protect. The moral obligation due to the fetus, however, is generally accepted within the context of medical ethics to be different from that owed to the mother.

It has also been generally accepted that the obligation owed to the fetus by the physician changes as the fetus advances in gestation, especially as it reaches and passes the threshold of viability. Chervenak and McCullough (see Further Reading) have written extensively on the subject of the fetus as patient, and propose that the viable fetus is a fetal patient and that the previable fetus is a fetal patient only when the woman confers such status on it.

Regardless of whether or not the fetus is viable and of whether or not it is considered to be a patient separate from the mother, the fetus, like a child, does not have independent moral status. Rather, the mother is regarded to have, throughout pregnancy, de facto decision-making authority for the fetus. This creates two areas in which ethical dilemmas arise: 1) situations in which protecting the best interest of one of these two patients will cause harm to the other, and 2) situations in which actions/decisions of the mother threaten the wellbeing of the fetus—these include both decisions to refuse a treatment or procedure that may be beneficial to the fetus and decisions or actions that may be directly harmful to the fetus.

The following two cases illustrate the ethical dilemmas in these areas.

Case 1

Ms. S. is a 31-year-old G2P1001 who is being seen for a prenatal care appointment. She is approximately 20 weeks estimated gestational age and the lab results from her first visit revealed that she is HIV-positive and has a high viral load. Ms. S. has been counseled extensively on the recommended care plan for her during pregnancy and postpartum, including the recommendation for highly active antiretroviral therapy in pregnancy and zidovudine during labor and birth to help prevent HIV transmission to the fetus. Despite multiple sessions with Ms. S., she refuses to take any medications.

Case 2

Ms. G. is a 28-year-old G4P2102 at 32 weeks' gestation who presents to the labor and delivery clinic with vaginal bleeding. A placental abruption in suspected. Cocaine use is a known risk factor for placental abruption. At her first prenatal care visit her urine tested positive for opioids. When she is counseled regarding these test results, Ms. G. refuses treatment and states that she does not want to be further tested for drugs during her pregnancy. On her presentation for delivery, she again refuses drug screening.

Discussion: In cases 1 and 2 there is a conflict between the duty to respect maternal autonomy and the duty to promote fetal wellbeing. The Ethics Committee of the ACOG has written a Committee Opinion devoted entirely to this conflict that should serve as a key reference to providers confronted with this clinical dilemma.

The recommended approach in a situation such as this is to counsel the woman on the reasoning behind the recommended course of action, including a review of the potential consequences to the fetus. The provider should draw on additional individuals, if necessary (such as members of an ethics committee), to ensure that the woman has the information she needs to make an informed decision. Once a reasonable effort has been made to give the patient the information, it is her responsibility to make an informed decision. According to the guidelines, "the obstetrician must respect the patient's autonomy, continue to care for the pregnant woman, and not intervene against the patient's wishes …"

There have been cases of such conflict between maternal and fetal interests in which providers have resorted to the courts or other legal action either to intervene against maternal wishes or to punish women for actions they have taken that endangered their fetuses. In some cases, women have been required to undergo court-ordered cesarean sections or have been incarcerated for substance abuse during pregnancy.

It is important to note, however, that in some key cases of this kind, appellate courts have vacated court-orders or dismissed criminal charges against the women. In these decisions, the appellate courts have ruled that a woman's right to self-determination, informed consent, and autonomous medical decision-making does not change due to her pregnant status.

In a 1990 decision by the District of Columbia Appellate Court, for example, the court stated that they could not think of a case in which the State might have an "interest sufficiently compelling to override a pregnant patient's wishes." In a subsequent case, the Appellate Court of Illinois reaffirmed the District of Columbia Appellate Court's assertion that "if a woman is a capable decision maker, her decision should control in virtually all cases."

Regardless of the legal precedents on this issue, it is important for the clinician to consider the ethical implications of legal action against a pregnant patient. Such cases, which tend to generate considerable media attention, can create barriers to access to health care.

Legislation that mandates testing of pregnant women for fetal indications can create similar barriers to care. In what is now a well-known study, researchers investigated the implications of mandatory HIV testing of pregnant women. This study compared health behaviors of pregnant women under a mandatory versus a voluntary HIV testing protocol. Based on their findings, these researchers calculated that enough women would choose to avoid prenatal care entirely in order to avoid mandatory testing, and that the expected number of perinatal HIV infections would actually increase rather than decrease under such a protocol.

Additional studies have confirmed that under voluntary protocols for HIV testing, where the mother is educating and engaged as the primary decision-maker for her fetus, a majority of women will consent to HIV testing. These studies underscore two important factors to consider: 1) even well-meaning legal action to protect the fetus can have broad, unintended consequences, and 2) most pregnant women, if counseled appropriately, will make decisions that promote fetal wellbeing.

Maternal Autonomy vs. Nonmaleficence

In the cases discussed above, there exists a conflict between maternal autonomy and fetal beneficence. Similar cases can arise in which there is a conflict between maternal autonomy and nonmaleficence to her or to the fetus. However, there are some important distinctions between these two types of cases, which are illustrated in Cases 3 and 4.

Case 3

Ms. J. is a 22-year-old G2P0010 admitted to a labor and delivery unit at 24 weeks estimated gestational age with severe pre-eclampsia and intrauterine growth retardation (IUGR). Ms. J. needs to be delivered. However, the obstetric team has determined that due to her medical status and the fact that she is obese, she is not a good candidate for surgery. Therefore, the optimal route of delivery for Ms. J. is vaginal. The neonatal team has counseled Ms. J. that due to the fact that the baby is extremely premature and has severe IUGR, there is an increased likelihood that labor will cause fetal asphyxia and or fetal death. Ms. J. has requested a cesarean section for the sake of the fetus. The obstetric team is not comfortable with this choice, however.

Case 4

Ms. B. is a 33-year-old G3P2002 at 12 weeks estimated gestational age. She had requested chorionic villus sampling (CVS) to obtain a fetal karyotype to "rule out birth defects." Blood test and ultrasound examination performed to screen for genetic defects do not reveal any increased risks, but Ms. B. still wants to proceed with CVS. During her visit with the genetic counselor immediately prior to the procedure, the counselor informs Ms. B. that her insurance may not pay for the procedure, since she is under 35 years old and her other tests results are within normal range. The patient reveals to the counselor that her reason for wanting CVS is not to rule out birth defects but to determine fetal gender. Ms. B. already has two other female children. The genetic counselor shares this information with the physician who is scheduled to perform the CVS. Although the physician has previously performed CVS without a clear medical indication to relieve patient anxiety related to genetic anomalies, she is unsure as to what to do in this case.

Discussion: In both of these cases, there is a conflict between respect for the patient's autonomy and nonmaleficence. The ethical dilemma in Case 3 does not lie in the decision to deliver the fetus prematurely. In this case, with worsening pre-eclampsia, the physician is obligated to protect maternal health by delivering the fetus, even if delivery at such premature gestation can have significant negative effect on the fetus. The ethical dilemma lies in determining the route of delivery.

Vaginal delivery is the preferred route of delivery in the face of severe pre-eclampsia due to an increased risk of perioperative morbidity and mortality (see Chapter 19). If the provider honored maternal autonomy by performing a cesarean section, he or she would have to violate the principle of nonmaleficence—or to "first, do no harm."

In Case 4, the patient is requesting a procedure that carries risks to her and to the fetus without a clear medical indication. Furthermore, from the information available, it seems possible that the patient may use the information gathered to seek a termination of her pregnancy based on gender.

What differentiates these cases from Cases 1 and 2 is that, unlike in the previous cases where the patient is asking the physician *to refrain* from doing something that will benefit the fetus, in these two scenarios the physicians are being asked by the patient *to do* something that could harm her or the fetus, which is against accepted standard practice in this situation.

As previously stated, although a woman has a right under almost all circumstances to refuse to have a treatment imposed on her against her will, "should she choose to exert her positive right to request on-demand a treatment or procedure that is not in accord with accepted medical practice, then that right can be denied...so that [the physician is] not forced to practice 'bad medicine'." This differentiation between the negative and positive rights of the patient is an important one in the field of medical ethics and has been written about extensively, especially as it relates to the difference between letting someone die versus euthanasia.

Similarly to the right of a woman to refuse interventions, the physician, as an independent moral entity, also is regarded as having rights to refuse to do, knowingly and purposely, something that will cause harm to the patient (e.g., allowing a woman to deliver vaginally in the face of a placenta previa). In the case of the fetal patient, the physician may do something to protect maternal wellbeing that will result in harm to the fetus (as in Case 3), but this is understood to be ethically different than doing something that will result in harm to the fetal patient for a maternal benefit that the provider determines does not outweigh the risk to the fetus.

A physician also has the right to decline to do something for which he or she has strong ethical, or even moral, objection. On the other hand, the physician has a professional responsibility to weigh these objections against his or her obligation to the patient. In situations where a patient is requesting a standard service provided by physicians in that specialty (e.g., a first trimester abortion, tubal ligation, or emergency contraception), this obligation may include assisting the patient in securing this service from another provider. In cases of medical emergency, the professional obligation to provide standard procedures supersedes personal moral objections. This topic is addressed in more detail later in this chapter.

Although in Case 4 the woman is asking for a procedure that is a standard service provided in obstetrics, her request is for a different indication than the one for which the procedure is intended. ACOG discourages sex determination for the purpose of sex selection for nonmedical reasons, as it promotes gender discriminatory behavior.

Ethical Dilemmas in Obstetrics: the Neonate as Patient

Once a baby is born, it has rights as a patient independent from the mother. However, the management of the extremely premature newborn can present particularly difficult dilemmas. Medical decision-making in the case of the newborn at the threshold of viability is further complicated by the need to take into account not only maternal wishes and the recommendations of the provider of obstetric care, but also the professional obligations of the pediatric team. Furthermore, once a baby has been born, the father also has decision-making authority. Case 5 illustrates these dilemmas.

Case 5

Ms. H. is admitted to the labor and delivery unit in preterm labor at 24 weeks estimated gestational age. She is on tocolysis, but her labor is progressing. The neonatology team has come to talk to her about the prognosis for a baby born so remote to term. Ms. H. and her husband, the father of the baby, state that they do not want aggressive resuscitation of the infant. The neonate is born later that same day. Per hospital protocol, the pediatric team intubates the newborn and takes him to the neonatal intensive care unit. Mr. H. is very angry and demands that the infant be taken off the ventilator and brought to his wife's bedside.

Discussion: Generally, parents are given medical decision-making authority for their children. Unlike in pregnancy, however, where maternal decision-making authority for the fetus is near absolute, once an infant is

born, providers of pediatric care can intervene, if they believe that the parents are not acting in the best interest of the child. In Case 5, this "best interest" becomes harder to identify clearly in the presence of extreme prematurity, when mortality and long-term morbidity rates are high despite aggressive resuscitation efforts and highly skilled neonatal intensive care.

Chervenak and McCullough argue that although aggressive resuscitation is warranted for the viable neonate, interventions should be viewed as experimental and, therefore, only undertaken with parental consent for the infant born near the threshold of viability. Thus, it is prudent to draft hospital guidelines for the management of parental requests for both resuscitation and "do not resuscitate" in the extremely premature neonate. Ideally, these guidelines should include a form to guide informed consent of parents, which will greatly facilitate decision-making and free the clinician at the bedside from having to make these critical decisions on an ad hoc basis when he or she may be unable to take into consideration all the relevant information.

Ethical Dilemmas in Gynecology

OB/GYN practitioners are in the eye of what is arguably the most tempestuous storm in medical ethics—that surrounding the issue of abortion. To address this topic appropriately is outside the scope of this chapter, but some important ethical questions regarding the role of medical providers are particularly relevant here, including the following questions:

- Should medical students be required to participate in the provision of abortions during their medical training?
- Should residents in obstetrics and gynecology be required to learn how to perform abortions? Should they be required to perform abortions as part of their residency training?
- Should obstetricians and gynecologists be required to counsel women on abortion when a woman presents with an unplanned/unwanted pregnancy?
- What, if any, is the obligation of a professional medical organization such as the AMA or ACOG to help ensure the availability and access to services that are within the legal rights of individuals to obtain?
- What is the responsibility of the individual provider of obstetric and gynecologic care to help ensure the availability and access to services that are within the legal rights of individuals to obtain?

Case 6 illustrates the difficult ethical dilemma OB/GYN practitioners face in deciding whether or not to provide abortion services.

Case 6

Ms. D. is a 25-year-old G3P2002. At 8 weeks estimated gestational age she presents to her gynecologist's office in a small rural town. Her husband is in the army reserves and was called back to duty and sent to fight in a war overseas. He came home unexpectedly for 2 weeks after a 10-month deployment. Ms. D. got pregnant at that time. He is now redeployed for another 10 months.

On military pay and without her husband's regular income, the family is struggling to make ends meet. They are in danger of losing their home, for which they saved for 6 years to be able to afford the down payment. To make ends meet, they have already sold the family car and taken their two children out of their private schools.

Mr. and Ms. D. have decided that they want to abort this pregnancy. Her gynecologist, due to moral objections, does not perform abortions and refuses to help Ms. D. find a safe and affordable place to have an abortion.

Discussion: The ACOG has recently released a Committee Opinion entitled, "The Limits of Conscientious Refusal in Reproductive Medicine," which tackles many of these questions and clearly outlines the organization's position on the ethical duty of physicians to fulfill their professional role in the face of conflict of conscience. In brief, it states that:

"Health care providers occasionally may find that providing indicated, even standard, care would present for them a personal moral problem ... Although respect for conscience is important, conscientious refusals should be limited if they constitute an imposition of religious or moral beliefs on patients, negatively affect a patient's health, are based on scientific misinformation, or create or reinforce racial or socioeconomic inequalities. Conscientious refusals that conflict with patient well-being should be accommodated only if the primary duty to the patient can be fulfilled. All health care providers must provide accurate and unbiased information so that patients can make informed decisions ... Physicians and other health care providers have the duty to refer patients in a timely manner to other providers if they do not feel that they can in conscience provide the standard reproductive services that patients request. In resource-poor areas, access to safe and legal reproductive services should be maintained."

Reproductive Services to Minors and Other Special Circumstances

Cases 7 through 9 illustrate the ethical dilemmas that OB/GYN practitioners often must deal with when providing reproductive services to minors or women with other special circumstances, such as conditions that might compromise their ability to make informed decisions on their own.

Case 7

Ms. L. is a 24-year-old G5P2032 seeing her gynecologist for her annual gynecologic exam. Her youngest baby is 6 months old. She has had two abortions and one miscarriage. She wants to have a tubal ligation. Her provider refuses to perform the procedure on the grounds that Ms. L. is "too young to decide that she never wants to be pregnant again."

Case 8

Ms. Q. is a 15-year-old G0P0 who is brought to the gynecologist by her mother for evaluation of irregular and painful periods. Once she is in the room alone with the gynecologist, Ms. Q. reveals during the medical history that she heard from her friend that the birth control pill "can make your periods regular." Further questioning reveals that Ms. Q. has recently become sexually active and is worried about getting pregnant. When asked if that is why she wants the pill, she replies, "Yes, but please don't tell my mother that I am having sex!"

Case 9

Ms. B. is a mentally retarded 25-year-old brought in by her mother, who has been contacted by the nurse at the group home where Ms. B. resides. The nurse believes that Ms. B. has become sexually active. Ms. B.'s mother wants the gynecologist to initiate provider-controlled birth control, such as Depo, Implanon, IUD, or sterilization, on her daughter.

Discussion: These three cases all involve contraception. However, the ethical principles involved in each are quite different. In Case 7, the ethical conflict is one of patient autonomy versus provider paternalism. Although evidence does clearly indicate that younger patients are most likely to regret the decision to undergo sterilization, women who meet the requirements of being an autonomous decision-maker (outlined earlier in the section on autonomy), and who are of adequate age to consent to surgical procedures, have the right to undergo sterilization.

In such cases where the provider truly believes that sterilization is not in the patient's best interest, the process of informed consent is particularly important, as it allows the provider to underscore the permanent nature of the procedure, the risks (including regret), and possible contraceptive options. Of note, in the landmark case of *Griswold vs. Connecticut* (1965) the Supreme Court ruled that the right to birth control is a constitutionally protected right under the right to privacy.

In contrast, in Case 8 the provider is being asked by a minor for a medication. In most realms of consent for medical treatment, minors are not considered fully autonomous decision-makers. Minors, it is argued, may not have the ability to fully understand what is in their best interest and, therefore, limits on their autonomy are warranted. This condition on limits to autonomy presupposes that the minor will undergo by proxy the process of informed consent and that the parents will act in a way that protects the best interest of their child.

The clinician in Case 8 has three potential choices:
1. To break with accepted norms regarding a minor's ability to provide informed consent and provide contraception to this patient
2. To deny this minor's request for contraception, even if it is the clinician's determination that providing contraception to this patient is in her best interest
3. To break patient confidentiality and inform the parent of the minor's sexual activity, so that the parent can consent for the minor

In most states this decision has been removed from the arena of the individual clinical encounter through legislation that clarifies a minor's ability to consent for contraceptive services. Thirty-one States and the District of Columbia allow either all minors, or minors of a certain age or maturity, to consent to contraceptive services. The rest of the States either have no explicit policy or limit a minor's ability to consent to contraceptive services to those minors who are married, already parents, pregnant or previously have been pregnant, or for whom there are health indications for contraceptive use.

In Case 9, since Ms. B. is not a minor, the clinician will likely have to obtain an official determination of Ms. B.'s competence to consent to the imposition of contraceptives, since mental retardation does not automatically equal inability to make medical decisions. Even if Ms. B. is deemed to be incompetent to make medical decisions, a court order may still be necessary in order to sterilize her.

The Rights of Third Parties

There are cases in which the clinician's professional obligations to respect an individual patient's confidentiality will conflict with the clinician's professional obligations to promote and protect the public's health. This conflict arises most frequently for OB/GYN physicians when there

is obligation to disclose to a patient's sexual partners the presence of a sexually transmitted disease, which is illustrated by Case 10.

Case 10

Ms. P. is a 27-year-old G1P0 who is pregnant and was recently diagnosed with HIV. She has started taking antiretroviral therapy to prevent transmission to her fetus. She tells her physician that nobody else, including her boyfriend, knows of her HIV status. She asks her obstetrician not to tell him.

Discussion: With the passage of the **Health Insurance Portability and Accountability Act** of 1996 and the ensuing media attention, many patients are now aware of their right to have their medical information kept confidential. Most patients, however, are not equally aware that there are limits to their right to confidentiality.

For example, physicians are obligated by law to report certain communicable diseases. The AMA *Code of Medical Ethics Opinion E-5.05* states that information disclosed to a physician by a patient is confidential but subject to certain exceptions to protect the public health or endangered third parties. Specifically with regard to HIV-infected patients, the AMA policy is one that:

> *"Promulgates the standard that a physician attempt to persuade an HIV-infected patient to cease all activities that endanger unsuspecting others and to inform those whom he/she might have infected. If such persuasion fails, the physician should pursue notification through means other than by reliance on the patient, such as by the Public Health Department or by the physician directly ..."*

In Case 10, the physician should also inform the patient that her HIV status will probably be revealed anyway, once the baby is born, owing to her pediatricians' obligation to inform parents (including the father) of any tests, medications, and procedures the child is being submitted to, and the indications for these interventions.

General Guidelines for Making Ethical Decisions

In summary, when confronted with an ethical dilemma in clinical practice, the clinician should take a consistent and systematic approach. Due to the nature of clinical encounters, including the fact that clinical scenarios can change quickly, it may not be feasible for the physician to conduct a thorough review of the literature and laws relevant to a case when an ethical dilemma arises.

However, there are steps that clinicians can take to help ensure that they are making informed recommendations and/or decisions. These include becoming familiar with:

- the role of the physician as an ethical actor in clinical practice
- the common ethical dilemmas that arise in the relevant field of practice
- the principles, rules, policies, and laws that should inform decision-making when these dilemmas arise

When an ethical clinical dilemma arises, the physician should:

- identify the relevant clinical and nonclinical facts regarding the case
- identify the relevant parties already involved and those that should be involved
- identify the question(s) or conflict(s) and state these clearly to ensure that everyone understands the issue
- gather available resources
- identify the principles and values involved
- identify the possible courses of action
- identify whether there are established laws or institutional guidelines that impact the decision as to which course of action should be chosen
- identify the preferable course(s) of action
- act
- re-evaluate each case once actions are taken

In their book *Clinical Ethics*, Jonsen et al. present a tool (**Table 56.4**) to help guide ethical decisions in clinical medicine.

Table 56.4 The Jonsen, Siegler and Winsdale Framework for Ethical Decisions in Clinical Medicine

Medical indications	Patient preferences
What is the patient's medical problem? History? Diagnosis? Prognosis?	Is the patient mentally capable and legally competent to make decisions?
Is the problem acute? Chronic? Critical? Emergent? Reversible?	Is there evidence of incapacity?
What are the goals of treatment?	**If patient is competent:**
What are the probabilities of success?	What is the patient stating about preferences for treatment?
What are the alternate plans?	Has the patient been informed of the benefits, risks, and alternatives to the proposed plan?
How can this patient be benefited by medical care?	Has the patient understood the information?
How can harm be avoided?	Has the patient given consent?
Quality of life	**Contextual features**
What are the prospects, with or without treatment, for a return to normal life?	Are there family issues that might influence treatment decisions?
What physical, mental, and social deficits is the patient likely to experience if treatment succeeds?	Are there provider issues that might influence treatment decisions?
Are there biases that might prejudice the provider's evaluation of the patient's quality of life?	Are there financial and economic factors?
Is the patient's present or future condition such that his or her continued life might be judged as undesirable?	Are there religious or cultural factors?
Is there any plan or rationale to forgo treatment?	Are there limits on confidentiality?
Are there plans for comfort and palliative care?	Are there problems of allocation of resources?
	How does the law affect treatment decisions?
	Is clinical research or teaching involved?
	Is there any conflict of interest on the part of the provider or institution?

Reproduced with permission from Jonsen AR, Siegler M, Winslade WJ. Clinical Ethics: a Practical Approach to Ethical Decisions in Clinical Medicine. New York: McGraw-Hill; 2006.

Key Points

- Because the field of obstetrics and gynecology deals with cases related to embryos, fetuses, birth, sex, contraception, sexually transmitted diseases, cancer, and death, ethical dilemmas are common.
- Many of these dilemmas are particular difficult for the clinician to help the patient work through, because they can challenge a provider's belief structure and moral core.
- Ethical dilemmas in obstetrics and gynecology are complex and often politically charged, and at times so sensitive that they can be catapulted into the national spotlight in news headlines or court cases.
- It is crucial for providers to learn to deal with these questions in a professional manner that appropriately subjugates personal biases and that promotes the wellbeing of the patient or patients involved.
- It is critical that education in ethical decision-making starts early in doctor's training and receives constant reinforcement.

Further Reading

American college of Obstetricians and Gynecologists. Maternal decision making, ethics, and the law. ACOG Committee Opinion No. 321. *Obstet Gynecol* 2005;106:1127–1137

American College of Obstetricians and Gynecologists. The limits of conscientious refusal in reproductive medicine. ACOG Committee Opinion No. 385. *Obstet Gynecol* 2007;110:1203–1208

American Medical Association. Code of Medical Ethics. Chicago, Ill: American Medical Association, 2008

American Medical Association. Opinion E-5.05 Confidentiality. Code of Medical Ethics: Current Opinions with Annotations, 2008–2009. Chicago, Ill: American Medical Association, 2008

Beauchamp TL, Childress JF. Principles of Biomedical Ethics. New York: Oxford University Press; 2008

Campbell A, Gillett G, Gareth J. Medical Ethics. Oxford: Oxford University Press; 2001

Chervenak FA, McCullough LB. Ethics in obstetrics and gynecology. An overview. *Eur J Obstet Gynecol Reprod Biol* 1997;75(1):91–94

Edelstein L. The Hippocratic Oath: Text, Translation, and Interpretation. Baltimore, Md: Johns Hopkins Press; 1943

Jonsen AR, Siegler M, Winslade WJ. Clinical Ethics: a Practical Approach to Ethical Decisions in Clinical Medicine. New York: McGraw-Hill; 2006

Nakchbandi IA, Longenecker JC, Ricksecker MA, Latta RA, Healton C, Smith DG. A decision analysis of mandatory compared with voluntary HIV testing in pregnant women. *Ann Intern Med* 1998;128(9):760–767

Pinkerton JV, Finnerty JJ. Resolving the clinical and ethical dilemma involved in fetal-maternal conflicts. *Am J Obstet Gynecol* 1996;175(2):289–295

57 Legal Issues in Obstetrics and Gynecology

Hugh E. Mighty and Jan Kriebs

Although it is easy to think of legal liability as based solely in clinical decision-making, it is not the case. Medicine is not practiced in isolation, but as part of a wider health care community. Thus, legal issues in obstetrics and gynecology are often concerned with relationships. In addition to the care provided, interpersonal aspects of that care also affect the patient's response to clinical events.

Legal requirements for practice and medicolegal interpretations of clinical outcomes are significant factors that are part of choosing a career in obstetrics and gynecology in most countries. Indeed, OB/GYN practitioners are among the specialists at highest risk when professional liability lawsuits are brought. In 2003, the average payout for a liability settlement in obstetrics lawsuits in the United States was more than a million dollars. A survey by the American College of Obstetricians and Gynecologists (ACOG) in 2006 found that doctors were stopping

obstetric practice, increasing the number of cesarean births, and reducing the number of gynecologic surgeries they performed, among other practice changes, due to worry about liability lawsuits (**Table 57.1**).

Indeed, involvement in a professional liability case is an emotionally and psychologically stressful event that can make one question one's own competence and make going to work everyday a challenge. This chapter discusses professional liability in general and steps that physicians and hospitals can take to communicate better with patients and their families and, ultimately, reduce the risk of adverse outcomes that have the potential to lead to medical malpractice lawsuits. At the end of the chapter is a discussion of two provisions of special note in the United States that have significant implications for medical liability in that country.

Table 57.1 Obstetric and gynecologic practice changes as a result of the risk or fear of professional liability claims or litigation

Practice changes	National	Greater than national		Less than national	
		District*		District*	
Increased number of cesarean deliveries	37.1%	III	44.4%	IX	30.5%
Stopped offering/performing VBAC	32.7%	VII	40.0%	I	23.7%
Decreased number of high-risk obstetric patients	33.1%	III	37.0%	I	27.1%
Decreased number of total deliveries	14.5%	III	16.7%	I	10.1%
		VII	16.8%		
Stopped practicing obstetrics	8.3%	III	10.5%	IX	6.4%
		IV	10.6%		
Decreased gynecologic surgical procedures	16.4%	III	24.3%	I	11.3%
Stopped performing major gynecologic surgery	4.9%	II	9.8%	VII	2.7%
Stopped performing all surgery	2.1%	III	2.9%	VII	1.3%

District V: Ind, Ky, Miss, and Ohio
District VI: Ill, Iowa, Minn, Neb, ND, SD, and Wis
District VII: Ala, Ark, Kan, La, Miss, Mo, Okla, Tenn, and Tex
District VIII: Alaska, Ariz, Colo, Hawai, Idaho, Mont, Nev, NM, Ore, Utah, Wyo, and Wash
District IX: Calif

VBAC, vaginal birth after cesarean.
*ACOG districts
District I: Conn, Me, Mass, NH, RI, and Vt
District II: NY
District III: Del, NJ, and Pa
District IV: DC, Fla, Ga, Md, NC, SC, Va, and WVa

Licensure, Certification, Credentialing, and Privileges

Taken together, licensing, certification, and credentialing serve to identify and specify qualifications for practice. *Licensing* is a jurisdictional process that confirms that the practitioner possesses certain educational qualifications, such as graduation from an accredited program, and passing an examination, or other requirements. *Certification* identifies those who have demonstrated specialized knowledge and is granted by a professional body, such as the Royal College of Pathologists in the United Kingdom. Certification may be required for licensing or credentialing. *Credentialing* is generally done at the institutional level. It verifies licensure and other qualifications for practice, including certification in a specialty or specific abilities. It may also require references to attest to interpersonal skills, ethical standards, and similar nonclinical measures.

Specific *privileges* may be granted by an institution based on licensure, certification, experience, or postgraduate training. These range from the right to admit patients to permission to perform specific surgical procedures. At the most basic level, being able to demonstrate that one has met the jurisdictional and institutional requirements for practice is essential to managing risk.

Standard of Care

Standard of care refers to the level or quality of care that any reasonable physician would provide in the same or similar circumstances. This does not mean that every professional must make identical recommendations to meet the standard. Indeed, clinical judgment will always be crucial for informing decisions about individual patient care. However, as the practice of medicine moves toward an increased reliance on evidence as the basis for decision-making, the standard of care is no longer local but reflects the understanding of health care professionals on a national or regional level. The concept of standard of care, thus, is the basis for judging whether a health care provider is at fault when there is an adverse event.

Adverse Outcomes

Adverse events in medicine can be defined by either the patient or the physician, based on their individual understanding of what "should have happened." These very different perspectives often lead to misunderstandings.

Objectively, an adverse outcome is an unintended or injurious event. It may be a wound infection, a delivery resulting in brachial plexus injury, a death, or any other negative result of patient care. Often, the adverse event will have been one that was mentioned, or should have been mentioned, while the patient was consenting to the procedure. However, an adverse outcome is not sufficient to lead to legal action. The best measure for preventing tension between patient and physician is open, honest communication.

Timing is critical in preventing adverse maternal obstetric outcomes. Although postpartum bleeding can kill a woman in a relatively short amount of time, for most other complications, a woman has between 6 and 12 hours or more to get life-saving emergency care. Similarly, most adverse outcomes occur during labor and delivery or the first 48 hours after delivery.

The United Nations Population Fund, an international development agency that provides funding and expertise to support emergency obstetric care around the globe, has developed the "three delays" model (**Fig. 57.1**), which has proven a useful tool for identifying the points at which delays can occur in the management of obstetric complications, and to design programs to address these delays.

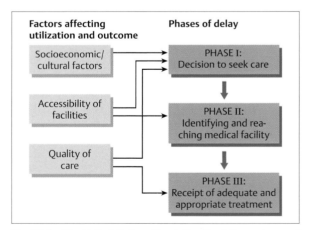

Fig. 57.1 The United Nations Population Fund three phases of delay.

Informed Consent

Informed consent is the process through which medical information is shared between physician and patient and provides documentation of the planned management of an illness or surgery. The elements of informed consent are:

1. The known or anticipated diagnosis or indication for a procedure
2. The recommended treatment—what it entails and why it is chosen
3. The benefits and risks of the recommended treatment
4. The potential side effects and complications associated with the procedure
5. The likelihood that the treatment will be successful
6. Any alternative treatments that are available including their benefits and risks
7. The potential consequences of not following the recommended plan
8. An assessment of the patient's understanding and agreement

The more significant that the diagnosis or planned treatment is, the more thorough the presentation of information must be. Risks, benefits, and side effects must be clearly stated. The major benefits of a procedure need to be balanced with the major risks, including the risks of doing nothing.

In addition, informed consent describes common and severe complications. Even if a complication is rare, if it is life-altering, then it should be disclosed. For example, paralysis is a rare risk of epidural anesthesia. Since paralysis would greatly affect the patient's quality of life, its potential should be disclosed. Alternative treatments must be identified and presented fairly. This requirement holds true even if the person providing the information is not able to offer the alternative treatment but would be referring the patient elsewhere for care.

Simply presenting information is not adequate for informed consent. The fact that someone has signed a form does not mean that they are well informed. The patient's questions need to be solicited and answered. The choice of words and illustrative examples used in the consent process need to be tailored to the patient's understanding and level of education. If the patient is not fluent in the physician's language, translation should not be left to a family member or friend. It is the physician's responsibility to assure that the patient understands the information being presented. The goal should be for the woman and her care provider to share in decisions about her care, based on adequate informed consent.

Discussing Unintended Outcomes

When an adverse outcome does occur, one of the most difficult tasks that a physician faces is to sit down and discuss what has happened with the patient and her family. Even if the event was not unexpected (e.g., the death of a fragile elderly woman following cancer surgery), a family's questions about what happened and why it happened need to be thoroughly answered.

Research has demonstrated that disclosure and honesty are protective. One survey that described possible scenarios after a medical error found that not disclosing the error increased the risk of being sued and of being reported to the licensing board. Patients who believe they have good communication with their provider are more likely to believe their provider is competent and not sue them. Or, such patients tend to sue the institution but not the provider. Another survey asked patients what information they want when there is a problem. Their responses were:

1. Being told promptly that there was a problem
2. Being told via personal communication, rather than telephone or other indirect methods (e.g., mail or e-mail)
3. Being told that something would be done to prevent this problem from happening to someone else
4. Being told that the doctor was sorry that there had been a problem
5. Having any financial charges to them related to this event canceled

Acknowledging a problem is not the same as making blaming statements about whom or what is at fault. In his book *What Do I Say*, Dr. James Woods discusses strategies for counseling patients. He advocates complete disclosure of adverse outcomes, writing that "full disclosure promotes the best qualities of medicine: honesty, integrity and compassion."

Although data indicate that patients want emotional support as well as information, physicians may be concerned that expressing sympathy will be interpreted as admitting guilt. State laws concerning legal protection after disclosure of a medical error vary widely. Risk management professionals at an institution or insurer can assist physicians in preparing for these conversations. They will have to be notified of the problem, in any event, and can serve as a support for organizing a response.

Risk Management

Risk management is both preventive and protective. Activities that fall under the heading of risk management include educating providers about elements of patient safety, informed consent, and other topics as well as monitoring trends and sentinel events, and discussing specific cases with individual practitioners to gain an understanding of the level of liability risk an adverse event creates.

Anytime there is a poor outcome, physicians should notify their risk manager, either with their employer or with their insurer. When the problem is reported in a timely fashion, the risk manager can review chart records and interview staff to gain their perspectives before time blurs memories. If there is significant risk of legal action, a file can be opened and money set aside to pay for future expenses related to the event.

Elements of Medical Negligence

Medical negligence is defined as failing to act in accordance with the standard of care, or acting in a way that a reasonably prudent professional would not. Negligence alone, however, does not define liability—it must lead to injury or damages.

There are four criteria that must be proved in a legal action for malpractice, or medical negligence. The first of these is *duty*. Duty is the responsibility of a physician to behave in such a way as to minimize risk of harm to the patient. That duty is created whenever there is a formal patient–physician interaction.

Duty extends beyond an actual visit to include responsibility for following up on tests that are ordered, facilitating further testing, and notifying the patient of abnormal findings. For example, a woman who is being seen for prenatal care at 28 weeks of pregnancy and has a 1-hour glucose challenge test that gives an elevated result requires a follow-up 3-hour glucose tolerance test to diagnose or rule out gestational diabetes. Failure to order the follow-up test could be construed as negligence.

The second requirement for a finding of negligence is a *breach of duty*. For example, if a test reveals a woman's blood glucose level is elevated but the results are misfiled and not reviewed, and the physician fails to notice the missing test results, the physician's duty to the patient has been breached. In other words, although the correct test was performed, the results were not acted upon.

Causation is the next link in the chain that leads to medical negligence. Infants of diabetic mothers are often heavier and have greater abdominal circumferences than do other infants. If such a woman, previously unsuspected of having diabetes, proceeds to labor and the infant is born with a birth-related injury after a difficult vaginal delivery, one of the factors in that injury would be the failure to diagnose gestational diabetes and treat it appropriately. Treatment includes assessing the potential for complications of birth.

Damage is the final requirement for a finding of medical negligence. Concerns about legal risk focus on major events such as childbirth or surgery. But medical errors that cause damage can also occur in the office setting. For example, a woman is seen for an annual examination and has a Papanicoloau (Pap) smear performed. The provider is responsible for knowing that the test results have been received and reviewed, and that the patient is notified of any abnormal findings. In this example, the test result is abnormal, suggesting cancer, but the laboratory fails to send the office a copy. No one notices the missing test result. Two years later, when the patient returns for her next examination, she has cervical cancer. A search for the previous result, still not in the chart, turns up an abnormal report from two years ago that had been misfiled without being reviewed. The breach of duty falls on the provider, since he or she is ultimately responsible for ensuring that staff members acting under their direction perform their jobs correctly.

Common Areas of Increased Liability Risk

In obstetrics, the major claims and largest awards are those for injured babies. Neurologic injuries, death, and shoulder dystocia claims are the most common. Gynecologic liability claims often relate to delays in treatment, or failure to diagnose breast or reproductive system cancers, reproductive pathology, and other medical complications. Many women or their families have unrealistic expectations of health care. The reality is that there are risks, even to being born. The need for providers to inform and educate the women they care for goes beyond providing informed consent at the time of a procedure.

Failure to communicate lies at the root of many adverse events. This includes communication between team members as well as between the woman and her provider. In the medical education setting, teamwork failures are just as important contributors to medical errors as are lack of knowledge or judgment. Thus, many patient-safety initiatives focus on the verbal communication between providers, documentation, and other communication strategies to reduce risk. These are an increasingly important part of medical training.

The Role of Documentation in Preventing Harm

Completeness, timeliness, accuracy, objectiveness, and legibility are the key requirements for clinical documentation. Just as oral communication between caregivers reduces the risk of misunderstanding or misinterpreting recommendations, clearly stated written material serves to help protect patients from medical errors.

The move to electronic medical records is seen as an important step toward decreasing the confusion sometimes caused by poorly written orders. Unfortunately, many electronic systems limit the amount of individualized information that can be provided. Just as it is the physician's responsibility to share information with patients, it is his or her responsibility to communicate effectively in writing.

When there is an adverse event, documentation of what happened, in what order, and who provided care helps defend against accusations of error or negligence. If necessary, a note describing a complicated process should be drafted before writing it into the patient record. Equally, legal risk can be reduced by avoiding finger-pointing or blame in the medical record and not making pejorative comments about the patient. Numerous organizations and companies provide customizable forms at relatively low cost, which facilitate capturing the records of all encounters with patients and the outcomes of those encounters.

Special Legal Provisions in the United States

The Emergency Treatment and Active Labor Act

In 1986, the US Congress passed the Emergency Treatment and Active Labor Act (EMTALA) amid growing concern over the limited availability of emergency health care services to the poor and uninsured. The statute was designed principally to address the problem of "patient dumping," whereby hospital emergency rooms deny uninsured patients the same treatment provided to paying patients, either by refusing care outright or by transferring uninsured patients to other facilities. EMTALA is often referred to as the "anti-dumping law."

Briefly, EMTALA requires that hospitals medically evaluate any patient who requests, or is presented for, emergency care and provide treatment for any emergent medical problems, regardless of ability to pay for services.

It also prevents hospitals from transferring patients with unstable medical conditions to another hospital, and requires that hospitals accept transfers from an emergency department unable to provide the necessary care, based only on the receiving hospital's ability to provide the needed services.

Finally, it requires that any woman presenting with a complaint of labor be evaluated and active labor ruled out before she can be discharged. The law is limited to hospitals that accept Medicare payments, but this limitation still includes almost all hospitals in the United States, except military facilities.

EMTALA defines an emergency condition as:

"a condition manifesting itself by acute symptoms of sufficient severity (including severe pain) such that the absence of immediate medical attention could reasonably be expected to result in placing the individual's health [or the health of an unborn child] in serious jeopardy, serious impairment to bodily functions, or serious dysfunction of bodily organs; or with respect to a pregnant woman who is having contractions that there is inadequate time to effect a safe transfer to another hospital before delivery, or that transfer may pose a threat to the health or safety of the woman or the unborn child."

The primary responsibility under EMTALA rests with the hospital, not the individual provider. However, a hospital may legitimately require that members of the medical staff participate in emergency room coverage or specialist consultations to the emergency room.

The passage of EMTALA in 1986, and its several revisions, has had both positive and negative effects. On the positive side, it guarantees access to emergency treatment for those roughly 47 million Americans without any health insurance. On the negative side, it means that the expenditures of hospitals to provide care for the uninsured or underinsured may never be repaid, since the patient may be unable to meet the financial cost of care. More than half of Emergency Department care is now uncompensated and written off as charity or bad debt.

The Health Insurance Portability and Accountability Act

Patient privacy is a legal issue not directly related to liability. The Health Insurance Portability and Accountability Act (HIPAA) privacy rule requires that patient information be protected from unintentional disclosure. This includes not discussing a patient's care or test results with those are not entitled to such information. For example, someone who is a co-worker of the patient or a nonfamily member visiting them in the hospital is not entitled to be briefed on the patient's personal medical information or care plan.

There are times when health care information is shared without a patient's specific permission. Reporting communicable diseases or child abuse, sending records to a consultant as part of a referral, or discussing a case for educational purposes are all allowed. In addition, the law clarifies the right of a patient or their personal representative to have access to the medical record. One place where this comes into play, specific to obstetrics and gynecology, is whether parents have a right to information about the reproductive care of their daughter (e.g., contraception, abortion, pregnancy). The HIPAA regulations defer to State law on the provision of care to minors and requirements for parental notification, consent to care, or access to records.

Key Points

- Fear of being sued has been shown to affect clinical practice, and many of the legal issues that affect health care providers relate to liability issues.
- OB/GYN practitioners are among the specialists at highest risk when professional liability lawsuits are brought.
- The more significant the diagnosis or planned treatment is, the more thorough must be the informed consent process.
- OB/GYN physicians can significantly reduce patient risks and protect themselves from legal challenges through effective communication and maintaining a high quality of clinical practice.
- Scrupulously documenting all treatments and interactions with the patient as well as with members of her family is also important for avoiding legal liability.

Further Reading

American College of Emergency Physicians. The Uninsured: Access to Medical Care. Available at: http://www.acep.org/patients.aspx?id=25932. Accessed July 17, 2008

American College of Obstetricians and Gynecologists. ACOG Committee Opinion No. 406: coping with the stress of medical professional liability litigation. *Obstet Gynecol* 2008;111(5):1257–1258

Chandra A, Nundy S, Seabury SA. The growth of physician medical malpractice payments: evidence from the National Practitioner Data Bank. *Health Aff (Millwood).* 2005;(Suppl Web Exclusives):W5-240–W5-249

DeNavas-Walt C, Proctor BD, Smith J. Income, Poverty and Health Insurance Coverage in the United States: 2006. US Census Bureau, 2007. Available at: http://www.census.gov/prod/2007pubs/p60-233.pdf. Accessed July 17, 2008

Department of Health and Human Services. OCR Privacy Brief. Summary of the HIPAA Privacy Rule. Available at: http://www.hhs.gov/ocr/privacysummary.pdf. Accessed July 9, 2008

Gallagher TH, Waterman AD, Ebers AG, Fraser VJ, Levinson W. Patients' and physicians' attitudes regarding the disclosure of medical errors. *JAMA* 2003;289(8):1001–1007

Moore PJ, Adler NE, Robertson PA. Medical malpractice: the effect of doctor-patient relations on medical patient perceptions and malpractice intentions. *West J Med* 2000;173(4):244–250

US Code Collection. Title 42, Chapter 7, Subchapter III, Part E § 1395dd. Examination and treatment for emergency medical conditions and women in labor. Available at: http://www4.law.cornell.edu/uscode/42/1395dd.html. Accessed July 17, 2008

West JR, Rozovsky FA. What Do I Say? Communicating Intended or Unanticipated Outcomes in Obstetrics. San Francisco, Calif: Jossey-Bass, 2003

Index

Notes: Entries in *italics* refer to figures whilst those in **bold** refer to tables/boxed material.